RETINA

Editor-In-Chief

Stephen J. Ryan MD

President, Doheny Eye Institute, Los Angeles, CA, USA

Senior Content Strategist: Russell Gabbedy
Content Development Specialist: Nani Clansey
Content Coordinators: Emma Cole/Trinity Hutton/Sam Crowe/Humayra Rahman
Project Manager: Caroline Jones
Design: Miles Hitchen
Illustration Manager: Jennifer Rose
Illustrator: Antbits
Marketing Manager: Helena Mutak
Cover image photographer: Tamera Schoenholz, CRA, OCT-C

Editor-In-Chief
Stephen J. Ryan MD
President
Doheny Eye Institute
Los Angeles, CA, USA

RYAN'S RETINAL IMAGING AND DIAGNOSTICS

Edited by
SriniVas R. Sadda MD
Associate Professor of Ophthalmology
Doheny Eye Institute
Associate Professor
Department of Ophthalmology
Keck School of Medicine
University of Southern California
Los Angeles, CA, USA

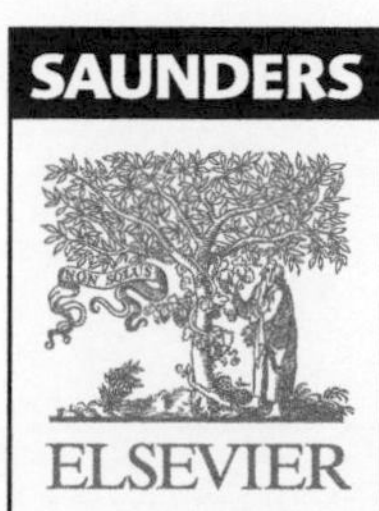

London New York Oxford St Louis Sydney Toronto 2013

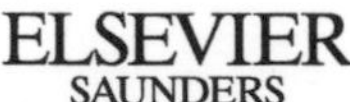

Notices

Knowledge and best practice in this field are constantly changing. As new research and experience broaden our understanding, changes in research methods, professional practices, or medical treatment may become necessary.

Practitioners and researchers must always rely on their own experience and knowledge in evaluating and using any information, methods, compounds, or experiments described herein. In using such information or methods they should be mindful of their own safety and the safety of others, including parties for whom they have a professional responsibility.

With respect to any drug or pharmaceutical products identified, readers are advised to check the most current information provided (i) on procedures featured or (ii) by the manufacturer of each product to be administered, to verify the recommended dose or formula, the method and duration of administration, and contraindications. It is the responsibility of practitioners, relying on their own experience and knowledge of their patients, to make diagnoses, to determine dosages and the best treatment for each individual patient, and to take all appropriate safety precautions.

To the fullest extent of the law, neither the Publisher nor the authors, contributors, or editors, assume any liability for any injury and/or damage to persons or property as a matter of products liability, negligence or otherwise, or from any use or operation of any methods, products, instructions, or ideas contained in the material herein.

Main edition 3-vol set Ryan Retina ISBN: 9781455707379

Ebook ISBN: 9780323223997
Print On Demand ISBN: 9780323262545

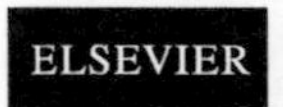

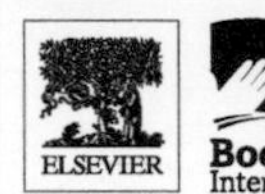

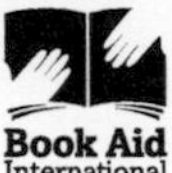

Printed and bound by CPI G roup (U K) Ltd, Croydon, CR0 4Y Y

Transferred to digital print 2013

Contents

Contributors

Michael Abràmoff MD, PhD
Associate Professor
Retina Service
Department of Ophthalmology and Visual Sciences
Biomedical Engineering, and Electrical and Computer Engineering
University of Iowa
Iowa City, IA, USA
Chapter 6

Everett Ai MD
Director, Ophthalmic Diagnostic Center
California Pacific Medical Center
San Francisco, CA, USA
Chapter 1

Ferdinando Bottoni MD, FEBO
Staff Member
Eye Clinic
Department of Clinical Science Luigi Sacco
Sacco Hospital, University of Milan
Milan, Italy
Chapter 2

Dingcai Cao PhD
Associate Professor
Department of Ophthalmology and Visual Sciences
University of Illinois at Chicago
Chicago, IL, USA
Chapter 10

Emmett T. Cunningham Jr MD, PhD, MPH
Director, The Uveitis Service
California Pacific Medical Center
San Francisco, CA
Adjunct Clinical Professor of Ophthalmology
Stanford University School of Medicine
Stanford, CA
West Coast Retina Medical Group
San Francisco, CA, USA
Chapter 1

Steven E. Feldon MD
Director, Flaum Eye Institute
Professor and Chair
Department of Ophthalmology
University of Rochester
Rochester, NY, USA
Chapter 12

Monika Fleckenstein MD
Ophthalmology Specialist
Department of Ophthalmology
University of Bonn
Bonn, Germany
Chapter 4

Laura J. Frishman PhD
Moores Professor, Vision Sciences
College of Optometry
University of Houston
Houston, TX, USA
Chapter 7

Arthur D. Fu MD
Clinical Professor of Ophthalmology
California Pacific Medical Center
San Francisco, CA, USA
Chapter 1

Carlos Alexandre de Amorim Garcia Filho MD
Post Doctoral Associate
Department Of Ophthalmology
Bascom Palmer Eye Institute
University of Miami Miller School of Medicine
Miami, FL, USA
Chapter 3

Andrea Giani MD
Ophthalmologist, Vitreo-Retinal Service
Eye Clinic
Department of Clinical Science Luigi Sacco
Sacco Hospital
University of Milan
Milan, Italy
Chapter 2

Giovanni Gregori PhD
Assistant Research Professor
Department of Ophthalmology
University of Miami
Miller School of Medicine
Miami, FL, USA
Chapter 3

Rudolf F. Guthoff MD
Head
University Eye Department
University of Rostock
Rostock, Germany
Chapter 9

Frank G. Holz MD, FEBO
Professor and Chairman
Department of Ophthalmology
University of Bonn
Bonn, Germany
Chapter 4

Robert N. Johnson MD
Clinical Professor of Ophthalmology
California Pacific Medical Center
San Francisco, CA, USA
Chapter 1

J. Michael Jumper MD
Retina Service Chief
California Pacific Medical Center
San Francisco, CA, USA
Chapter 1

Christine N. Kay MD
Assistant Professor
Department of Ophthalmology
University of Florida
Gainesville, FL, USA
Chapter 6

Pearse A. Keane MD, MRCOphth, MRCSI
Clinical Lecturer in Ophthalmic Translational Research
NIHR Biomedical Research Centre for Ophthalmology
Moorfields Eye Hospital NHS Foundation Trust
UCL Institute of Ophthalmology
London, UK
Chapter 5

Leanne T. Labriola DO
Clinical Assistant Professor of Ophthalmology
Medical Retina Service
University of Pittsburgh School of Medicine
Pittsburgh, PA, USA
Chapter 9

Brandon J. Lujan MD
Associate
West Coast Retina
San Francisco, CA, USA
Chapter 1

H. Richard McDonald MD
Clinical Professor of Ophthalmology
California Pacific Medical Center
Director, Vitreoretinal Fellowship Program
California Pacific Medical Center
Director, San Francisco Retina Foundation
San Francisco, CA, USA
Chapter 1

Yozo Miyake MD, PhD
Chairman of the Board of Directors
Aichi Medical University
Aichi, Japan
Chapter 8

Carmen A. Puliafito MD, MBA
Dean
Keck School of Medicine
May S and John Hooval Dean's Chair in Medicine
Professor of Ophthalmology and Health Management
Doheny Eye Institute
University of Southern California
Los Angeles, CA
Voluntary Professor of Ophthalmology
Bascom Palmer Eye Institute
University of Miami
Miami, FL, USA
Chapter 3

Rajeev S. Ramchandran MD
Assistant Professor
Retinal Services
Flaum Eye Institute
University of Rochester Medical Center
Rochester, NY, USA
Chapter 12

Philip J. Rosenfeld MD, PhD
Professor of Ophthalmology
Bascom Palmer Eye Institute
Miami, FL, USA
Chapter 3

Gary S. Rubin PhD
Helen Keller Professor of Ophthalmology
UCL Institute of Ophthalmology
London, UK
Chapter 11

Humberto Ruiz-Garcia MD
Retina Specialist
Clinica Santa Lucia
Universidad de Guadalajara
Guadalajara, Mexico
Chapter 5

SriniVas R. Sadda MD
Associate Professor of Ophthalmology
Doheny Eye Institute
Associate Professor
Department of Ophthalmology
Keck School of Medicine
University of Southern California
Los Angeles, CA, USA
Chapter 5

Steffen Schmitz-Valckenberg MD, FEBO
Professor
Department of Ophthalmology
University of Bonn
Bonn, Germany
Chapter 4

Kei Shinoda MD, PhD
Associate Professor
Department of Ophthalmology
Teikyo University School of Medicine
Tokyo, Japan
Chapter 8

Oliver Stachs PhD
Physicist
Department of Ophthalmology
Faculty of Medicine
University of Rostock
Rostock, Germany
Chapter 9

Giovanni Staurenghi MD
Professor of Ophthalmology
Chairman Eye Clinic
Department of Clinical Science Luigi Sacco
Sacco Hospital
University of Milan
Milan, Italy
Chapter 2

Zohar Yehoshua MD, MHA
Assistant Research Professor
Department of Ophthalmology
University of Miami
Miller School of Medicine
Miami, FL, USA
Chapter 3

Preface

The Fifth Edition of Ryan *Retina* represents the most extensive and comprehensive revision to the text since the first edition. The text has been completely reorganized and updated through the efforts of an international group of 338 expert authors from 21 countries. The diagnostics section in particular has been expanded to include the latest innovations in ophthalmic imaging which have transformed the practice of retina. The electronic edition of the text also includes a wealth of additional figures, tables, and text which could not be included in the print version due to space limitations. *Ryan's Retinal Imaging and Diagnostics* e-book presents the first 12 chapters from *Retina* Fifth Edition as a vital standalone resource featuring over 1000 figures and covering the full spectrum of modalities and new technologies including optical coherence tomography (OCT), fundus imaging, and autofluorescence imaging.

The Fifth Edition of *Retina* represents the last edition of the book to be assembled and edited under the leadership of the late Dr Stephen J. Ryan, editor-in-chief, and *Ryan's Retinal Imaging and Diagnostics* e-book is dedicated to his memory. Dr Ryan has unquestionably been a true visionary leader for the field of retina in our time. In addition to his far reaching contributions through this textbook which continues to honor his name, the astonishing magnitude of his impact on retina and the field of ophthalmology as a whole are difficult to quantify or capture in words. He was a tireless leader and advocate, protecting the interests and future of ophthalmology at the national and international level. He mentored and inspired countless ophthalmologists, retina specialists, and vision scientists around the world. He helped thousands of grateful patients and allowed them to keep their precious eyesight. He was a mentor, colleague, and loyal friend to me and to so many others. He can never be replaced, but will also never be forgotten. Ryan's *Retina,* into which he has poured so much love and energy, will also remain as part of his monumental legacy.

SriniVas Sadda

Chapter 1

Fluorescein Angiography: Basic Principles and Interpretation

Robert N. Johnson, Arthur D. Fu, H. Richard McDonald, J. Michael Jumper, Everett Ai, Emmett T. Cunningham Jr, Brandon J. Lujan

For nearly 50 years, fundus photography and fluorescein angiography have been valuable in expanding our knowledge of the anatomy, pathology, and pathophysiology of the retina and choroid.[1] Initially, fluorescein angiography was used primarily as a laboratory and clinical research tool; only later was it used for the diagnosis of fundus diseases.[1-5] An understanding of fluorescein angiography and the ability to interpret fluorescein angiograms are essential to accurately evaluate, diagnose, and treat patients with retinal vascular and macular disease.

This chapter discusses the basic principles of fluorescein angiography and the equipment and techniques needed to produce a high-quality angiogram. Potential side-effects and complications of fluorescein injection are also discussed. Finally, interpretation of fluorescein angiography, including fundus anatomy and histology, the normal fluorescein angiogram, and conditions responsible for abnormal fundus fluorescence are described.

BASIC PRINCIPLES

To understand fluorescein angiography, a knowledge of fluorescence is essential. Likewise, to understand fluorescence, one must know the principles of luminescence. Luminescence is the emission of light from any source other than high temperature. Luminescence occurs when energy in the form of electromagnetic radiation is absorbed and then re-emitted at another frequency. When light energy is absorbed into a luminescent material, free electrons are elevated into higher energy states. This energy is then re-emitted by spontaneous decay of the electrons into their lower energy states. When this decay occurs in the visible spectrum, it is called luminescence. Luminescence therefore always entails a shift from a shorter wavelength to a longer wavelength. The shorter wavelengths represent higher energy, and the longer wavelengths represent lower energy.

Fluorescence

Fluorescence is luminescence that is maintained only by continuous excitation. In other words, excitation at one wavelength occurs and is emitted immediately through a longer wavelength. Emission stops at once when the excitation stops. Fluorescence thus does not have an afterglow. A typical example of fluorescence is television. In the television tube, the excitation radiation is the electron beam from the cathode ray tube. This beam excites the phosphors of the screen, which re-emit the beam as a glow that constitutes a television picture.

Sodium fluorescein is a hydrocarbon that responds to light energy between 465 and 490 nm and fluoresces at a wavelength of 520–530 nm. The excitation wavelength, the type that is absorbed and changed, is blue; the resultant fluorescence, or emitted wavelength, is green–yellow. If blue light between 465 and 490 nm is directed to unbound sodium fluorescein, it emits a light that appears green–yellow (520–530 nm).

This is a fundamental principle of fluorescein angiography. In the procedure, the patient, whose eyes have been dilated, is seated behind the fundus camera, on which a blue filter has been placed in front of the flash. Fluorescein is then injected intravenously. Eighty percent of the fluorescein becomes bound to protein and is not available for fluorescence, but 20% remains free in the bloodstream and is available for fluorescence. The blue flash of the fundus camera excites the unbound fluorescein within the blood vessels or the fluorescein that has leaked out of the blood vessels. The blue filter shields out (reflects or absorbs) all other light and allows through only the blue excitation light. The blue light then changes those structures in the eye containing fluorescein to green–yellow light at 520–530 nm. In addition, blue light is reflected off the fundus structures that do not contain fluorescein. The blue reflected light and the green–yellow fluorescent light are directed back toward the film of the fundus camera. Just in front of the film a filter is placed that allows the green–yellow fluorescent light through but keeps out the blue reflected light. Therefore the only light that penetrates the filter is true fluorescent light (Fig. 1.1).

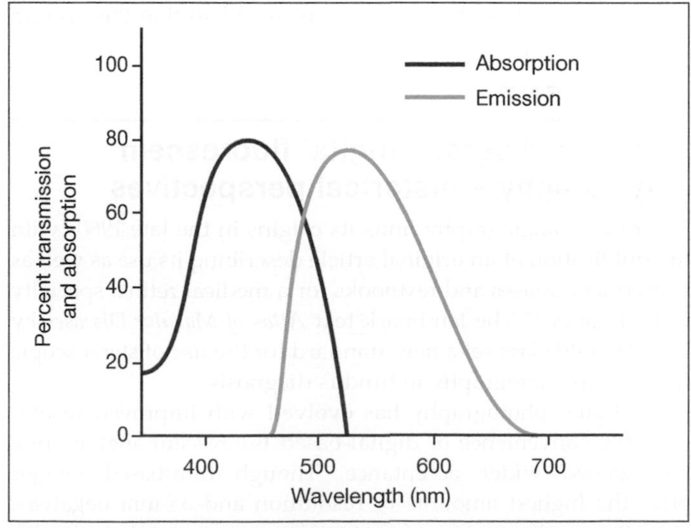

Fig. 1.1 Absorption and emission curves of sodium fluorescein dye. The peak absorption (excitation) is at 465–490 nm (blue light). The peak emission occurs at 520–530 nm (yellow–green light).

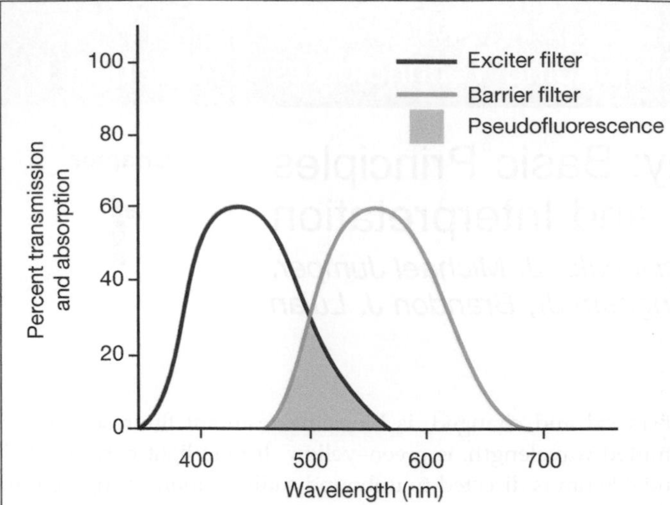

Fig. 1.2 Pseudofluorescence. The blue exciter filter overlaps into the yellow–green zone, and the yellow–green barrier filter overlaps into the blue zone. The combination results in pseudofluorescence.

Pseudofluorescence

Pseudofluorescence occurs when nonfluorescent light passes through the entire filter system. If green–yellow light penetrates the original blue filter, it will pass through the entire system. If blue light reflected from nonfluorescent fundus structures penetrates the green–yellow filter, pseudofluorescence occurs (Fig. 1.2). Pseudofluorescence (i.e., fake fluorescence) causes nonfluorescent structures to appear fluorescent. It can confuse the physician interpreting the fluorescein angiogram and lead him or her to think that certain fundus structures or materials are fluorescing when they are not. Pseudofluorescence also causes decreased contrast, as well as decreased resolution. Because fluorescein angiography uses black-and-white film, the nonfluorescent or pseudofluorescent light appears as a background illumination. The background illumination from pseudofluorescence is especially heightened if there are white areas of the fundus, such as highly reflective, hard exudates. Pseudofluorescence must be avoided. Therefore the excitation (blue) and barrier (green–yellow) filters should be carefully matched so that the overlap of light between them is minimal.

EQUIPMENT

Film-based versus digital fluorescein angiography – historical perspectives

Fluorescein angiography finds its origins in the late 1960s with the publication of an original article describing its use as well as subsequent atlases and textbooks for a medical retinal specialty in its infancy.[1,6] The landmark text *Atlas of Macular Diseases* by Dr J. Donald Gass set a new standard for the use of stereoscopic fluorescein angiography in fundus diagnosis.[7]

As digital photography has evolved with improved resolution, the convenience of digital-based fluorescein angiography has gained wider acceptance. Though film-based images offer the highest amounts of resolution and 35-mm negatives are often easier to view for stereo, images are relatively difficult to manipulate, and training and effort are required to process and duplicate film. Transmitting or sharing film-based images is also time-consuming compared with digital images (Box 1.1).[8]

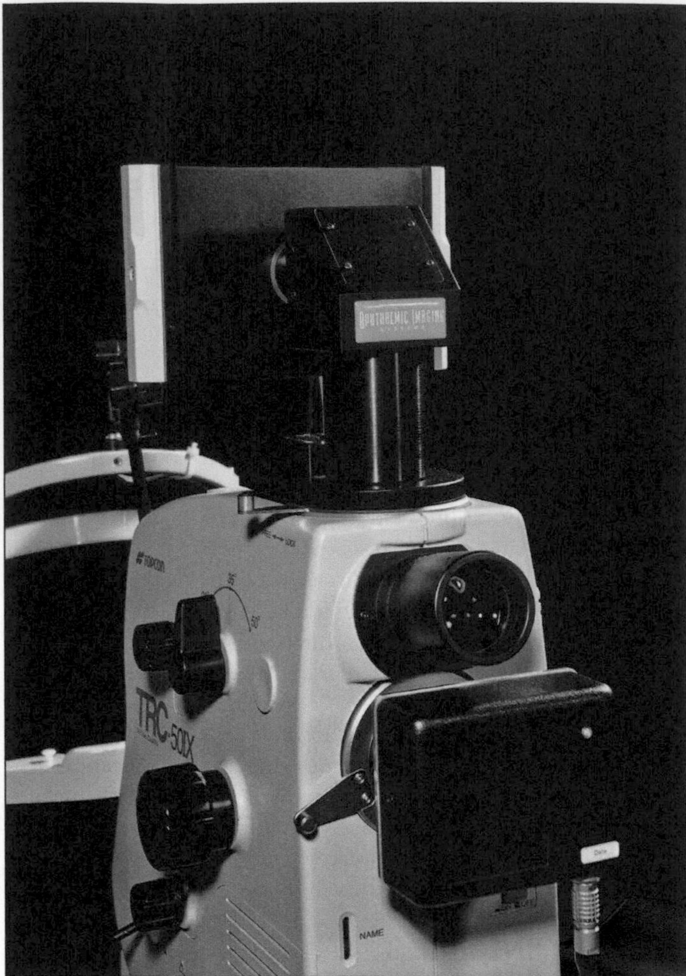

Fig. 1.3 Digital fundus camera for color fundus and fluorescein angiography.

Box 1.1 Equipment and materials needed for angiography

- Fundus camera and auxiliary equipment
- Matched fluorescein filters (barrier and exciter)
- Digital photoprocessing unit (computer-based) and software user interface
- 23-gauge scalp vein needle
- 5 mL syringe
- 5 mL of 10% fluorescein solution
- 20-gauge, 1½-inch needle to draw the dye
- Armrest for fluorescein injection
- Tourniquet
- Alcohol swabs
- Bandage
- Standard emergency equipment

Camera and auxiliary equipment

Cameras differ in the degree of fundus area included in the photographs. Fundus cameras may range from 35° to 200° wide-field camera systems such as Optos.[9,10] In clinical retinal practice, cameras ranging from 35° to 50° are routinely used (Fig. 1.3). Regardless of range, a camera with the ability to yield high

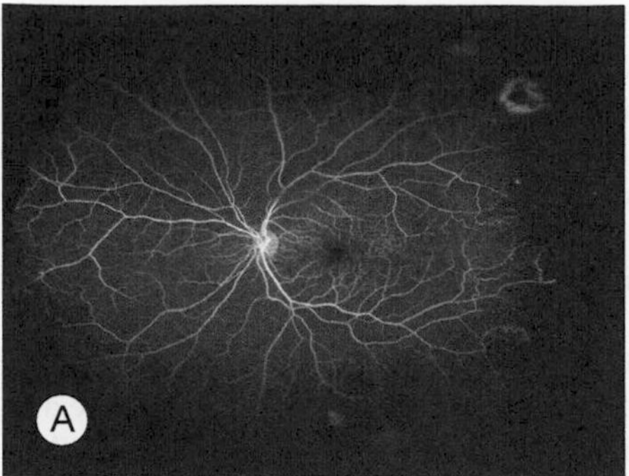

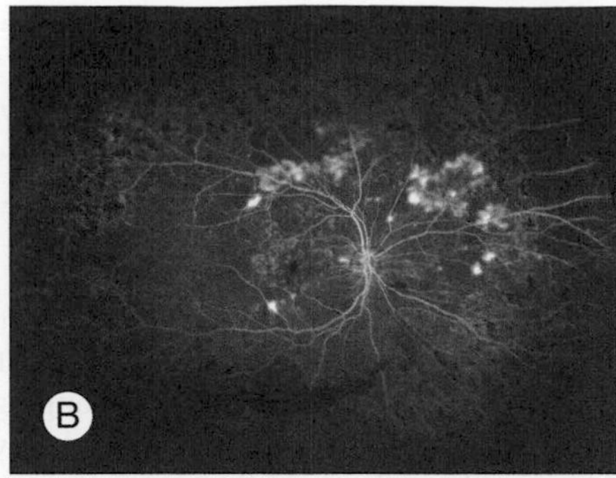

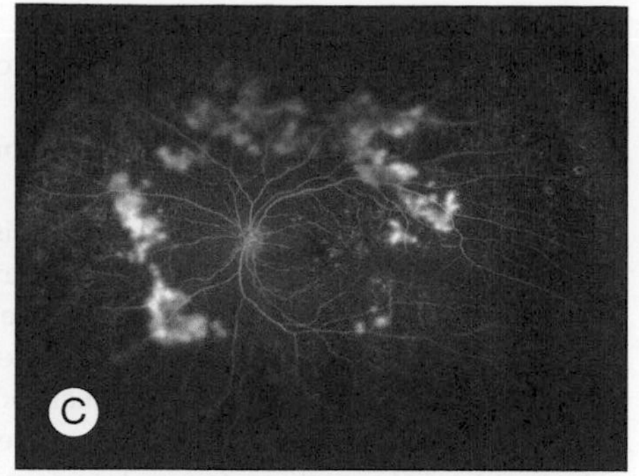

Fig. 1.4 Optos wide-field images. (A) Nonperfusion detected in the left eye with wide-field fluorescein imaging. (Courtesy of Umar Mian, MD. Image taken by Carolina Costa.) (B, C) Wide-field angiography of the right and left eyes of a patient with diabetic retinopathy. Note the multiple areas of leakage corresponding to areas of retinal neovascularization associated with capillary nonperfusion. It is often difficult in certain wide-field images to determine the presence of small neovascular complexes versus leakage from capillary nonperfusion, unless areas are magnified further. (Courtesy of Szilárd Kiss, MD.)

resolutions of the posterior pole is essential for most macular problems, especially when laser treatment is to be done, as with background diabetic retinopathy, branch-vein occlusion, or choroidal neovascularization.

Wide-angle angiography has the benefit of capturing a single image of the retina in high resolution well beyond the equator. The potential for clinical efficiency and sensitivity in detecting neovascularization in the far periphery as well as acquiring an excellent clinical picture of the degree of capillary retinal nonperfusion is an exciting development in fluorescein angiography (Fig. 1.4).

Stereophotography

A subtle joystick movement, by a trained photographer, from right to left photographing from one side of the pupil to the opposite side of the pupil produces a stereoscopic image when combined through hand-held stereo viewers. It is important to note that, in the process of acquiring images for stereophotography, individual images may be blurred or may contain artifacts. The photographer should not attempt to discard images until viewed with the stereo viewers.

Matched fluorescein filters

Typically included in modern camera units, fluorescein angiography uses both exciter and barrier filters. The exciter filter must transmit blue light at 465–490 nm, the absorption peak of fluorescein excitation. The barrier filter transmits light at 525–530 nm, the fluorescent, or emitted, peak of fluorescein. The filters should allow maximal transmission of light in the proper spectral range to achieve a good image without the use of an excessively powerful flash unit. Most new cameras come with filters. When choosing a camera, one should request the transmission curves of the filter combination to be sure that no significant overlap exists; pseudofluorescence results when there is overlap.

After several years, filters become thin, emitting more light and increasing the incidence and degree of pseudofluorescence. The clinician should always check the control photograph of each angiogram for excessive pseudofluorescence. Filters should be replaced once pseudofluorescence reduces the quality of the angiophotograph.

Light sources (viewing bulb and flash strobe)

In film-based cameras, bulbs burn out, but are easily replaced. A supply of each should always be kept on hand (Fig. 1.5).

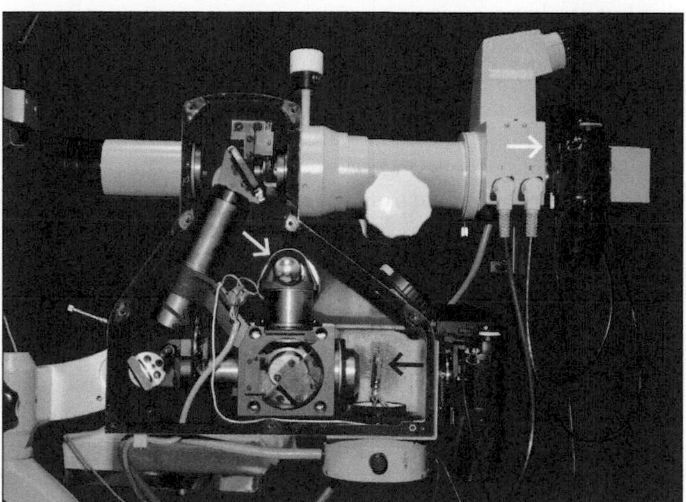

Fig. 1.5 Fundus film camera with side wall removed to view inside parts. Yellow arrow, viewing bulb; black arrow, flash bulb; red arrow, exciter filter wheel. The light from the flash goes through the system in this photograph from right to left. The light is reflected off a mirror and travels upward to another mirror; it is then reflected to the left, into the patient's eye. From there it is reflected directly to the right of the fluorescein camera back (white arrow).

Fluorescein solution

Sodium fluorescein, an orange-red crystalline hydrocarbon ($C_{20}H_{12}O_5Na$), has a low molecular weight (376.27 Da) and readily diffuses through most of the body fluids and through the choriocapillaris, but it does not diffuse through the retinal vascular endothelium or the pigment epithelium.

Solutions containing 500 mg fluorescein are available in vials of 10 mL of 5% fluorescein or 5 mL of 10% fluorescein. Also available are 3 mL of 25% fluorescein solution (750 mg). The greater the volume, the longer the injection time will be; the smaller the volume, the more likely a significant percentage of fluorescein will remain in the venous dead space between the arm and the heart (see Injecting the fluorescein, below). For this reason we prefer 5 mL of 10% solution (500 mg fluorescein).

Fluorescein is eliminated by the liver and kidneys within 24 hours, although traces may be found in the body for up to a week after injection. Retention may increase if renal function is impaired. The skin has a yellowish tinge for a few hours after injection, and the urine has a characteristic yellow–orange color for most of the first day after injection.

Various side-effects and complications can occur with fluorescein injection (Box 1.2).[11–15]

A serious complication of the injection is extravasation of the fluorescein under the skin. This can be extremely painful and may result in a number of uncomfortable symptoms. Necrosis and sloughing of the skin may occur, although this is extremely rare. Superficial phlebitis also has been noted. A subcutaneous granuloma has occurred in a few patients after fluorescein extravasation. In each instance, however, the granuloma has been small, cosmetically invisible, and painless. Toxic neuritis caused by infiltration of extravasated fluorescein along a nerve in the antecubital area can result in considerable pain for up to a few hours. The application of an ice pack at the site of extravasation may help relieve pain. For extremely painful reactions an injection of a local anesthetic at the site of extravasation is effective but rarely necessary.

If extravasation occurs, the physician must decide whether to continue angiography. Extravasation may occur immediately, and thus the serum concentration of the fluorescein will be insufficient for angiography. In this case it usually is best to place the needle in another vein and reinject a full dose of fluorescein, starting the process again from the beginning. Occasionally, only a small amount of fluorescein is extravasated at the end of the injection. In this case photography can continue without stopping or reinjecting.

A common cause of extravasation is the use of a large, long needle directly attached to a syringe. It is difficult to hold the syringe in the dark. For this and other reasons we have discussed earlier, a scalp-vein needle attached to a syringe by a flexible tube is the best choice for this procedure. Also, the patient's own blood can be drawn back into the tubing of the scalp-vein needle, with the blood going all the way up to but not into the syringe. When it is time to inject, the person giving the injection can look at the tip of the needle to ensure that extravasation has not occurred. If it has, the patient's own blood is extravasated, and little chance of complication exists if the injection is stopped at this point so that no fluorescein is injected.

It is always important to watch for extravasation at the beginning of the injection so that, should it occur, the process can be halted; thus only a minimal amount of fluorescein will have been injected and extravasated. The amount of extravasated fluorescein can be minimized by slow injection and constant observation of the needle with a hand-held light or if injection is done before turning off the room lights.

Box 1.2 Side-effects and complications of fluorescein injection

- Extravasation and local-tissue necrosis[13]
- Inadvertent arterial injection
- Nausea[11–13]
- Vomiting
- Vasovagal reaction (circulatory shock, myocardial infarction)[12]
- Allergic reaction, anaphylaxis (hives and itching, respiratory problems, laryngeal edema, bronchospasm)
- Nerve palsy
- Neurologic problems (tonic–clonic seizures)
- Thrombophlebitis
- Pyrexia
- Death

Nausea is the most frequent side-effect of fluorescein injection, occurring in about 5% of patients. It is most likely to occur in patients under 50 years of age or when fluorescein is injected rapidly. When nausea occurs, it usually begins approximately 30 seconds after injection, lasts for 2–3 minutes, and disappears slowly.

Vomiting occurs infrequently, affecting only 0.3–0.4% of patients.[11,13] When it does occur, it usually begins 40–50 seconds after injection. By this time most of the initial-transit photographs of the angiogram will have been taken. A receptacle and tissues should be available in case vomiting does occur. When patients experience nausea or vomiting, they must be reassured that the unpleasant and uncomfortable feeling will subside rapidly. Photographs can be taken after the vomiting episode has passed. A slower, more gradual injection may help to prevent vomiting.

Patients who have previously experienced nausea or vomiting from fluorescein injection may be given an oral dose of 25–50 mg of promethazine hydrochloride (Phenergan) by mouth approximately 1 hour before injection. Promethazine has proved to be helpful in preventing or lessening the severity of nausea or vomiting. We have recently found that we can also reduce the incidence of nausea by warming the vial of fluorescein to body temperature and drawing it into the syringe through a needle with a Millipore filter. Restriction of food and water for 4 hours before the fluorescein injection may reduce the incidence of vomiting; an empty stomach may prevent vomiting but will not affect nausea. If the patient still has a tendency to vomit despite taking all these measures, a lesser amount of fluorescein can be given and injected more slowly if the photographic results will not be compromised.

Vasovagal attacks occur much less frequently during fluorescein angiography than nausea and are probably caused more by patient anxiety than by the actual injection of fluorescein. We have seen vasovagal attacks even when the patient sees the needle or immediately after the skin has been penetrated by the needle but before the injection has begun. Occasionally a vasovagal reaction causes a patient to faint, but consciousness is regained within a few minutes. If early symptoms of a vasovagal episode are noted, smelling salts usually reverse the reaction. The photographer must be alert for signs of fainting because the patient could be injured if he or she falls.

Shock and syncope (more severe vasovagal reaction) consist of bradycardia, hypotension, reduced cardiovascular perfusion, sweating, and the sense of feeling cold. If the photographer and person injecting see that the patient is getting "shocky" or light-headed, the patient should be allowed to bend over or lie down with their feet elevated. The patient's blood pressure and pulse should be carefully monitored. It is important to differentiate this from anaphylaxis, in which hypotension, tachycardia, bronchospasm, hives, and itching occur.

Hives and itching are the most frequent allergic reactions, occurring 2–15 minutes after fluorescein injection. Although hives usually disappear within a few hours, an antihistamine, such as diphenhydramine hydrochloride (Benadryl), may be administered intravenously for an immediate response. Bronchospasm and even anaphylaxis are other reactions that have been reported, but these are extremely rare. Epinephrine, systemic steroids, aminophylline, and pressor agents should be available to treat bronchospasm or any other allergic or anaphylactic reactions. Other equipment that should be readily available in the event of a severe vasovagal or anaphylactic reaction includes oxygen, a sphygmomanometer, a stethoscope, and a device to provide an airway. The skilled photographer observes each patient carefully and is alert to any scratching, wheezing, or difficulty in breathing that the patient may have after injection.

There are a few published and unpublished reports of death following intravenous fluorescein injection. The mechanism may be a severe allergic reaction or a hypotensive episode induced by a vasovagal reaction in a patient with pre-existing cardiac or cerebral vascular disease. The cause of death in each case may have been coincidental. Acute pulmonary edema following fluorescein injection has also been reported.

There are no known contraindications to fluorescein injections in patients with a history of heart disease, cardiac arrhythmia, or cardiac pacemakers. Although there have been no reports of fetal complications from fluorescein injection during pregnancy, it is current practice to avoid angiography in women who are pregnant, especially those in the first trimester.

TECHNIQUE

Aligning camera and photographing

To align the fundus camera properly, the photographer must first assess the "field of the eye." The camera is equipped with a joystick with which the photographer can adjust the camera laterally and for depth. The camera is also equipped with a knob for vertical adjustment. The photographer finds the red fundus reflex, which is an even, round, sharply defined, pink or red light reflex. If the camera is too close to the eye, a bright, crescent-shaped light reflex appears at the edge of the viewing screen or a bright spot appears at its center. If the camera is too far away, a hazy, poorly contrasted photograph results.

The photographer moves the camera from side to side to ascertain the width of the pupil and the focusing peculiarities of the particular cornea and lens. The photographer studies the eye through the camera lens, moving the camera back and forth and up and down, looking for fundus details (e.g., retinal blood vessels). The photographer then determines the single best position from which to photograph (Figs 1.6 and 1.7).

Occasionally, a patient has a peculiar corneal reflex or central lens opacity, and it may be impossible to follow the usual procedure of aligning the camera through the central axis of the eye. Moving the camera slightly off axis may help improve focus and resolution.

Any abnormalities, such as an unusual light reflex or a poorly resolved image that the photographer sees through the camera system, will appear on the photograph. If the ophthalmoscopic view seen through the camera is not optimal, the photograph will not be optimal (Fig. 1.8). If the view is optimal, well aligned, in focus, and without reflexes, the photograph can be optimal. A helpful concept for the photographer is "what you see is what you get (or worse – never better)."

Focusing

Achieving perfect focus is a major factor in the photographic process. Both the eyepiece crosshairs and the fundus details must be in sharp focus to obtain a well-resolved photograph. The proper position of the eyepiece is determined by the refractive error of the photographer and the degree to which he or she accommodates while focusing the camera.

The photographer first turns the eyepiece counterclockwise (toward the plus, or hyperopic, range) to relax his or her own accommodation; this causes the crosshairs to blur. The photographer then turns the eyepiece slowly clockwise to bring the crosshairs into sharp focus. The eyepiece is focused properly when the crosshairs appear sharp and clear (Fig. 1.9). They must remain perfectly clear while the photographer focuses on the fundus with the camera's focusing detail. With experience, the photographer becomes expert in adjusting the eyepiece and in keeping the crosshairs in focus throughout the entire photographic sequence.

The best position for the eyepiece is the point at which the crosshairs are in focus while the photographer's accommodation is relaxed. Photographers learn to relax accommodation by keeping both eyes open. The photographer focuses the eyepiece with one eye and, with the other eye, keeps a distant object, such as the eye chart, in sharp focus. This skill may be difficult for technicians without ophthalmic training, but it is seldom impossible to learn.

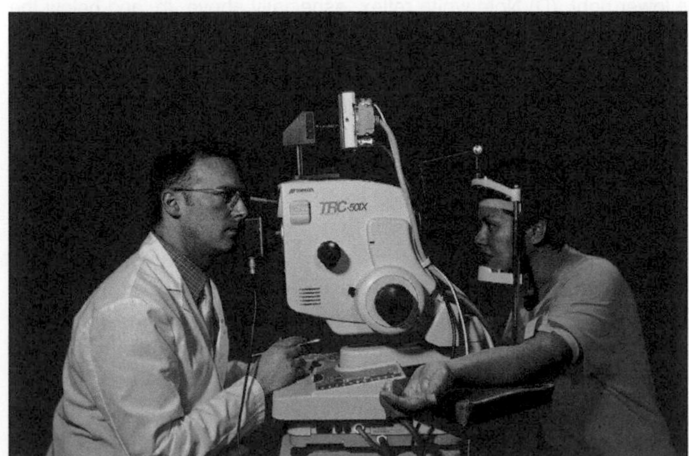

Fig. 1.6 The patient's arm rests on an adjustable armrest that is elevated so that the patient's arm is at or above the level of her heart. The armrest also facilitates easy placement of the intravenous needle and injection of fluorescein.

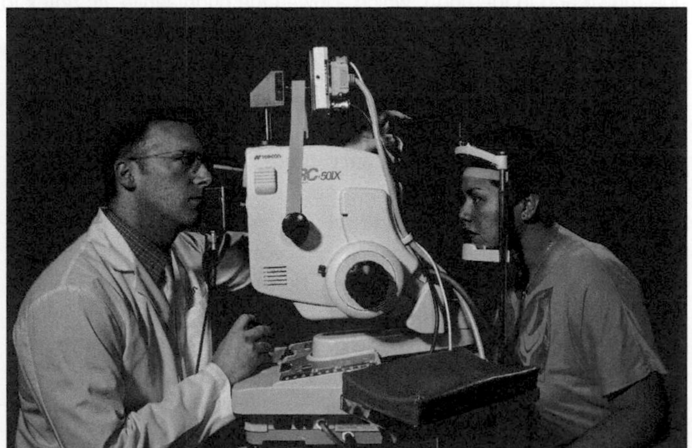

Fig. 1.7 The patient's head is kept steady in the chinrest and headrest of the fundus camera. The photographer aligns the camera and focuses on the patient's right fundus. Each is in a comfortable position, facilitating the stability necessary to achieve a good fluorescein angiogram.

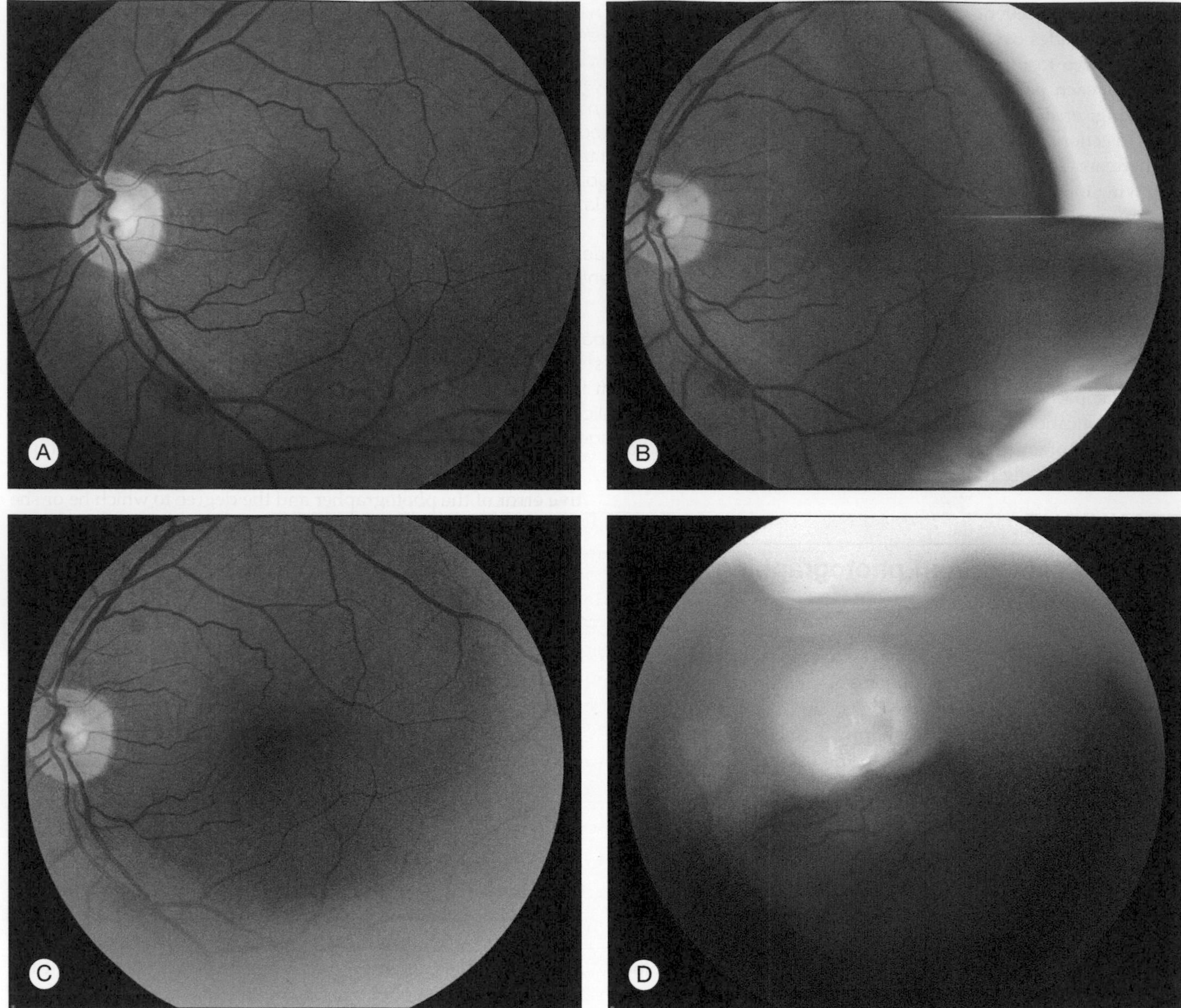

Fig. 1.8 Fundus photograph and reflexes. (A) Photograph of right fundus without reflexes. The camera was properly aligned and focused. (B) Note the bright red, yellow and blue arc on the right side. The flash is reflecting off the iris. This can be remedied by repositioning the camera slightly to the right or left. (C) In this case the camera was placed at the proper distance from the fundus but was placed too far to one side (down and to the right), which allowed the bright white arc reflex to the lower right. (D) Note white reflex, especially above, in, and below the papillomacular bundle. In this case the camera was in proper alignment but was placed too far away from the patient's eye.

Keeping the crosshairs in sharp focus, the photographer then turns the focusing dial on the camera to focus the fundus detail. Some photographers focus the crosshairs just once at the beginning of each day and control their accommodation throughout the day. This is not a good idea because the photographer's accommodation may change during a photographic session; the photographer should be aware of this possibility and regularly check and readjust the eyepiece for focus. With the camera properly aligned and focused, the photographer is ready to start the preliminary photographs and angiograms.

Digital angiography

In theory, film-based photography has advantages over digital imaging: image resolution and stereoscopic viewing.[8] Film-based images contain 10 000 lines of resolution, in contrast to digital imaging, which may have as little as 1000 lines of resolution.[8] However, some argue that, despite higher resolution in film, the greater ability to magnify digital images makes the disadvantage of digital photography less clinically relevant.[8] Digital angiography offers advantages, including the instantaneous availability of the angiogram, and the avoidance of the equipment and time necessary to develop film. With instantaneous images, digital angiography facilitates education and discussion concerning the patient's condition and treatment options. Also, digital angiography facilitates training of ophthalmic personnel. We have found that it is useful to stay in the room during the initial frames of the angiogram to ensure that the desired pathology is photographed. Any changes can be promptly made, and the photographer can also learn from this prompt feedback. Digital angiography, however, necessitates an ongoing investment of money both in software updates and storage of digital electronic files. Also, excessive image manipulation with image-editing software may result in artifacts. Specifically, some areas may appear overly hyperfluorescent due to limited dynamic range in images and software manipulation. Care should be taken in avoiding misinterpretation of hyperfluorecence and hypofluorescence in digital images.

Using stereophotography

Stereophotography separates, photographically, the tissues of the eye for the observer. Stereo fluorescein angiography facilitates interpretation by separating in depth the retinal and choroidal circulation.[16,17] Stereo angiography is considered absolutely essential in certain situations.[18] The photographic protocol for the Macular Photocoagulation Study required stereo fluorescein angiography. Without well-resolved stereo images, interpretation of angiograms with, for instance, choroidal neovascularization associated with age-related macular degeneration, can be extremely difficult, if not impossible (Fig. 1.10). On the other hand, stereophotography, although extremely helpful in cases that are difficult to interpret, is not always absolutely necessary because other fundus features and characteristics usually indicate the level at which abnormal fluorescence is located.

Adequate stereophotographs can be achieved with a pupillary dilation of 4 mm, although dilation of 6 mm or more is best. The first photograph of any stereo pair is taken with the camera positioned as far to the photographer's right (the patient's left) of the pupil's center as possible (of course, without inducing reflexes). The second photograph of the stereo pair is taken with the camera held as far to the photographer's left (the patient's right) of the pupil's center as possible. This order is extremely important because the photographs are taken and positioned on the film so that the angiogram is read from right to left. Thus the first photograph in the stereo sequence appears on the right on the contact sheet to correspond with the interpreter's right eye; the second is printed on the left for his or her left eye. It follows, then, that the first view of a stereo pair should be taken from the photographer's right, followed by a view from the left.

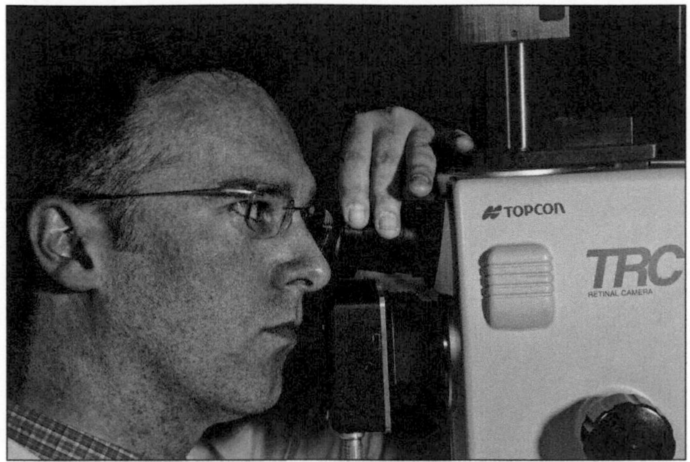

Fig. 1.9 The photographer focuses the eyepiece of the camera by initially turning the eyepiece counterclockwise, then clockwise, and stopping when it is in exact focus. The photographer must be sure that the eyepiece crosshairs remain in perfect focus throughout the photographic procedure.

Photographing the periphery

Photographing the peripheral retina with a standard 50° fundus camera demands precision and skills acquired only after many hours of practice. Problems with patient position and camera alignment and focus are compounded by marginal corneal astigmatism, unsteadiness of patient fixation, light reflexes, and awkward camera placement. All steps necessary for taking posterior photographs, such as alignment and focusing, must be employed to achieve good peripheral fundus photography. The Zeiss camera comes with an astigmatic dial to help neutralize the induced astigmatism. A tilt mechanism, now standard on most cameras, helps position the camera for extreme superior and inferior peripheral photography (Fig. 1.11).

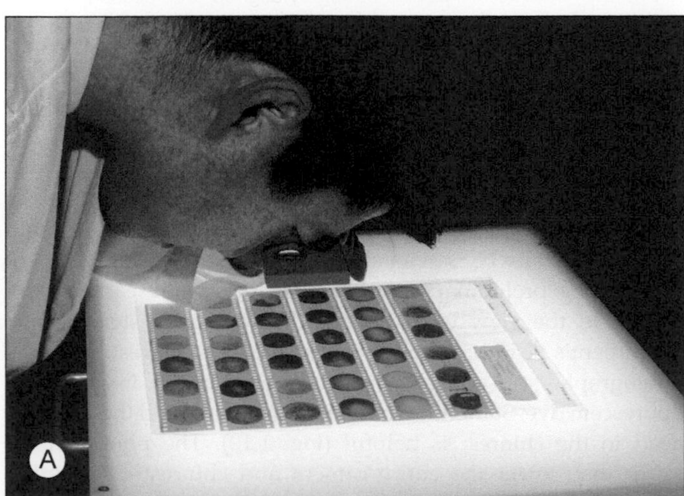

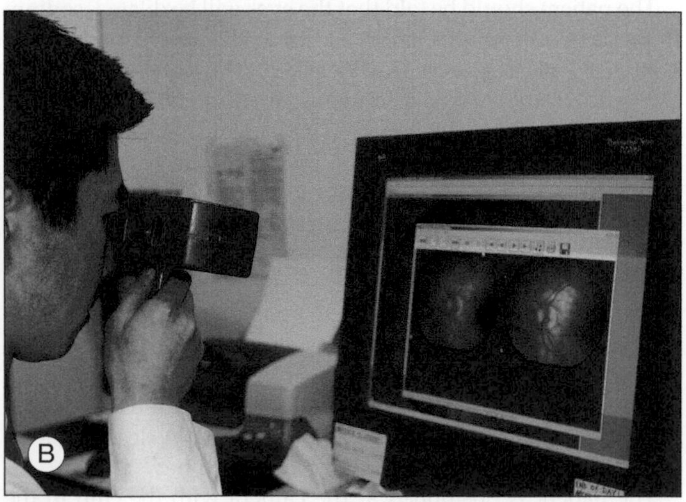

Fig. 1.10 Viewing stereo fundus photographs. (A) Negatives are placed on a viewing back-lit display. Two negative images are then viewed with an adjustable stereo lens. Reading the contact print of the angiogram. The stereo viewer can be easily made up using a trial frame. In viewing negative images, "hyperfluorescence" corresponds to dark objects while corresponding "hypofluorescent" objects are lighter. (B) Reading a stereo pair of digital angiograms. The special viewer allows the observer to focus both images. The software displayed is Ophthalmic Imaging Systems.

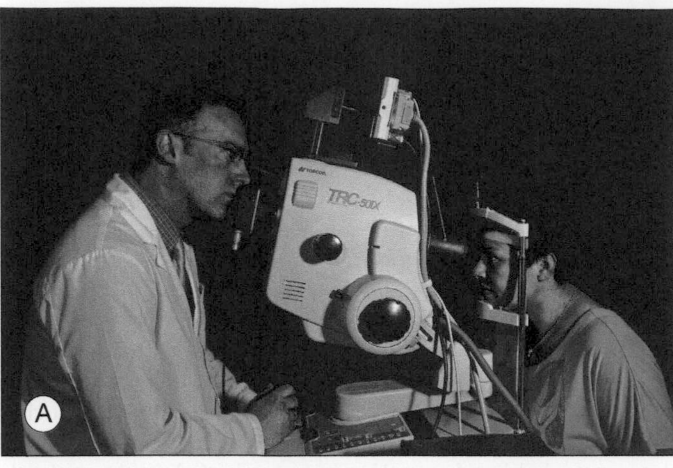

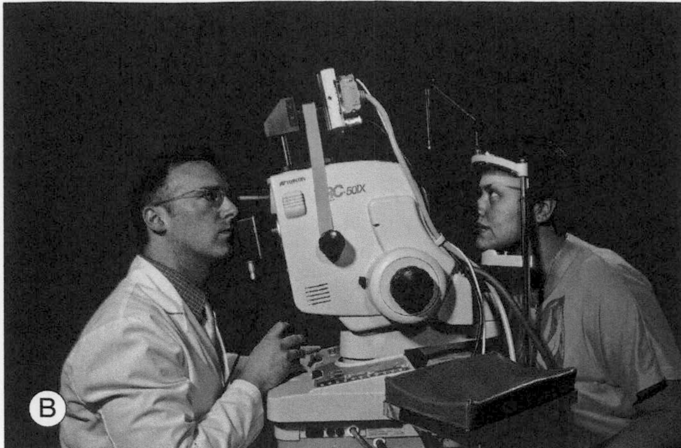

Fig. 1.11 Photographing the periphery. (A) The tilt mechanism of the camera allows the back of the camera to be lifted up (tilted to aim downward) for photography of the inferior periphery. The same tilt mechanism can be used to bring the camera far down (tilted to aim upward) to take pictures of the superior periphery (B). In photographing the inferior periphery, the photographer must sometimes stand. This photograph was a mock situation. In a real situation, the photographer or an assistant would have to lift the patient's upper lid to view the inferior periphery properly.

During photography of the periphery, the patient tends to turn or move his or her head. Unsatisfactory photographs caused by the movement of the head away from the camera or to the side can be avoided if the photographer is alert to these possibilities and takes the necessary steps to prevent them. On the whole, achieving good peripheral photographs depends on photographic skill, of course, but also on patience on the part of both photographer and patient.

Informing the patient

An important step toward a successful angiogram is to inform the patient about the procedure. An informed patient is generally less anxious and more cooperative than one who is unsure of the situation. Some institutions routinely provide a consent form to be signed by patients who are to have angiograms. However, this practice cannot replace the duty of the physician to inform the patient about the procedure and its potential complications and to answer all questions.

The patient should be told that the eyes will be dilated, sodium fluorescein will be injected in a vein in the arm or back of the hand, and photographs will be taken. The patient should be assured that the flash is a harmless, bright light (not an X-ray) and that fluorescein dye is safe. The patient should be told that injection of the dye can cause complications but that such occurrences are rare. If the patient requests further details about complications, the physician is obligated to supply the information.

Positioning the patient

Before the patient is seated at the camera, the photographer makes sure that the front lens is free of any dirt or dust. The lens should always be covered by a lens cap when the camera is not in use. The front of the lens should be kept clean using chloroform and a tightly rolled rod of lens tissue. To clean the lens, begin at the center and rotate out to the periphery.

The patient is positioned at the camera with the chin in the chinrest and the forehead against the head bar. Because the most common cause of poor fluorescein photographs is involuntary movement of the patient's head, the photographer should prepare and make adjustment for this before the fluorescein is injected. The photographer should aim and focus the camera on the specific area of primary interest, at the same time noting the patient's responses. If the photographer finds that the camera must continually be moved closer to the patient while aligning it or taking preliminary photographs, or if reflexes suddenly appear in the view even though the camera is steady, then the patient's head has moved away from the chinrest. If so, the photographer can make some adjustment before injecting the fluorescein dye. Sometimes having an assistant hold the patient's head in the chinrest is helpful (Fig. 1.12). The photographer either may lower the entire camera and chinrest or raise the patient's chair. This causes the patient to lean forward in the chinrest and against the forehead bar, making it more difficult for the patient to pull back.

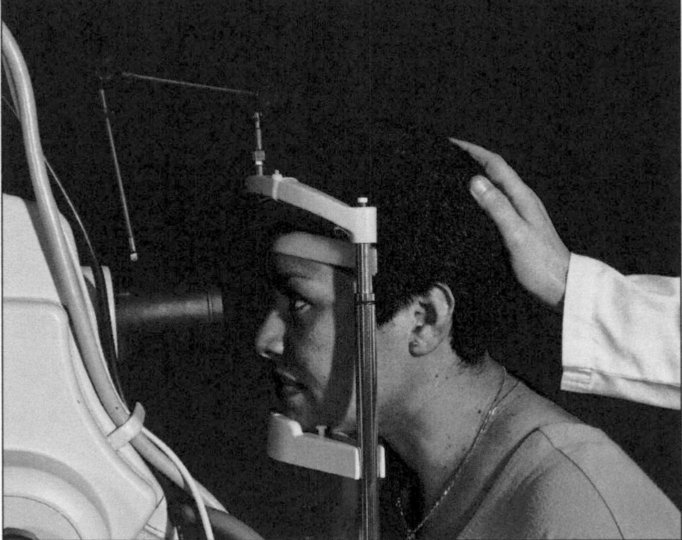

Fig. 1.12 An assistant holds the patient's head as a reminder to the patient to keep the chin in the chinrest and forehead against the bar.

Before photography begins, and between shots, the photographer may ask the patient to blink several times. This usually makes the patient more comfortable and also moistens the cornea and keeps it clear. When the pictures are actually being shot, the patient should be instructed to blink as infrequently as possible.

The photographer should talk to the patient frequently during the procedure, informing the patient of the progress of the testing and assuring him or her that all is going well. Explanation and reinforcement help produce better photographs.

Injecting the fluorescein

The color stereoscopic fundus photographs are taken first, before the fluorescein is injected. For injection, we recommend a syringe with a 23-gauge scalp-vein needle (Fig. 1.13). The scalp-vein needle has several advantages: it is small enough to enter most visible veins, and an intravenous opening is then available in the event of an emergency. Once in the vein, it requires no further attention, and although it can be taped in place, this usually is unnecessary. Whenever an antecubital vein is not visible or accessible, the vein in the back of the hand or radial (thumb) side of the wrist can usually be used for injection. Injecting the fluorescein into a hand or wrist vein increases the circulation time by a few seconds, but this seldom makes any difference.

Injection of the fluorescein is coordinated with the photographic process and is done after the first photographs (color fundus and control photographs; see next section) have been taken. With the needle in place, angiography can begin. By a predetermined, preferably silent, signal (such as a nod of the head), the photographer indicates to the physician to begin injecting fluorescein. The photographer starts the timer on the camera simultaneously with the start of injection and takes one photograph. This frame will show zero time on the photograph. In this way, the time from the beginning of injection is recorded on each subsequent angiographic photograph. When the injection is finished, the photographer may take another picture, which shows how long the injection took.

A rapid injection of 2 or 3 seconds delivers a high concentration of fluorescein to the bloodstream for a short time and probably yields somewhat better photographs than does a slower injection. However, the more rapid the injection, the greater the incidence of nausea from a highly concentrated bolus of fluorescein. For this reason a slower injection (4–6 seconds) is preferable; the photographs will still be of good quality. Because some fluorescein dye remains in the tubing, the scalp-vein needle should have short, rather than long, tubing to ensure that more of the dye is injected.

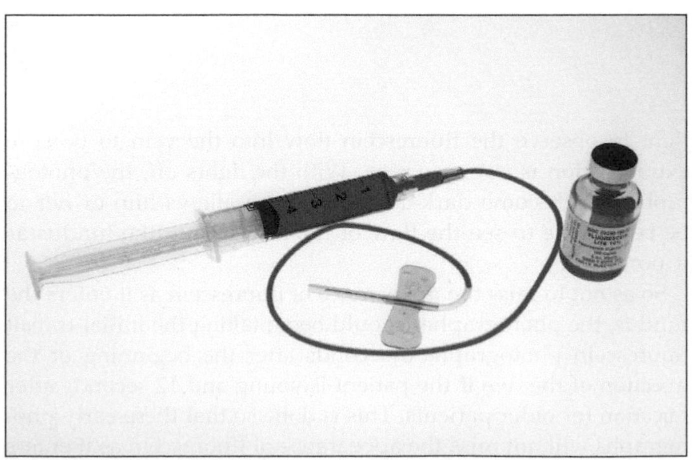

Fig. 1.13 Ten percent fluorescein solution, 5 mL syringe, and 23-gauge scalp-vein needle.

Developing a photographic plan

To photograph and print the fluorescein angiogram, we suggest the following comprehensive plan, designed to yield maximal angiographic information from each fundus and to facilitate a thorough and complete interpretation (Fig. 1.14). In contrast to film-based angiograms which required multiple duplicate attempts to assure at least one image would be optimal, fewer photographs are necessary in digital angiography. Although most angiograms will be complete by following this procedure, there will be exceptions. This plan must be modified if abnormalities occur in areas other than the macula and disc.

The photographic strategy essentially begins when the clinician has identified a condition or finding that requires angiographic study. The pathology dictates whether the photographic approach should image a magnified highly detailed finding versus a wider field of view for a more diffuse disease. Narrower field limits with higher magnification yield optimal images for focal pathology in conditions such as maculopathies, optic nerve disorders, and small focal lesions. Wider field of view often sacrifices magnification, but is effective in documenting conditions involving the periphery, such as diabetic retinopathy and vascular occlusive disease. Peripheral retinal scans for areas of neovascularization, as well as consideration for images that can be later montaged for wide-field reproductions, must also be incorporated into certain photographic plans. Elevated lesions such as tumors require great care in capturing high-quality stereo images.

It is both essential and extremely cost-effective for the physician to indicate specifically what areas to photograph. The photographer should be directed as to where to start the angiogram and the issues important for each specific angiogram. It is most efficient to use a photographic instruction slip that indicates the specific number of color photographs to take of each area, where to start the angiogram, what the diagnosis is, and any other information about the patient or fundus that is pertinent to the photographic process (Fig. 1.15). Although digital color and angiograms avoid the issue of wasted film and developing costs, unnecessary computer storage of images and patient inconvenience can be avoided with good technique and a repeatable, accurate algorithm for angiography.

Historically, because the roll of 35-mm negative film used for fluorescein angiography has 36 frames, it was convenient to think of the photograph session in terms of six rows of six frames each. Thus frame 1 appears in the upper right-hand corner and frame 36 in the lower left-hand corner. The angiogram developed from 36-mm negatives thus reads from right to left and from top to bottom. With the advent of digital imaging, theoretically, an unlimited number of frames can be acquired. However, to maximize efficiency of resources, digital storage of 20 frames per digital proof sheet is typically more than adequate for most clinical scenarios.

The first frame of the angiographic series is the color photograph of each eye. Then, a preinjection "control" photograph checks the dual-filter system for autofluorescence and pseudofluorescence.

	Inject fluorescein, when injection ends, begin angio-photography of primary macula Youth: 10 sec Elderly 12 sec	Pre-injection photograph with fluorescein filters secondary macula	Pre-injection photograph with fluorescein filters primary macula	Left eye macula	Right eye macula
Stereo pair Secondary macula	1–2 sec later primary macula	1–2 sec later primary macula	1–2 sec later primary macula	1–2 sec later primary macula	1–2 sec later primary macula
Stereo pair Secondary macula	Stereo pair Secondary macula	Stereo pair Primary disc	Stereo pair Primary disc	Stereo pair Primary macula	Stereo pair Primary macula
Patient rest period unless peripheral scans indicated	Angiophotograph other areas of importance in either eye according to fluorescein angioscopy or nature of case	Post-venous filling Secondary macula and disc	Post-venous filling Primary macula and disc	Stereo pair Secondary disc	Stereo pair Secondary disc
Late angiophotographs of other areas of importance		Late secondary disc	Late secondary macula	Late primary disc	Late primary macula

Fig. 1.14 Photographic plan for fluorescein angiography of macular disease. Film-based images printed upside down because the fundus camera inverts the image of the fundus, and, to read the angiogram upright, the film is printed with the frame numbers upside down. In digital photography, no inversion is required.

At this point the fluorescein injection is begun. The needle is inserted in a vein in the patient's arm (Fig. 1.16). The photographer waits for confirmation of successful venous access and awaits verbal confirmation that infusion is about to begin. Once the injecting clinician starts the infusion of fluorescein, the photographer begins the initial "injection" image. When the injecting clinician has completed infusion, he or she announces "injection complete" and the photographer takes the "end-of-injection" image. Because it is important to observe the site of the needle tip for extravasation of fluorescein, the lights are turned off only at the end of the injection. An alternative method is to turn the lights off after the needle has been inserted in the vein. The person injecting can hold a hand light to observe the fluorescein flow into the vein to be sure extravasation is not occurring. With the lights off, the photographer can become dark-adapted, which allows him or her to be better able to see the flow of fluorescein into the fundus as it occurs.

So as not to miss the appearance of fluorescein as it enters the fundus, the photographer should begin taking the initial-transit fluorescein photographs 8 seconds after the beginning of the injection of the dye if the patient is young and 12 seconds after injection for older patients. This is done so that these early photographs will not miss the appearance of fluorescein as it enters the fundus. Then, at intervals of 1.5–2 seconds, approximately 6 photographs should be taken in succession.

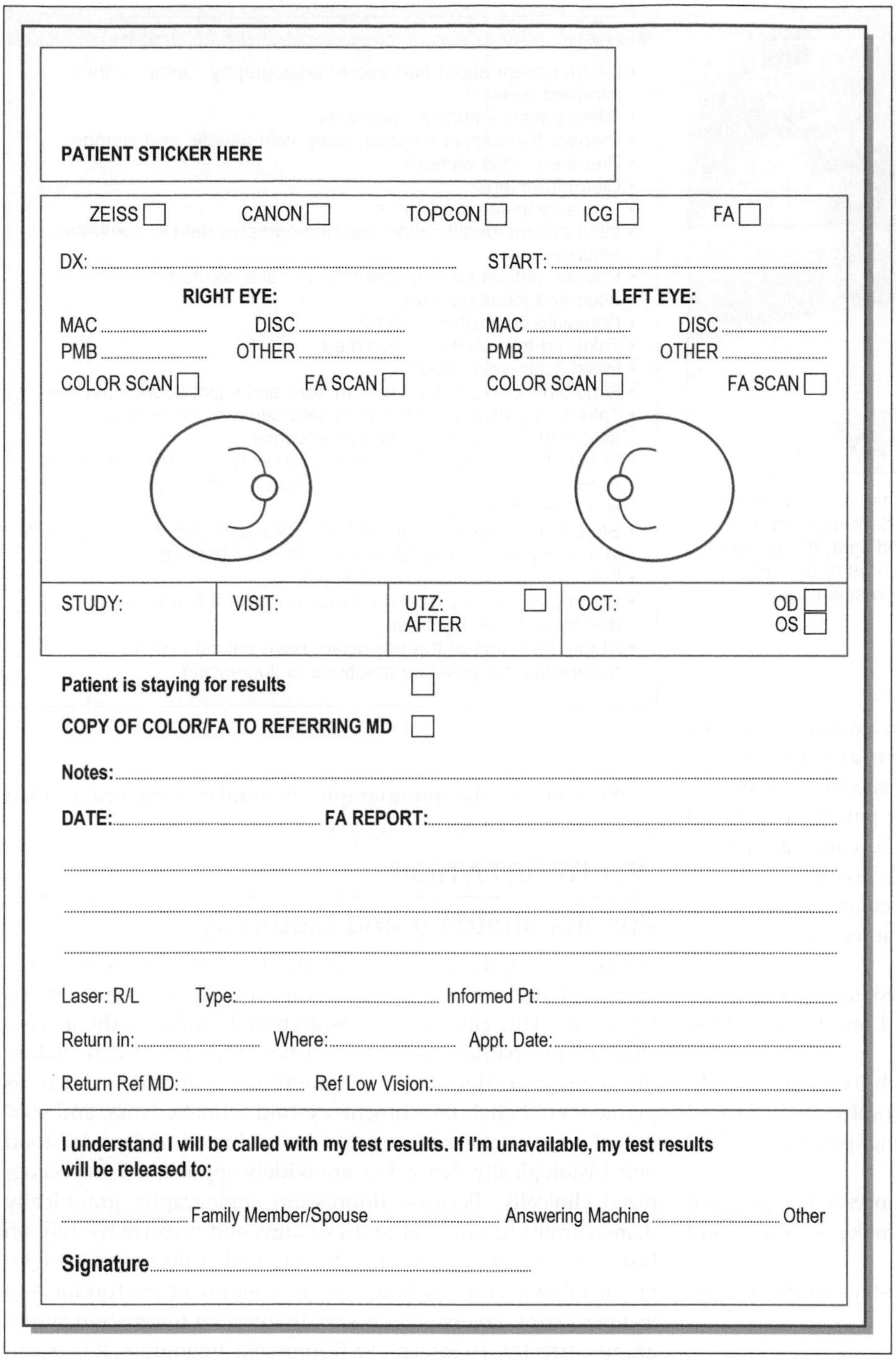

PATIENT STICKER HERE

ZEISS ☐ CANON ☐ TOPCON ☐ ICG ☐ FA ☐

DX: .... START: ....

RIGHT EYE: **LEFT EYE:**

MAC .... DISC .... MAC .... DISC ....

PMB .... OTHER .... PMB .... OTHER ....

COLOR SCAN ☐ FA SCAN ☐ COLOR SCAN ☐ FA SCAN ☐

STUDY:	VISIT:	UTZ: ☐ AFTER	OCT:	OD ☐ OS ☐

Patient is staying for results ☐

COPY OF COLOR/FA TO REFERRING MD ☐

Notes: ....

DATE: .... **FA REPORT:** ....

Laser: R/L Type: .... Informed Pt: ....

Return in: .... Where: .... Appt. Date: ....

Return Ref MD: .... Ref Low Vision: ....

I understand I will be called with my test results. If I'm unavailable, my test results will be released to:

.... Family Member/Spouse .... Answering Machine .... Other

Signature ....

Fig. 1.15 Photographic request form. In the top left portion of the form, the physician indicates the number of color photographs required for each area in the fundus. The physician also indicates the diagnosis because experienced photographers will know which type of photographs to take for each particular diagnosis. The physician also indicates in which location of the fundus the initial-transit phase of the angiogram should take place or, in other words, where the photographer should start the angiogram. In the lower right portion of the photographic request form, the physician can indicate to the photographer specifics about the patient that will facilitate the photographic process and save the photographer time. The physician can indicate whether an eye can fixate on a light, whether the media are clear (so that if the photographer cannot get a clear view, he or she can immediately understand that it is caused by a problem of the eye), and what the patient's refraction is so that the photographer can know which special lenses to use in the photographic process.

If the photographer does not see fluorescein entering and filling the retinal vessels while the six initial-transit photographs are taken, he or she must continue to photograph the fundus until filling takes place and also should check to see why no fluorescein is present.

After the first six initial-transit photographs and approximately 20–30 seconds after injection, with sufficient fluorescein concentration in the eye, the photographer should take a photograph of the fellow eye, a stereoscopic pair of photographs of the primary area of interest, followed by a stereoscopic pair of other pertinent areas. For example, in the suggested photographic plan, after stereophotographs of the right macula are taken, stereophotographs of the right disc are taken. The photographer should then photograph in stereo the macula and disc of the fellow eye.

Late-stage angiographs, preferably in stereo, are taken of the pertinent areas of each eye. It is important to photograph both discs and macula and any other areas of abnormal fluorescence and to note any areas that could not be photographed. This ensures that the interpreter will have adequate information for a complete interpretation of the angiogram.

The entire photographic process lasts 5–10 minutes. Angiophotographs taken more than 10 minutes after injection are usually not necessary. In some cases of central serous

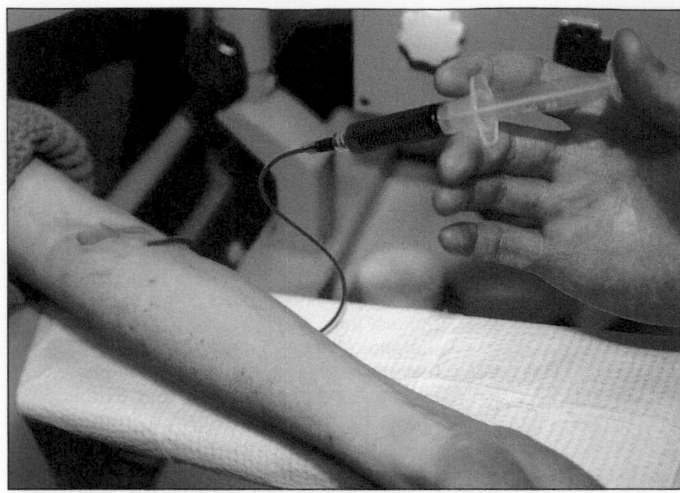

Fig. 1.16 After the needle is placed in the vein, the lights can be turned off so that the photographer can become dark-adapted and see fluorescein flow in the eye. With the use of a hand light, the person injecting can carefully observe the injection site so as to be sure extravasation is not occurring. In this way the fluorescein solution can be injected while the room lights are out.

Box 1.3 Checklist for fluorescein angiography

- Inform patient about fluorescein angiography. Obtain written informed consent
- Dilate patient's pupil if necessary
- Prepare fluorescein solution, scalp-vein needle, and syringe
- Prepare fundus camera
- Clean front lens
- Focus eyepiece crosshairs
- Input patient identification and demographic data in computer database
- Position patient for alignment, focus, and comfort
- Align and focus camera
- Complete color photography
- Take red-free photos if indicated
- Insert scalp-vein needle
- Simultaneously start timer from zero and inject fluorescein dye
- Take preinjection photograph: these serve as controls in detecting auto- and pseudofluorescence
- Shoot at exact start of injection as timer is turned on and shoot second shot at exact finish of injection (length of time of injection is automatically recorded)
- Start fluorescein photograph 8 seconds after the start of injection in young patients and 12 seconds in older patients
- Follow fluorescein angiography plan
- When photography is done, reassure patient that urine will be discolored for a day or so
- At the discretion of the physician, have patient wait for observation for possible reactions to fluorescein

chorioretinopathy, or other rare situations, angiophotographs taken longer than 10 minutes after injection are helpful. This photographic algorithm is modified for specific conditions. For instance, in an angiogram of a diabetic patient, peripheral scans may be included at the request of the clinician surveying for neovascularization. In a patient with possible choroidal neovascularization due to age-related macular degeneration, additional angiophotographs of the suspicious lesion may be useful.

At the end of the session the patient is asked regarding any sensations related to an allergic reaction and reminded that the urine will be discolored for about a day.

In the event of a technical difficulty, such as camera breakdown, repeat fluorescein injection or photography can be carried out with satisfactory results after a waiting period of 30–60 minutes.

The plan we have suggested allows the fluorescein angiogram to yield all the information necessary to make a proper and thorough interpretation.

Box 1.3 provides a checklist of important steps in the fluorescein angiography procedure.

Diabetic retinopathy

Diabetic retinopathy presents a unique challenge for the photographer as significant pathology may be located both within the macula and the periphery. A photographic plan must yield information regarding leakage contributing to diabetic macular edema and nonfilling from capillary nonperfusion. At the same time, peripheral scans confirming the presence of neovascularization in preproliferative and proliferative diabetic retinopathy must also be obtained. In this setting, rather than stereo pairs of macula and disc of the fellow eye, photographs of the nasal, superior, temporal, and inferior quadrants, respectively, of the primary eye are studied. For the purpose of orientation, interpretation, and uniformity, the nasal, superior, and inferior photographs are taken with the edge of the disc at the edge of the photograph and the temporal photograph with the fovea at the edge of the photograph. A similar sequence is then performed on the secondary eye.

INTERPRETATION

Fundus anatomy and histology

Fluorescein angiography has greatly increased our knowledge of retinal and choroidal circulatory physiology and fundus pathology. This clinical and research tool facilitates the in vivo study of histopathologic characteristics of fundus disease. Before the advent of fluorescein angiography, conditions such as pigment epithelial detachment, cystoid retinal edema, and subretinal neovascularization could be evaluated and understood only histologically. Now they are widely appreciated and recognized clinically. Because fluorescein angiography graphically demonstrates fundus pathophysiology, and because we rely on histologic points of reference to interpret a fluorescein angiogram, a thorough knowledge of the anatomy of the fundus and its microscopic layers is necessary to interpret fluorescein angiograms correctly. To interpret a fluorescein angiogram, it is essential to understand the microscopic layers of the fundus (i.e., the histology).

A logical place to begin this study is at the vitreous. In its normal state, and in a normal angiogram, the vitreous is clear and nonfluorescent. However, when it contains opacities that block the view of retinal and choroidal fluorescence, hypofluorescence occurs. The vitreous is also an important point of reference when intraocular inflammation or retinal neovascularization is present. In these cases fluorescein leaks into the vitreous, causing fluffy fluorescence as fluorescein molecules disperse into fluid vitreous and vitreous gel.

For the purpose of fluorescein angiographic interpretation, it is convenient to divide the sensory retina into two layers: the inner vascular half and the outer half, which is avascular. The inner vascular half extends from the internal limiting membrane to the inner nuclear layer. This portion of the retina contains the retinal blood vessels, which are located in two separate planes: the larger retinal arteries and veins are located in the nerve fiber layer; the retinal capillaries are located in the inner nuclear layer. In a well-focused stereoscopic fluorescein angiogram, these two vascular layers can be seen as distinct planes in the retina. An extremely important fluorescein angiographic concept is that normal retinal blood vessels are impermeable to fluorescein leakage; that is, fluorescein flows through the normal retinal vessels without leakage into the retina.

The outer avascular half of the sensory retina comprises the outer plexiform layer, the outer nuclear layer, and the rods and cones. The outer plexiform layer is the primary interstitial space in the retina. When the retina becomes edematous, it is in this layer that fluid accumulates, causing cystoid spaces. Deep retinal hemorrhages and exudates (lipid deposits) may also be deposited in the outer plexiform layer.

The rods and cones are very loosely attached to the pigment epithelium, especially in the macular region, whereas the pigment epithelium is very firmly attached to Bruch's membrane. In fluorescein angiographic interpretation the pigment epithelium is an extremely important tissue because it prevents fluorescein leakage from the choroid and blocks, to a greater or lesser extent, visualization of choroidal fluorescence.

Bruch's membrane separates the pigment epithelium from the choriocapillaris, which is permeable to fluorescein. Fluorescein passes freely from the choriocapillaris and diffuses through Bruch's membrane up to, but not into, the pigment epithelium. Beneath the choriocapillaris are the larger choroidal vessels, which are impermeable to fluorescein. Melanocytes are dispersed throughout the choroid but are most heavily concentrated in the lamina fusca, the thin layer between the choroid and sclera. The sclera lies beneath the choroidal vessels.

The ophthalmic artery gives rise usually to two main posterior ciliary arteries: the lateral and medial. However, three posterior ciliary arteries may be present, in which case the medial artery is the one usually duplicated less frequently. In rare instances there may be a superior posterior ciliary artery.

The posterior ciliary arteries supply the lateral and medial halves of the disc and choroid. During angiography a vertical zone of slightly delayed filling may be seen passing through the papillomacular region, including the disc. Occasionally, there is an oblique orientation to this supply or even a superoinferior distribution. This border between the main posterior ciliary arteries has been termed the watershed zone, where patchy choroidal filling often can be seen on fluorescein angiograms.

Each main posterior ciliary artery divides into numerous short arteries and one long artery. On the temporal side the short posterior ciliary arteries supply small, variously sized, wedge-shaped choroidal segments, whose apices are centered near the macula. The lateral long posterior ciliary artery passes obliquely through the sclera. It supplies a wedge of choroid that begins temporal to the macular region and participates in the formation of the greater circle of the iris.

The choriocapillaris is made up of discrete units called lobules, thought to be approximately one-fourth to one-half of a disc diameter in size. The center of each lobule is fed by a precapillary arteriole (terminal choroidal arteriole), which comes from a short posterior ciliary artery. Each lobule functions independently in the normal state. It has been assumed that angiographic zones of delayed or patchy choroidal filling gradually fill in a transverse fashion, with one lobule spilling over into another. Careful inspection, however, indicates that these filling defects generally remain the same size, indicating a delayed filling from a posterior origin (its own arteriolar feeder). In the abnormal state, as when a choroidal vascular occlusion occurs, there is a freely connecting "spilling over" of blood flow from well-perfused choroid to the occluded area.

Around the margin of each lobule is a ring of postcapillary venules that drain each lobule. These postcapillary venules drain into the vortex veins, which drain the entire choroid. There are usually four vortex veins, and each functions as a well-defined quadrantic segmental drainage system for the entire uvea. In the case of a posterior ciliary artery obstruction, this occluded portion of the choroid can fill by a retrograde mechanism from an adjacent posterior ciliary artery by way of the choroidal venous system. This mechanism may provide adequate nourishment to prevent extensive ischemic changes until the occluded artery reopens.

Knowledge of each of these layers of the fundus is important in understanding fundus histopathology. The following six areas, however, are more important than others in the interpretation of abnormal fundus fluorescence:

1. preretinal area, where contraction from an epiretinal membrane may influence the retinal circulation and where hemorrhage may be located
2. vascular layers of the sensory retina, both superficial and deep
3. avascular portion of the sensory retina, particularly the outer plexiform layer, the principal site of intraretinal edema and exudate
4. retinal pigment epithelium, which has the potential for many manifestations, including proliferation, depigmentation, hyperpigmentation, and detachment
5. choroidal circulation, including the choriocapillaris and the large choroidal vessels
6. sclera, which lies beneath the choroid.

Throughout this chapter a modified schematic drawing relates various fluorescein angiographic abnormalities to fundus histopathologic changes (Fig. 1.17). The size and proportion of these various layers have been modified to include various pathologic manifestations and to illustrate the effects of these abnormalities on the angiogram. Because of its importance and various pathologic changes, the pigment epithelium is drawn to a larger scale in relation to other fundus structures. Only the inner portion of the sclera is represented because the outer portion of the sclera is usually of little importance to angiographic interpretation. The retinal and choroidal vessels are drawn larger and more numerous than they appear in a normal histopathologic section to emphasize the contribution of circulatory pathophysiologic interpretation.

Two specialized areas of the fundus warrant more detailed discussion: the macula (Fig. 1.18) and the optic nerve head. The fovea is the center of the macula and contains only four layers of the retina: (1) the internal limiting membrane; (2) the outer plexiform layer; (3) the outer nuclear layer; and (4) the rods and cones. No intermediate layers exist between the internal limiting

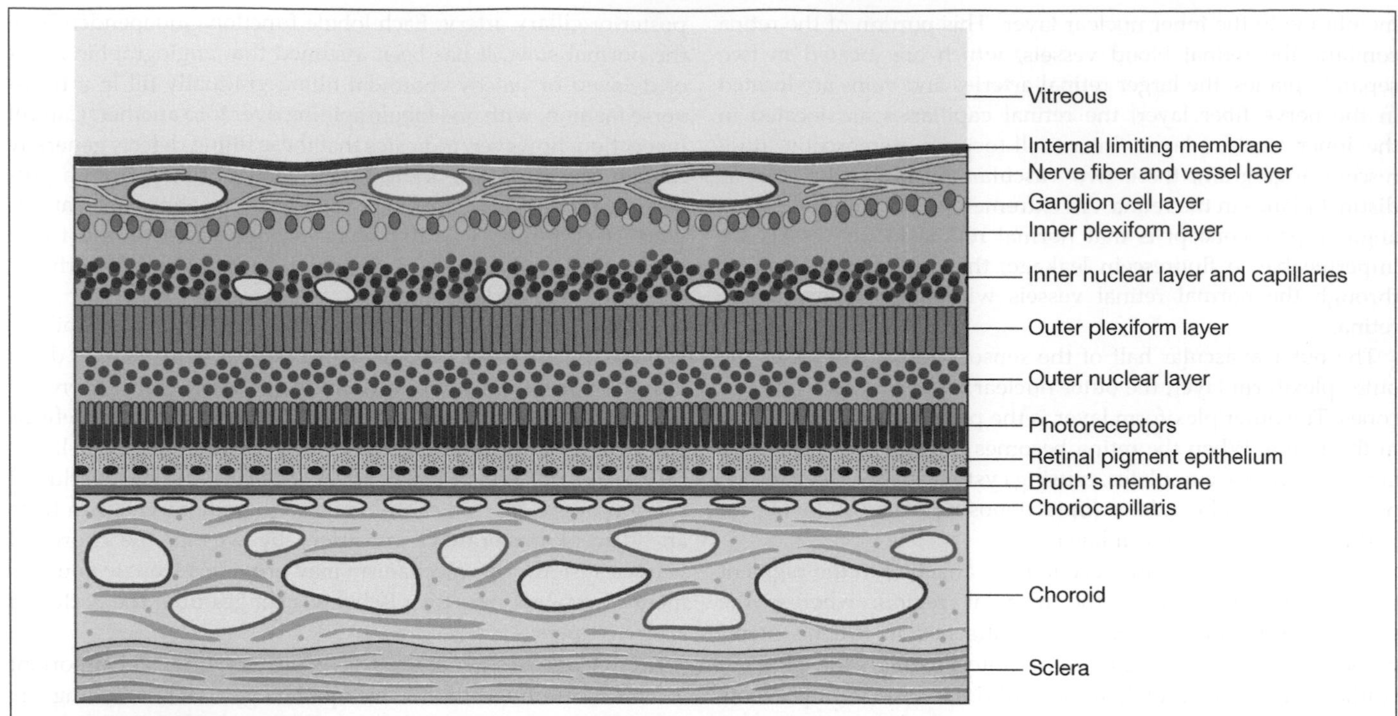

Fig. 1.17 Modified schematic drawing of a microscopic section of retina, pigment epithelium, and choroid.

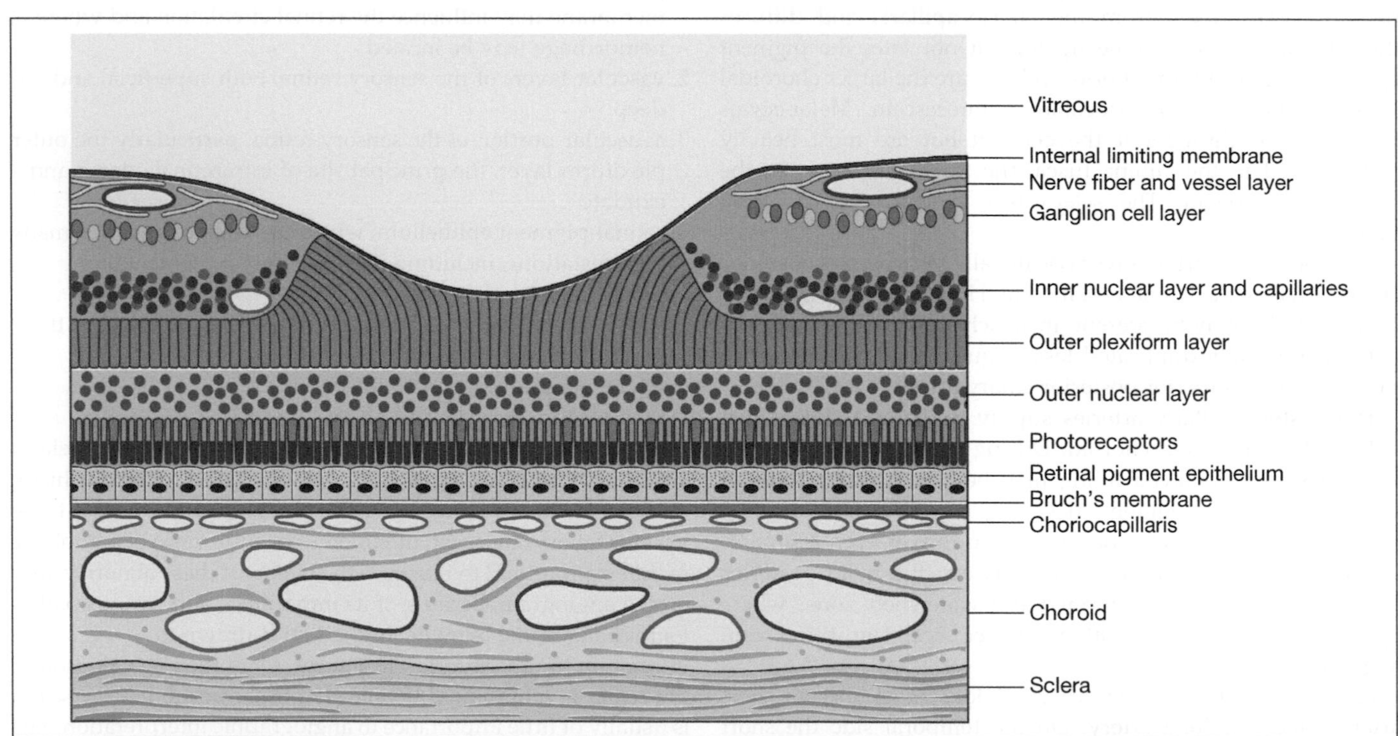

Fig. 1.18 Modified schematic drawing of a microscopic section of the macula.

membrane and the outer plexiform layer in the fovea, which in the macula is oblique. This is an important factor in understanding the stellate appearance of cystoid edema in the macula as opposed to the honeycomb appearance of cystoid edema outside the macula. Beyond the macular region the outer plexiform layer is perpendicular rather than oblique.

The pigment epithelial cells in the macula are more columnar and have a greater concentration of melanin and lipofuscin granules than in the remainder of the fundus.

Xanthophyll is present in the fovea, located probably in the outer plexiform layer. These differences in pigmentation are the chief factors responsible for producing the characteristic dark zone in the macular region on normal angiograms. The absence of retinal vessels in the fovea (i.e., the perifoveal capillary-free zone), in most cases approximately 400–500 mm in diameter in the center of the fovea, is another cause of the dark appearance of the macula.

The optic nerve head, or disc, is the other highly specialized tissue of the posterior pole. The disc is fed by two circulatory systems: the retinal vascular system and the posterior ciliary vascular system. Widespread anastomotic channels exist between the posterior ciliary vasculature and the optic nerve and retinal vasculature and become exaggerated in certain pathologic conditions. The disc is made up of many layers of nerve fibers and glial supporting columns that contain the large retinal vessels.

The central retinal artery arises from the ophthalmic artery in close proximity to the main posterior ciliary arteries. In about 45% of the population, the central retinal artery and the medial posterior ciliary artery arise from a common trunk. In 12% of persons the central retinal artery originates from the ciliary artery. Therefore it is impossible to have a choroidal infarction, anterior ischemic optic neuropathy, and a central retinal artery occlusion all due to a single site of obstruction.

The central retinal artery provides a major source of blood supply to the axial portion of the anterior orbital portion of the optic nerve. In the intraneural or axial course, short centrifugal branches arise but usually end a short distance behind the lamina cribrosa. There are then no further branches from the central retinal artery until it reaches the retina. If a cilioretinal artery is present, it supplies the corresponding segment of the disc.

The peripapillary nerve fiber layer is supplied by small, recurrent branches from the retinal arterioles at the peripapillary region. Emanating from these arterioles at the disc are the radial papillary capillaries. These capillaries are rather straight and long, have few anastomoses, and lie in the superficial portion of the peripapillary nerve fiber layer. The capillaries to the disc are continuous with these retinal peripapillary capillaries.

The short posterior ciliary arteries, or the recurrent branches from the peripapillary choroid, supply the retrolaminar portion of the optic nerve. The laminar cribrosa portion of the nerve is supplied by centripetal branches of the short posterior ciliary arteries. In this region a partial, or, rarely, a complete Zinn's vascular circle is occasionally found. The prelaminar portion is supplied by centripetal branches from the peripapillary choroid.

Because most of the disc is fed by the ciliary system, fluorescein appears simultaneously at the optic nerve head and the choroid and before it is apparent in the retinal arteries.

The main venous drainage of the disc is into the central retinal vein. The prelaminar portion empties into both the central retinal vein and the peripapillary choroid, thus providing potential collateral drainage in the case of obstruction of the central retinal vein behind the lamina cribrosa. Such large dilated collaterals are frequently seen following central retinal vein occlusion and are called retinociliary veins. Some mistakenly call them opticociliary shunts, a misnomer because they are not true shunts (defined as a congenital artery that empties into a vein and that skips the capillary bed, sometimes part of the Wyburn–Mason syndrome), and they are not optico because they emanate from the retina. They are, most accurately, retinovenous to ciliovenous collaterals.

In summary, fluorescein angiography provides an in vivo understanding of the histopathologic and pathophysiologic changes of various fundus abnormalities. Therefore an anatomic and, more specifically, a histologic understanding of important fundus landmarks is essential to fluorescein angiographic interpretation.

Normal fluorescein angiogram

The normal fluorescein angiogram is distinguished by certain specific characteristics. Knowledge of these characteristics provides an essential frame of reference for interpreting abnormal fluorescein angiograms.

In the normal fluorescein angiogram (Fig. 1.19), the first true fluorescence begins to show in the choroid approximately 10–12 seconds after injection in young patients (e.g., adolescents) and 12–15 seconds after injection in older patients.

Fluorescence can appear even earlier than 8 seconds in very young patients. The choroid occasionally begins to fluoresce 1 or 2 seconds before the initial filling of the central retinal artery. Early choroidal fluorescence is faint, patchy, and irregularly scattered throughout the posterior fundus. It is interspersed with scattered islands of delayed fluorescein filling. This early phase is referred to as the choroidal flush. When adjacent areas of choroidal filling and nonfilling are quite distinct, the pattern is designated as patchy choroidal filling.

Within the next 10 seconds (approximately 20-25 seconds after injection), the angiogram becomes very bright for about 5 seconds because of the extreme choroidal fluorescence. Choroidal fluorescence, however, is not visible in the macula because of the taller, more pigmented epithelium present in the fovea (retina). Therefore the macula remains dark throughout the angiogram.

If present, a cilioretinal artery usually begins to fluoresce as the choroid fluoresces, rather than as the retina fluoresces. Within 1-3 seconds after choroidal fluorescence is visible, or approximately 10–15 seconds after injection, the central retinal artery begins to fluoresce. The less dense the concentration of pigment in the pigment epithelium, the greater the time between the visibility of the choroidal fluorescence and the filling of the retinal vessels. The lighter pigment presents less interference to choroidal fluorescence, allowing it to be evident earlier in its filling phase. With a more densely pigmented pigment epithelium, the blockage barrier effect is greater. Therefore choroidal fluorescence appears somewhat later because a greater concentration of fluorescein is required to overcome the increased density of the pigment epithelial barrier.

Because no barrier exists in front of the retinal vessels, the patient's pigmentation has no effect on the visibility of the retinal vessels, although the degree of pigmentation does affect the contrast of the angiophotographs. The darker the pigment epithelium is, the less visible the choroidal fluorescence will be and the greater the contrast of the retinal vascular fluorescence (i.e., the better they stand out). The lighter the pigment epithelium is, the more visible the choroidal fluorescence will be and the less the contrast of the fluorescence from the retinal vessels.

After the central retinal artery begins to fill, the fluorescein flows into the retinal arteries, then into the precapillary arterioles, the capillaries, the postcapillary venules, and finally the retinal veins. Because the fluorescein from the venules enters the veins along their walls, the flow of fluorescein in the veins is laminar. Because vascular flow is faster in the center of a lumen (tube) than on the sides, the fluorescein seems to stick to the sides, creating the laminar pattern of retinal venous flow. The dark (nonfluorescent) central lamina is nonfluorescent blood that comes from the periphery, which takes longer to fluoresce because of its more distant location.

In the next 5–10 seconds, fluorescence of the two parallel laminae along the walls of the retinal veins becomes thicker. At the junction of two veins, the inner lamina of each vein may merge. This creates three laminae: one in the center and one on each side of the vein. As fluorescein filling increases in the veins, the laminae eventually enlarge and meet, resulting in complete fluorescence of the retinal veins.

Fluorescence of the disc emanates from the posterior ciliary vascular system, both from the edge of the disc and from the tissue between the center and the circumference of the disc. Filling also comes from the capillaries of the central retinal artery on the surface of the disc. Because healthy disc tissue contains many capillaries, the disc becomes fairly hyperfluorescent on the angiogram.

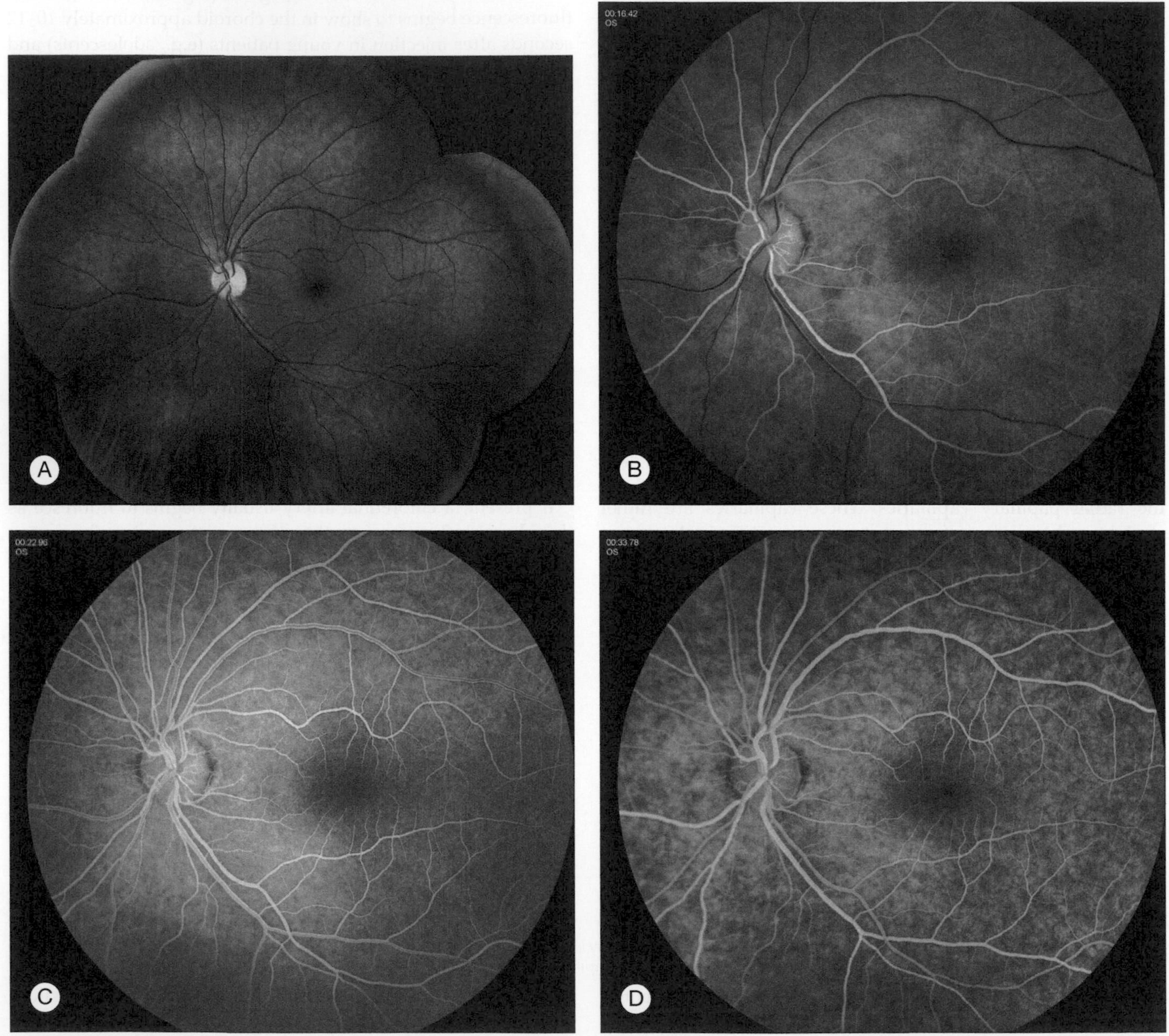

Fig. 1.19 Normal fundus photos and fluorescein angiogram of left disc and macula taken with a 50° camera. (A) Montage photograph of multiple fields shows normal macula, fovea, and retinal vessels. (B) Early arterial phase of the fluorescein angiogram. Note the ground-glass fluorescence of the choriocapillaris. There is very little fluorescence in the retinal veins; just the margins of the veins are fluorescent. This is the earliest portion of the laminar filling phase of the vein. Note some hyperfluorescence of choriocapillaris. These dark patches of the choroid are areas that have not fully filled, referred to as patchy choroidal filling. (C) The retinal arteries and capillaries have filled and the retinal veins have filled more substantially. Note the laminar flow in the retinal veins; this is indicated by the white line of fluorescence along the walls of the retinal veins. (D) Late venous phase. Laminar filling is no longer detectable and uniform filling is seen in both arterial and venous circulation.

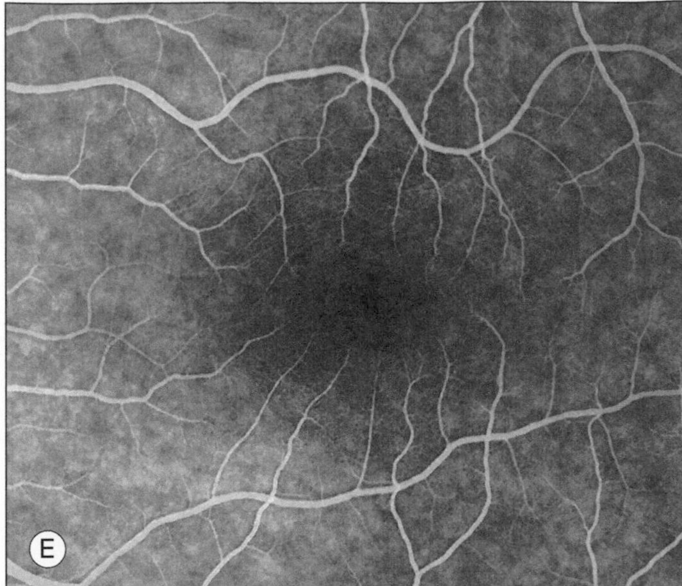

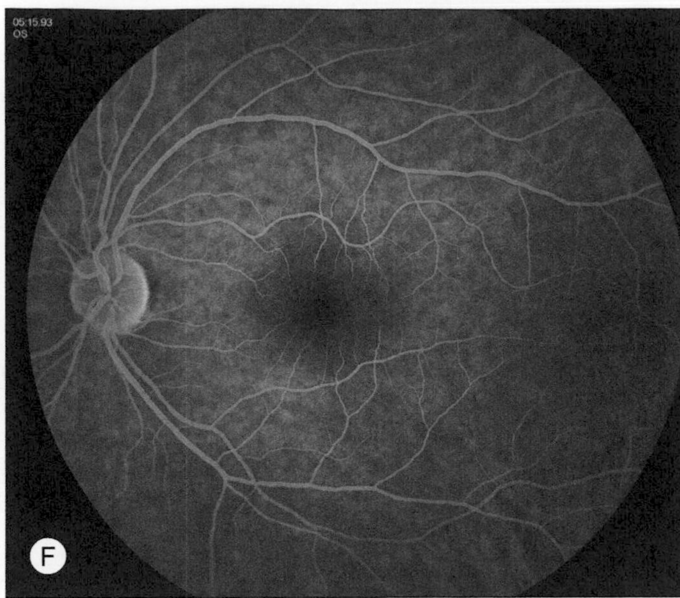

Fig. 1.19 Cont'd (E) Mid to later arteriovenous phase of fluorescein angiogram. Note that the ground-glass fluorescence of the choriocapillaris is complete. The retinal arteries and veins are completely filled. (F) Arteriovenous phase of fluorescein angiogram showing the disc. Again, there is diffuse fluorescence of the choriocapillaris. The arteries and veins have completely filled, and optic nerve fluorescence is normal.

The perifoveal capillary net cannot always be seen on the fluorescein angiogram. It can be seen best in young patients with clear ocular media about 20–25 seconds after a rapid fluorescein injection. This is called the "peak" phase of the fluorescein angiogram. The photographer should be aware of this phase and be sure not to miss it by shooting as rapidly as possible as the fluorescein concentration increases and by continuing to shoot rapidly until the concentration of fluorescein begins to decrease.

Approximately 30 seconds after injection, the first high-concentration flush of fluorescein begins to empty from the choroidal and retinal circulations. Recirculation phases follow, during which fluorescein in a lower concentration continues to pass through the circulation of the fundus.

Generally, 3–5 minutes after injection, the choroidal and retinal vasculatures slowly begin to empty of fluorescein and become gray. Vessels of most normal patients almost completely empty of fluorescein in approximately 10 minutes. The large choroidal vessels and the retinal vessels do not leak fluorescein. However, because of large gaps in its endothelium, the choriocapillaris does leak fluorescein. The extravasated fluorescein diffuses through the choroidal tissue, Bruch's membrane, and sclera. Leakage of fluorescein with retention in tissues is designated as staining. In the later phase of the angiogram, staining of Bruch's membrane, the choroid, and especially the sclera may be visible if the pigment epithelium is lightly pigmented. The disc and adjacent visible sclera remain hyperfluorescent because of staining. When the retinal pigment epithelium is especially lightly pigmented, the large choroidal vessels can be seen in silhouette against the fluorescent (fluorescein-stained) sclera. The lamina cribrosa within the disc also remains hyperfluorescent because of staining. This depends on the cup-to-disc ratio and the presence of any visible sclera, such as occurs within a conus adjacent to the disc. The edge of the disc stains from the adjacent choriocapillaris, which normally leaks.

To summarize, the angiogram is initially dark; choroidal and retinal filling is seen 10–15 seconds after fluorescein injection. The retinal and choroidal vasculatures fill maximally about 20–30 seconds after injection. Late angiophotographs show fluorescence of the choroid and sclera (if the pigment epithelium is light) and fluorescence of the optic cup and the edge of the disc, but otherwise the fundus is dark (nonfluorescent in the late phase).

ABNORMAL FLUORESCEIN ANGIOGRAM

The purpose of this section is to offer a schema by which the interpretation of the fluorescein angiogram follows a simple and logical progression. The first step is to recognize areas of abnormal fluorescence and determine if they are hypofluorescent or hyperfluorescent (Fig. 1.20).

Hypofluorescence

Hypofluorescence is a reduction or absence of normal fluorescence, whereas hyperfluorescence is abnormally excessive fluorescence. A systematic series of decisions follows this initial differentiation to arrive at a proper diagnosis. These decisions relate to: (l) the anatomic location of various abnormalities; (2) the quality and quantity of the abnormal fluorescence; and (3) other unique characteristics, as indicated in Fig. 1.20.

Hypofluorescence is any abnormally dark area on the positive print of an angiogram. There are two possible causes of hypofluorescence: blocked fluorescence or a vascular filling defect.

Blocked fluorescence is sometimes referred to as masked, obscured, or negative fluorescence or transmission decrease. Each of these terms indicates a reduction or absence of normal retinal or choroidal fluorescence because of a tissue or fluid barrier located anterior to the respective retinal or choroidal circulation. For example, blood in the vitreous or a layer of blood in front of the retina obscures the view of the retinal and choroidal circulations and therefore blocks fundus fluorescence from

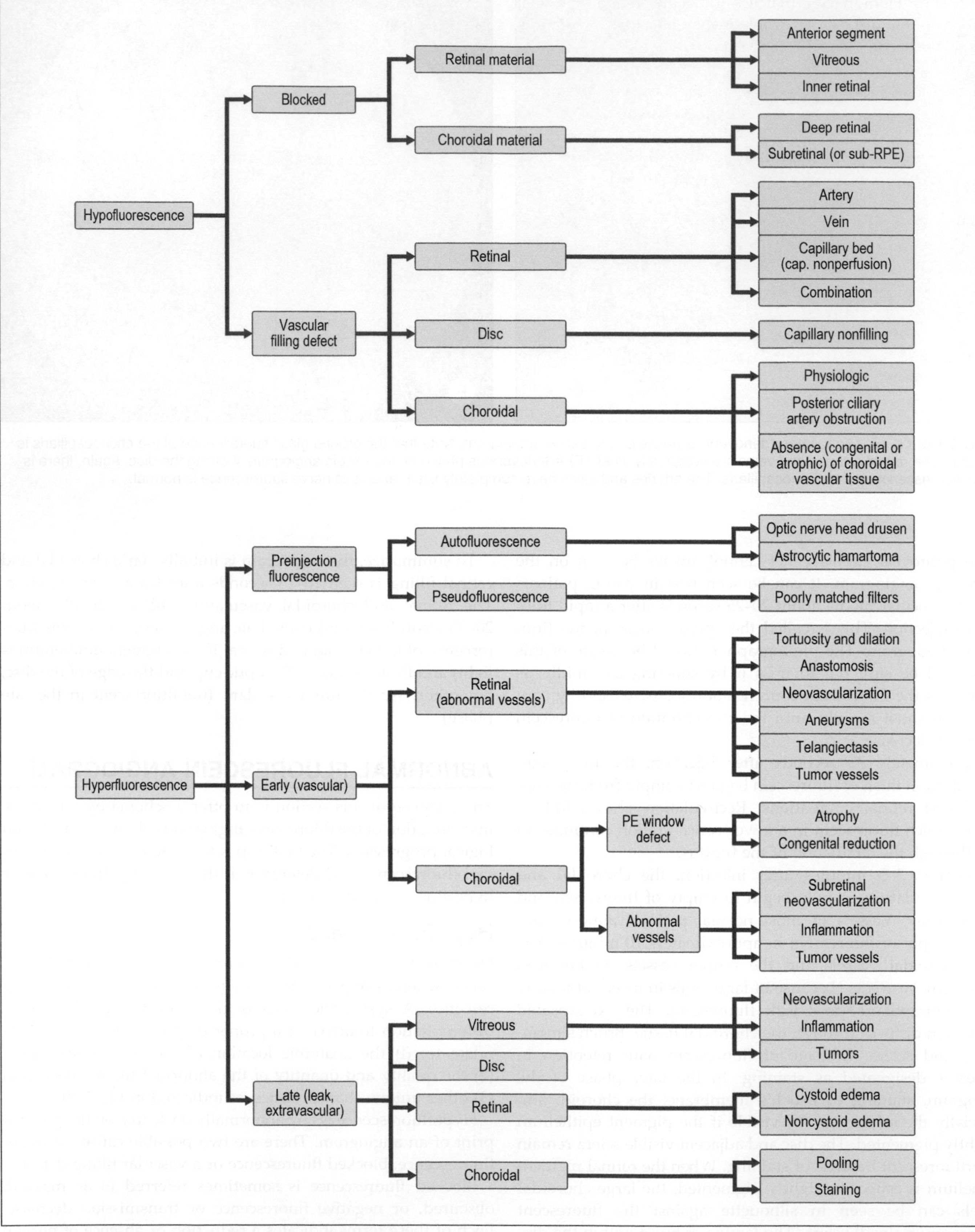

Fig. 1.20 Flow sheet for abnormal fluorescein angiography.

these tissues. Hemorrhage that lies under the retina or retinal pigment epithelium, but in front of the choroidal circulation, does not obstruct visibility of the retinal circulation but does block the view of the choroidal circulation. Therefore the approximate histologic location of blocking material can be determined by the presence or absence of visibility of one or both fundus circulations.

Fluorescein is present but cannot be seen in blocked fluorescence. With vascular filling defects, however, fluorescein cannot be seen because it is not present.

The key to differentiating blocked fluorescence from a vascular filling defect is to correlate the hypofluorescence on the angiogram with the ophthalmoscopic view. If there is material visible ophthalmoscopically that corresponds in size, shape, and location to the hypofluorescence on the angiogram, then blocked fluorescence is present. If there is no corresponding material on the color photograph, then it must be assumed that fluorescein has not perfused the vessels and that the hypofluorescence is caused by a vascular filling defect.

Hypofluorescence resulting from a vascular filling defect occurs when either of the two fundus circulations is not perfusing normally. This is caused by an absence of the vascular tissue or by a complete or partial obstruction of the particular vessels. In these situations an absence or delay of fluorescence of the involved vessels will occur. This type of hypofluorescence has a pattern that follows the geographic distribution of the vessels involved. Although the ophthalmoscopic picture will demonstrate the material blocking fluorescence, it may show nothing if the hypofluorescence is the result of a vascular filling defect.

To summarize, after an area of hypofluorescence is recognized, one must refer to the ophthalmoscopic photograph to determine the cause. If material is visible ophthalmoscopically and corresponds to the area of hypofluorescence, this is blocked fluorescence. If no corresponding blocking material exists, the hypofluorescence is therefore a vascular filling defect.

Anatomic location of hypofluorescence

After determining the cause of the hypofluorescence, the next step is: (1) to determine the anatomic location of the material that is blocking fluorescence or (2) to determine which of the two fundus circulations is involved in the filling defect. Blocking material affects the retinal and choroidal circulations if it is located in front of the retina. The material blocks only the choroidal circulation if it is located beneath the retinal circulation and in front of the choroid. Similarly, vascular filling defects occur in either the retinal or the choroidal vasculature or in the vessels of the optic nerve head.

Blocked retinal fluorescence

Blocked retinal vascular hypofluorescence is caused by anything that reduces media clarity. An opacification in front of the retinal vessels involving the cornea, anterior chamber, iris, lens, vitreous, or the most anterior portion of the retina or disc produces hypofluorescence.

The further the opacification is in front of the fundus, the less it will block fluorescence and the more it will affect the overall quality of the photographs. The closer the material is to the fundus, the more it will block, causing hypofluorescent images on the angiogram. Any material that blocks retinal vascular fluorescence will, of course, block choroidal fluorescence as well.

Any anterior-segment material, such as a corneal opacity, anterior-chamber haziness, or lens opacity, obscuring the view of the ocular fundus will result in an angiogram of reduced brilliance, contrast, and resolution. This affects the quality of the angiogram and is, in a sense, a type of blocked fluorescence.

Many conditions of the vitreous produce a hazy medium that prevents visualizing fundus detail. The most common vitreous opacity to cause blockage is hemorrhage. Whether diffusely dispersed in the vitreous gel or more densely accumulated, vitreous hemorrhage reduces or completely blocks fundus fluorescence. In addition to hemorrhage, media haze may be caused by a variety of opacifications, including asteroid hyalosis, vitreous condensation resulting from vitreous degenerative disease, inflammatory debris, vitreous membranes, or opacification secondary to amyloidosis. When anterior-segment and vitreous opacities are present, the angiogram may be of higher resolution and quality than the color photograph because the light scattered from the nonfluorescing opacities is not transmitted through the barrier filter and therefore has no effect on the angiographic photograph.

Any translucent or opacified material in the retina or in the nerve fiber layer blocks fluorescence from both planes of retinal vessels, as well as from the choroidal vessels. The large retinal vessels and precapillary arterioles are located in the nerve fiber layer in the anterior plane of the retina. The capillaries and postcapillary venules are located deeper in the retina, in the inner nuclear layer. If a blocking material lies in front of the nerve fiber layer, it blocks both planes of retinal vessels (Fig. 1.21). However, if the material lies beneath the nerve fiber layer but within or in front of the inner nuclear layer (where the smaller retinal vessels are located), it blocks only the retinal capillaries (and choroidal vessels), leaving the view of the large retinal vessels unobstructed. If a blocking material lies deeper than the retinal vascular structures, deep to the inner nuclear layer, it does not block the vessels but will block the choroidal vascular fluorescence. In other words, deep intraretinal blocking material, such as hemorrhage or exudate, does not obstruct retinal vascular fluorescence, since the retinal vessels are located in the inner half of the retina (Fig. 1.22).

Therefore one can determine the location of a retinal abnormality, such as hemorrhage, by the vessels that are blocked by it and by the fluorescence of the vessels that are not blocked.

The most common cause of blocked retinal vascular fluorescence is hemorrhage. Subinternal limiting membrane hemorrhage blocks fluorescence of all underlying retinal vessels and choroidal vasculature. Nerve fiber layer hemorrhage, which usually is flame-shaped, blocks the smaller retinal vessels lying deeper in the retina but only partially blocks the larger retinal vessels in the nerve fiber layer. Blockage from hemorrhage is usually complete, as opposed to the partial blockage caused by the myelinated nerve fibers.

Various retinal vascular (arteriolar) occlusive diseases may cause white ischemic thickening (nerve fiber edema), which results in some opacification of the retina and blockage of the remaining retinal vascular and choroidal fluorescence. Conditions such as arterial occlusion in hypertension or Purtscher's retinopathy cause enough intracellular "cloudy" swelling and opacification to block fluorescence. It should be noted that, because there is occlusion in this type of hypofluorescence, the hypofluorescence is caused partly by the vascular filling defect. However, the opacified ischemic retina

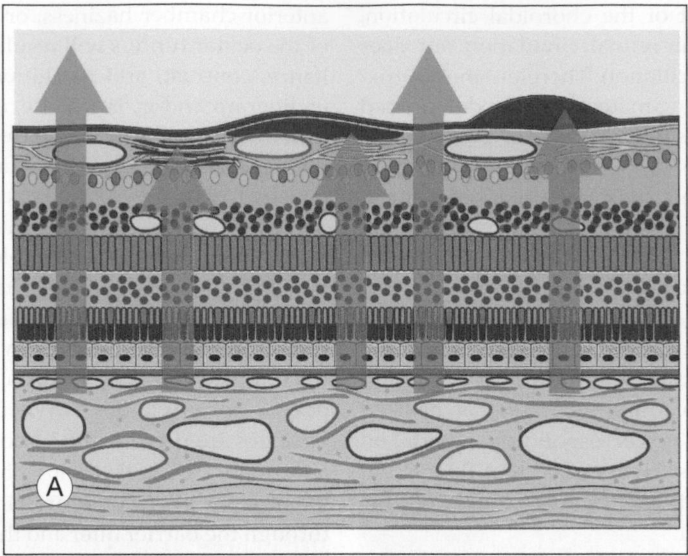

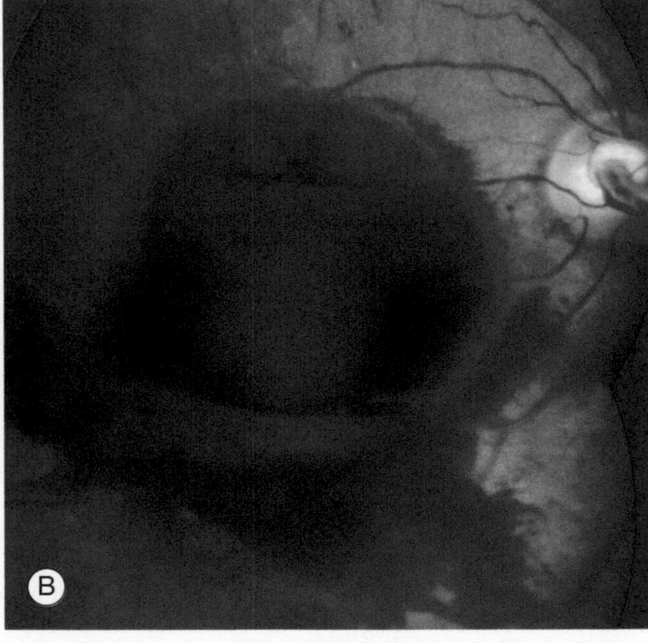

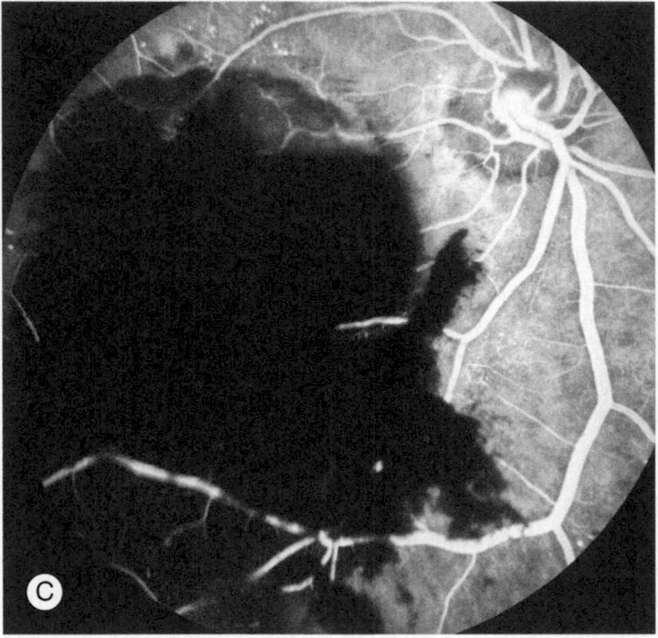

Fig. 1.21 Preretinal hemorrhage causing hypofluorescent blockage of all retinal and choroidal fluorescence. (A) Schematic drawing of subhyaloid (right), subinternal limiting membrane (central), and nerve fiber layer (left) hemorrhages. Each hemorrhage lies in front of the retinal, and therefore choroidal, vasculature, causing hypofluorescence-blocked fluorescence. (B) Color photograph of the right disc showing substantial preretinal hemorrhage. (C) Fluorescein angiogram of the right disc showing hypofluorescence caused by blockage as a result of the preretinal hemorrhage. Comment: all fluorescence of the fundus is blocked because the hemorrhage lies in front of the retinal vasculature.

effectively blocks fluorescence from underlying retinal and choroidal vasculature.

In summary, the concept of blocked retinal vascular hypofluorescence is fairly easy to understand and to identify on the angiogram. When the retinal vessels do not fluoresce, the ophthalmoscopic view should be studied to determine if blocking material is located in front of the retinal vessels.

If blocking material is present, the next step is to determine its anatomic location.

Blocked choroidal fluorescence

Hypofluorescence caused by blocked choroidal vasculature occurs when fluid, exudate, hemorrhage, pigment, scar, inflammatory material, or the like accumulates in front of the choroidal vasculature and deep to the retinal vasculature (Fig. 1.23).

Deep retinal material

Materials deposited in the deep retina that cause blockage of choroidal fluorescence are fluid, hard exudate, hemorrhage, and pigment.

Fluid that accumulates in the deep retina has a predilection for the tissue of least resistance, the outer plexiform layer. Deposition of edema fluid, originating from leaking retinal vessels or migrating from subretinal space into the retina, most frequently occurs in the outer plexiform layer. After reaching a certain volume, the fluid tends to form spaces, or pockets, between

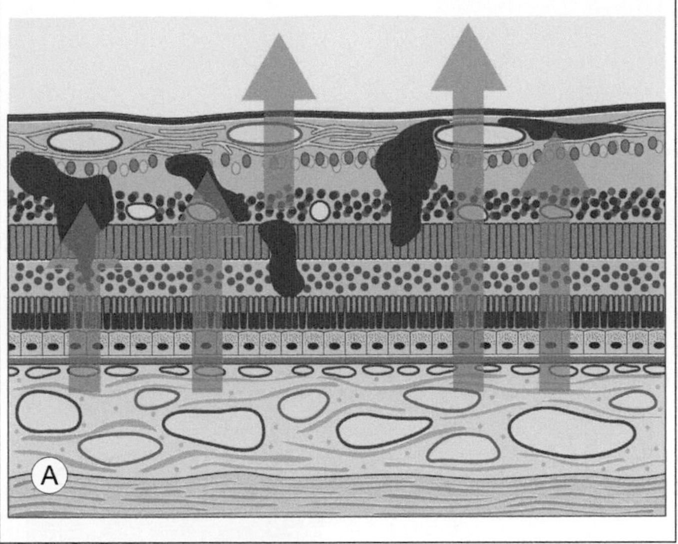

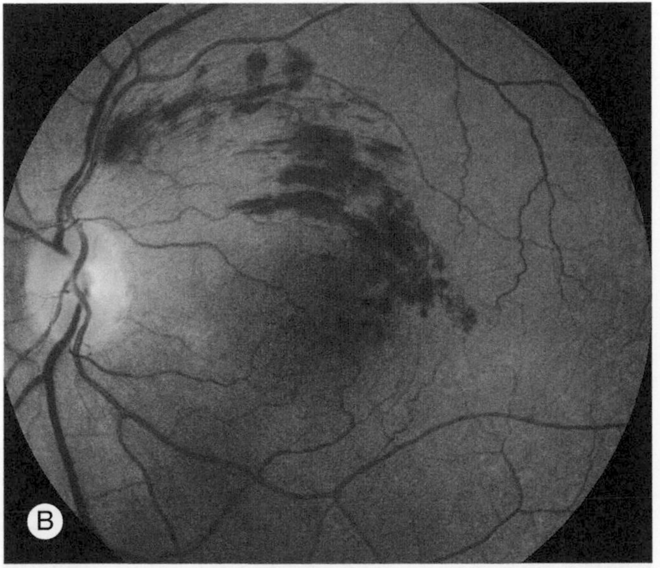

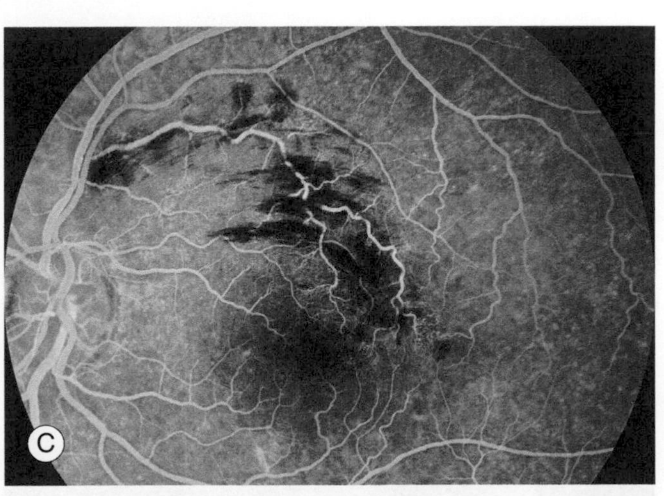

Fig. 1.22 Intraretinal hemorrhages causing hypofluorescent blockage. (A) Schematic of retina showing hemorrhages located in most of the layers of the retina from the internal limiting membrane to the outer nuclear layer. (B) Color photograph of left macula shows dot-and-blot, as well as flame-shaped hemorrhages just above the fovea. This is a case of branch-vein occlusion. (C) Fluorescein angiogram of left macula shows that the hemorrhage causes irregular hypofluorescent blockage. The flame-shaped hemorrhage located in the nerve fiber layer blocks all the retinal vasculature. The dot-and-blot hemorrhages do not block the large retinal vessels and therefore can be localized deeper in the retina. The hemorrhages that do not block retinal capillary fluorescence can be located deeper to the capillary layer, which is in the inner nuclear layer. Comment: Once hypofluorescent blockage is determined, an anatomic localization of the blocking material can be made by determining which fluorescent structures can be seen normally and which are being blocked.

compressed nerve and Müller's fibers, which are pushed aside in the process. This pattern of fluid accumulation in the outer plexiform layer is called cystoid retinal edema. Noncystoid retinal edema occurs when the volume of extracellular fluid is insufficient to produce pockets, or spaces, in the outer plexiform layer or other layers of the retina. A significant amount of retinal edema, whether cystoid or noncystoid, especially if turbid or containing lipid-laden macrophages, partially blocks choroidal fluorescence in the early phase of the fluorescein angiogram. Later in the angiogram, retinal edema fluoresces. Intraretinal hard exudates and lipid-laden macrophages, usually located in the outer plexiform layer, partially block choroidal fluorescence. When retinal vessels bleed, the blood can be deposited anywhere in the retina. When located deep to the retinal vessels beneath the inner nuclear layer, retinal vascular fluorescence is visible, whereas choroidal fluorescence is blocked.

Subretinal material

Any opaque or translucent substance located beneath the retina but in front of the choroid blocks fluorescence of the choroidal vasculature but does not block retinal vascular fluorescence (Fig. 1.23). Blood located under the retina causes complete blockage of choroidal fluorescence, with the retinal fluorescence showing through normally. Subretinal hemorrhage appears red,

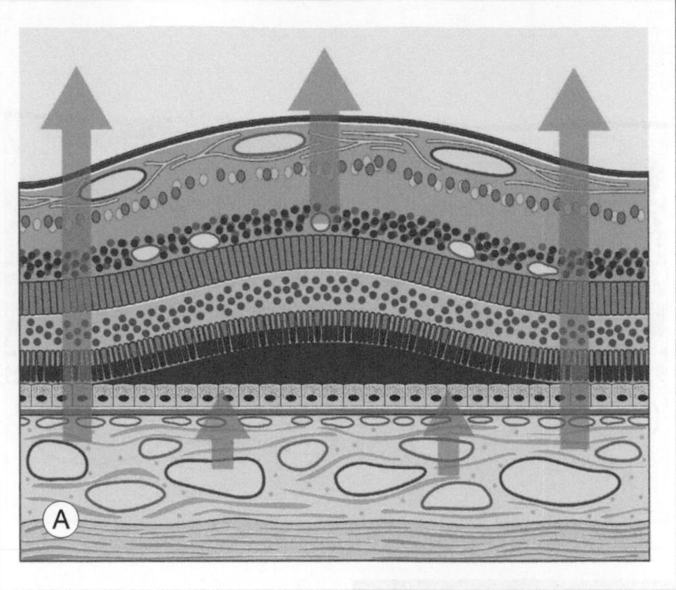

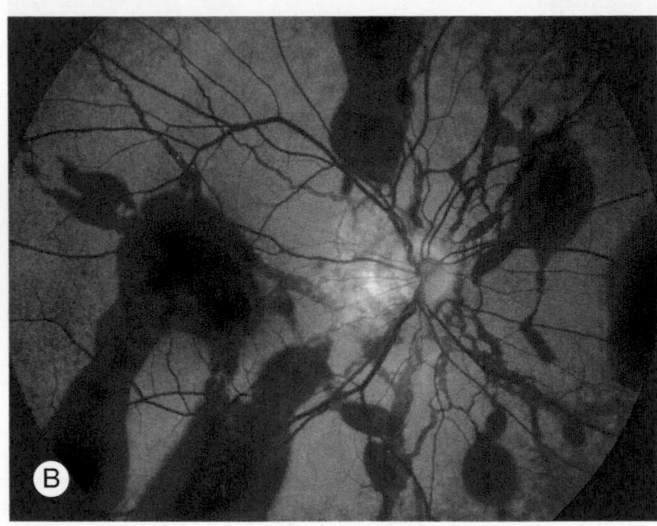

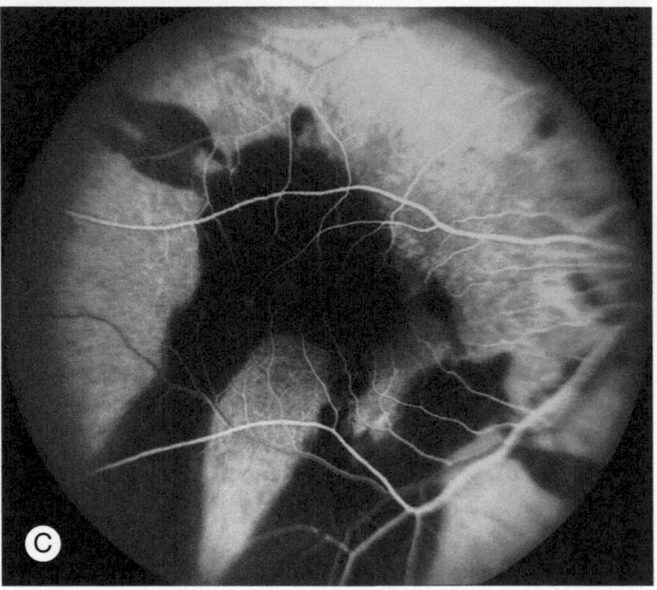

Fig. 1.23 Subretinal hemorrhage causing hypofluorescence, specifically, blockage of choroidal fluorescence. (A) Schematic of retina with subretinal hemorrhage (blood located between photoreceptors and pigment epithelium). (B) Color photograph of right macula of an eye with angioid streaks showing large scattered areas of subretinal hemorrhage. (C) Fluorescein angiogram of right macula shows marked hypofluorescence caused by blocked choroidal fluorescence (the retinal vessels are visible) that is due to the subretinal hemorrhage. Comment: The subretinal hemorrhage completely obscures fluorescence from the choroid. The retinal vessels are clearly seen overlying the subretinal hemorrhage.

and subpigment epithelial hemorrhage is dark. Subretinal hemorrhage is generally scalloped with somewhat irregular margins, whereas subpigment epithelial hemorrhage is often quite round and well demarcated (Fig. 1.23).

Accumulated pigment (melanin and lipofuscin) from diseased retinal pigment epithelium causes blocked choroidal fluorescence (Fig. 1.24). Any hyperpigmentation of the pigment epithelium causes blocked choroidal fluorescence. Xanthophyll, the pigment present in the outer layers of the fovea, blocks choroidal fluorescence by selectively absorbing the blue exciting light, which results in less fluorescence. Finally, a choroidal nevus may block much of the choroidal fluorescence (Fig. 1.25) and especially blocks the later hyperfluorescent staining of the sclera. The choriocapillaris may be seen normally over the nevus.

To summarize, various materials located in the deep retinal layers, or beneath the retina, block choroidal fluorescence and are evident ophthalmoscopically. These materials result from a variety of disease processes.

Vascular filling defect

The second cause of abnormal hypofluorescence is vascular filling defect. With blocked fluorescence, the fluorescein is

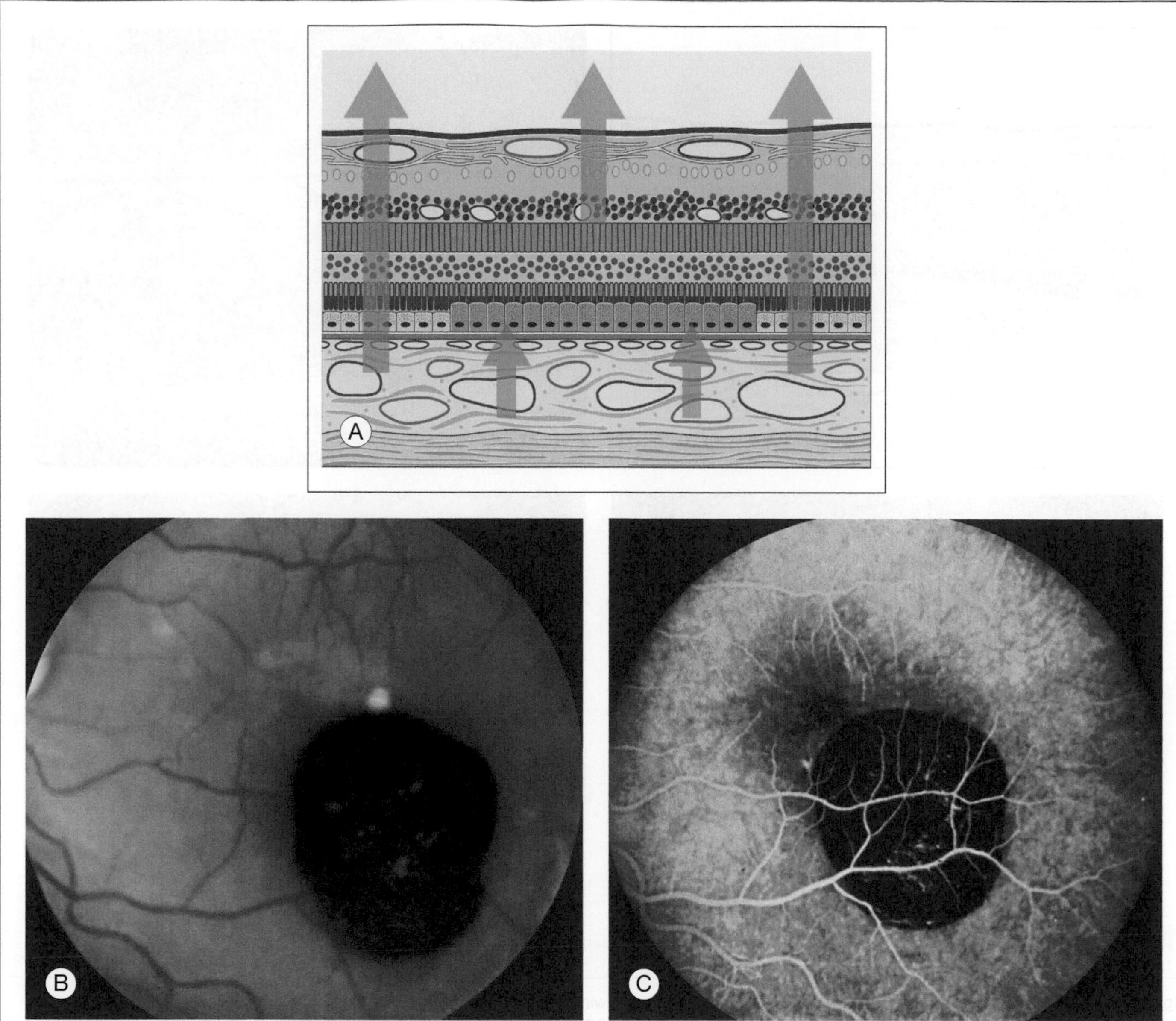

Fig. 1.24 Hypertrophy of the retinal pigment epithelium. (A) Schematic showing hypertrophic pigment epithelial cells. (B) Color photograph of the macula shows a well-demarcated hyperpigmented lesion. (C) Fluorescein angiogram of the same area shows marked hypofluorescence of the choroid resulting from blocked fluorescence. Comment: This patient had marked hypertrophy of the retinal pigment epithelium, which allowed normal retinal fluorescence; it completely blocked choroidal fluorescence.

present in the circulations of the fundus but is not visible because a tissue or fluid barrier conceals it. With vascular filling defect, fluorescein cannot be seen because it is not present. Since fluorescein reaches the retina and choroid by way of vessels, lack of the fluorescein dye in either vascular system indicates an obstructive problem or a lack of vessels (i.e., a vascular filling defect).

As previously indicated, when a hypofluorescent area is seen on an angiogram, the best way to differentiate blocked fluorescence from a vascular filling defect is to compare the angiogram with the ophthalmoscopic picture. When blood, pigment, or exudate can be seen ophthalmoscopically corresponding to the area of hypofluorescence, the material is causing blocked fluorescence. When no material is visible ophthalmoscopically (on the color photograph), one must assume that fluorescein has not perfused the vessels and that the abnormal hypofluorescence is caused by a vascular filling defect. In some instances both forms of hypofluorescent mechanisms play a role simultaneously, as with retinal arteriolar occlusion, when the retina is not only not perfused (vascular filling defect) but is ischemic and therefore white and opaque, causing blocked fluorescence.

Vascular filling defects result from vascular obstruction, atrophy, or absence (congenital or otherwise) of vessels. Any of these conditions can be total or partial. When the obstruction is complete (occlusion) or the vascular tissue is atrophied completely, the hypofluorescence is complete and lasts throughout the angiogram. When the obstruction is only partial or the vascular tissue is not entirely atrophied, the vascular fluorescein filling is delayed or reduced relative to corresponding areas that fill normally. Whatever the cause of a partial vascular filling defect, hypofluorescence will be seen in the early phases of the

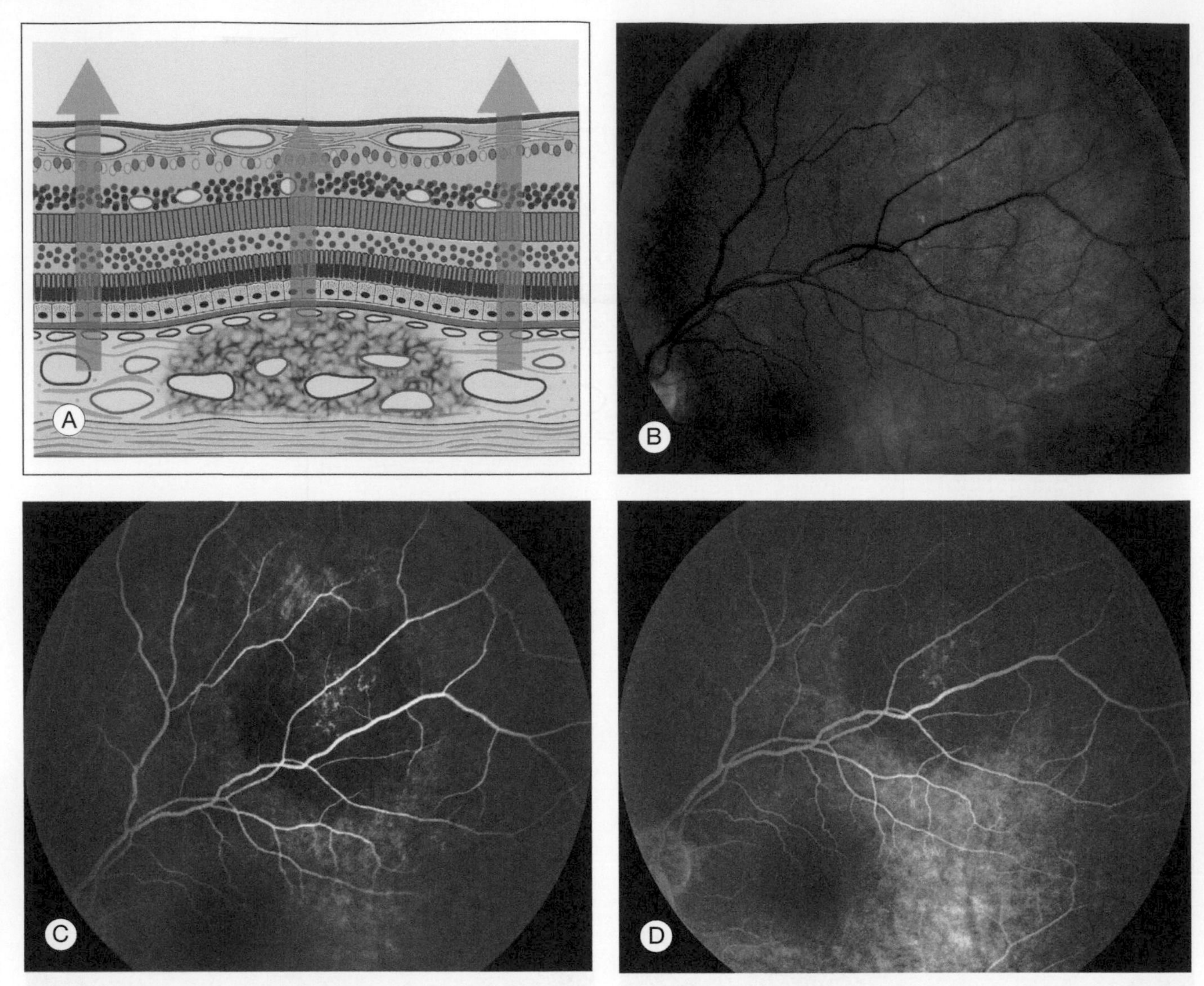

Fig. 1.25 Choroidal nevus hypofluorescent blockage. (A) Schematic drawing of retina showing choroidal nevus. Note that the choriocapillaris is intact. (B) Color photograph of nevus. (C) Arteriovenous phase of fluorescein angiogram shows hypofluorescence corresponding to the area of the nevus. (D) Later arteriovenous phase of fluorescein angiogram shows that the nevus is still hypofluorescent, although the choriocapillaris ground-glass fluorescence can be seen surrounding.

angiogram but may not persist throughout the entire angiogram. Some vascular filling, although delayed or reduced, will eventually occur.

Once it is determined that a vascular filling defect is the cause of an area of hypofluorescence, the next step is to determine which of the retinal, disc, or choroidal vessels are involved. A vascular filling defect of the disc is easy to discern angiographically. Determining whether a vascular filling defect is retinal or choroidal can be more difficult. Since retinal vessels are normally present, however, the absence of retinal vessels is usually readily apparent. If, on the other hand, a vascular filling defect is found but the retinal vessels are full and visible, the hypofluorescence must be choroidal in origin. Stereoscopic angiophotographs allow one to distinguish between the planes of the retina and choroid and enable exact determination of the location of the hypofluorescence.

Retinal vascular filling defect

If a retinal vascular filling defect is present, the clinician then considers whether the defect results from obstruction of a retinal artery or vein, capillary bed, or any combination of these. Distinguishing the cause of the obstruction is not difficult because the fluorescein angiographic process is dynamic and timed. When nonfilling of a specific retinal vessel occurs, it is easy to differentiate an arterial occlusion from a venous occlusion because the retinal arteries fill first, then the retinal capillary bed, followed by the retinal veins. In addition, retinal vascular filling defects can be localized by tracing the course of a particular vessel; these defects correspond anatomically to the normal distribution of the retinal vasculature (Figs 1.26 and 1.27). Thus retinal vascular filling defects result from a variety of disease processes, but most are commonly associated with atherosclerosis and diabetes.

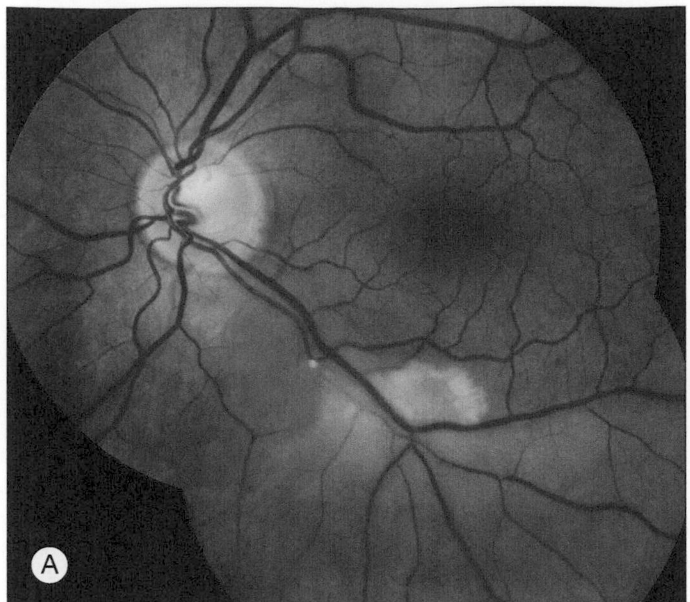

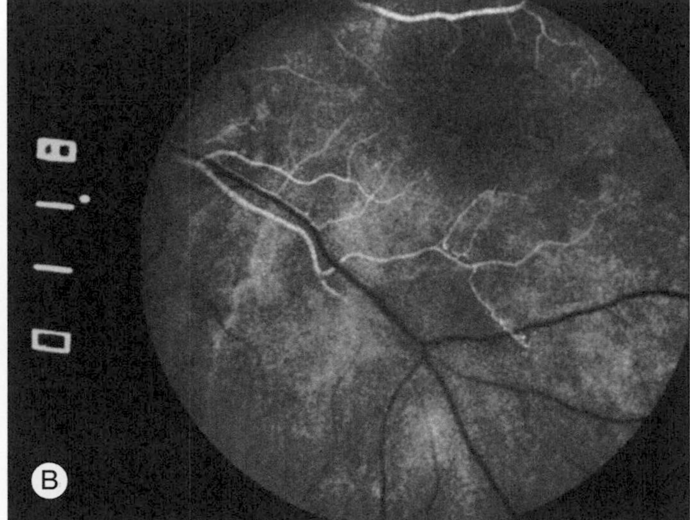

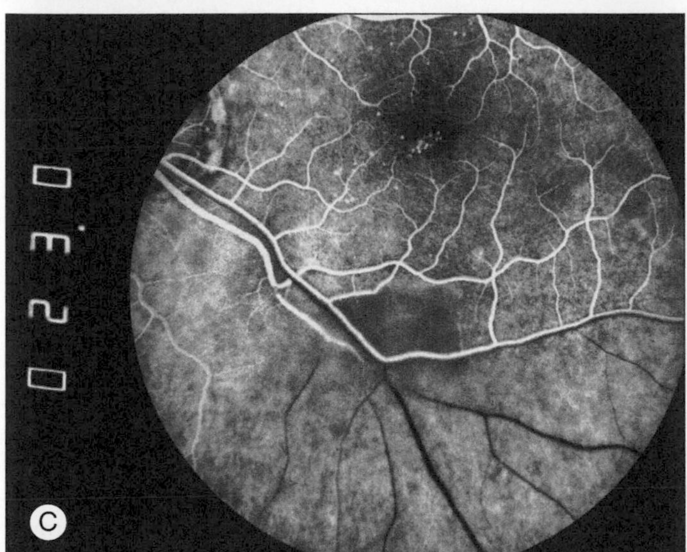

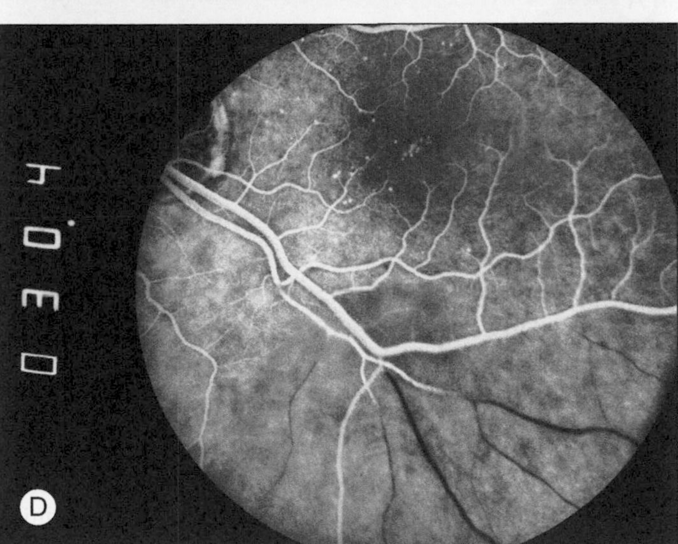

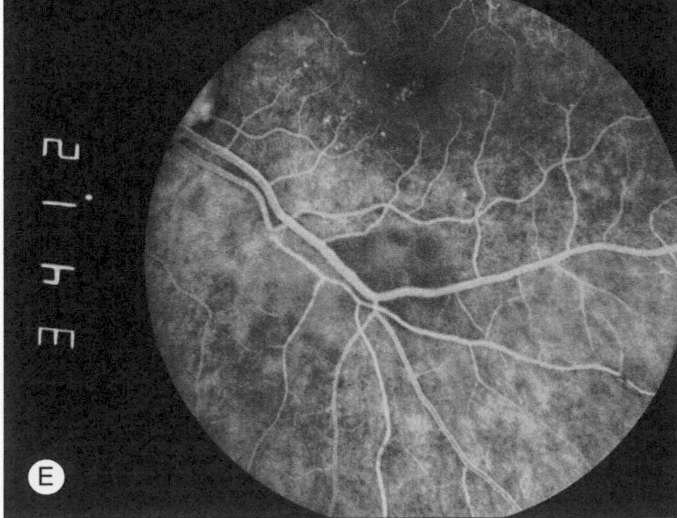

Fig. 1.26 Branch retinal artery occlusion. (A) Color photograph showing areas of retinal whitening inferior to the macula. An intra-arterial embolus is seen proximal to the whitened retina. (B) Earliest arterial filling. An area of hypofluorescence is located inferior to the macula. A small retinal artery feeding this area is occluded at the site of the embolus previously identified on Figure 1.26A. (C) Midarterial venous filling with a small area of intra-arterial hyperfluorescence distal to the site of embolic obstruction. (D) Late arteriovenous phase of fluorescein angiogram shows that the occluded artery is still mostly hypofluorescent. (E) Portions of the area did fill with fluorescein due to retrograde filling from surrounding areas. There is some mild staining of the occluded retinal artery.

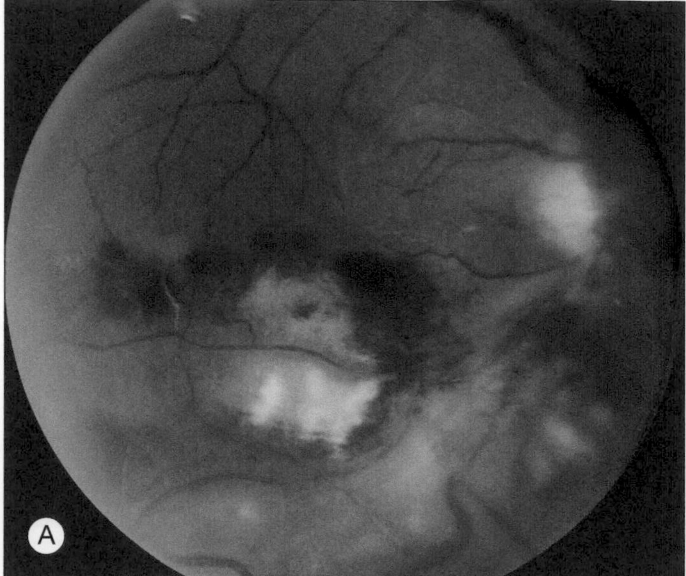

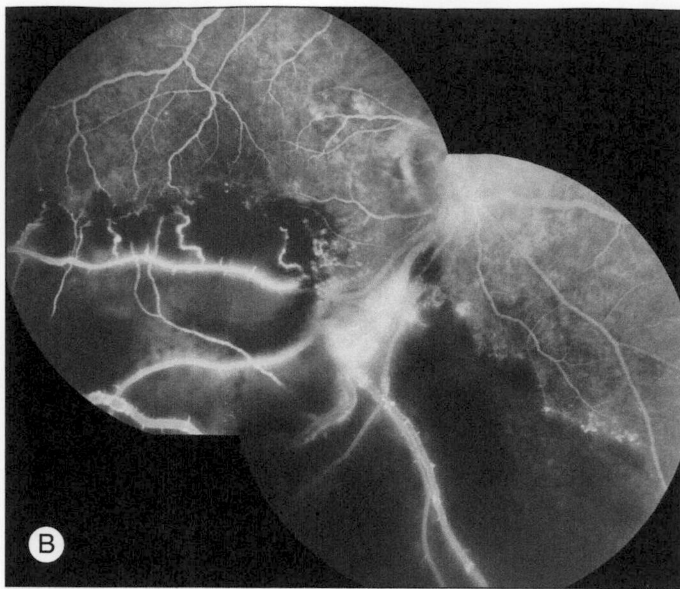

Fig. 1.27 Retinal branch-vein occlusion. (A) Color photograph of the right macula and disc. There are areas of retinal hemorrhage, retinal whitening, and cotton-wool spots. (B) The fluorescein angiogram of the right disc and macula shows normal fluorescence of the superior portion of the macula. The inferior portion shows substantial hypofluorescence due to retinal capillary nonperfusion. The very bright hyperfluorescent areas are due to neovascularization. Comment: This patient had a very ischemic inferotemporal branch retinal vein occlusion of the right eye. This was a severe occlusion, as evidenced by closure of large areas of the capillary bed. The hypofluorescence was caused not only by vascular filling defect but also by the nonperfused retina, which becomes partially opaque and caused hypofluorescence of the choroid. (In other words, there was blockage of choroidal fluorescence by the opaque retina, which was caused by the retinal capillary nonperfusion.)

Vascular filling defects of the disc

Vascular filling defects of the disc occur because of the failure of the capillaries of the optic nerve head to fill. This failure can be caused by: (1) congenital absence of disc tissue, as in an optic pit or optic nerve head coloboma (Fig. 1.28); (2) atrophy of the disc tissue and its vasculature, as in optic atrophy; or (3) vascular occlusion, as in an ischemic optic neuropathy.[19,20] Each condition is characterized by early hypofluorescence caused by nonfilling and late hyperfluorescence resulting from staining of the involved tissue.

Choroidal vascular filling defect

The normal choroidal vasculature is usually difficult to document with fluorescein angiography because of the pigment epithelial barrier. If chronic choroidal vascular filling defects exist, the pigment epithelium is often secondarily depigmented or atrophied. In these cases the hypofluorescence caused by a vascular filling abnormality of the choroid and choriocapillaris can be documented angiographically.

When choroidal vessels do not fill, dark patches of hypofluorescence beneath the retina appear early in the angiogram. The distribution and morphology of the hypofluorescence vary according to the disease process. Because the choroidal circulation is completely separate from the retinal circulation, choroidal vascular filling defects do not correlate with the retinal vascular distribution. If the choriocapillaris is absent and the large choroidal vessels are still present, the choroidal and retinal vessels fluoresce, but hypofluorescent gaps appear because of the loss of the diffuse "ground-glass" fluorescence from the choriocapillaris (Fig. 1.29). When the choroidal vasculature does not fill, as in total occlusion or in atrophy, hypofluorescence occurs early in the angiogram. The hypofluorescence remains throughout the late stages of the procedure, although leakage from surrounding areas of normal choriocapillaris extends into the occluded area. When sufficient leakage occurs, the sclera retains fluorescein (stains) late in the angiogram. When the involved area is large and the leakage is minimal, the hypofluorescence remains throughout the later stages.

A normal physiologic condition exists in many patients in which the choroid fills in a patchy manner. Areas adjacent to the foci that are filling show early hypofluorescence but eventually fill normally, usually 2–5 seconds later. This has been termed patchy choroidal filling, and it is the most common form of choroidal vascular filling defect. This form of filling follows a pattern in which the short posterior ciliary arteries enter the eye perpendicularly through the sclera. These vessels then feed the choriocapillaris lobules.

The prechoriocapillaris arterioles and lobules are end, or terminal, vessels demonstrating no anastomoses with adjacent choriocapillaris arterioles or lobules. Each choriocapillaris lobule is connected to adjacent lobules on the venous, or emptying, side of the circulation. Fluorescence in each choriocapillaris segment or lobule is in the form of a round, irregular, or hexagonal patch. When some of the channels fill late, a heterogeneous filling pattern results. The choriocapillaris fills most areas, whereas dark hypofluorescent patches are present in other areas. These dark areas are lobules from separate end channels that are not filled simultaneously with adjacent choriocapillaris lobules. They are filled in a delayed fashion by the single feeder choroidal arteriole.

In general, vascular filling defects of the choroid are caused by obstructive disorders or absence of tissue with the following fluorescein angiographic characteristics: (1) normal retinal vascular flow; (2) depigmentation of the pigment epithelium; (3) reduction of choroidal blood flow; and (4) hypofluorescence in

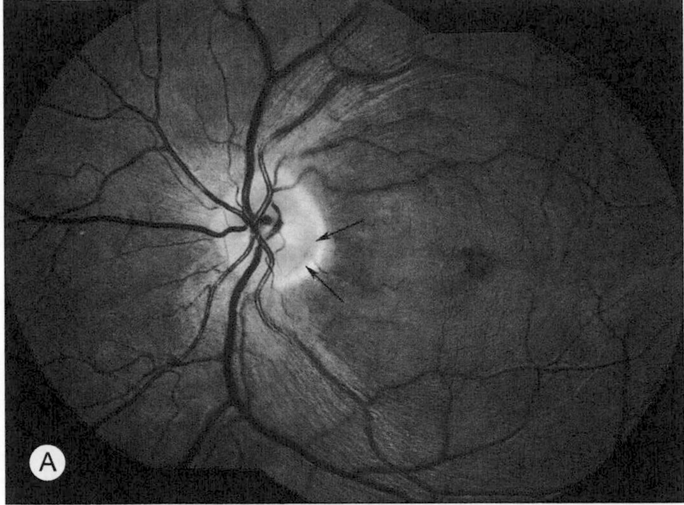

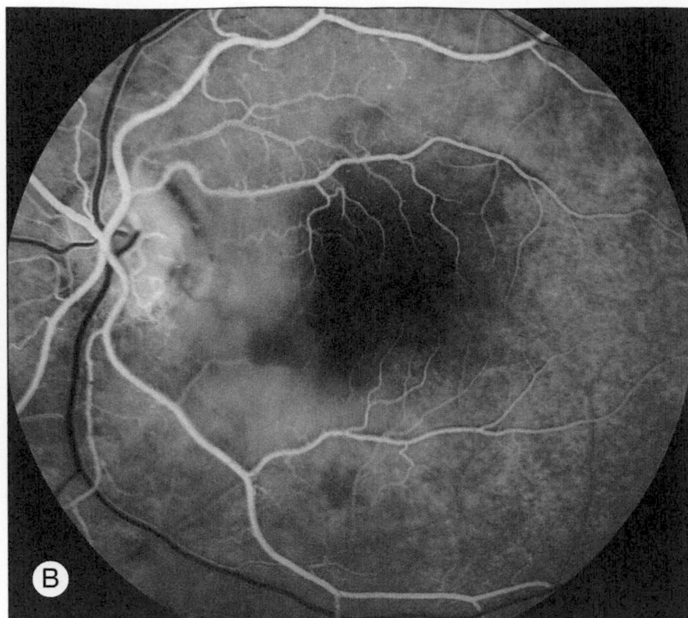

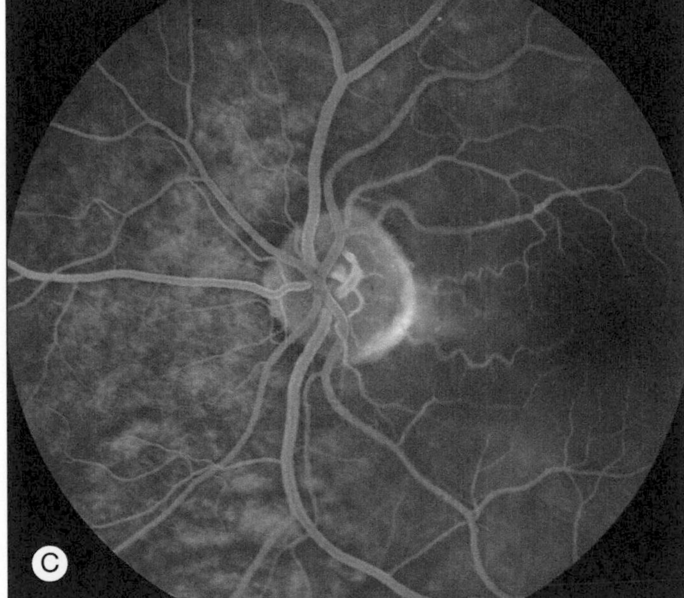

Fig. 1.28 Optic pit and sensory macula detachment. (A) Color photograph of left macula. Note the dark area of the optic pit (arrows). Cystic edema is present in the macula secondary to the macular schisis detachment from the optic pit. (B) Early arteriovenous phase of fluorescein angiogram shows hypofluorescence of the disc in the area of the pit due to absence of tissue and vessels. (C) In the late arteriovenous phase fluorescein angiogram, the hypofluorescent area of the pit is evident.

the early phases of angiography caused by loss of the normal ground-glass choriocapillaris fluorescence. In some conditions the large choroidal vessels are also absent, resulting in total early hypofluorescence in the affected area, with scleral staining only on the circumference of the lesion because of the adjacent patent choriocapillaris. Choroidal vascular defects result from a variety of disease processes (Figs 1.30 and 1.31).

Hyperfluorescence

Hyperfluorescence is any abnormally light area on the positive print of an angiogram, that is, an area showing fluorescence in excess of what would be expected on a normal angiogram. There are four possible causes of abnormal hyperfluorescence: (1) preinjection fluorescence; (2) transmitted fluorescence; (3) abnormal vessels; and (4) leakage. The appearance of fluorescence depends in part on the relationship of its appearance to the timing of the fluorescein injection.

Preinjection fluorescence is hyperfluorescence that can be seen before fluorescein is injected and is caused by structures that naturally fluoresce (autofluorescence) or by poorly matched filters (pseudofluorescence).

Transmitted fluorescence and abnormal vascular fluorescence occur in the early, or vascular, stage of the angiogram, when fluorescein fills patent blood vessels. Transmitted fluorescence appears when fluorescein fills the normal choriocapillaris, but it is more noticeable when there is reduced pigment in the pigment epithelium or loss of retinal pigment epithelium. This is designated pigment epithelial window defect.

When abnormal retinal, disc, or choroidal vessels are present and fill with fluorescein, hyperfluorescence occurs. This type of hyperfluorescence, abnormal vascular fluorescence, is also seen in the early, or vascular, phase of the angiography.

Hyperfluorescence caused by leakage is seen predominantly in the later, or extravascular, phase of angiography. In this phase, fluorescein has emptied from normal and abnormal vessels. Any significant fluorescein that remains in the eye is fluorescein that has escaped or leaked from vascular or tissue barriers and is thus extravascular.

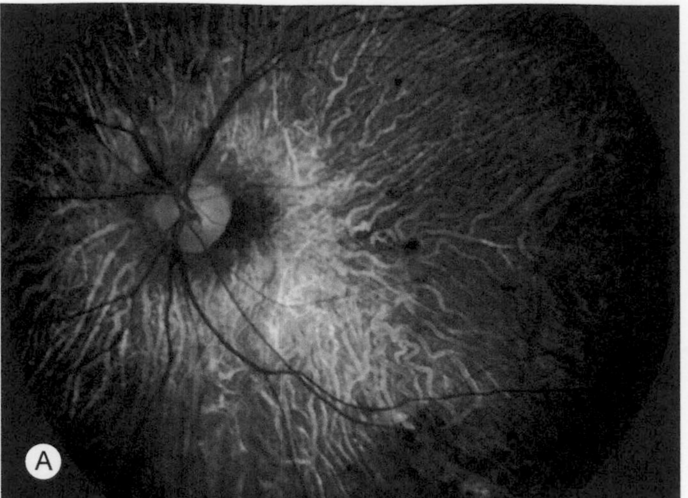

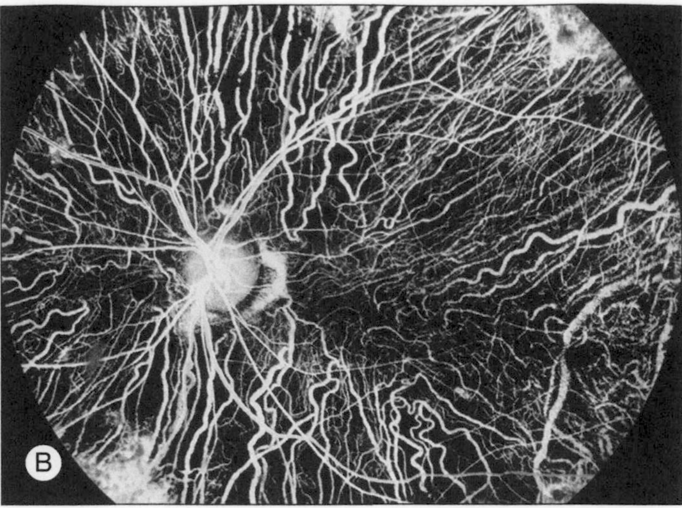

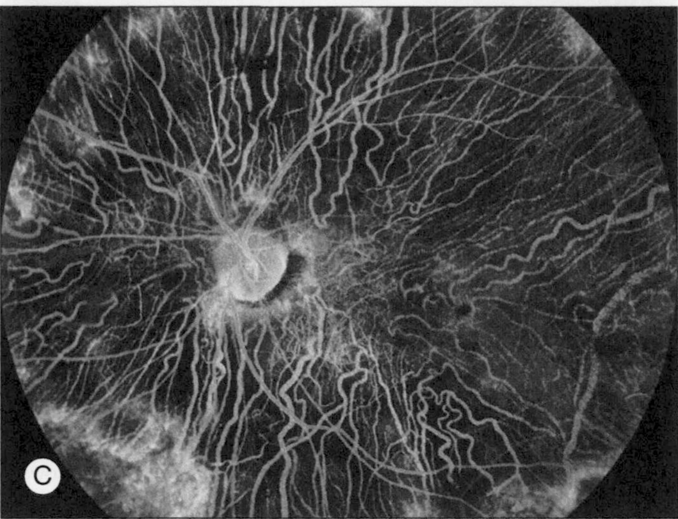

Fig. 1.29 Choroideremia: total loss of retinal pigment epithelium (RPE) and choriocapillaris with much of the large choroidal vasculature remaining. (A) Color photograph of the left disc and macula. The large choroidal vasculature can be seen as pale, irregular lines. Dark patches of pigment are located in the macula and around the disc. (B) Late venous phase of fluorescein angiogram of the left disc and macula. The large choroidal vessels can be seen filling, as can the retinal arteries. The choriocapillaris is not seen. (C) Recirculation phase of fluorescein angiogram. The large choroidal vessels and retinal vessels can be seen, but the choriocapillaris (usually seen as ground-glass fluorescence) is not seen except in the far edges of the view. Comment: This patient had a total loss of RPE and choriocapillaris in most areas of the fundus. The ground-glass choroidal fluorescence was absent from most areas. The large choroidal vessels could be seen. The large choroidal vessels do not leak fluorescein, and therefore the sclera did not stain in these areas. The RPE and choriocapillaris were partially intact in a few areas. These can be seen at the far extremes, where there is some mild ground-glass appearance.

Therefore, to ascertain the type of hyperfluorescence, one must determine the time at which the hyperfluorescence appears in relation to when the fluorescein was injected. Once the hyperfluorescence is determined to be caused by preinjection fluorescence, transmitted fluorescence, the presence of abnormal vessels, or by leakage, the next step is to determine the anatomic location of the hyperfluorescence. Abnormal blood vessels may come from the retina and disc or from the choroid. Leakage can occur in the vitreous, disc, retina, or choroid.

Preinjection fluorescence

Each angiographic study should include one photograph of the fundus taken with the fluorescein filters in place and before fluorescein is injected. This exposure is called the preinjection, or control, fluorescein photograph. In normal situations this photograph is totally dark; it is completely hypofluorescent. When the photograph is not dark, autofluorescence or pseudofluorescence is present. The conditions that cause autofluorescence occur infrequently, and the filter problems that produce pseudofluorescence have in recent years been minimized by the development of more precisely matched filter systems.

Autofluorescence

Autofluorescence is the emission of fluorescent light from ocular structures in the absence of sodium fluorescein. Conditions that cause autofluorescence are optic nerve head drusen and astrocytic hamartoma (Fig. 1.32).

Pseudofluorescence occurs when the blue exciter and green barrier filters overlap. The blue filter overlaps into the green range, allowing the passage of green light, or the green barrier filter overlaps into the blue range, allowing the passage of blue light (Fig. 1.2). The overlapping light passes through the system, reflects off highly reflective surfaces (light-colored or white structures), and stimulates the film. This reflected nonfluorescent light is called pseudofluorescence.

Conditions that tend to produce pseudofluorescence include any light-colored or white (reflective) fundus change (e.g., sclera, exudate, scar tissue, myelinated nerve fibers, foreign body).

Currently, fluorescein angiographic filters are usually very well matched; overlap is minimal, so pseudofluorescence is faint and rarely a major problem. However, filters do tend to get thin with time. The frequent flashes of light from the fundus camera wear them down, and most filter pairs eventually allow pseudofluorescence. Therefore, depending on frequency of use, fluorescein filters must be changed occasionally.

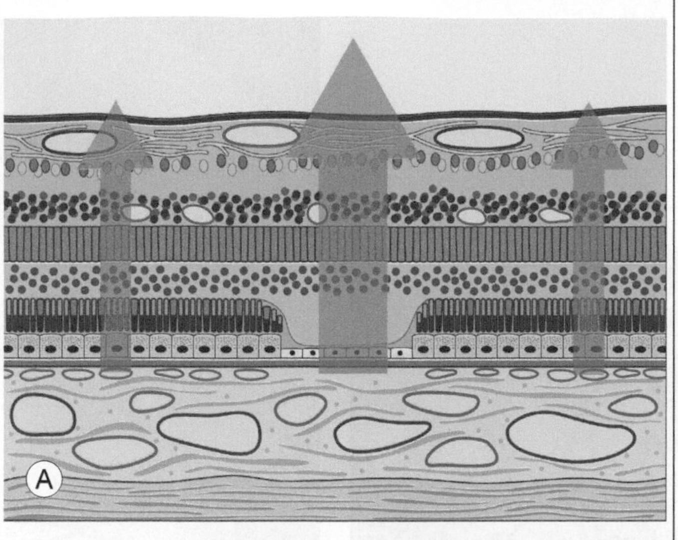
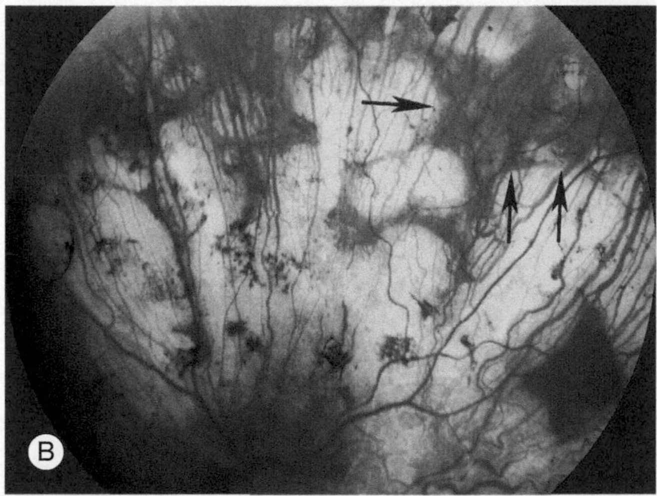
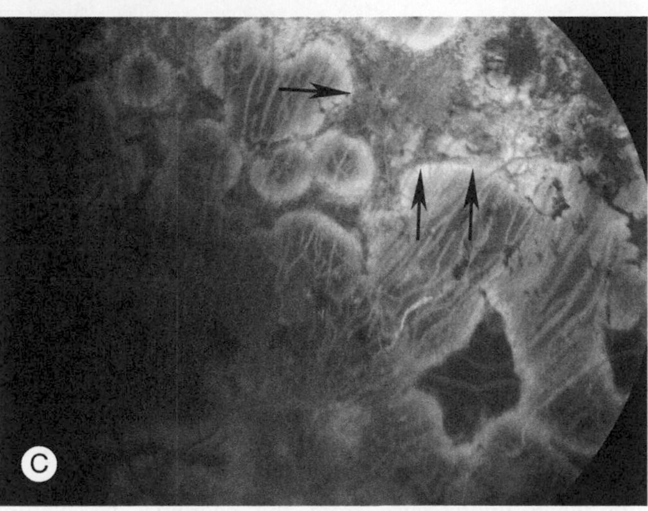

Fig. 1.30 Choroidal atrophy, with some remaining islands of choriocapillaris, due to choroideremia. (A) Schematic of retina shows loss of pigment epithelium and choriocapillaris and some of the outer retina (especially photoreceptors). (B) Color photograph of left superior retina showing areas of severe atrophy and more intact areas of retinal pigment epithelium (RPE) peripherally. Arrows delineate margins between normal RPE and RPE atrophy producing window defect. (C) The arteriovenous phase of fluorescein angiogram shows normal fluorescence of the retinal arteries. The large choroidal vessels can be seen temporally on the right side of the photograph. The ground-glass fluorescence of the choriocapillaris can be seen more peripherally on the left side of the angiogram, where the RPE and choriocapillaris are more intact. Comment: This patient had severe atrophy of the RPE and choriocapillaris. Large choroidal vessels could be seen causing hypofluorescence in relationship to absence of ground-glass choroidal fluorescence. Some areas of choriocapillaris remained and showed normal hyperfluorescence (perhaps increased hyperfluorescence caused by loss of overlying RPE).

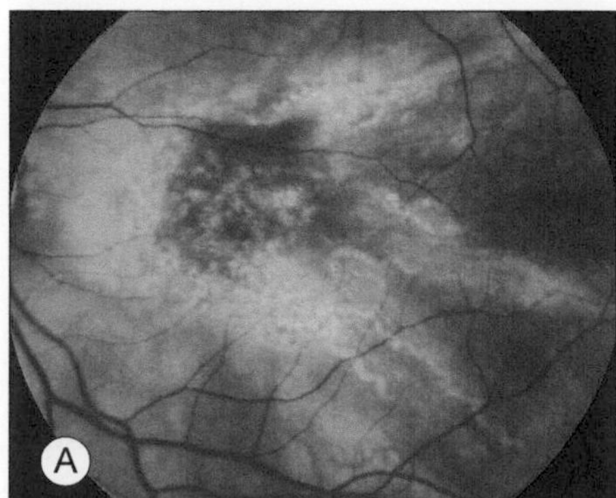
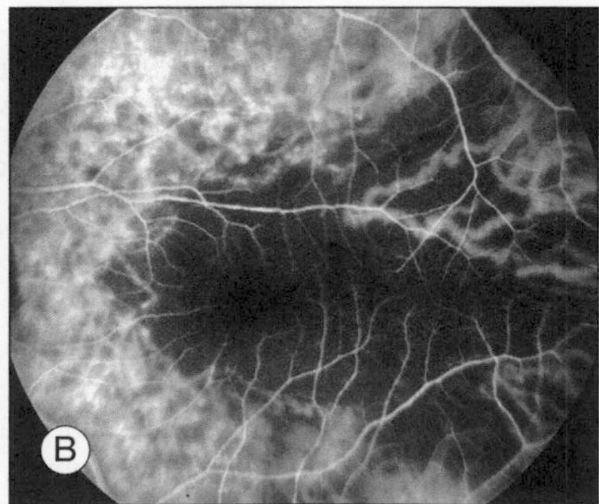
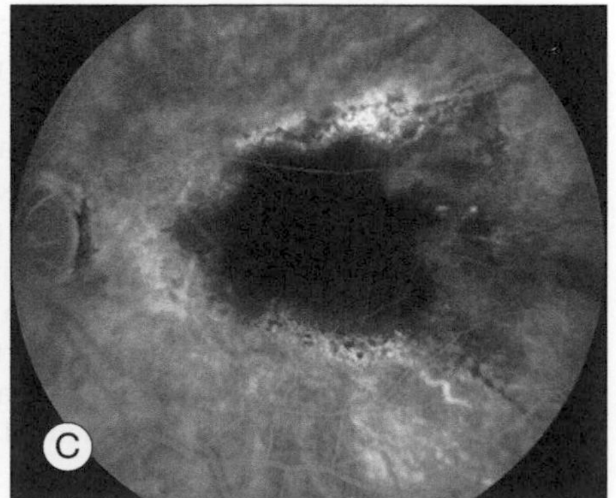

Fig. 1.31 Choroidal hypoperfusion caused by photodynamic therapy with verteporfin. (A) Left macula. Color photograph shows widespread retinal pigment epithelial alterations and drusen secondary to an occult choroidal neovascular membrane secondary to age-related macular degeneration. This treatment was considered standard therapy prior to the advent of intraocular antivascular endothelial growth factor medications. (B) The late arteriovenous phase of the fluorescein angiogram of the left macula shows hypofluorescence of the macula and a large area temporally. Larger choroidal vessels are perfused. The macular hypofluorescence corresponds to the laser treated area. The large area of hypofluorescence temporally represents an area of choroidal nonperfusion caused by selective choriocapillaris occlusion from photodynamic therapy. (C) Later phase of the fluorescein angiogram shows continued hypofluorescence of the area temporal to the macula despite relative restoration of perfusion to choriocapillaris temporal to macula.

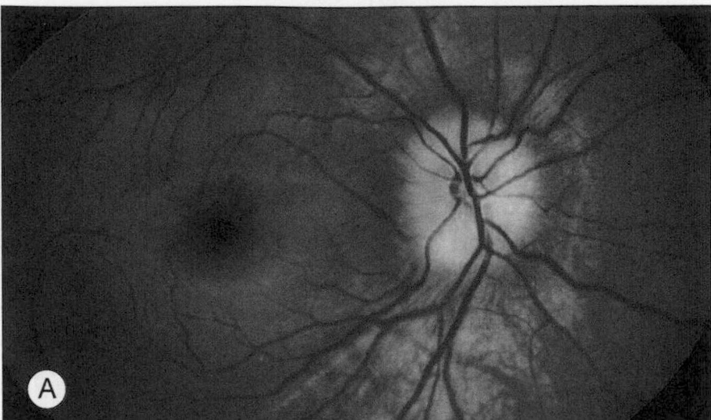

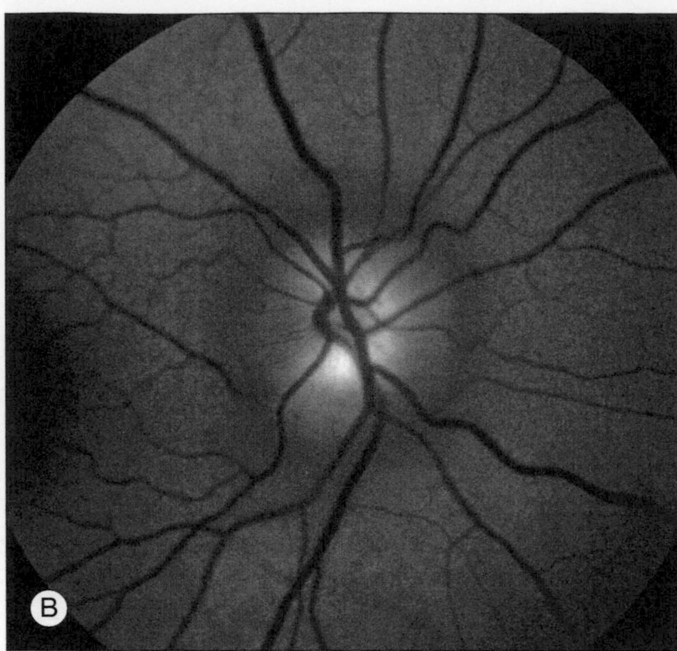

Fig. 1.32 Autofluorescence of optic nerve drusen. (A) Right disc and macula show a blurred disc margin with nonhyperemic vessels. Blurring of the central optic nerve is consistent with disc edema noted on stereophotos. (B) Preinjection or "control" photos are performed with filters in place, prior to any injection of fluorescein. This allowed for the identification of optic nerve drusen, which autofluoresce.

Our experience indicates that change is required approximately every 5 years.

Transmitted fluorescence (pigment epithelial window defect)

This fluorescence is an accentuation of the visibility of normal choroidal fluorescence. Transmitted fluorescence occurs when fluorescence from the choroidal vasculature appears to be increased because of the absence of pigment in the pigment epithelium, which normally forms a visual barrier to choroidal fluorescence. The major cause of pigment epithelial window defect is atrophy of the pigment epithelium (Figs 1.33–1.36).

When the pigment epithelium is dense, choroidal fluorescence is not clearly visible because the pigment blocks the view of the choroid and acts as a barrier to fluorescein. The density of the pigment determines the degree to which transmission of the normal choroidal fluorescence is blocked. The visibility of choroidal fluorescence is inversely proportional to the concentration of pigment in the pigment epithelium. If the pigment epithelium contains less than the normal amount of pigment or is defective, the choriocapillaris appears to fluoresce more brightly. The presence of hyperfluorescence caused by a defect in the pigment epithelium depends on the state of both the pigment epithelium and the choriocapillaris. The choriocapillaris must be intact for a depigmented area of the pigment epithelium to be apparent. If the choriocapillaris does not fill, a depigmented area of the pigment epithelium does not fluoresce.

Transmitted fluorescence has the following four basic characteristics:

1. It appears early in angiography, coincidental with choroidal filling.

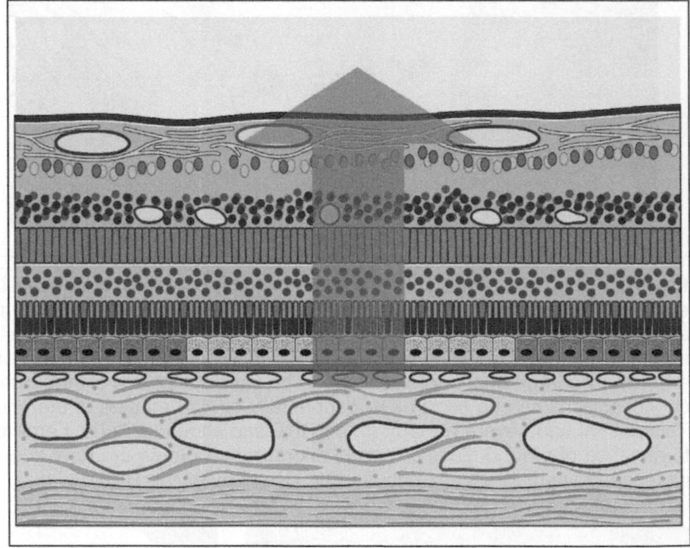

Fig. 1.33 Pigment epithelial window defect. This schematic of the retina shows that the pigment epithelium in the center of the section is less pigmented than the normal pigment epithelium. This allows the normal choroidal and choriocapillaris fluorescence to show through; that is, this pathologic condition would create a typical pigment epithelial window defect.

2. It increases in intensity as dye concentration increases in the choroid.
3. It does not increase in size or shape during the later phases of angiography.
4. It tends to fade and sometimes disappear as the choroid empties of dye at the end of angiography.

In short, transmitted fluorescence appears, peaks early, and fades late without changing size or shape, as would any normal

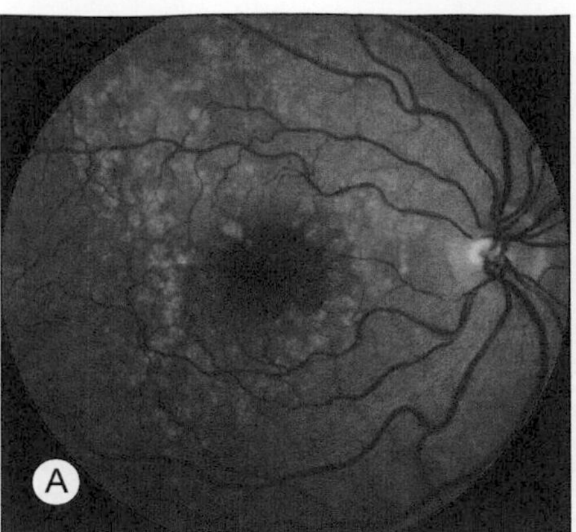

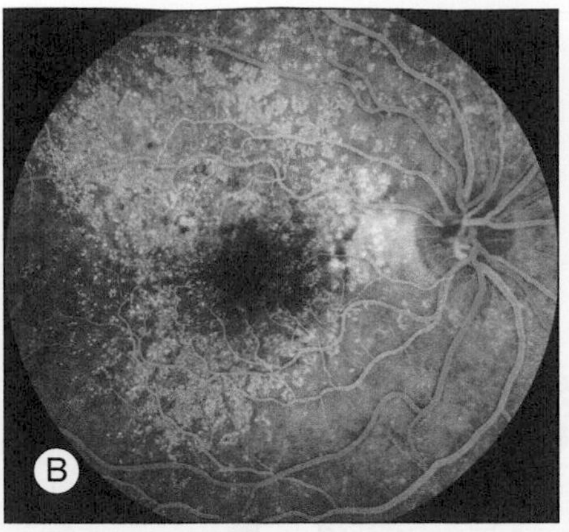

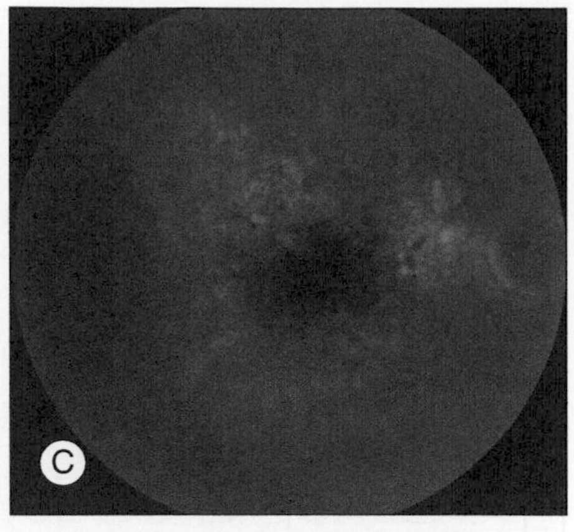

Fig. 1.34 An eye with drusen demonstrating pigment epithelial window defects. (A) Color photograph: right macula shows multiple drusen temporally. (B) Late arteriovenous phase of fluorescein angiogram shows marked hyperfluorescence in the areas of the drusen. (C) Late recirculation phase of fluorescein angiogram shows fading of fluorescence. Comment: Note the degree of fluorescence of the entire fundus vasculature. This is typical of a pigment epithelial window defect, which is a type of vascular fluorescence. The drusen allow a better view to the choriocapillaris because of the thinning of the pigment epithelium overlying them.

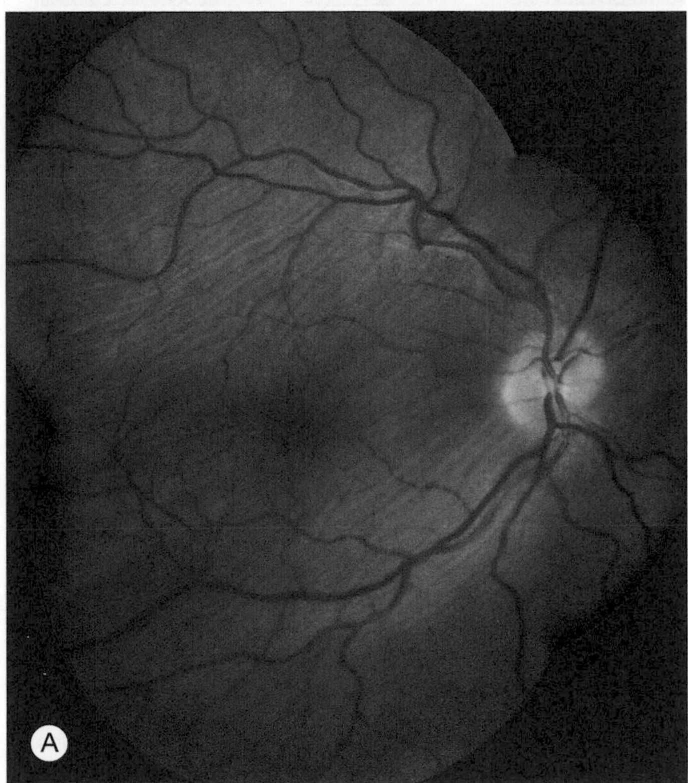

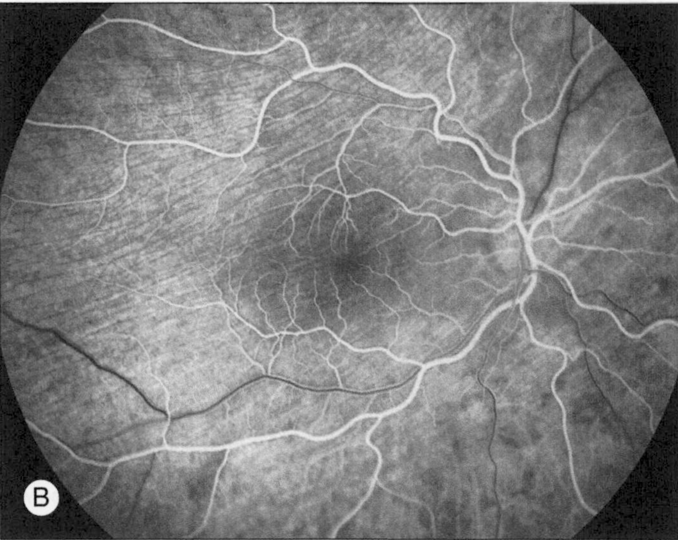

Fig. 1.35 Pigment epithelial window defect: choroidal folds. (A) Montage color photograph of right disc and macula. Note the pale lines (choroidal folds) scattered throughout the posterior pole. (B) Arteriovenous phase of fluorescein angiogram of the disc and macula. Hyperfluorescent lines correspond to the folds, and adjacent hypofluorescent lines are present throughout the macula and surrounding the disc. Comment: This patient had pigment epithelial folds caused by prolonged hypotony from a filtering bleb. The hyperfluorescent lines are thought to be the hills of the folds, in the apices of which the pigment epithelium is thinned, allowing hyperfluorescence in the early phases of the fluorescein angiogram (pigment epithelial window defect). The dark lines are thought to be the valleys of the folds, with an increase in pigmentation causing blockage of choroidal fluorescence. The later phases of fluorescein angiograms often show fading of fluorescence. Choroidal folds represent a type of pigment epithelial window defect with early vascular fluorescence and late fading of fluorescence.

vascular fluorescence. When pigment epithelial depigmentation is extensive, late fluorescein staining of the choroid and sclera may be visible, although it is less intense than the fluorescence of the window defect.

Abnormal retinal and disc vessels

Abnormal vascular fluorescence occurs when abnormal vessels are present. Such pathologic vessels may be in the retina, on the disc, or at the level of the choroid. Normal and abnormal retinal and disc vessels are clearly visible on the angiogram because no barrier obscures them from view. Gross abnormalities of the retinal and disc vasculature and subtle microvascular changes that cannot be appreciated adequately by ophthalmoscopic examination will be well defined and easily distinguished by fluorescein angiography. These changes in the retinal vasculature can be classified into six morphologic categories:

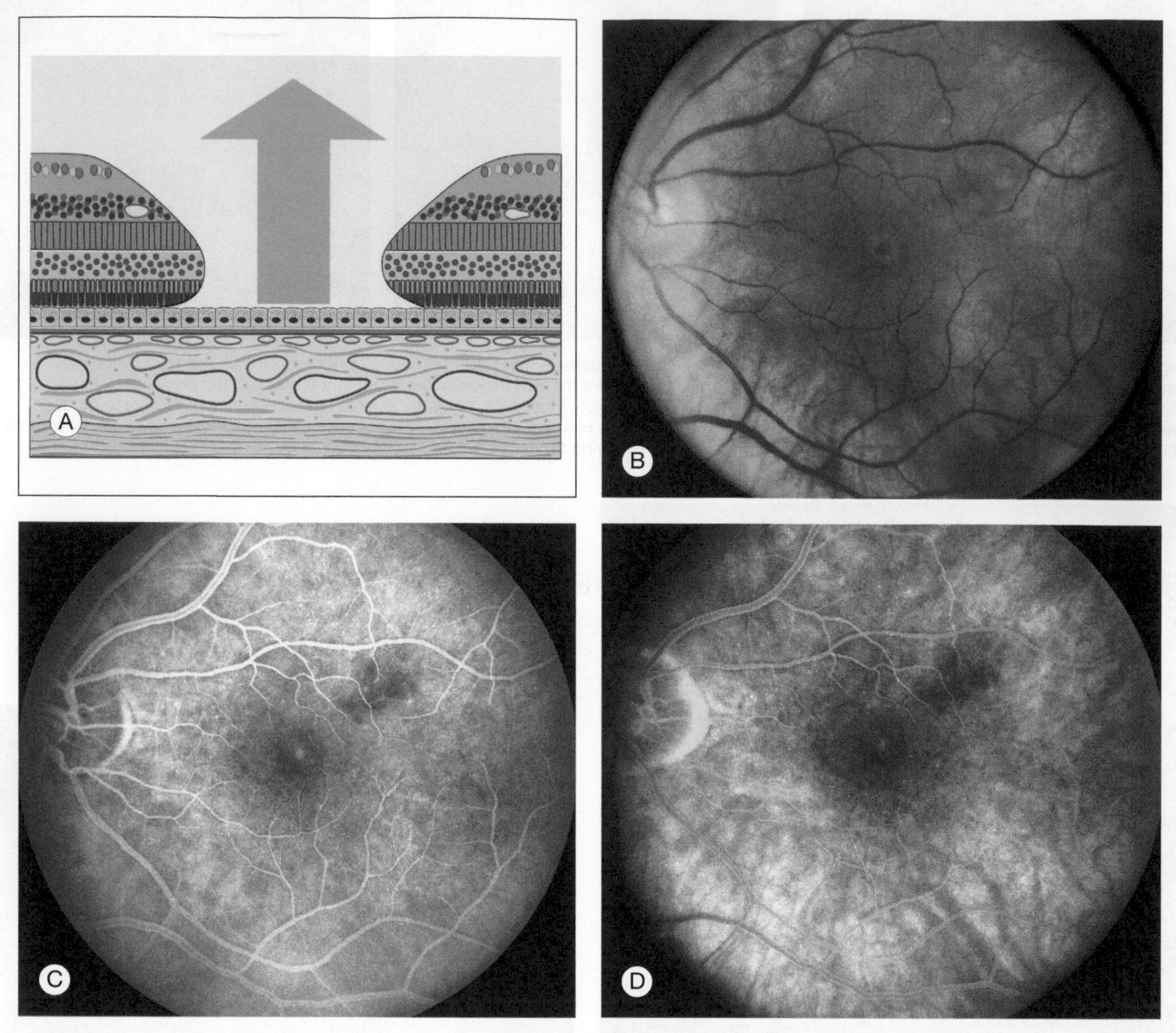

Fig. 1.36 Pigment epithelial window defect: macular hole. (A) Schematic drawing of macula showing loss of entire central foveal tissue. (B) Color photograph of the left macula. This patient has a macular hole. Note a corona of lighter detached, swollen retinal tissue surrounding the foveal center where the hole is located. (C) Late phase of fluorescein angiogram shows hyperfluorescence within the macular hole. (D) Later phase of the fluorescein angiogram shows some fading of the hyperfluorescence within the macular hole. Comment: The choriocapillaris was intact. Therefore the angiogram showed normal fluorescence of the choriocapillaris (early hyperfluorescence within the center of the fovea) and fading in the late phase of the angiogram.

(1) tortuosity and dilation (Figs 1.37 and 1.38); (2) telangiectasis (Figs 1.39 and 1.40); (3) neovascularization (Fig. 1.41); (4) anastomosis (Fig. 1.38); (5) aneurysms (Figs 1.38 and 1.39); and (6) tumor vessels (Figs 1.42 and 1.43).

These aforementioned changes can be viewed in the early (vascular) phases of angiography. Later, as the vessels empty, some of these vascular abnormalities leak fluorescein, whereas others do not.

Vascular abnormalities of the retina and disc are readily apparent on the fluorescein angiogram. The changes are characterized by early vascular-appearing hyperfluorescence. Each of the six morphologic types indicates specific disease processes that aid the clinician in making a diagnosis, determining the degree of the distinct pathologic process, and understanding the pathophysiology of retinal vascular disease.

Abnormal choroidal vessels

Abnormal vessels that may be present under the retina and originate from the choroid are subretinal neovascularization and vessels within a tumor. When subretinal neovascularization is present, the early angiogram often shows a lacy, irregular, and nodular hyperfluorescence (Figs 1.44 and 1.45). With a choroidal tumor, the abnormal hyperfluorescence is a similar, early vascular-type fluorescence, although it may be coarser, as seen in choroidal hemangioma (Fig. 1.46) and malignant melanoma (Fig. 1.47).

Text continued on p. e39

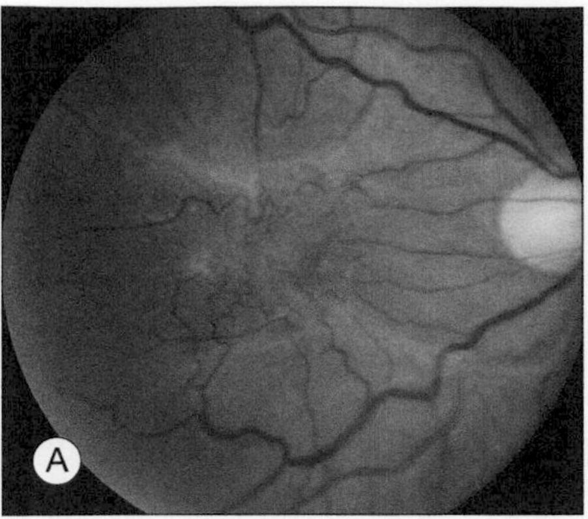

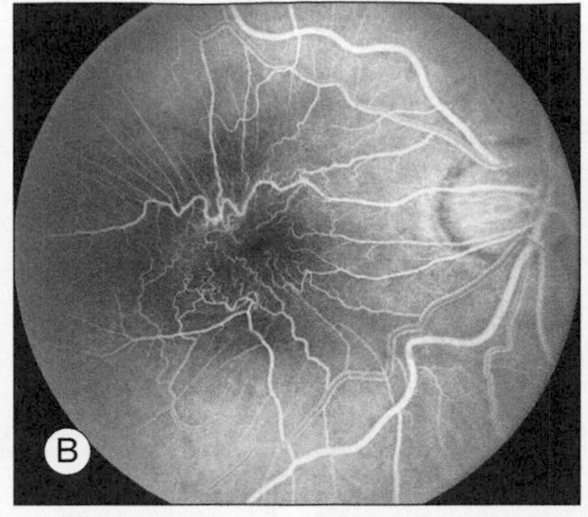

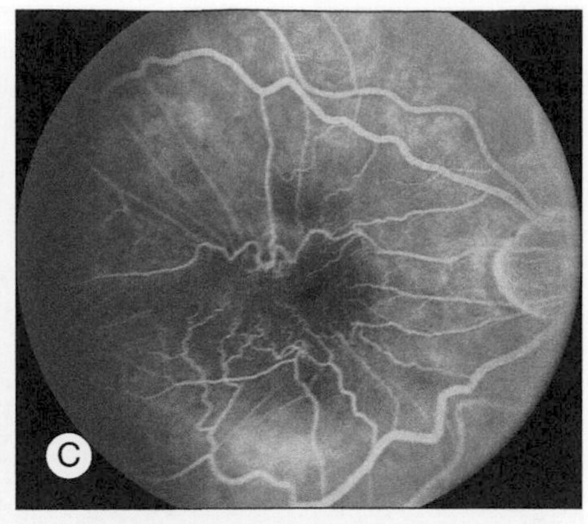

Fig. 1.37 Abnormal retinal vessels, tortuosity, and dilation: internal limiting membrane contraction. (A) Color photograph of right macula shows a pale membrane overlying the right macula, producing contraction of the retina and tortuosity of the retinal vessels. (B) Arteriovenous phase of fluorescein angiogram shows marked irregularity and tortuosity of the retinal vessels in association with the preretinal membrane (macular pucker). (C) Late phase of fluorescein angiogram shows a small amount of vascular leakage due to contraction of the membrane and pulling on the retinal vessels. Comment: This is tortuosity and dilation, a type of abnormal retinal vascular fluorescence. It is caused by the mechanical traction of an epiretinal membrane.

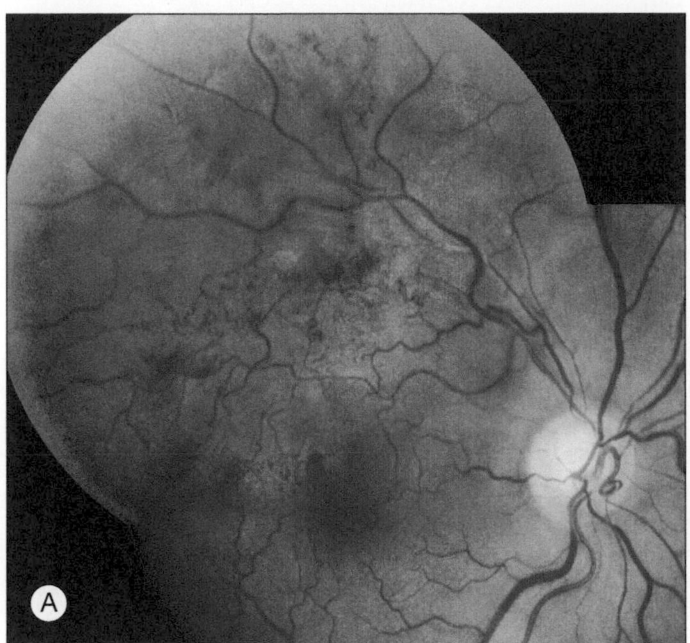

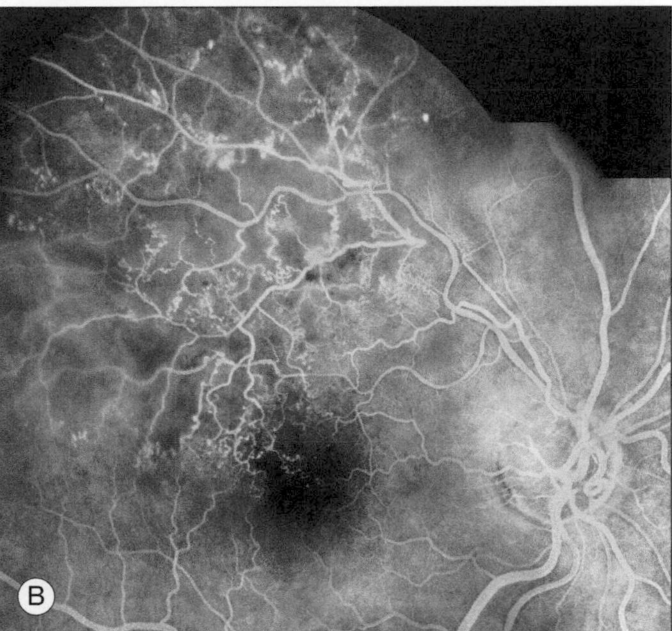

Fig. 1.38 Abnormal retinal vascular fluorescence: retinal vascular microaneurysms, telangiectasis, and anastomoses. (A) Color photography of right eye shows numerous telangiectatic retinal vessels due to a superotemporal branch-vein occlusion. (B) Arteriovenous-phase fluorescein angiogram shows multiple areas of smaller and larger microaneurysms and telangiectasis. Several small venous–venous anastomoses can be seen just temporal to the macula. The venous system of the occluded area has collateralized with patent vessels in uninvolved areas.

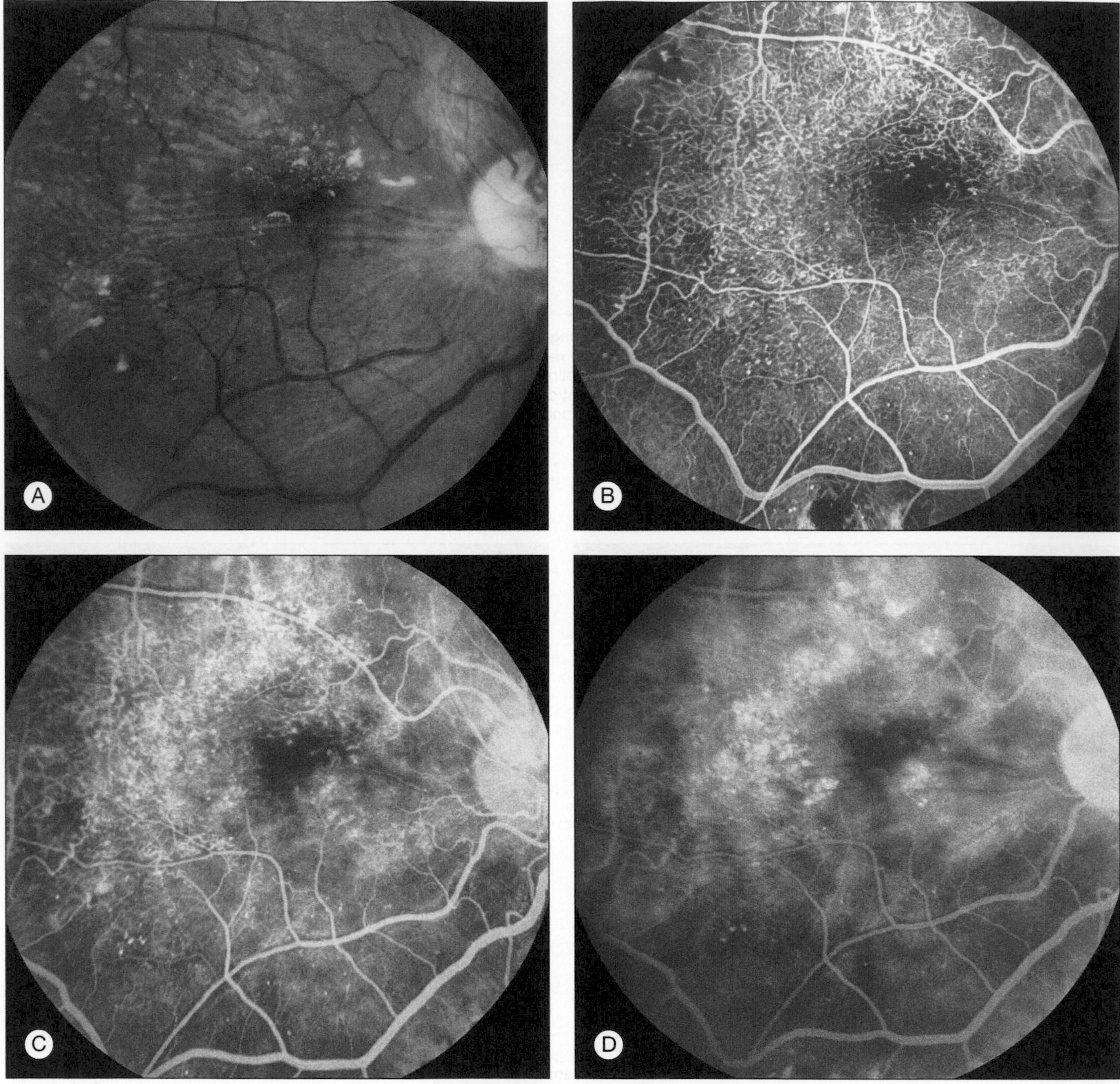

Fig. 1.39 Retinal telangiectasis and microaneurysms secondary to diabetic retinopathy. (A) Color photography of right macula showing retinal exudate, retinal striae, and irregularly dilated retinal vessels (telangiectasis). (B) Arteriovenous-phase fluorescein angiogram shows extensive hyperfluorescence from the numerous microaneurysms, and telangiectatic retinal vessels. (C) Later arteriovenous-phase fluorescein angiogram of right macula showing leakage from many of these vessels. (D) Late-phase fluorescein angiogram of right macula shows multiple circular areas of hyperfluorescence due to accumulation of dye in extensive cystoid spaces. Comment**:** This patient had significant retinal microvascular changes due to diabetic retinopathy.

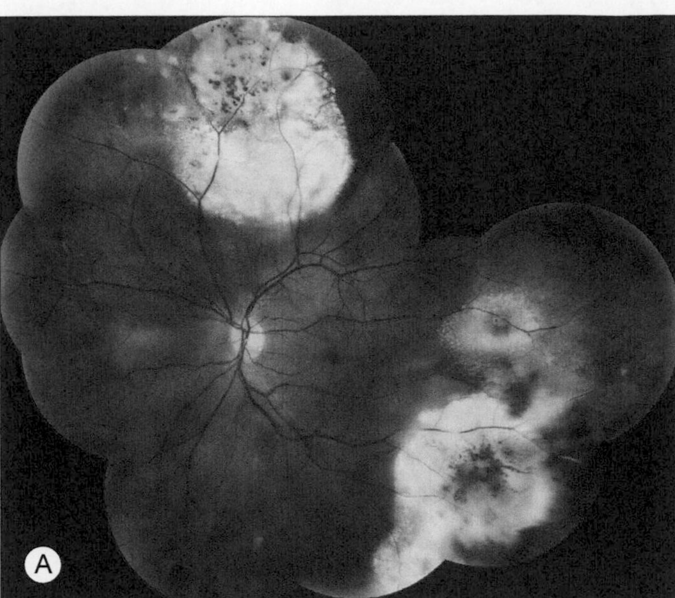

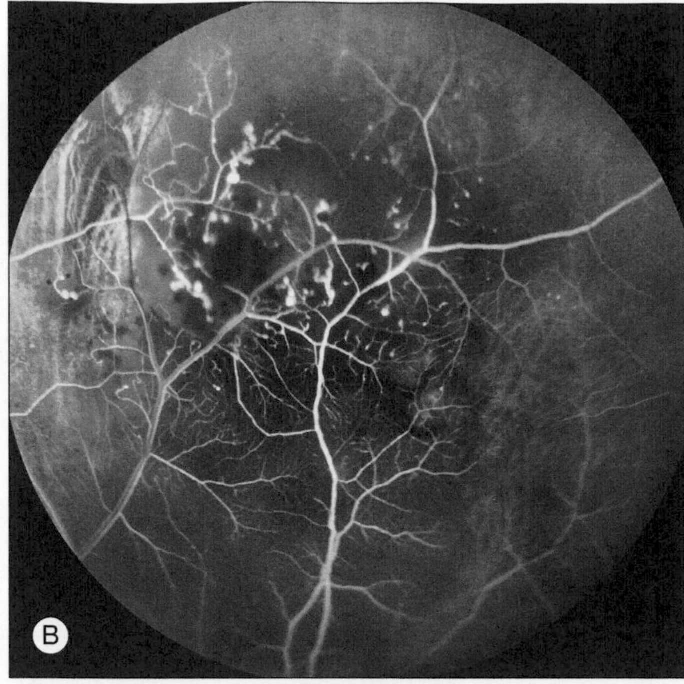

Fig. 1.40 Abnormal retinal vessels: telangiectasis. (A) Color montage photograph demonstrating severe areas of exudation, as well as dilated and telangiectatic vessels. The retina is very edematous. (B) Arteriovenous phase of fluorescein angiogram shows marked irregularity of the retinal vasculature. There are areas of capillary nonperfusion, telangiectasis, and tortuosity. Comment: This patient had Coats disease with a markedly abnormal retinal capillary bed, including telangiectasis and dilated vessels.

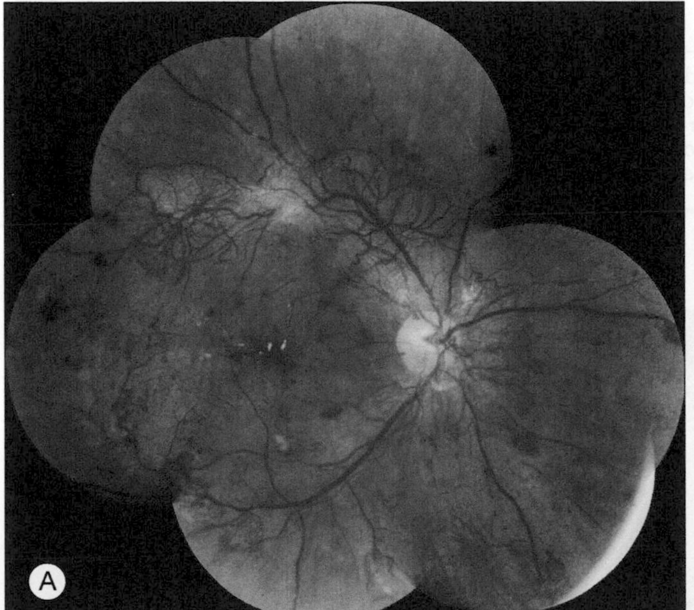

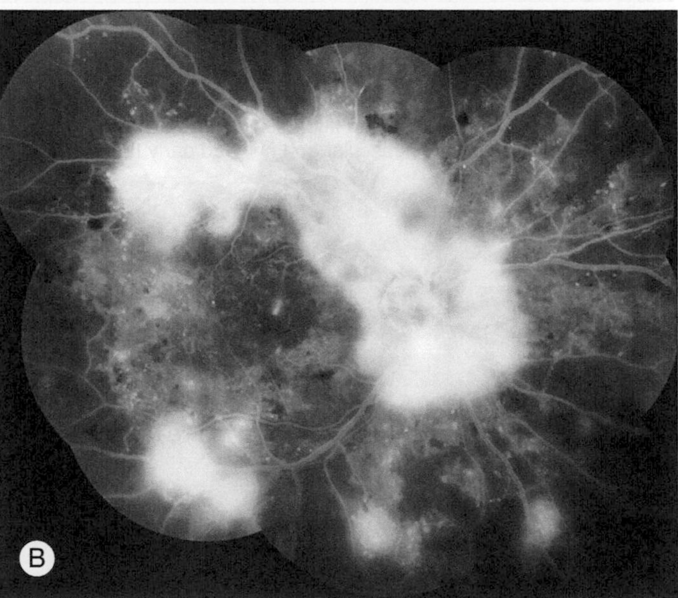

Fig. 1.41 Abnormal retinal vessels: retinal neovascularization due to proliferative diabetic retinopathy. (A) Montage color photograph of the posterior pole of the right eye. Extensive irregular tortuous vessels extend from the optic nerve along the vascular arcades and nasally. These vessels lie on the surface of the retina. (B) Later arteriovenous phase of fluorescein angiogram montage shows increasing hyperfluorescence of the retinal neovascularization. Comment: This patient had severe proliferative diabetic retinopathy with extensive neovascularization of the right disc. The vessels fluoresced early (vascular fluorescence) and leaked late. This is very typical of retinal or disc neovascularization.

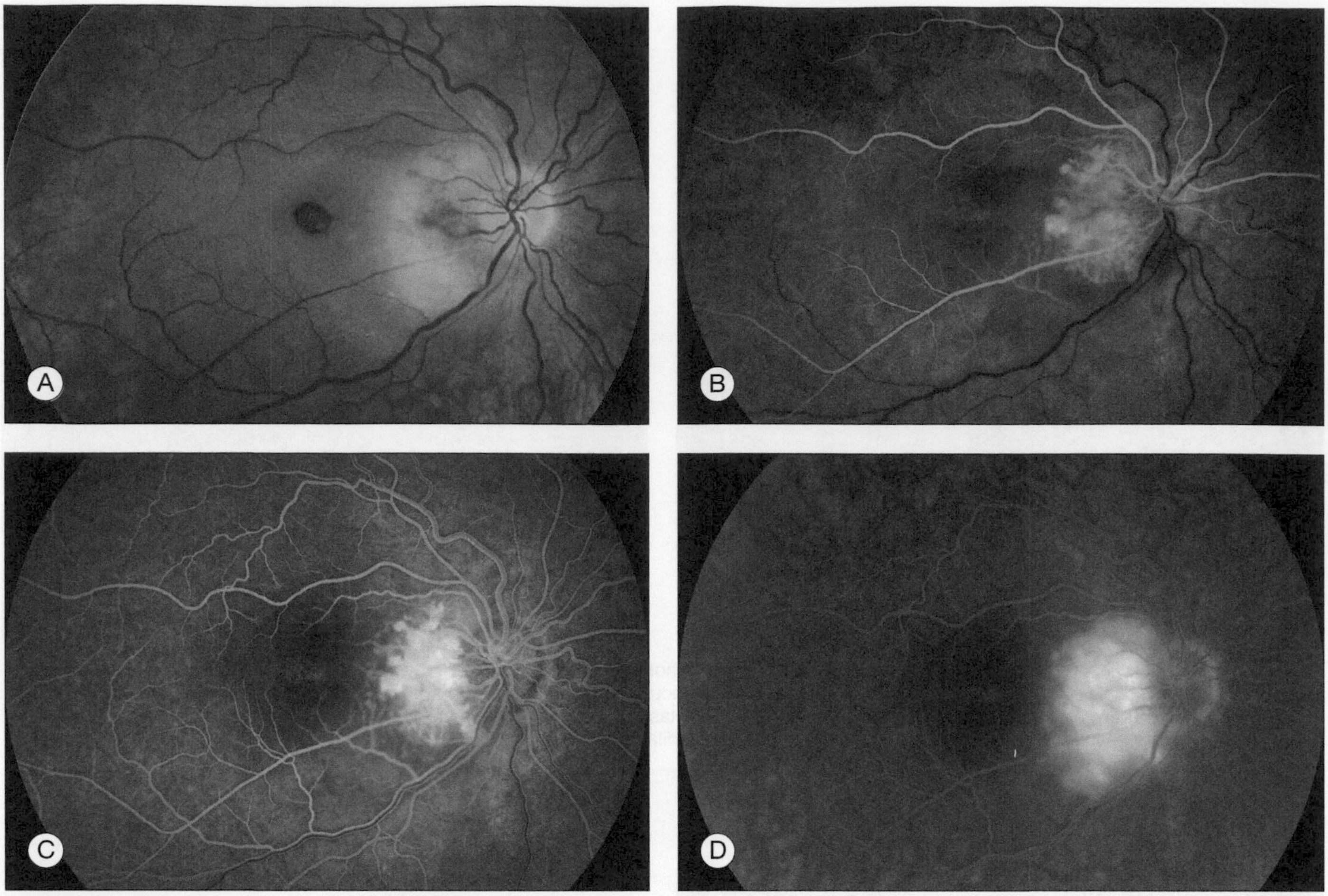

Fig. 1.42 Abnormal retinal vessels: tumor–retinal angioma as part of von Hippel's disease. (A) Color photograph of right macula and disc shows exudate temporal and inferior to the disc. A very vascular, slightly elevated mass was noted on the temporal border of the disc. Ophthalmoscopy showed that it has a reddish appearance. A large full-thickness macular hole is also observed. (B) Early arterial phase of the fluorescein angiogram shows marked fluorescence of the mass. (C) Midarteriovenous phase of the fluorescein angiogram shows an increased fluorescence of the mass. (D) Late phase of the fluorescein angiogram shows leakage of fluorescein within the mass. Comment**:** This patient had a peripapillary retinal angioma. It was very vascular and showed early fluorescence and extensive late leakage.

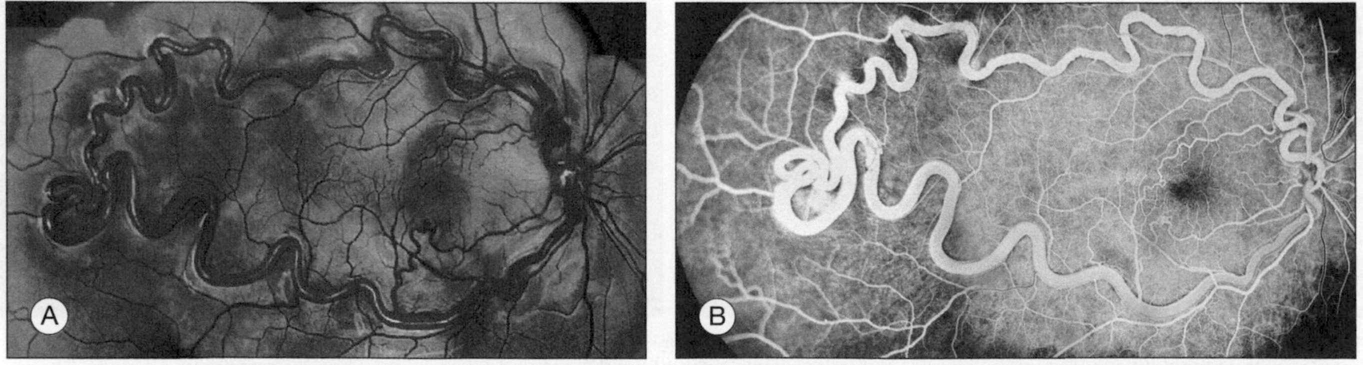

Fig. 1.43 Arteriovenous malformation: Wyburn–Mason type. (A) Color montage photograph of right macula and temporal retina showing enlarged, dilated retinal artery, with direct connection to an engorged draining vein. There is no intervening capillary bed. (B) Fluorescein angiogram showing marked hyperfluorescence of the abnormal, dilated retinal artery and vein. Two smaller arteriovenous malformations appear to be present, one just above the macula, and the other just below.

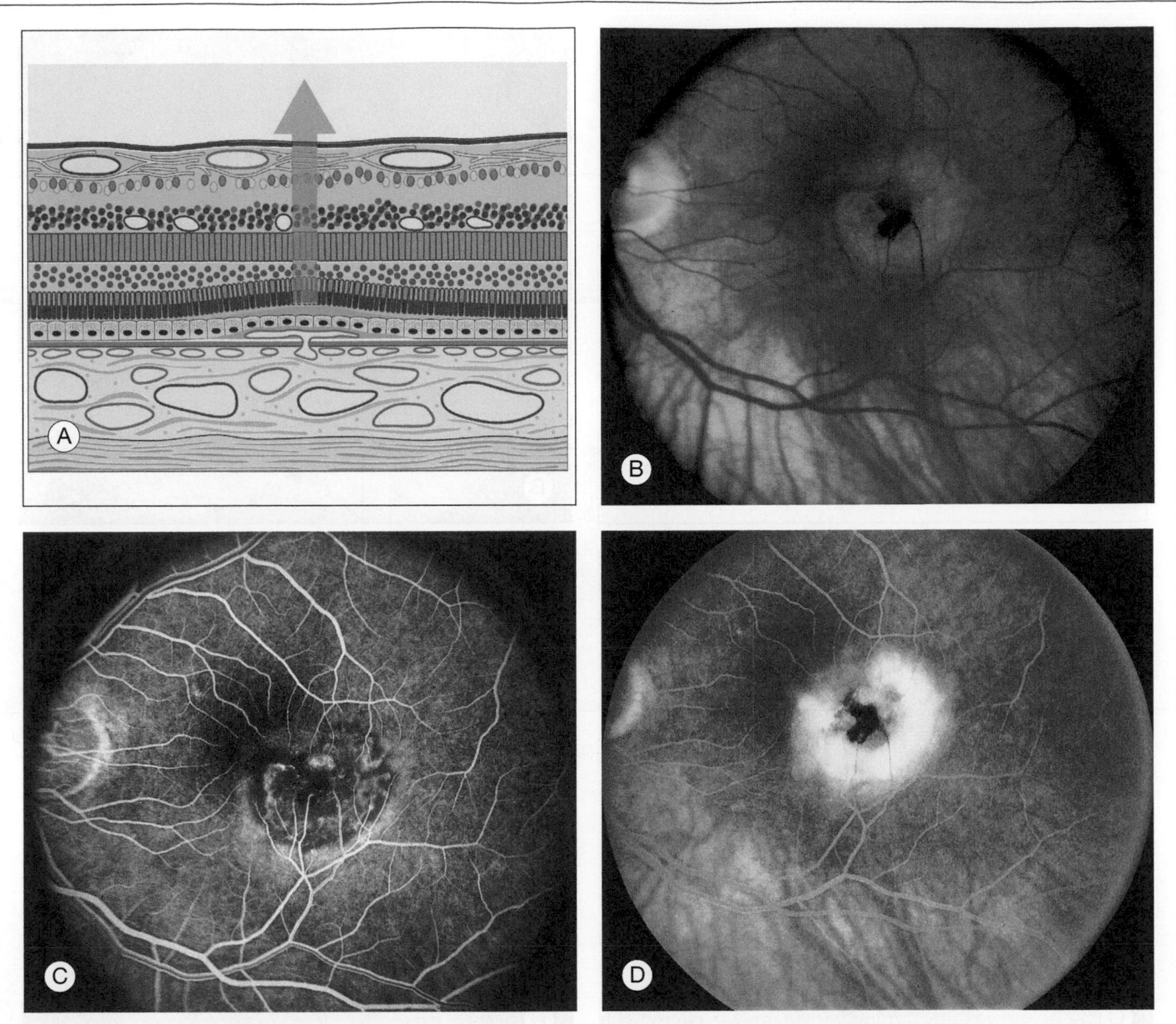

Fig. 1.44 Abnormal choroidal vessels: subretinal neovascularization. (A) Schematic view of the retina shows a small break in Bruch's membrane, with a fine proliferation of capillaries through the break dissecting under and lifting up the pigment epithelium. There is a shallow sensory retinal detachment. (B) Color photograph of the left macula. There is a dirty-gray membrane involving the central macula. Note the small area of subretinal hemorrhage. There is a shallow sensory retinal detachment. (C) The arteriovenous phase of fluorescein angiogram shows fine, lacy, irregular hyperfluorescence corresponding to a small, fine patch of subretinal neovascularization. (D) Late phase of fluorescein angiogram shows leakage of these vessels into the subpigment epithelial and subretinal spaces. Comment: This patient had a small patch of subretinal neovascularization involving the central fovea. The angiogram shows typical, early vascular fluorescence (in a nodular, irregular, lacelike fashion) and late hyperfluorescent leakage.

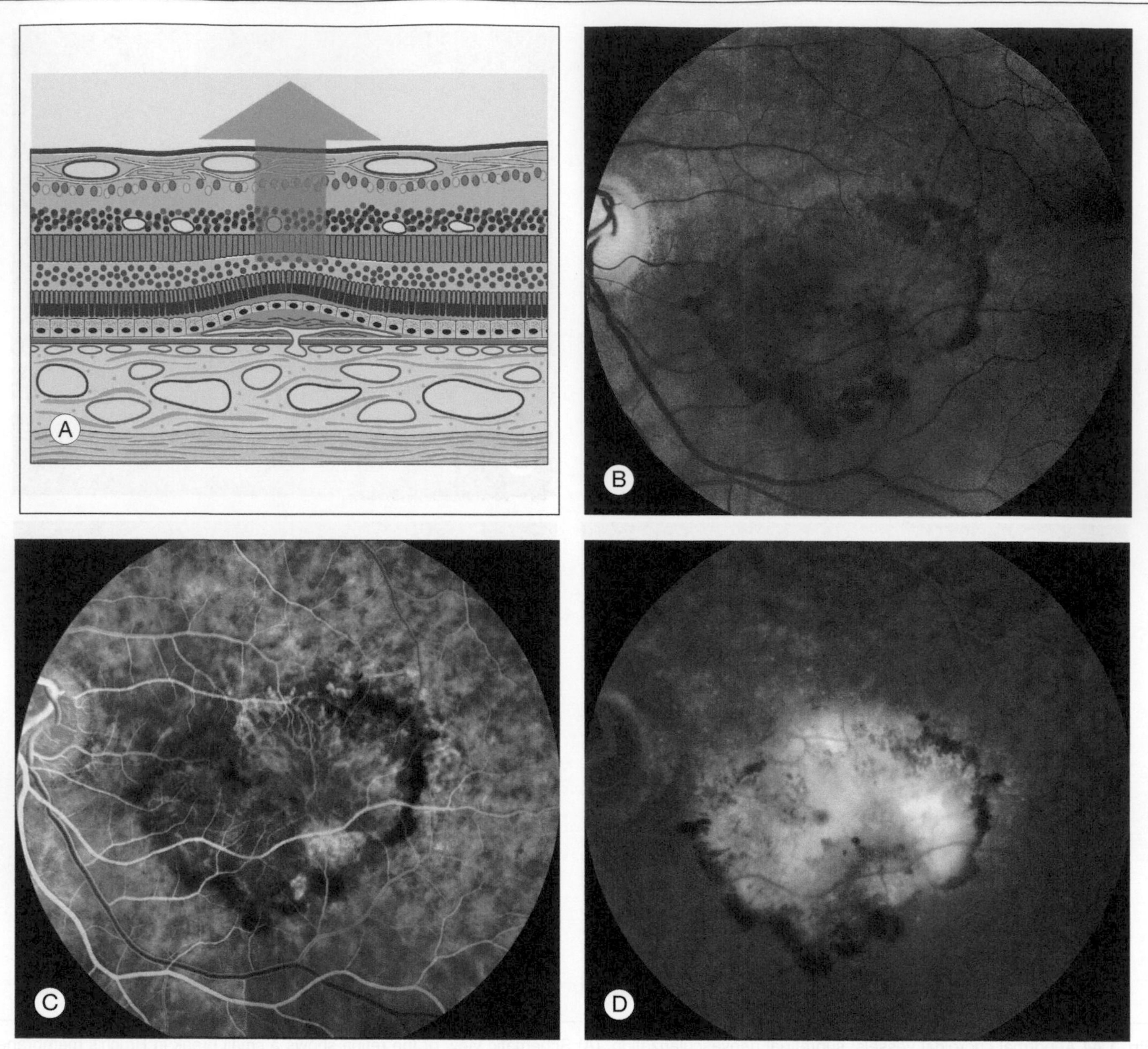

Fig. 1.45 Abnormal choroidal vessels: subretinal neovascularization. (A) Schematic drawing of retina shows vascular proliferation from the choriocapillaris dissecting under the pigment epithelium, with associated fibrous tissue. The pigment epithelium has become thinned and the sensory retina detached. The outer plexiform layer of the sensory retina shows cystic spaces. (B) Red-free photograph of left macula shows some hemorrhage and exudate. On the color photograph and slit-lamp biomicroscopy, a dirty-gray membrane was noted in the inferotemporal portion of the macula. This is seen as a slightly pale lesion in the inferotemporal macula. (C) Early arteriovenous phase of fluorescein angiogram shows a lacy, irregular, nodular area of hyperfluorescence in the inferotemporal macula. This is a flat patch of vessels that has proliferated from the choriocapillaris under the pigment epithelium. (D) Late phase of the fluorescein angiogram shows leakage from the patch of subretinal neovascularization. Most of the fluorescence is pooling of fluorescein under the sensory retinal detachment, although there is some cystic change in the fovea. Comment: This patient had a patch of subretinal neovascularization that was nearly 4 disc diameters in size. It fluoresced early with the vascular phase of the angiogram (typical for subretinal neovascularization) and leaked late. Actually, "subretinal neovascularization" is a misnomer because the new vessels are initially located in the subpigment epithelial space.

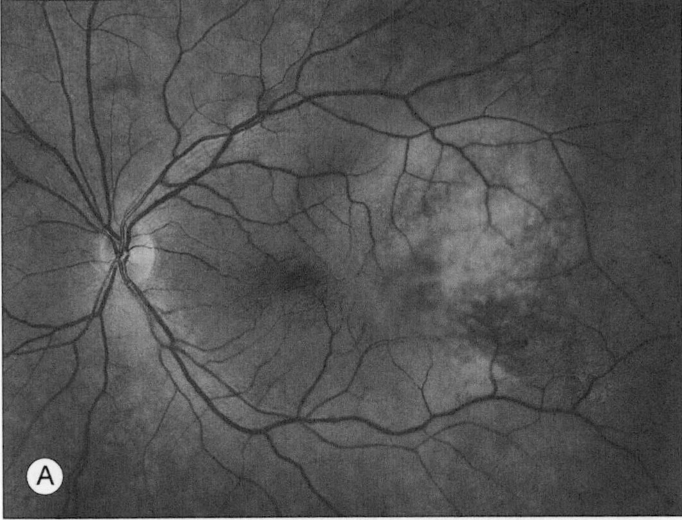
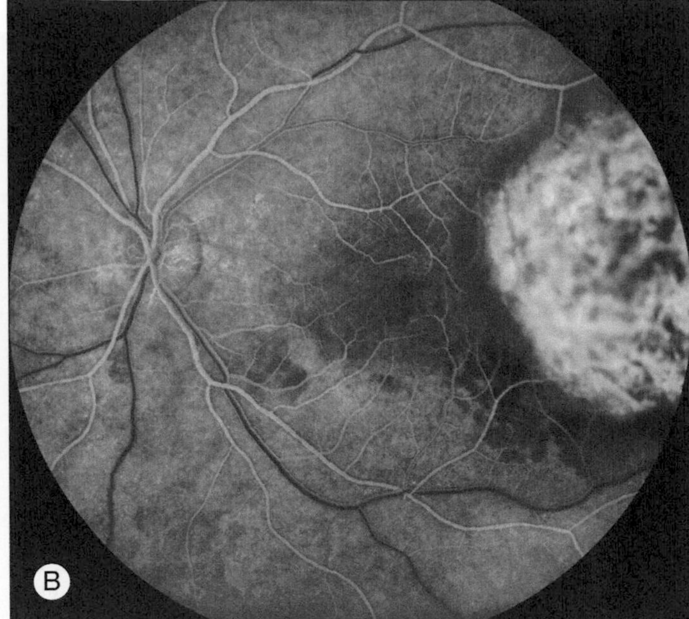
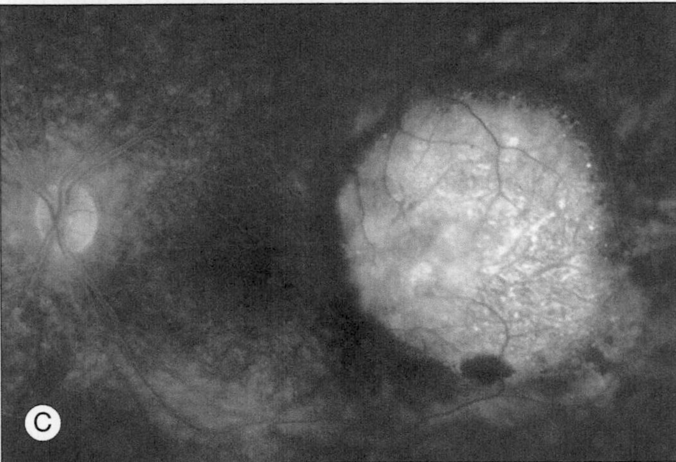

Fig. 1.46 Abnormal choroidal vessels in a patient with choroidal hemangioma. (A) Color photo of left macula and disc with elevated choroidal hemangioma. (B) Arteriovenous phase of the fluorescein angiogram shows prominent hyperfluorescence in this area demonstrating the tumor vessels. (C) Late phase of the fluorescein angiogram shows marked leakage in this area. Comment: This patient had a choroidal hemangioma, which is a very vascularized choroidal mass. The vascularity in this mass causes the marked hyperfluorescence and leakage.

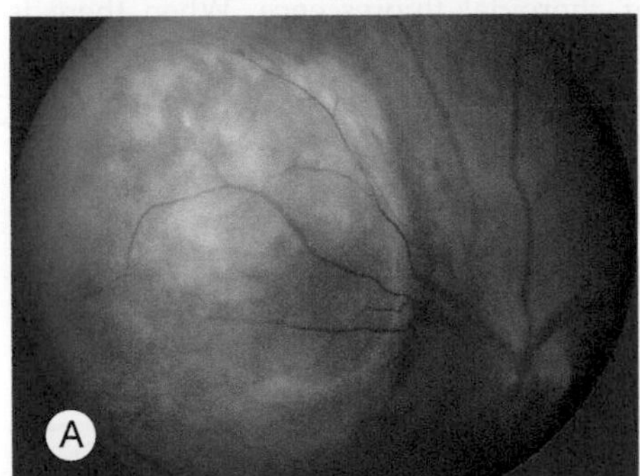
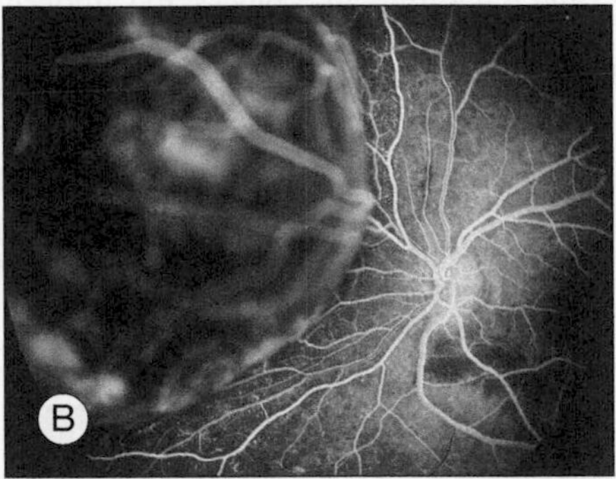
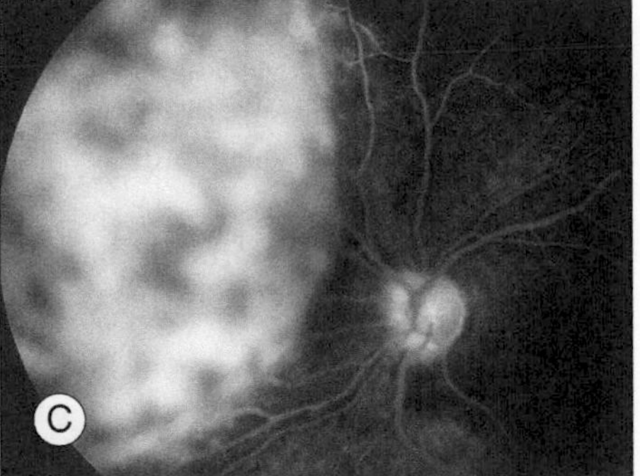

Fig. 1.47 Abnormal choroidal vascular fluorescence due to malignant melanoma. (A) Color photograph of left eye. Note the darkly pigmented mass nasal to the optic nerve. There is some orange lipofuscin pigment overlying the surface of this as well. (B) Arteriovenous phase of fluorescein angiogram of the mass shows hyperfluorescence over the surface of the tumor. This patient also had some macular drusen, which show some early hyperfluorescence in the macula. (C) Late phase of the fluorescein angiogram shows leakage from the mass. There are multiple "hot spots" overlying the tumor. Comment: This patient had a choroidal malignant melanoma. This was a medium-sized tumor that showed the typical early fluorescence that is seen in a medium-sized melanoma.

Leak

Fluorescence of the retinal and choroidal vessels begins to diminish about 40–60 seconds after injection. Fluorescein empties almost completely from the retinal and choroidal vasculature about 10–15 minutes after injection. Any fluorescence that remains in the fundus after the retinal and choroidal vessels have emptied of fluorescein is extravascular fluorescence and represents leakage.

Four types of late extravascular hyperfluorescent leakage occur in the normal eye: (1) fluorescence of the disc margins from the surrounding choriocapillaris; (2) fluorescence of the lamina cribrosa; (3) fluorescence of the sclera at the disc margin if the retinal pigment epithelium terminates away from the disc, as in an optic crescent; and (4) fluorescence of the sclera when the pigment epithelium is lightly pigmented. These are the only forms of late hyperfluorescence or leakage that can be considered "normal." Any other hyperfluorescence observed 15 minutes after the fluorescein injection represents extravascular fluorescein and is referred to as leakage.

Either or both of the two vascular systems of the fundus can produce abnormal late hyperfluorescence (leakage) if defects are present in their respective barriers to fluorescein. The barrier to fluorescein leakage from the retinal vessels is the retinal vascular endothelium. The barrier to leakage from the choroidal circulation is the pigment epithelium. An abnormality of the retinal vascular endothelium can result in permeability to fluorescein and leakage of fluorescein into the retinal tissue. Similarly, an abnormality of the pigment epithelium can result in permeability to fluorescein, and fluorescein will leak from the choroidal tissue through the pigment epithelium. Abnormal late hyperfluorescence of the choroid, however, can occur without damage to the pigment epithelium, as in cellular infiltrates of the choroid that occur in choroidal inflammation or tumor.

There are two other types of late abnormal fluorescence: one occurs when fluorescein enters the vitreous, and the other when fluorescein leaks into the optic nerve head.

Vitreous leak

Leakage of fluorescein into the vitreous creates a diffuse, white haze in the late phase of the fluorescein angiogram. In some instances the haze is generalized and evenly dispersed, and in other cases the white haze is localized.

Leakage of fluorescein into the vitreous is due to three major causes: (l) neovascularization growing from the retinal vessels on to the surface of the retina or disc or into the vitreous cavity; (2) intraocular inflammation; and (3) intraocular tumors.

Vitreous hyperfluorescence secondary to retinal neovascularization is usually localized and appears as a cotton-ball type of fluorescence surrounding the neovascularization (Fig. 1.41B). The vitreous fluorescence secondary to intraocular inflammation is often generalized, giving a diffuse, white haze to the vitreous because of generalized leakage of fluorescein from the iris and ciliary body. The vitreous fluorescence secondary to tumors is most often localized over the tumor.

Disc leak

The optic nerve head normally has some fluorescein leakage (late hyperfluorescence) as a result of staining of the lamina cribrosa and the surrounding margins of the disc (from the normally leaking peripapillary choriocapillaries). The difference between normal and abnormal leakage at the disc may be subtle.

Papilledema and optic disc edema

Papilledema is swelling of the optic nerve head as a result of increased intracranial pressure. Edema of the optic disc is defined as swelling of the optic nerve head secondary to local or systemic causes (Fig. 1.48). The angiogram is similar in each case, demonstrating leakage associated with swelling of the optic nerve head. In the early phases of the angiogram, dilation of the capillaries on the optic nerve head may be seen; in the late angiogram, the dilated vessels leak, resulting in a fuzzy fluorescence of the disc margin.

Retinal leak

In the late stages of the normal angiogram, the retinal vessels have emptied of fluorescein and the retina is dark. Any late retinal hyperfluorescence is abnormal and indicates leakage of retinal vessels. When the leakage is severe, the extracellular fluid may flow into cystic pockets, and the angiogram shows fluorescence of the cystic spaces. Fluorescein flows out of the patent retinal vessels to lie in pools in the cystoid spaces or stains the edematous (noncystic) retinal tissue. Cystoid retinal edema is apparent as the fluorescein pools in small loculated pockets. In the macula, cystoid edema takes on a stellate appearance (Fig. 1.49); elsewhere in the retina, it has a honeycombed appearance (Fig. 1.50). Fluorescent staining of noncystoid edema is diffuse, irregular, and not confined to well-demarcated spaces (Figs 1.51 and 1.52).

The amount of fluorescein leakage depends on the dysfunction of the retinal vascular endothelium (Fig. 1.52). When leakage is not pronounced, the cystoid spaces fill slowly and become visible only late in angiography. When this occurs, the area of cystoid retinal edema may be somewhat hypofluorescent early in the angiogram because the fluid in these spaces acts as a barrier and blocks the underlying choroidal fluorescence. When there is heavy fluorescein leakage, the cystoid spaces fill rapidly, in some cases within a minute after injection. The large confluent cysts seen with severe cystoid macular edema may fill late in the angiogram. The large retinal vessels can also leak. This is called perivascular staining and is seen in three distinct situations: inflammation (indicating a perivasculitis), traction (severe pulling on a large retinal vessel, Fig. 1.52), and occlusion. When a large retinal

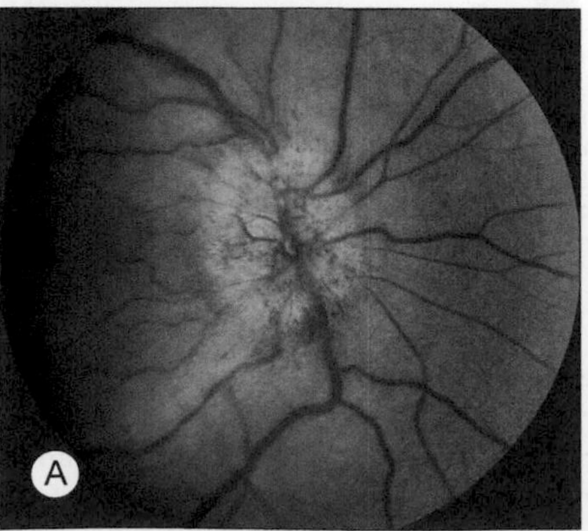

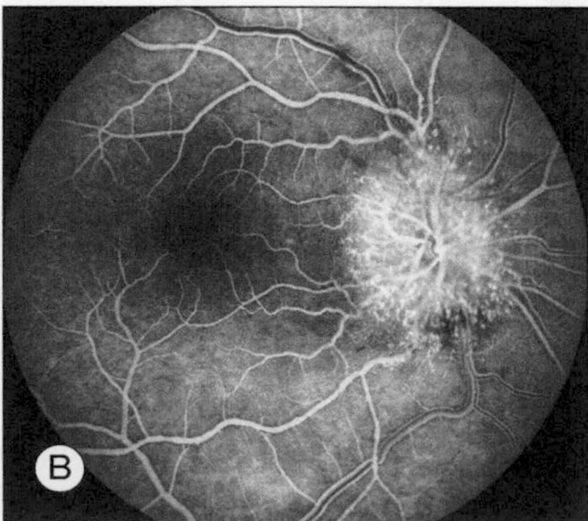

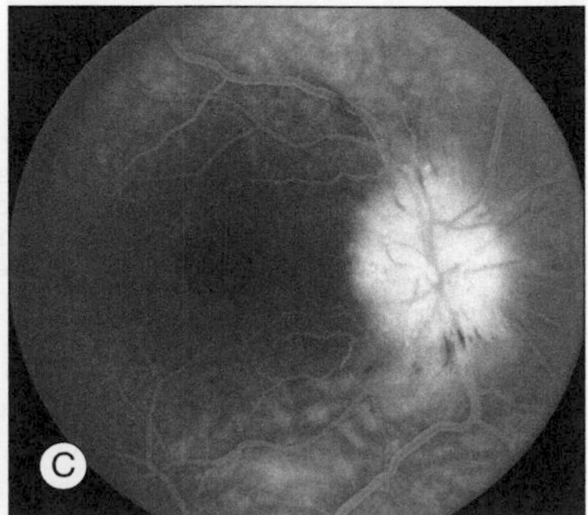

Fig. 1.48 Disc leakage. (A) Color photograph of right optic nerve. Note the dilation of the disc capillaries. (B) The arteriovenous-phase angiogram of the right disc and macula shows the hyperfluorescence due to these dilated disc capillaries. (C) The late phase of the angiogram shows significant leakage from these dilated optic disc capillaries. Comment: This patient had a papillopathy related to diabetes. This produced significant dilation of the disc capillaries. The leakage from this abnormal disc is quite obvious.

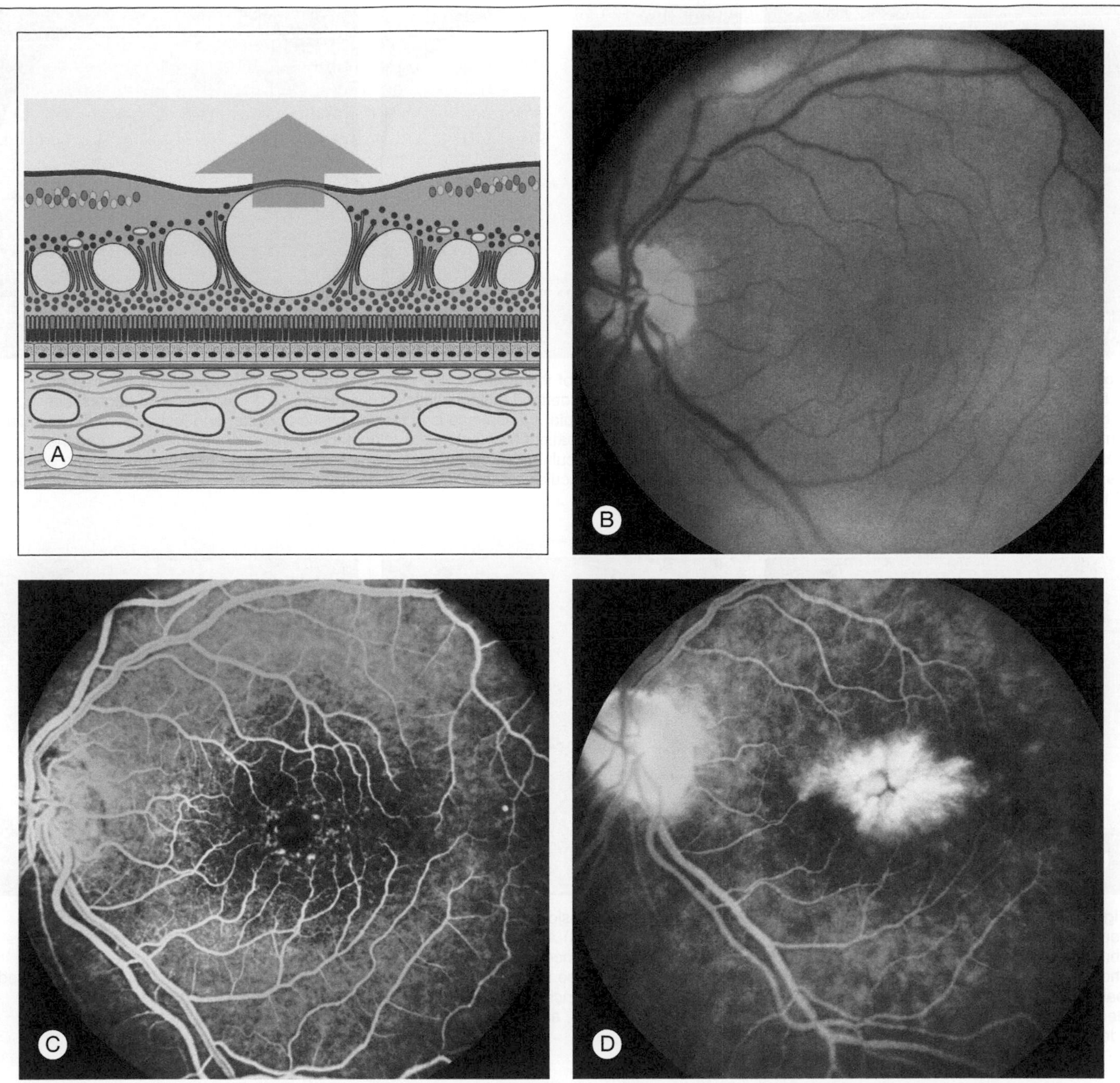

Fig. 1.49 Retinal leak: cystoid macular edema. (A) Schematic drawing of the macula shows large cystic spaces in the outer plexiform layer. There are some cystic spaces in the inner nuclear layer. (B) Color photograph of left macula. Careful inspection of the retina is often necessary on biomicroscopy to detect intraretinal cystoid. (C) Arteriovenous phase of fluorescein angiogram shows some dilation of the fine capillary network around the fovea. (D) Late phase of fluorescein angiogram shows hyperfluorescence from the accumulation of dye filling the cystic spaces. Note the stellate appearance of the cystoid macular edema. Comment: This patient had late hyperfluorescence (i.e., leakage) into the retina that was severe enough to create cystic spaces. This is a typical example of cystoid macular edema.

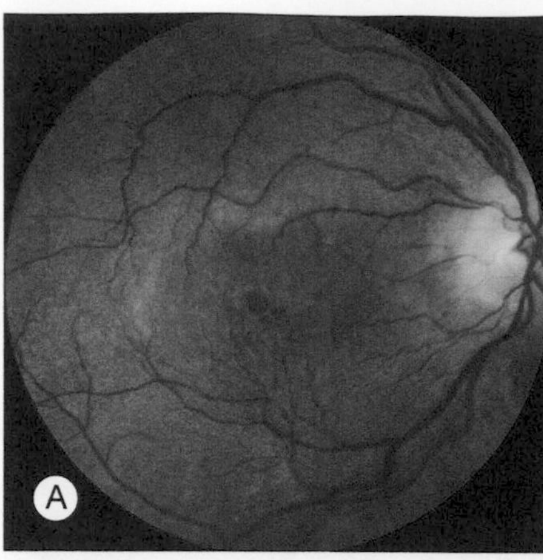

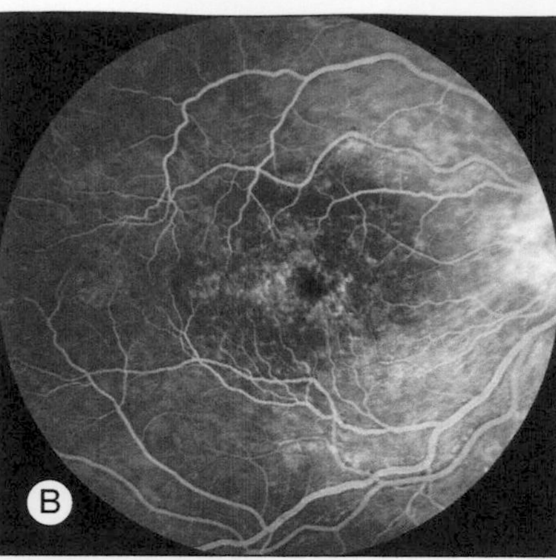

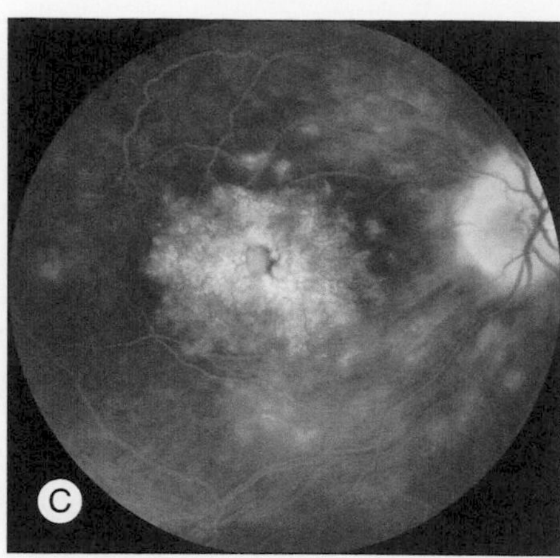

Fig. 1.50 Retinal leakage: cystoid retinal edema. (A) Color photograph of the right macula. Large central cystoid cavity is seen corresponding to fovea. (B) Arteriovenous phase of fluorescein angiogram shows well-defined telangiectatic retinal vessels. (C) Late phase of fluorescein angiogram shows leakage from these vessels. In the center of the macula, the leakage is in stellate cystic pockets, and just outside the macula, temporally, the leakage has taken a honeycomb form. Comment: This patient had leakage of telangiectatic vessels into the retina, and the leakage formed cystoid spaces. Cystoid edema in the center of the macula takes on a stellate form because of the oblique nature of the outer plexiform layer. The cystic spaces take on a honeycomb form in nonmacular areas of the retina because of the perpendicular nature of the fibers of the outer plexiform layer.

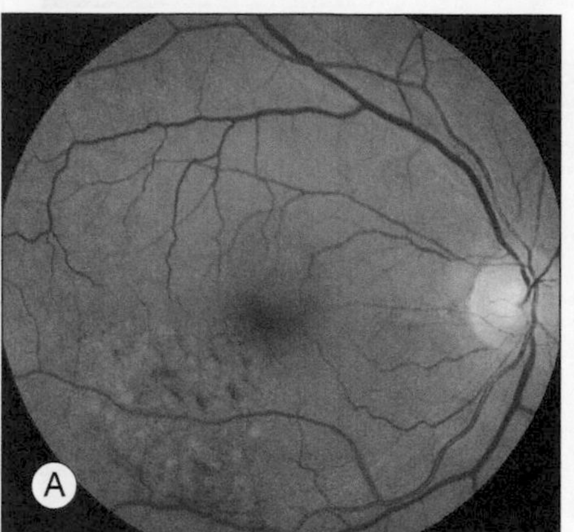

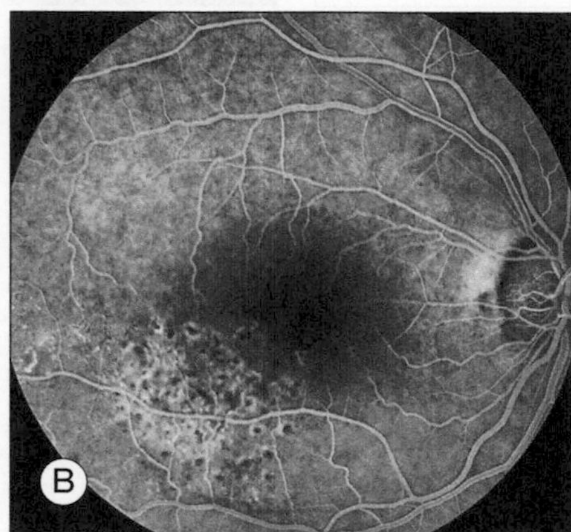

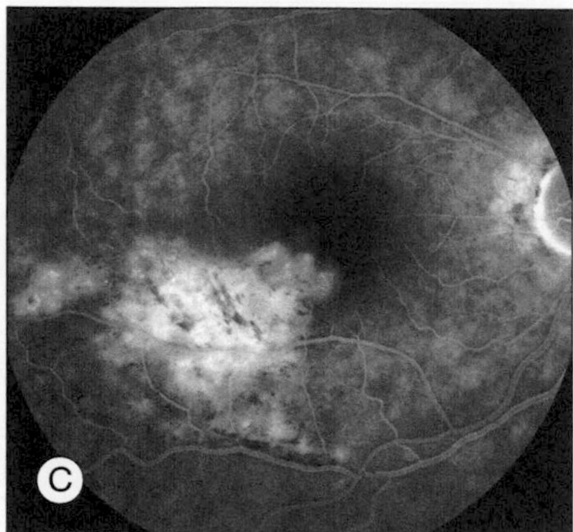

Fig. 1.51 Retinal leakage, severe noncystoid edema. Branch-vein occlusion. (A) Color photograph of right macula shows multiple retinal hemorrhages inferotemporally due to a retinal branch-vein occlusion. (B) Arteriovenous phase of fluorescein angiogram shows the vascular abnormalities associated with the branch-vein occlusion. Hypofluorescence corresponds to areas previously treated with grid pattern laser photocoagulation. (C) Late phase of fluorescein angiogram shows diffuse leakage of the fluorescein dye. Comment: This patient had generalized leakage of the retinal vascular bed in the distribution of the blocked branch vein. The leakage was not yet severe enough, however, to form clearly defined cystic spaces. Late hyperfluorescence indicates leakage, and this fluorescence is located in the retina; thus this was retinal edema.

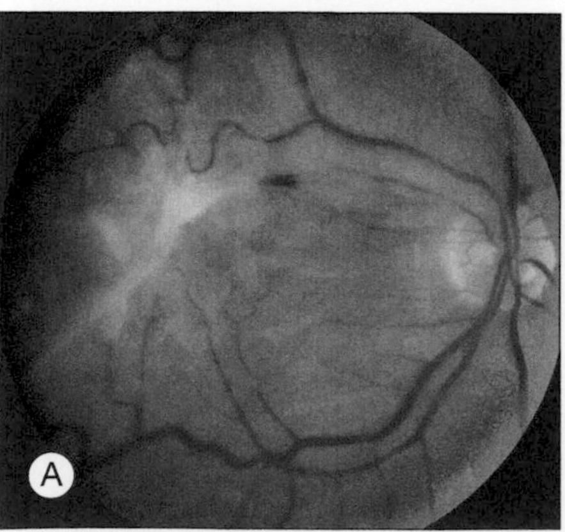

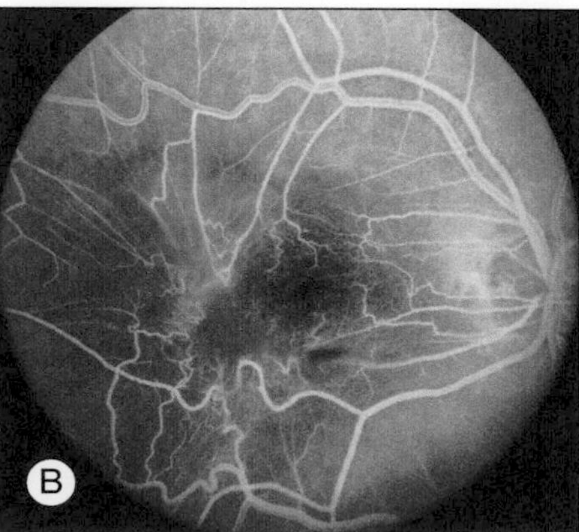

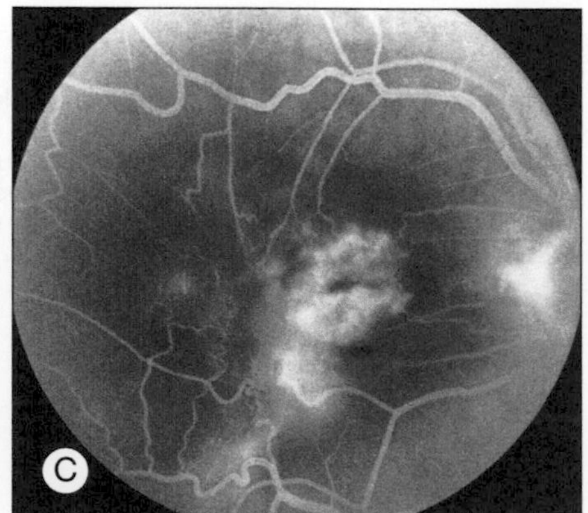

Fig. 1.52 Late hyperfluorescence, retinal leakage: severe epiretinal membrane contraction. (A) Color photograph of right macula showing thick epiretinal membrane overlying the macula and producing severe traction and contraction of the retina and vessels. (B) Arteriovenous phase of fluorescein angiogram shows that the retinal vasculature is tortuous and irregular. (C) Late arteriovenous phase of fluorescein angiogram shows leakage from the retinal vessels. Comment: The marked preretinal membrane caused sufficient traction on the retina, resulting in marked retinal vascular leakage.

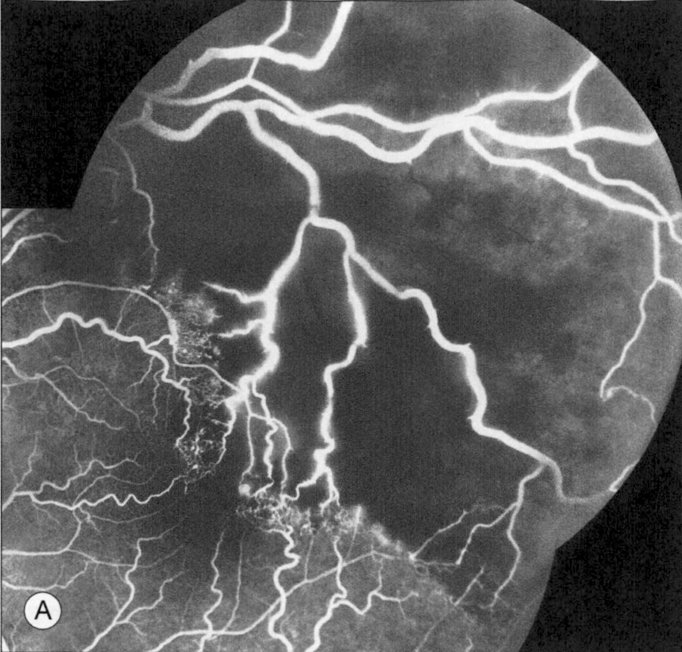

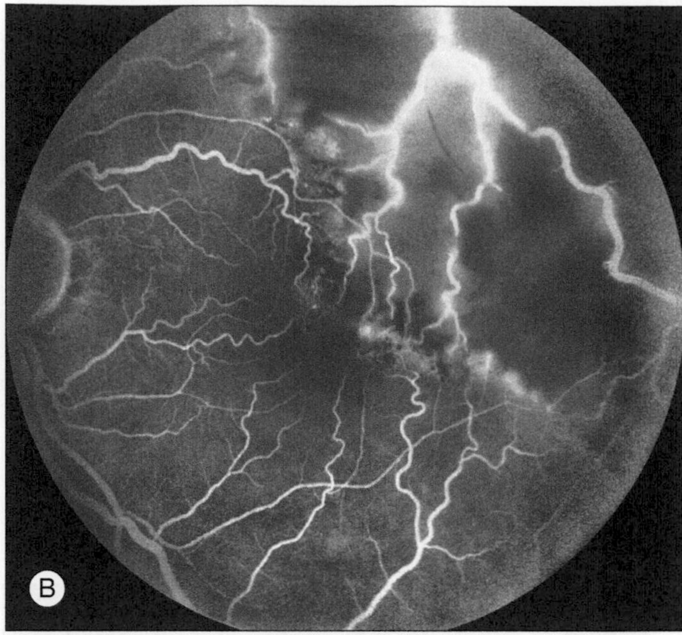

Fig. 1.53 Retinal leakage: perivascular staining. (A) In this late arteriovenous-phase fluorescein angiogram, note the beading of the large retinal veins. There is also associated leakage from these vessels. (B) Later phase of fluorescein angiogram shows perivascular staining (leakage) from the large retinal vessels that are traversing large zones of capillary nonperfusion. Comment: Typically, when a large retinal vessel (artery or vein) is perfused but traverses an area of capillary nonperfusion, ischemic retinal factors will act adversely on the endothelium of the large vessel and cause it to leak. This is called perivascular staining. Perivascular staining also occurs with traction or inflammation.

vessel leak is partially occluded, or when it traverses an area of occlusion (and capillary nonperfusion), it will leak (Fig. 1.53).

Choroidal leak

Late hyperfluorescence under the retina can be classified as either pooling or staining (Fig. 1.54). Pooling is defined as leakage of fluorescein into a distinct anatomic space; staining is leakage of fluorescein diffused into tissue.

Fluorescein pools in the spaces created by detachment of the sensory retina from the pigment epithelium or in the space created by detachment of the pigment epithelium from Bruch's membrane. The posterior layer of the sensory retina is made up of rods and cones that are loosely attached to the pigment epithelium. When a sensory retinal detachment occurs, the detached segment separates with little force, forming a very gradual angle at the point of attachment to the pigment epithelium. Because of this narrow angle, the exact limits of a sensory retinal detachment are difficult to locate ophthalmoscopically or by slit-lamp biomicroscopy.

Depending on the specific disease, the late angiogram may or may not portray the full fluorescent filling of the subretinal fluid. For example, in central serous chorioretinopathy the leakage is gradual, and fluorescence of the subsensory retinal fluid will not be complete. In other conditions, such as subretinal neovascularization, fluorescein leakage is profuse, and the subsensory fluid often completely fluoresces (Fig. 1.55).

In contrast to the attachment of the sensory retina, the basement membrane of the pigment epithelium adheres firmly to the collagenous fibers of Bruch's membrane. The firm adhesion and wide angle of detachment make it easy to discern a pigment epithelial detachment ophthalmoscopically. Occasionally a light-orange ring appears around the periphery of a pigment epithelial detachment, further facilitating identification (Fig. 1.56).

The differences in the adherence and the angle of detachment between a sensory retinal detachment and a pigment epithelial detachment result in specific differences in fluorescent pooling patterns. The hyperfluorescent pooling of a sensory retinal detachment tends to fade gradually towards the site where the sensory retina is attached. This makes fluorescein angiographic determination of the extent of a sensory retinal detachment difficult. In contrast, the hyperfluorescent pooling under a pigment epithelial detachment extends to the edges of the detachment, making the entire detachment and its margins hyperfluorescent and clearly discernible.

Pooling of fluorescein under a sensory retinal detachment in central serous retinopathy takes place slowly, since the dye passes through one or more points of leakage in the defective pigment epithelium (Fig. 1.54). When leakage comes from subretinal neovascularization (Fig. 1.55) or a tumor (Fig. 1.47), it is more rapid and complete. When the pigment epithelium is detached from Bruch's membrane, fluorescein passes freely and rapidly through Bruch's membrane from the choriocapillaris into the subpigment epithelial space (Fig. 1.56).

In some cases of central serous chorioretinopathy, there is an associated pigment epithelial detachment, and pooling under each (sensory retinal detachment and the pigment epithelial detachment) is evident. Occasionally, the edge of a pigment epithelial detachment may tear, or rip, and allow fluorescein dye to pass freely into the subretinal space (Fig. 1.57). Drusen may also show late hyperfluorescence similar to that seen with a pigment epithelial detachment (Fig. 1.58). In some cases of pigment epithelial detachment, especially in older patients, subretinal neovascularization is also present. This combination of subretinal neovascularization and pigment epithelial detachment results in an interesting angiogram that can be challenging to interpret (Fig. 1.59).

Text continued on p. e50

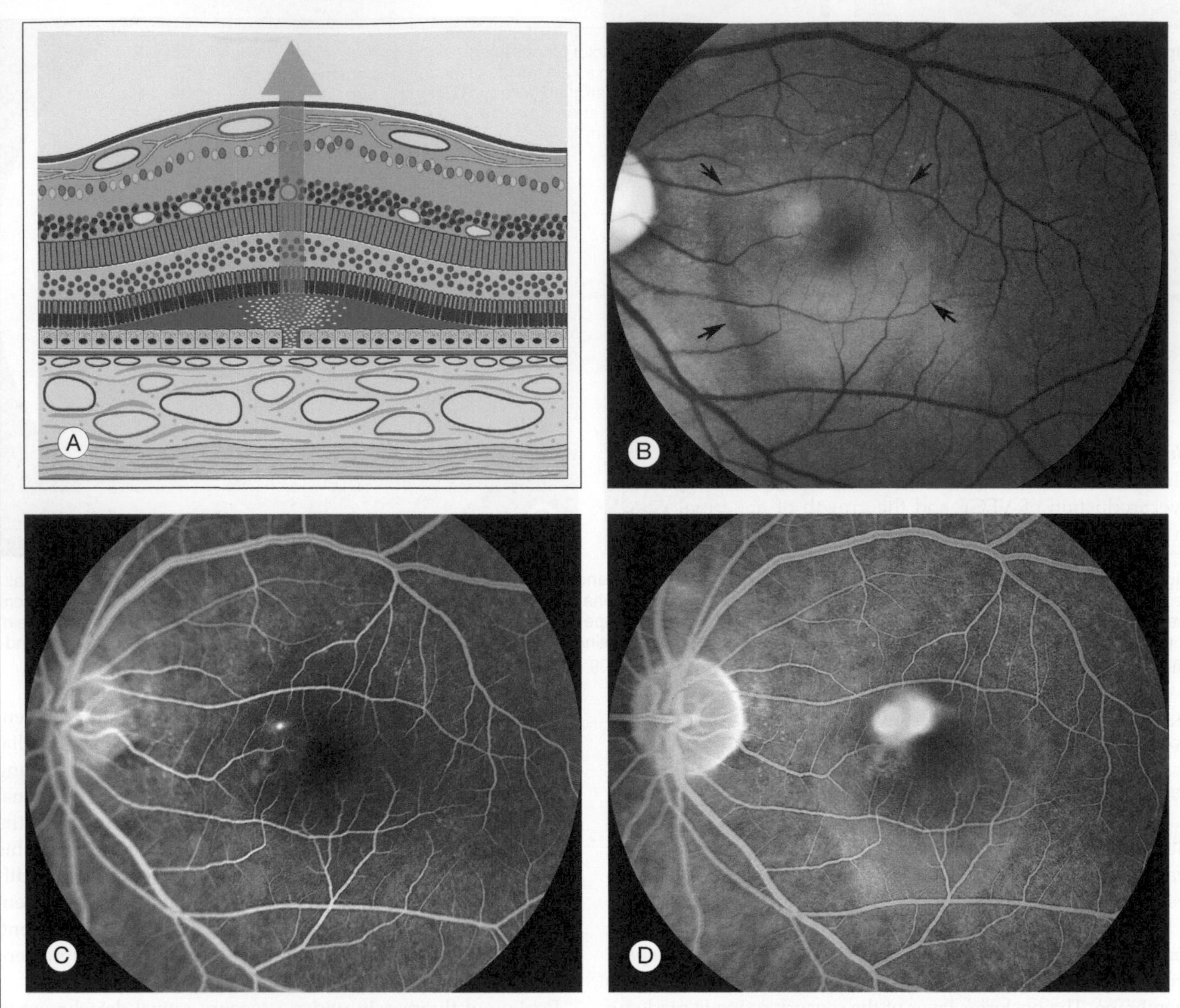

Fig. 1.54 Late hyperfluorescence, subretinal pooling: central serous chorioretinopathy. (A) Schematic drawing of retina shows a sensory retinal detachment. There is a break in the pigment epithelium. Fluorescein flows from the choriocapillaris through Bruch's membrane, through the break in the pigment epithelium, and into the subretinal space, under the detached retina. (B) Color photograph of left macula shows a shallow sensory detachment (arrows). Just superonasal to the fovea is a small white area with a gray center. The fluorescein angiogram will reveal that this is the area of the leak. (C) Arteriovenous phase of fluorescein angiogram shows a hyperfluorescent spot that was seen on stereoangiography to be leakage of fluorescein coming from the pigment epithelium. (D) Late phase of fluorescein angiogram shows that the spot of pigment epithelial leakage has enlarged and become fuzzy. This is the release of fluorescein molecules into the fluid under the detached sensory retina. Comment: This patient had central serous chorioretinopathy. There was a break in the pigment epithelium that allowed leakage of fluorescein through it and into the subretinal space. Late hyperfluorescence means leakage, and in this case, there is pooling of fluorescein under the detached retina.

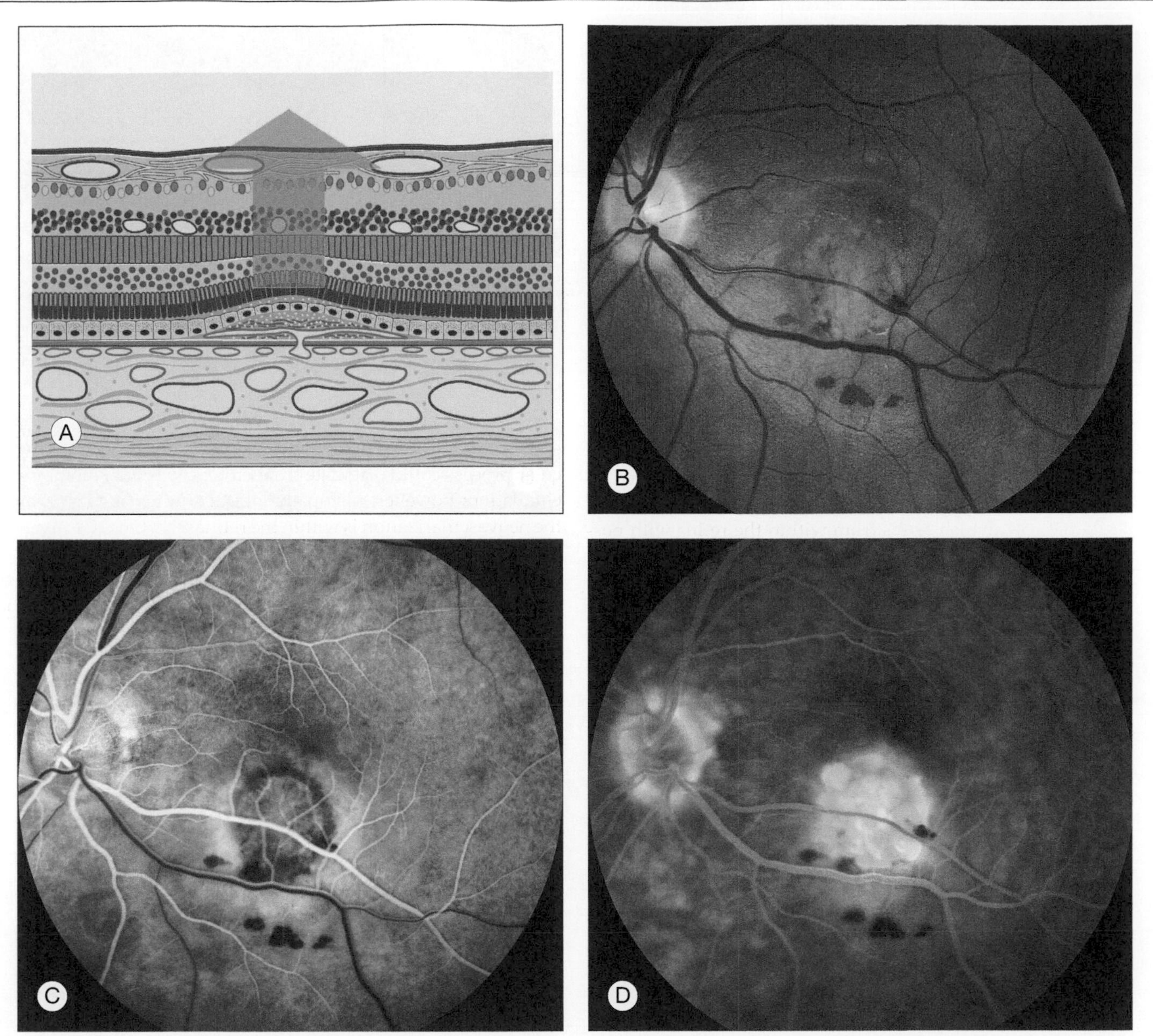

Fig. 1.55 Late hyperfluorescence, leakage, and pooling under the sensory retina caused by subretinal neovascularization, resulting in a sensory retinal detachment. (A) Schematic of the retina showing that it has detached (photoreceptors are separated from pigment epithelium). Vessels have proliferated from the choriocapillaris through Bruch's membrane. There is a fibrovascular scar involving the pigment epithelium. The sensory retina is detached. (B) Color photograph of left macula shows a pale gray lesion in the inferior portion of the macula with some associated hemorrhage. (C) Arteriovenous phase of fluorescein angiogram shows a patch of subretinal neovascularization inferior to the fovea; this is evidenced by the lacy, irregular hyperfluorescence in this area. (D) Late phase of fluorescein angiogram shows fuzzy fluorescence. There is pooling of fluorescein under the detached retina and some staining of the fibrous tissue associated with the subretinal neovascularization. Comment: This patient had a patch of subretinal neovascularization with a great deal of leakage, causing a sensory detachment. The early-phase angiogram showed the vascular nature of the lesion, and the late-phase angiogram showed the leakage and pooling in the subretinal space.

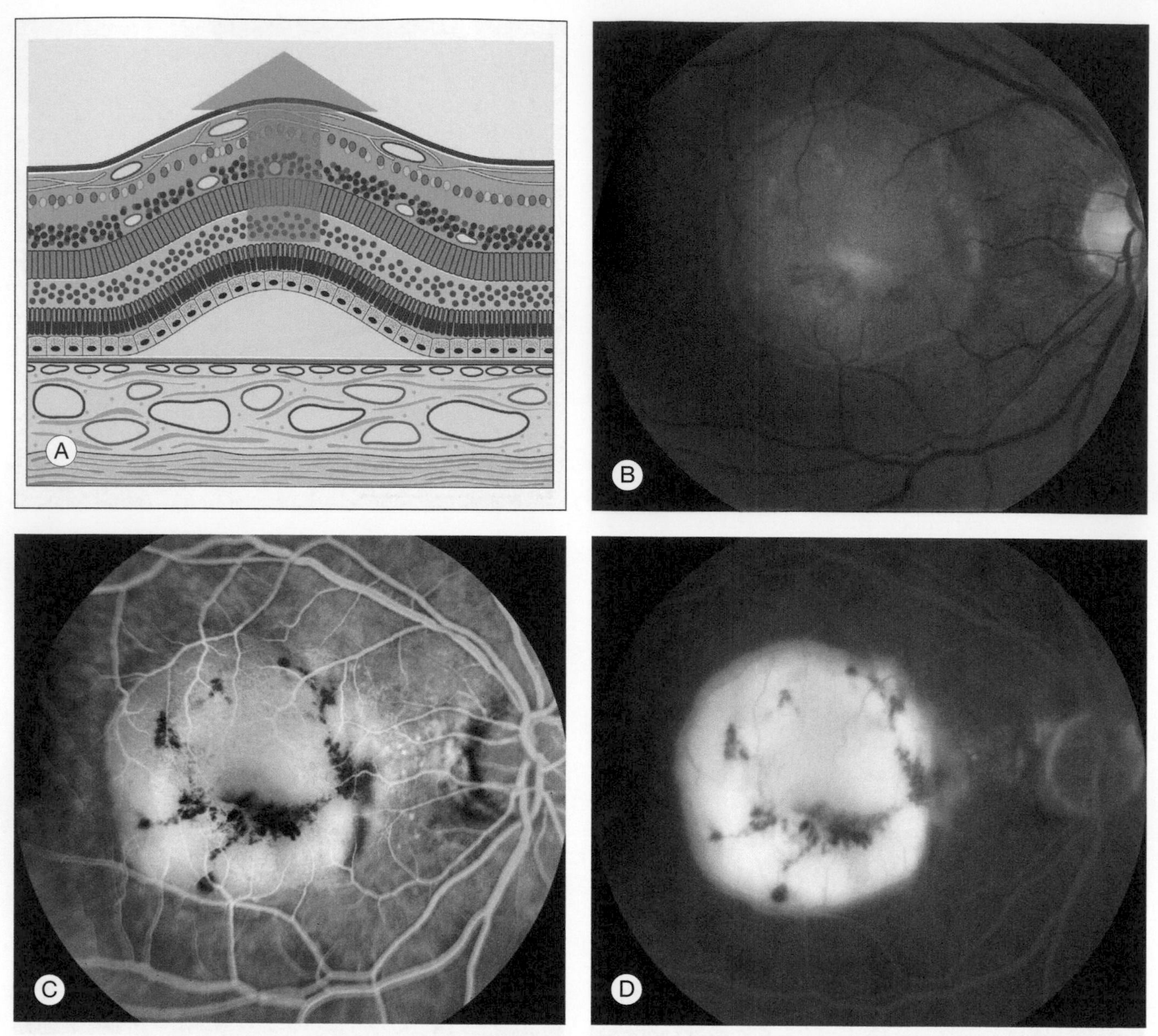

Fig. 1.56 Late hyperfluorescent pooling under the retinal pigment epithelium (pigment epithelial detachment). (A) Schematic diagram illustrating detachment and elevation of the pigment epithelium; the pigment epithelium is separated from Bruch's membrane. Because the attachment of the pigment epithelium to Bruch's membrane is quite firm, the angle of detachment is quite large. (B) Color photography of right macula shows a round detachment of the pigment epithelium. (C) Early arteriovenous phase of fluorescein angiogram shows early fluorescence from the area of detachment pigment epithelium. (D) Late-phase angiogram of right macula shows well-demarcated hyperfluorescent pooling of fluorescein under the detached pigment epithelium. Comment: Fluorescein flows freely through Bruch's membrane and stops at the pigment epithelium. When the pigment epithelium is detached, the fluorescein flows right through Bruch's membrane into the space made by the detached pigment epithelium. Therefore a pigment epithelial detachment fluoresces evenly and slowly (like a light bulb on a rheostat) and shows intense hyperfluorescent pooling that is well demarcated (indicating its well-defined angle of attachment) late in the angiogram.

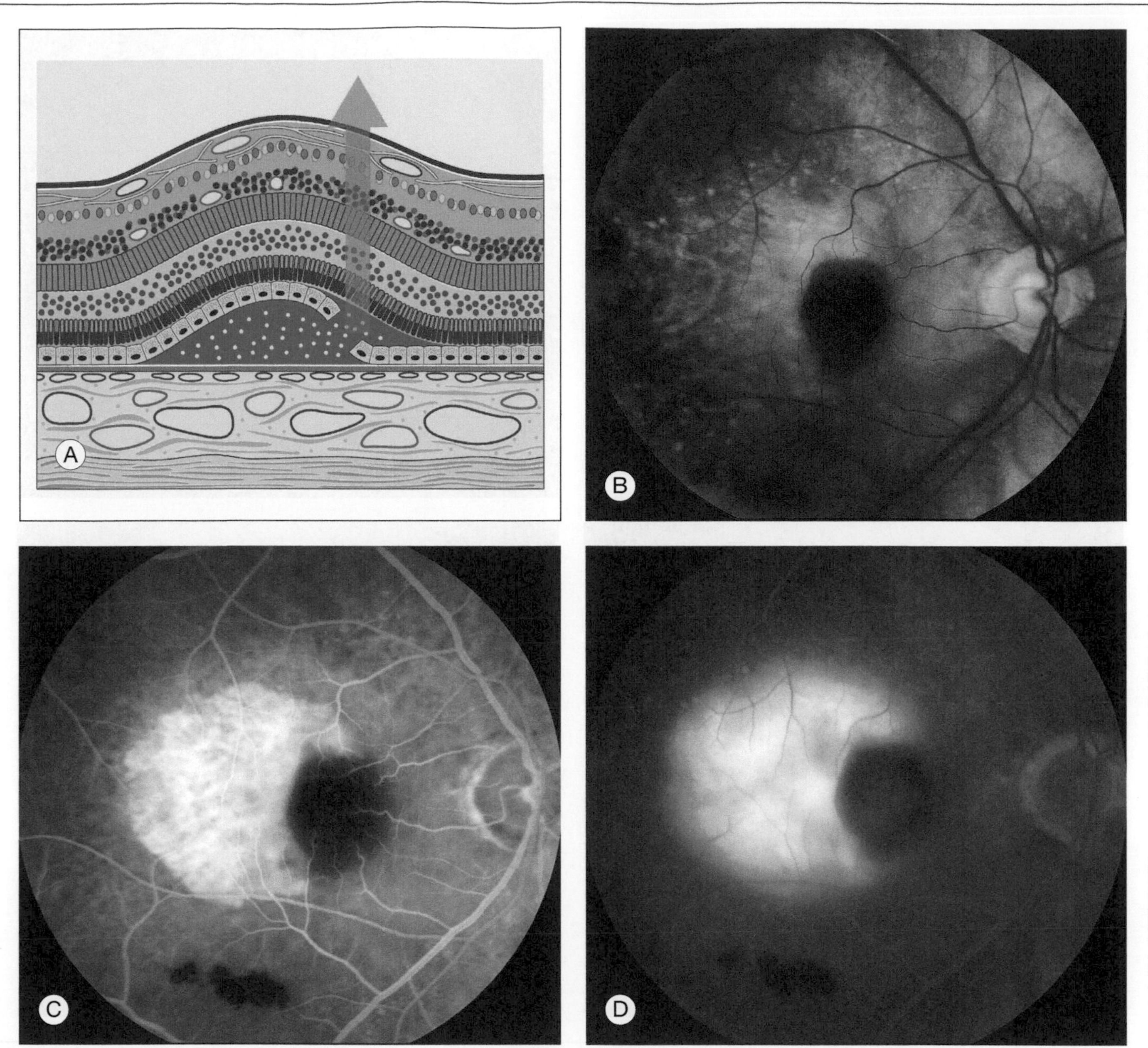

Fig. 1.57 Late hyperfluorescence under the retina – leakage from the choroid due to a retinal pigment epithelial (RPE) rip. (A) Schematic of a pigment epithelial detachment that has developed a tear along one edge. The barrier function of the pigment epithelium is lost and fluorescein dye can diffuse easily and rapidly in the subretinal space. (B) Color photography of right macula showing a round dark area under the fovea, and light (depigmented) area extending temporally. In the inferior portion of the macula, some subretinal hemorrhage is seen. (C) Early arteriovenous-phase fluorescein angiogram shows bright hyperfluorescence of the depigmented area temporally, and hypofluorescence under the fovea as well as inferiorly in the area of the subretinal blood. (D) Late-phase fluorescein angiogram shows pooling of fluorescein under the retina where the dye has been able to diffuse freely through Bruch's membrane in the sensory retinal detachment. Comment: This patient developed a tear of the pigment epithelial detachment. The dark area under the fovea is where the pigment epithelium has rolled up after tearing away from the area temporally. The area temporal to the macula appears light due to absence of the RPE in this area. Since the RPE barrier is absent in this area, the dye diffuses readily and rapidly into overlying sensory retinal detachment, producing late pooling of fluorescein.

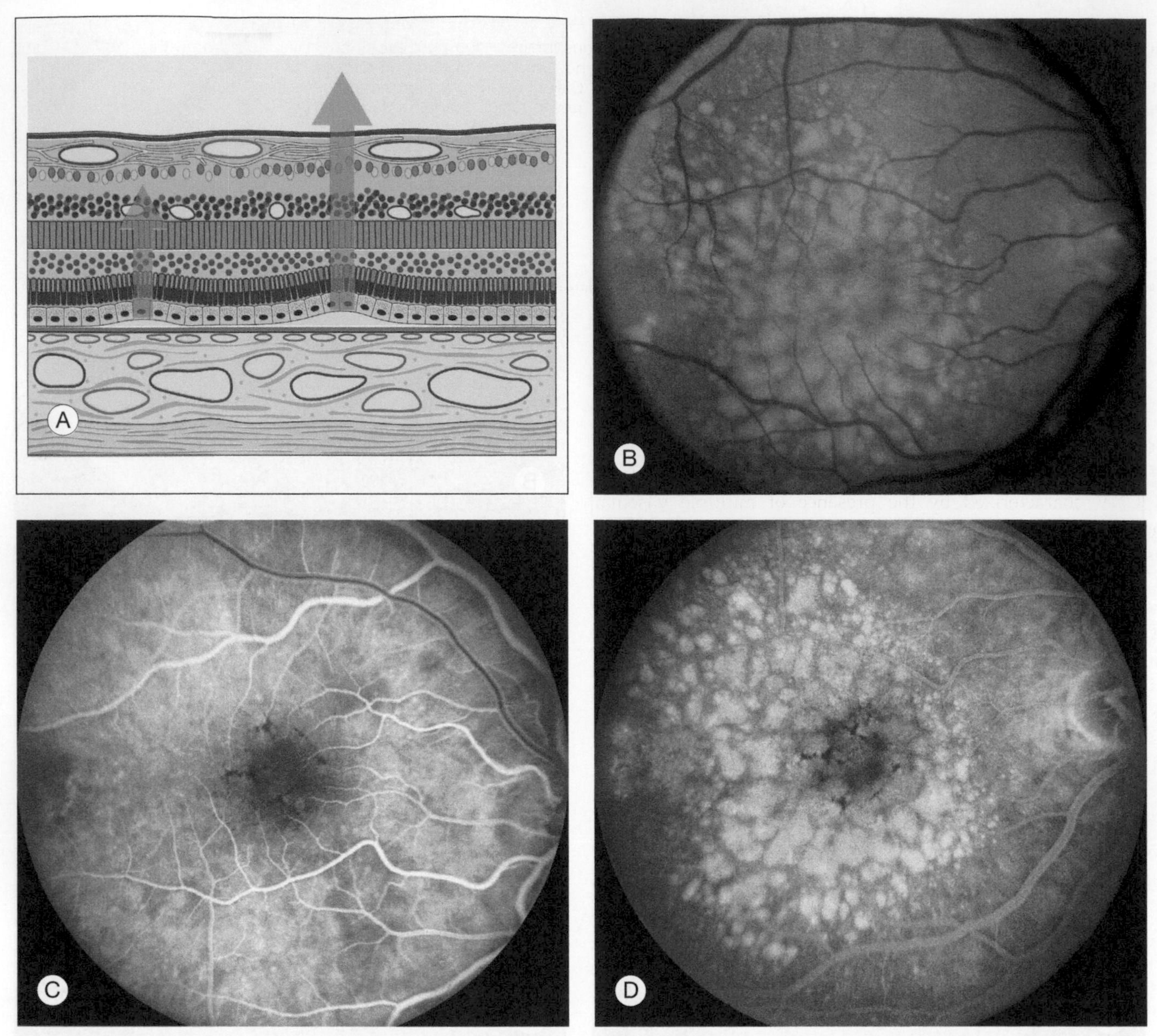

Fig. 1.58 Late hyperfluorescent pooling (or staining) of large drusen. (A) Schematic section of retina shows progressively larger detachments of pigment epithelium. Drusen deposit between the pigment epithelium and Bruch's membrane and lift the pigment epithelium up, forming small or large pigment epithelial detachments, depending on the size of the drusen. (B) Color photograph of right macula shows multiple, pale, round, and variably sized drusen. (C) Arteriovenous phase of fluorescein angiogram shows some early hyperfluorescence of the areas of the drusen. (D) Late phase of fluorescein angiogram shows marked hyperfluorescence of the drusen. The larger drusen take longer for the hyperfluorescence to develop. Comment: The larger the drusen, the more similar they are to pigment epithelial detachments, and therefore the more likely it is that they will show pooling of fluorescein (or staining of the drusen material).

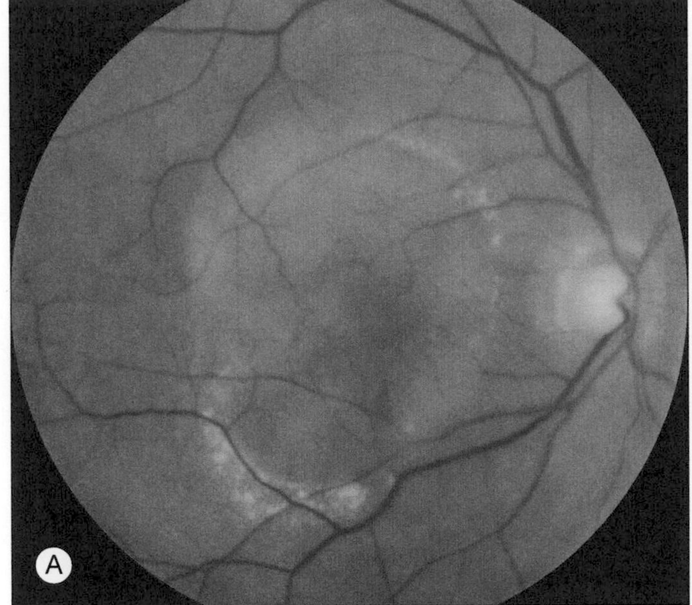

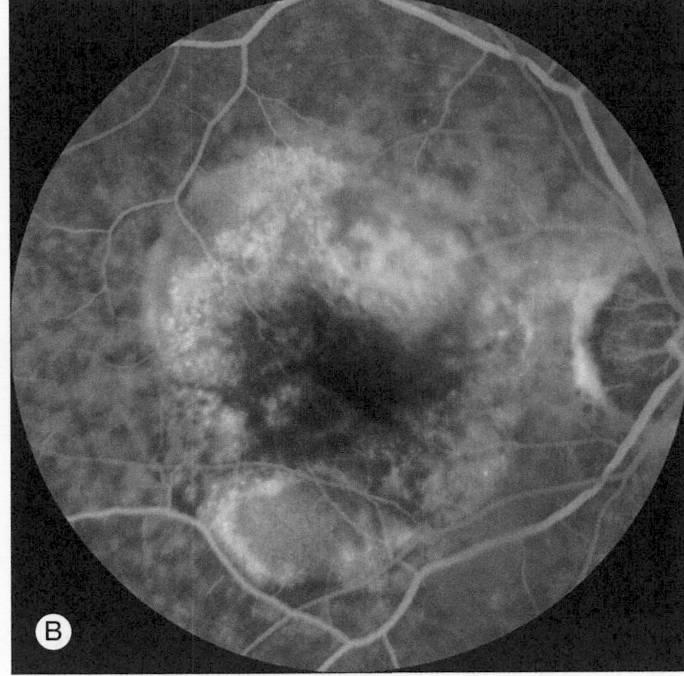

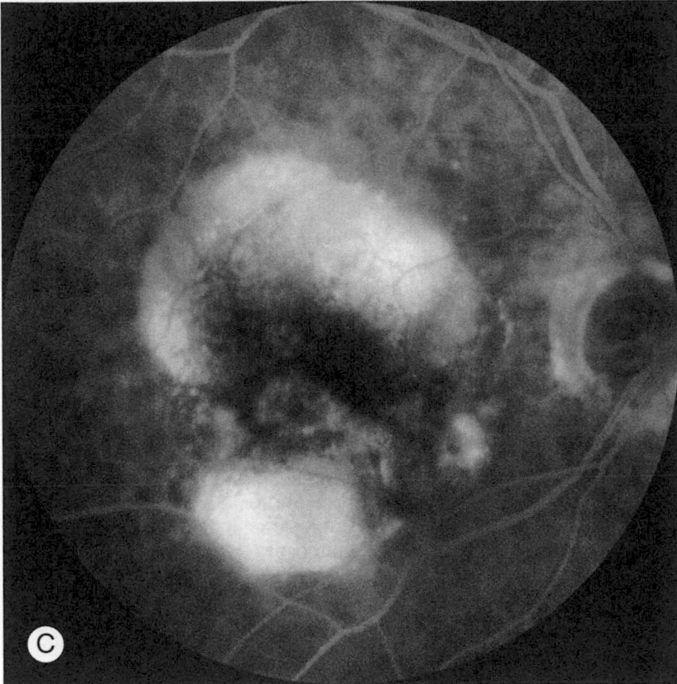

Fig. 1.59 Pigment epithelial detachment with associated (suspicious) subretinal neovascularization. (A) Color photograph of right macula. Note the pigment epithelial detachment temporally and sensory retinal detachment. (B) Arteriovenous-phase fluorescein angiogram shows early hyperfluorescence of the superotemporal pigment epithelial detachment. (C) Late-phase fluorescein angiogram of left macula shows that the fluorescence of the pigment epithelial detachment temporally has increased significantly. Comment: This patient had an irregularly shaped pigment epithelial detachment, which is a sign of possible choroidal neovascularization. The irregular, fuzzy hyperfluorescence is due to likely occult choroidal neovascularization.

In summary, late hyperfluorescence beneath the retina should first be distinguished as pooling of fluorescein into a space or as tissue staining with fluorescein. When pooling is present, one must determine whether a sensory retinal or a pigment epithelial detachment is present. Similarly, if staining is present, one must find out whether the tissue involved is the retinal pigment epithelium and Bruch's membrane, choroid, or sclera. From this anatomic determination a more specific diagnosis can be determined.

Staining

Staining refers to leakage of fluorescein into tissue or material and is contrasted with pooling of the fluorescein into an anatomic space. Many abnormal subretinal structures and materials can retain fluorescein and demonstrate later hyperfluorescent staining.

Drusen

The most common form of staining occurs with drusen. Most drusen hyperfluoresce early in the angiogram because choroidal fluorescence is transmitted through defects in the pigment epithelium overlying the drusen (Fig. 1.34). Fluorescence from most small drusen diminishes as the dye leaves the choroidal circulation. However, some larger drusen display later hyperfluorescence or staining (Fig. 1.58). The larger the drusen, the more likely they will retain fluorescein and staining will occur. When drusen are large and have smooth edges, the late staining on the angiogram is similar in appearance to that of pooling of fluorescein under a pigment epithelial detachment. In many cases it is difficult, if not impossible, to differentiate large drusen from small pigment epithelial detachments: they have a similar ophthalmoscopic, fluorescein angiographic, and even microscopic appearance.

Scar

Scar tissue retains fluorescein and usually demonstrates well-demarcated hyperfluorescence because little, if any, fluid surrounds the scar. Later in the healing process, when only a few vessels remain, the early angiogram is hypofluorescent because of the paucity of vessels and blockage by the scar tissue. The most commonly seen scar tissue is the disciform scar, which is the endstage of subretinal neovascularization. Scarring is also seen following numerous other insults to the pigment epithelium and choroid, especially inflammation (Fig. 1.60).

Sclera

In several situations the sclera is visible ophthalmoscopically and exhibits late hyperfluorescent staining on fluorescein angiography. Scleral staining is best seen when the retinal pigment epithelium is very pale (as in a blonde patient) or when the

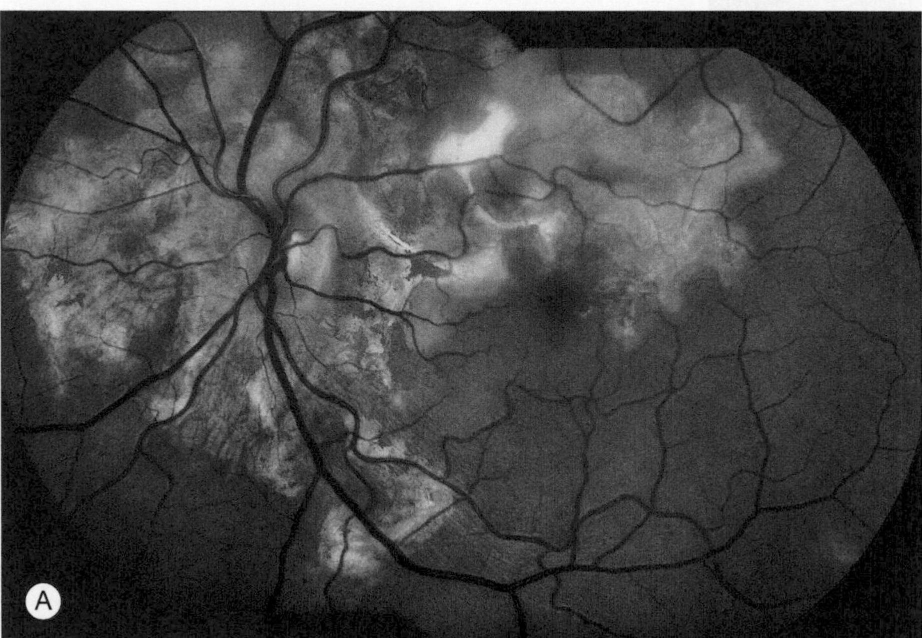

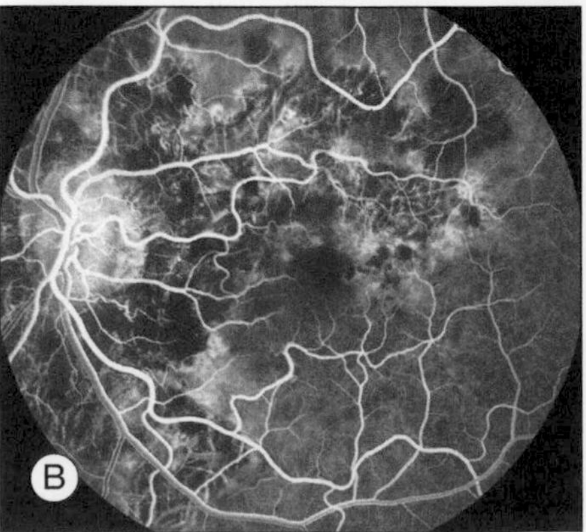

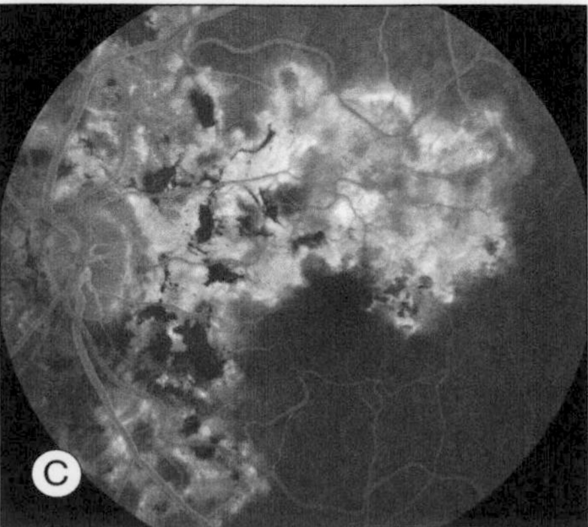

Fig. 1.60 Late hyperfluorescence and leakage – staining in geographic helicoid peripapillary choroidopathy (GHPC). (A) Color montage of left disc and macula shows large geographic areas of atrophy of pigment epithelium and choriocapillaris. There is some hyperplasia of the pigment epithelium noted as hyperpigmentation (especially in the macula and papillomacular bundle). Some fibrous scar tissue is present. (B) Arteriovenous-phase fluorescein angiogram shows that the geographic lesions are mostly hypofluorescent; they are caused by loss of pigment epithelium and choriocapillaris. Note that the large choroidal vessels can be seen within these lesions, indicating that the pigment epithelium and choriocapillaris are both gone. There is some hyperfluorescence along the edges of the geographic lesions. The pigment epithelial hyperplasia causes blocked fluorescence. (C) Late fluorescein angiogram of left macula shows hyperfluorescent staining along the edges of the geographic lesion. Comment: This patient had GHPC; inflammation of choroid and pigment epithelium resulted in a loss of the pigment epithelium and choriocapillaris and some of the choroid. The angiogram showed that only large choroidal vessels remained within these lesions. The choriocapillaris was intact, however, in the normal tissue adjacent to the geographic atrophic tissue. The normal choriocapillaris leaked into the atrophic area in a horizontal fashion, causing late hyperfluorescence of areas of scar tissue and some scleral staining.

choriocapillaris is fully intact. When the choriocapillaris is not intact, fluorescein staining of the sclera can occur from the edges of the atrophic area where fluorescein leaks from the intact choriocapillaris inward toward the atrophy (Fig. 1.60).

In conditions such as physiologically light-colored (blonde) fundus or in myopia, the choriocapillaris is usually sufficient to stain the sclera completely. After the choroidal vessels have emptied of fluorescein in the later phases of angiography, the large hypofluorescent choroidal vessels appear as dark lines in silhouette against the stained sclera.

When a loss of choroid and choriocapillaris has occurred, there is a consequent diminution of fluorescein flow in the choroid. When this occurs, the sclera stains with fluorescein only from adjacent normal patent choriocapillaris vasculature. These vessels stain the sclera on the borders of the lesion because the dye tends to diffuse toward the center of the lesion. The entire lesion may not stain if the distance from the edge of the sclera is more than 1 mm. When the choriocapillaris is intact or the lesion is not expansive, the sclera will stain completely.

In summary, late hyperfluorescence beneath the retina should first be distinguished as pooling of fluorescein into a space or as tissue stained with fluorescein. When pooling is present, it must be determined whether a sensory retinal or a pigment epithelium detachment is present. Similarly, if staining is present, it must be determined whether the tissue involved is the retinal pigment epithelium and Bruch's membrane, choroid, or sclera. From this anatomic differentiation, a more specific diagnosis can be determined.

ACKNOWLEDGMENTS

This work was supported by the San Francisco Retina Research Fund. The authors would like to thank Sean Grout, head of photography at West Coast Retina Medical Group, for his assistance in acquiring many of the images used in this text.

REFERENCES

1. Novotny HR, Alvis DL. A method of photographing fluorescence in circulating blood in the human retina. Circulation 1961;24:82–6.
2. Rabb MF, Burton TC, Schatz H, et al. Fluorescein angiography of the fundus: a schematic approach to interpretation. Surv Ophthalmol 1978;22:387–403.
3. Schatz H. Letter: flow sheet for the interpretation of the fluorescein angiograms. Arch Ophthalmol 1976;94:687.
4. Gass JD, Sever RJ, Sparks D, et al. A combined technique of fluorescein funduscopy and angiography of the eye. Arch Ophthalmol 1967;78:455–61.
5. Haining WM, Lancaster RC. Advanced techniques for fluorescein angiography. Arch Ophthalmol 1968;79:10–5.
6. Novotny HR, Alvis D. A method of photographing fluorescence in circulating blood of the human eye. Tech Doc Rep SAMTDR USAF Sch Aerosp Med 1960;60-82:1–4.
7. Gass JD. Atlas of macular diseases: diagnosis and treatment. St Louis: Mosby; 1970.
8. Yannuzzi LA, Ober MD, Slakter JS, et al. Ophthalmic fundus imaging: today and beyond. Am J Ophthalmol 2004;137:511–24.
9. Friberg TR, Gupta A, Yu J, et al. Ultrawide angle fluorescein angiographic imaging: a comparison to conventional digital acquisition systems. Ophthalmic Surg Lasers Imaging 2008;39:304–11.
10. Manivannan A, Plskova J, Farrow A, et al. Ultra-wide-field fluorescein angiography of the ocular fundus. Am J Ophthalmol 2005;140:525–7.
11. Moosbrugger KA, Sheidow TG. Evaluation of the side-effects and image quality during fluorescein angiography comparing 2 mL and 5 mL sodium fluorescein. Can J Ophthalmol 2008;43:571–5.
12. Pacurariu RI. Low incidence of side-effects following intravenous fluorescein angiography. Ann Ophthalmol 1982;14:32–6.
13. Lipson BK, Yannuzzi LA. Complications of intravenous fluorescein injections. Int Ophthalmol Clin 1989;29:200–5.
14. Lu VH, Ho IV, Lee V, et al. Complications from fluorescein angiography: a prospective study. Clin Exp Ophthalmol 2009;37:826–7.
15. Zografos L. [International survey on the incidence of severe or fatal complications which may occur during fluorescein angiography.] J Fr Ophtalmol 1983;6:495–506.
16. Chen LJ, Yeh SI. Computer-assisted image processing for a simulated stereo effect of ocular fundus and fluorescein angiography photographs. Ophthalmic Surg Lasers Imaging 2010;41:293–300.
17. Watzke RC, Klein ML, Hiner CJ, et al. A comparison of stereoscopic fluorescein angiography with indocyanine green videoangiography in age-related macular degeneration. Ophthalmology 2000;107:1601–6.
18. Patz A, Finkelstein D, Fine SL, et al. The role of fluorescein angiography in national collaborative studies. Ophthalmology 1986;93:1466–70.
19. Arnold AC, Hepler RS. Fluorescein angiography in acute nonarteritic anterior ischemic optic neuropathy. Am J Ophthalmol 1994;117:222–30.
20. Segato T, Piermarocchi S, Midena E. The role of fluorescein angiography in the interpretation of optic nerve head diseases. Metab Pediatr Syst Ophthalmol 1990;13:111–4.

Section 1 Optical Imaging Technologies

Chapter 2

Clinical Applications of Diagnostic Indocyanine Green Angiography

Giovanni Staurenghi, Ferdinando Bottoni, Andrea Giani

INTRODUCTION

Intravenous fluorescein angiography provides excellent spatial and temporal resolution of the retinal circulation, with a high degree of fluorescence efficiency and minimal penetration of the retinal pigment epithelium (RPE). Unfortunately, imaging of the choroidal circulation is prevented by secondary poor transmission of fluorescence through ocular media opacities, pathologic manifestations such as serosanguineous fluid or lipid exudation, and fundus pigmentation, including that from the RPE layer.

In medicine, a core principle for diagnostic imaging is the selection of a technique that best visualizes the disease undergoing investigation. Indocyanine green (ICG) has several advantages over sodium fluorescein in imaging the choroidal vasculature. Its physical characteristics allow for visualization of the dye through overlying melanin, xanthophyll pigment, serosanguineous fluid, or lipid exudates. The use of high-resolution infrared digital fundus cameras and confocal scanning laser ophthalmoscopes (SLO), specifically designed for ICG angiography (ICGA), has reflected a growing awareness and interest in choroidal vascular lesions, and has facilitated the rapid diffusion of ICGA in the ophthalmic community.

Even in the era of anti-vascular endothelial growth factor (VEGF) intravitreal injections, a therapy for which accurate localization of the choroidal neovascular membrane is not as critical, ICGA, among other imaging techniques, is still extremely useful in clinical practice.[1]

HISTORY

ICGA was developed by Kodak Research Laboratories,[2] on request by cardiologists to be used as an indicator of cardiac output which was not influenced by variations in blood oxygen saturation.[3,4] Hepatologists subsequently began to use ICGA to evaluate hepatic blood flow[5] and hepatocellular function.[6]

In 1969, Kogure and Choromokos first used ICGA for studying the cerebral circulation in a dog.[7] The following year, Kogure et al. reported on intra-arterial ICG absorption of the choroid in monkeys.[8] The first human ICG angiogram was of the carotid artery.[9] In 1971, Hochheimer modified the system for ICGA by changing the color film which had previously been used to black-and-white infrared film.[10]

In 1972, Flower and Hochheimer performed the first intravenous ICGA to image the human choroid.[11] In the following years, Flower and coworkers evaluated the potential utility of ICGA in the investigation of the normal and pathologic eye.[11,12] The relatively poor fluorescence efficiency of the ICG molecule and its limited ability to produce high-resolution images on infrared film initially restricted its angiographic application. The resolution of ICGA was improved in the mid-1980s by Hayashi and de Laey, who developed improved filter combinations with sufficient sensitivity for near-infrared wavelengths.[13] They were also instrumental in the transition from still-frame to dynamic imaging by introducing videoangiography.[14,15]

Although the sensitivity of the initial video camera system was a vast improvement over previous techniques, its inability to study individual images and the potential light toxicity using a 300-W halogen bulb restricted the duration and quality of the technique. In 1989, Destro and Puliafito[16] performed ICGA using a system very similar to that described by Hayashi. In the same year, the use of the SLO for ICG videoangiography was introduced by Scheider and Schroedel.[17] In 1992, Guyer et al. introduced the use of a 1024 × 1024-line digital imaging system to produce high-resolution ICGA.[18] However, this system lacked flash synchronization with the video camera.

Finally, Yannuzzi and coworkers described a 1024-line resolution system, which was synthesized with the appropriate flash synchronization and image storage capability, permitting high-resolution, long-duration ICGA.[19]

CHEMICAL AND PHARMACOKINETICS

ICG is a tricarbocyanine, anionic dye. Its structural formula is 2,2′-indo-6,7,6′,7′-dibenzocarbocyanine sodium salt[20] with a molecular weight of 774.96 Da.[2] ICG is soluble in highly distilled water,[21] even though in protein-free buffer it is difficult to obtain stable and simple ICG solutions, because of the formation of reversible dimers/polymers.[2] Binding to albumin or plasma proteins improves the stability of ICG solutions.[2] ICG is supplied with a solvent consisting of sterile water at pH 5.5–6.5. The final product contains 5–9.5% sodium iodine,[22] to prevent recrystallization.[23]

ICG absorbs light in the near-infrared region of the spectrum. The maximum absorption is at 790 nm,[23] while the maximum emission occurs at approximately 835 nm.[24] These optical properties allow penetration through macular pigment, melanin,[25] blood, and pigment.

About 98% of ICG is bound to plasma protein, in particular to globulins, such as A1-lipoproteins.[22] In pig plasma, lipoprotein HDL3 is the major binding protein.[2] ICG is excreted by the liver,[5,26] with negligible extrahepatic removal.[5,27] The presumed mechanism is active[27] and depends on both liver blood flow and hepatocellular function.[28] ICG is excreted into the bile without metabolic process or enters the enteropathic circulation,[27] through three steps: (1) uptake over the hepatocyte sinusoidal (basolateral) membrane (Na^+-mediated); (2) passage through the cell, with some role of the microfilaments and vesicular transport; and (3) excretion over the canalicular (apical) membrane.[2] Rate of ICG disappearance from vascular compartment is 18–24% per minute, and after 20 minutes no more than 4% remains in the plasma.[29] Plasma decay curve is initially exponential, then decelerates.[26] No peripheral uptake has been described, in kidney,[26] lungs, or placenta.[30]

ICG's high molecular weight, in combination with the high percentage of dye bound to plasma proteins, reduces the amount of dye that exits from fenestrations in choroid vessels. This feature and its optical properties make ICG suitable for choroidal vascular network visualization. Although it has been reported that ICG can diffuse through the choroid and can accumulate in RPE cells, no dye should remain in the late phases (30–40 minutes) of the angiogram.[29]

Toxicity

ICG is considered a safe and well-tolerated dye. Its LD_{50} is 60 mg/kg in mice.[20] Constant infusions over a 3-hour period with dosages as high as 50 mg/kg of body weight were well tolerated.[27] Subcutaneous extravasation also does not produce significant local effects.[26,31] Overall, the side-effect rate is low: 0.15% with mild events (nausea, vomit, sneezing, pruritus), 0.2% with moderate events (urticarial, syncope, pyrexia, nerve palsy), 0.05% with severe events (bronchospasm, laryngospasm, anaphylaxis).[31]

The mechanism of these various adverse side-effects is uncertain. For some, a dose-dependent pseudoallergic mechanism has been proposed,[32] though there does not appear to be correlation with iodide or shellfish intolerance, suggesting that the sodium iodide component is of little significance.[22,33] Nevertheless patients with a history of definite iodine allergy should not be given the dye, because of concerns for possible anaphylaxis.[31] Caution should also be observed in patients affected by liver diseases[29] and kidney diseases, since a 9.3% incidence of adverse reactions has been reported in dialysis patients.[22,34]

ICG was extensively used as a chromodiagnostic agent in the evaluation of hemodynamic changes during pregnancy.[35] Nevertheless there are concerns among ophthalmologists, since the Food and Drug Administration has classified ICG as a pregnancy category C drug, meaning that adequate studies of safety have not been conducted.[30]

Instrument comparison

There are several instruments at present that can be used to perform ICGA. All of them can be divided into two main categories: digital flash fundus cameras and SLOs.

At the time of writing, the flash camera group includes the TRC-50DX ICG (Topcon, Tokyo, Japan), the FF 450plus (Carl Zeiss Meditec, Dublin, CA, USA), and the VX-10i (Kowa, Tokyo, Japan). ICG-capable SLO systems include the Spectralis HRA (Heidelberg Engineering, Heidelberg, Germany) and the F10 (Nidek, Gamagori, Japan).

The differences between these instruments are largely related to the acquisition modality (Fig. 2.1). The light source for a digital camera is a white light with an excitation filter (640–780 nm) and a barrier filter (820–900 nm). In an SLO a laser monochromatic light is used to excite (785–790 nm) with a barrier filter at 805 nm. The laser light for an SLO system is moved on the fundus by two rotating mirrors and the image is acquired point by point. For a typical 30° image, this takes approximately 60–200 ms. The presence of a confocal aperture in SLO systems allows selective acquisition of light from a particular tissue layer (from the focal plane), and blocks the light that is coming from the surrounding tissue.[36,37] Flash systems, in contrast, do not use a confocal aperture, and thus the fluorescent light returning to the camera will emanate from multiple layers. However, even for clinical confocal SLO ICG systems, the confocal aperture is much larger than one would choose for optimum z-resolution imaging. The reason for this is that fluorescence light from different depth planes (i.e., from the choroid and from the retinal vessel) needs to be imaged simultaneously for many clinical applications.

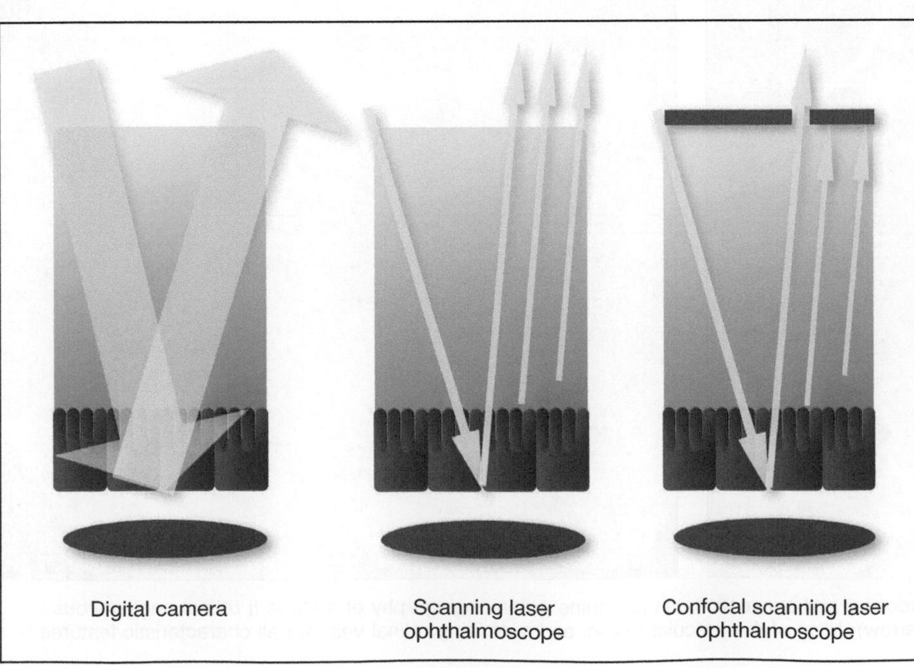

Fig. 2.1 Schematic representation of the differences between digital flash fundus cameras (A), scanning laser ophthalmoscopes (SLO) (B), and confocal SLO instruments (C). In digital flash fundus cameras, white light (with or without excitation/barrier filters) is used. In SLO systems the light source is a monochromatic laser. In SLO confocal systems a pinhole aperture blocks the reflected or fluorescent light from areas outside the focal plane.

These characteristics are important to recognize the different appearance of ICGA images obtained by different instruments (Fig. 2.2). Another difference is the number of images acquired per second. With SLO systems the frame rate may reach 12 images per second, thus permitting dynamic ICGA (Fig. 2.2). With digital fundus cameras the maximum rate is one frame per second.

Injection technique

The concentration and preparation for intravenous injection of ICG vary with the instrument used. For fundus cameras the standard concentration is 25 mg of ICG dissolved in 5 mL solvent.[38] The dosage may be increased to 50 mg in patients with poorly dilated pupils and heavy pigmentation.[39] For SLOs the

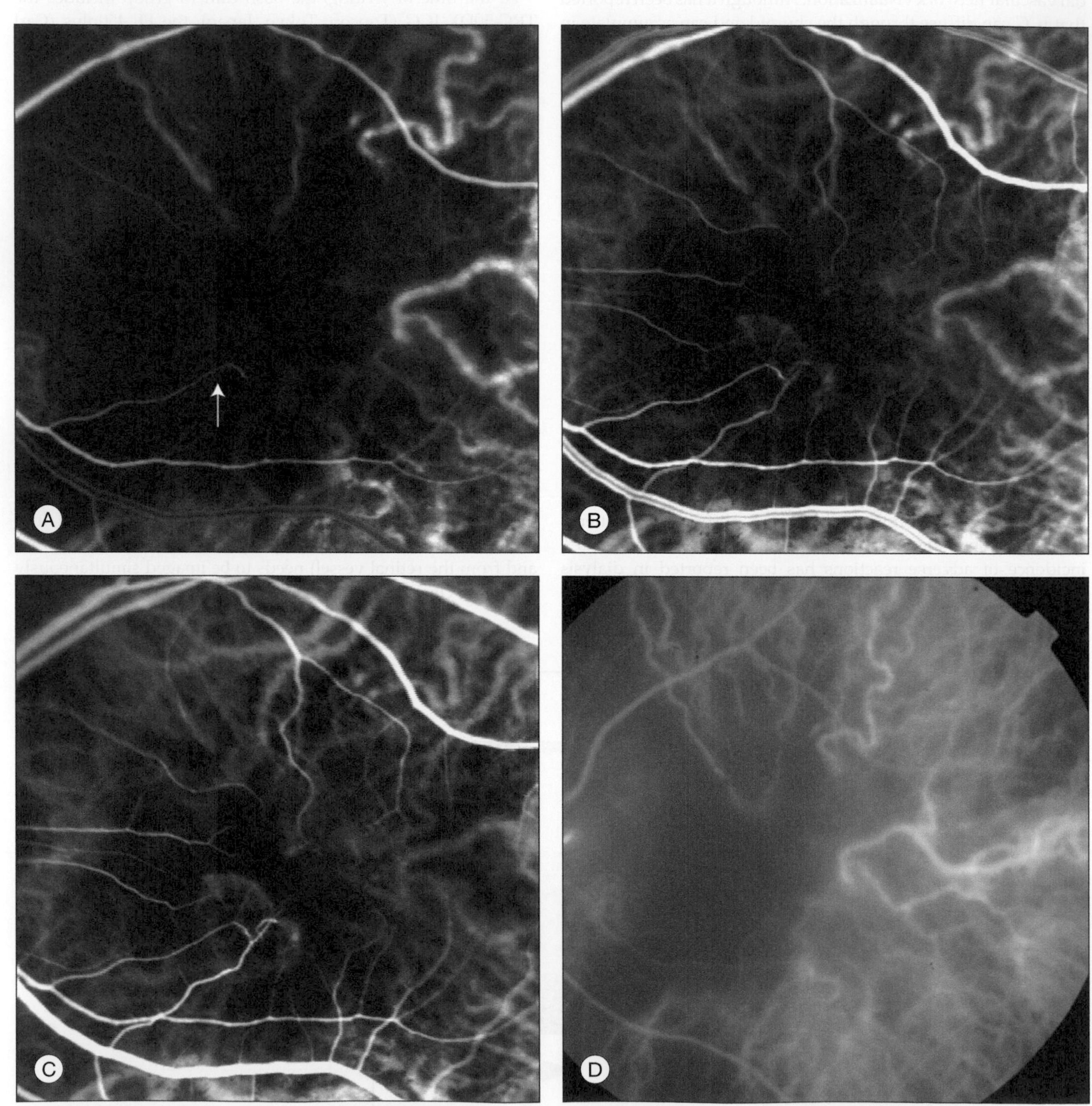

Fig. 2.2 Comparison of dynamic (six frames per second) and conventional indocyanine green angiography of a stage II retinal angiomatous proliferation lesion. A feeding retinal arteriole (A, arrow), filling of the vascular lesion, and a draining retinal vein are all characteristic features visible in the dynamic sequences (A–C).

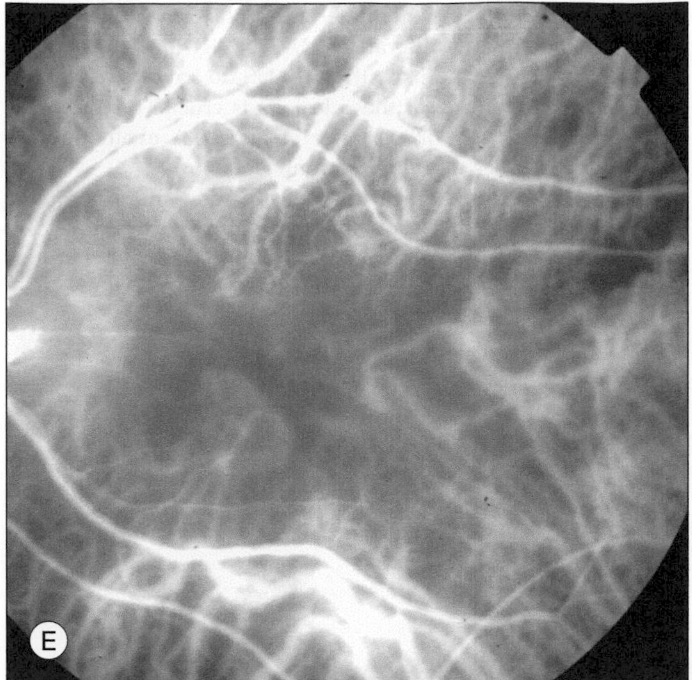

Fig. 2.2 Cont'd The filling sequence is missed during the first two images captured with a conventional flash fundus camera system (D, E).

standard dosage is 25 mg of ICG dissolved in 3 mL, and 1 mL of the solution is injected. The solvent may be either saline alone or fluorescein sodium solution at 10–20–25% concentrations, for combined fluorescein and ICGA. Intravenous ICG injection should be rapid and immediately followed by a 5-mL saline flush.

In patients with iodine allergy, infracyanine green is available: this is the iodine-free formula of ICG. The technique of injection is equivalent, but a glucosate solvent should be used for preparation. As a result, combined fluorescein angiography and infracyanine green angiography is not possible.

INDOCYANINE GREEN ANGIOGRAPHY INTERPRETATION

Normal eye

To understand the manifestations of disease on ICGA, a recognition of the normal appearance of ICGA in normal subjects is essential.

Since ICGA is a dynamic examination, the characteristic findings may vary depending on the time after dye injection or the phase of the angiogram. It is well known that fluorescein angiography has an arterial retinal phase, an arteriovenous, and a venous phase. Similarly for ICGA, one can recognize an early phase when the retinal artery is not yet filled, a midphase when both arteries and veins are filled, and a late or recirculation phase more than 10 minutes after injection.

In ICGA, the early filling phase may best be correlated with the filling of different layers of the choroid. The first choroidal vessels to be filled are the ones of the deeper Haller's layer, followed by the intermediate Sattler's layer (Fig. 2.3). The choriocapillaris is the last layer to be filled (therefore the sequence progresses from the biggest and outermost to the smallest and innermost vessels). However, the choriocapillaris is typically quite difficult to visualize, since the resolution of the cameras is insufficient to resolve the size of its small lobular morphology. Therefore the choriocapillaris is visualized as a diffuse indistinct haze, more evident in the posterior pole and less evident in the peripheral retina (Fig. 2.3).

Choroidal vessels are usually first observed emanating from the posterior ciliary arteries. A well-defined watershed zone is present between the medial and lateral posterior ciliary artery (Fig. 2.4).[40] Compared to fluorescein, the watershed zone is more difficult to visualize, since there is less contrast between perfused and nonperfused choroid.

Choroidal vortex veins are visible in the late phase of ICGA and are usually four in number (Fig. 2.5). They drain the corresponding segment of the iris, ciliary body, and choroid. Sometimes, especially in myopic eyes, a vein may be seen passing from the choroid through the sclera closely adjacent to the optic nerve head and draining into the venous plexus of the pial sheath of the optic nerve (choriovaginal vein) (Fig. 2.5).[40]

In case of a thin sclera, such as in the setting of a choroidal staphyloma, extrabulbar vessels may be visualized. These can be distinguished from normal choroidal vessels because they pulsate in accordance with the heartbeat. Moreover, they change shape and position with eye movements.[41,42]

Exudative age-related macular degeneration

Exudative age-related macular degeneration (AMD) is generally classified based upon the axial location of the choroidal neovascularization (CNV). A type 1 CNV is a neovascular membrane that is located under the RPE, whereas a type 2 CNV has passed through the RPE and lies under the neurosensory retina.[43] According to the Macular Photocoagulation Study, type 1 CNV is generally considered to correspond to "occult" CNV on fluorescein angiography (as defined by the Macular Photocoagulation Study), and type 2 CNV generally corresponds to "classic" CNV.[44,45] More recently, type 3 CNV has been defined to be CNV with a definite intraretinal component.[46]

The fact that occult CNV accounts for the vast majority of the exudative complications in AMD[47] explains in part why ICGA, with its ability to delineate occult CNV, has become part of standard care in exudative AMD for many clinicians.[19,48,49] Nonetheless, in peer-reviewed journals, the number of articles published whose title included the terms "indocyanine green angiography (or videoangiography)" decreased between 1995 and 2010.[1] One likely explanation might be the advent of anti-VEGF therapy which inaugurated a new era in the management of exudative AMD: it was the first therapy to improve the mean visual acuity of eyes treated with monthly injections of ranibizumab, regardless of whether the CNV lesion was predominantly classic[50] or occult.[51] Thus, the management of CNV has changed from the use of therapy for which accurate localization of the membrane was crucial (i.e., laser photocoagulation, photodynamic therapy) to the nonspecific intravitreal delivery of active and highly effective biologic drugs. Nonetheless, we would still argue that the gold-standard diagnostic procedure should be the one which best visualizes the disease (CNV) under investigation.

Type 1 choroidal neovascularization

This type of CNV is by definition under the RPE, and corresponds to the occult neovascular network on fluorescein angiography. The Macular Photocoagulation Study recognized two forms of occult CNV: (1) a fibrovascular pigment epithelial detachment (PED); and (2) a late-phase leakage of an undetermined source (LLUS).[44] As for the fibrovascular PED, its prevalence may vary from 22% to 50%[47–49,52] of occult CNV lesions; dynamic ICGA may delineate the presence of a neovascular network usually located along the edges of the PED[49,53,54] (Fig. 2.6). Moreover, dynamic ICGA may reveal a feeder vessel that can be successfully treated with laser photocoagulation, when it is located outside the foveal region[55,56] (Fig. 2.7). In case of LLUS, which may represent 36–78% of occult CNV,[47,48,52] dynamic ICGA may differentiate an occult form of CNV from retinal angiomatous proliferation (RAP)[52] (Fig. 2.8). Considering that one-fourth of patients with an LLUS do have a RAP,[52] and that an early diagnosis of these lesions is crucial for the functional prognosis,[57] the importance of an ICGA evaluation for these cases becomes readily apparent.

In conclusion, ICGA faciliates a better and more complete classification of occult CNV subtypes, compared to fluorescein angiography. Of note, Yannuzzi et al.[19] found that 39% of lesions classified as poorly demarcated occult lesions by fluorescein angiography were well defined by ICGA.

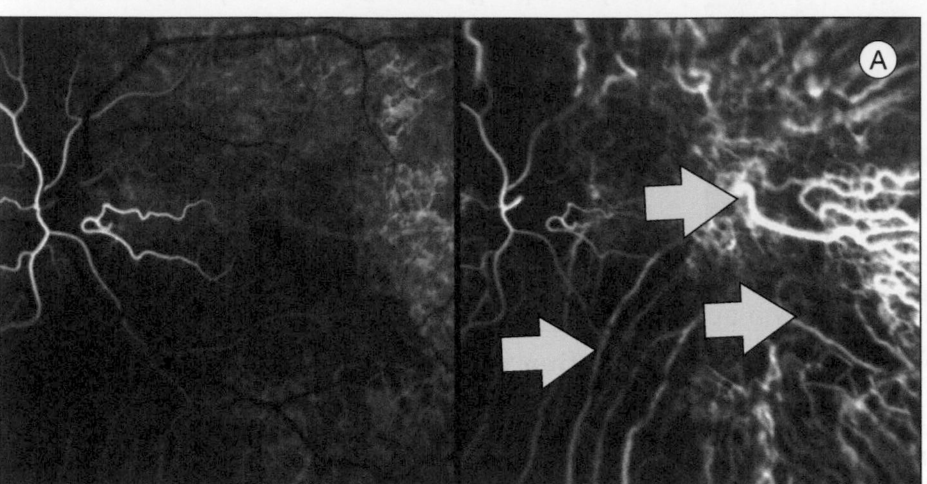

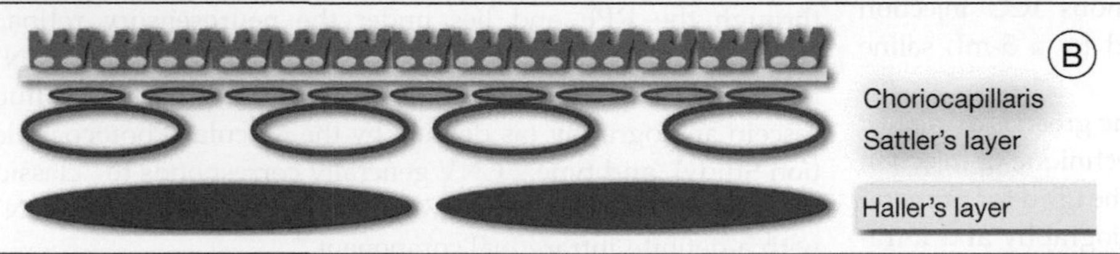

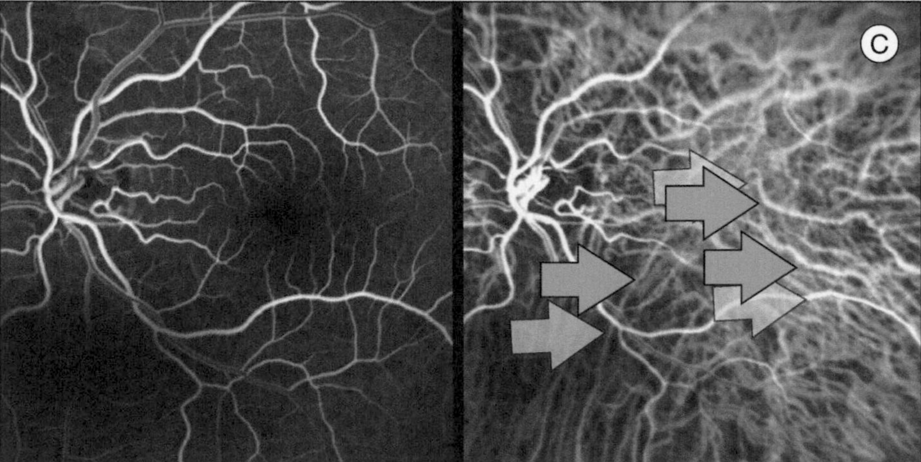

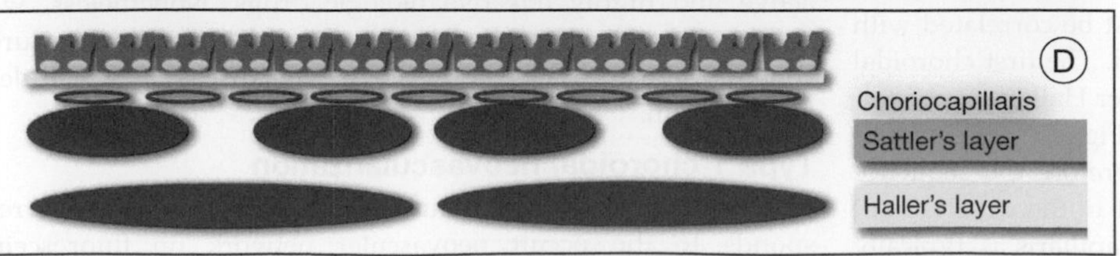

Fig. 2.3 The filling of vessels during an indocyanine green angiogram follows a precise sequence. The first layer to be filled is Haller's layer (A, B), followed by Sattler's layer (C, D).

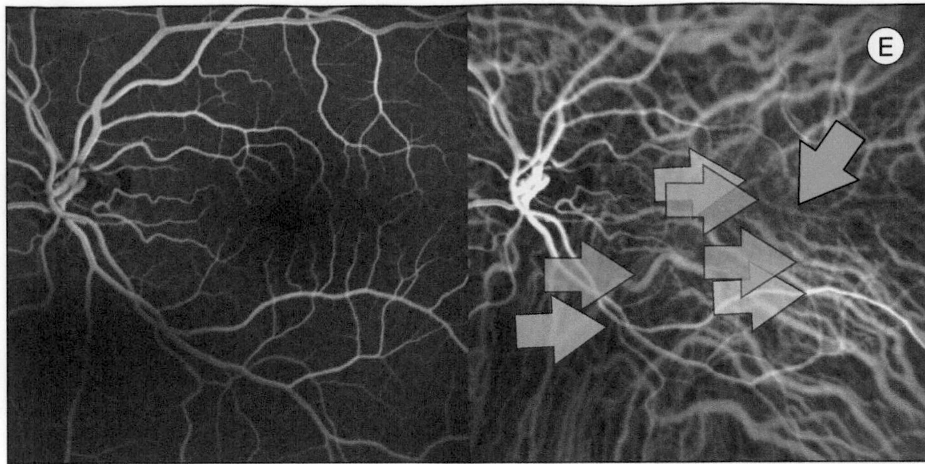

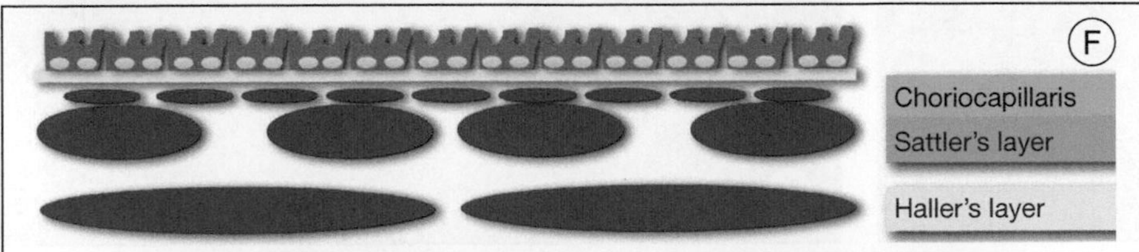

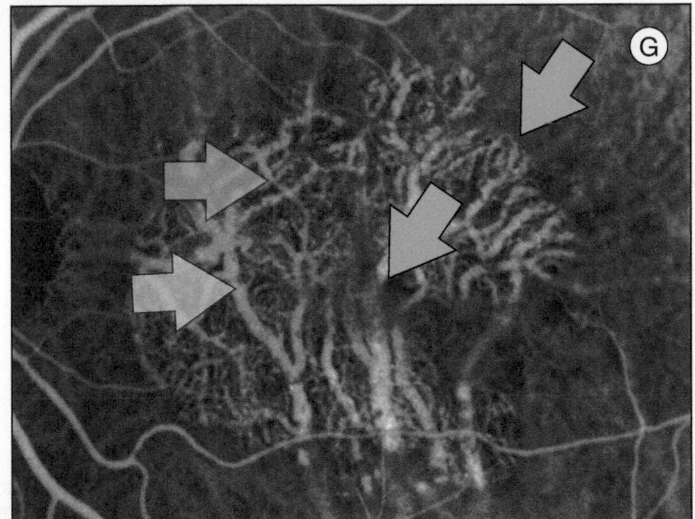

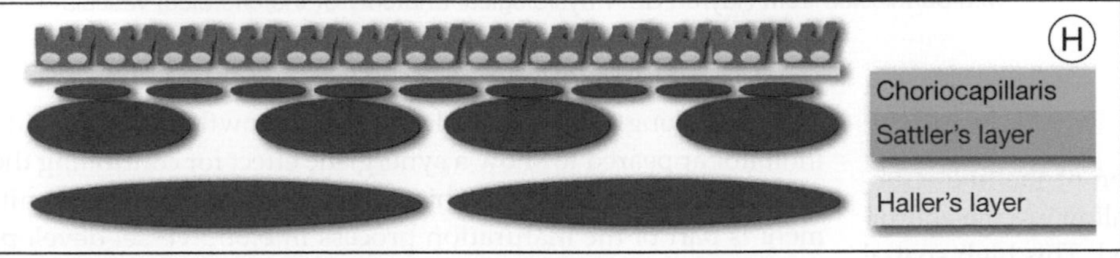

Fig. 2.3 Cont'd After Haller's layer and Sattler's layer, the choriocapillaris is filled next (E, F). Simultaneous dynamic fluorescein and indocyanine green angiography (A, C, E) permits the different phases to be resolved. The choriocapillaris may be better appreciated when there are adjacent areas of focal loss, as in the example of geographic atrophy shown in panels (G) and (H).

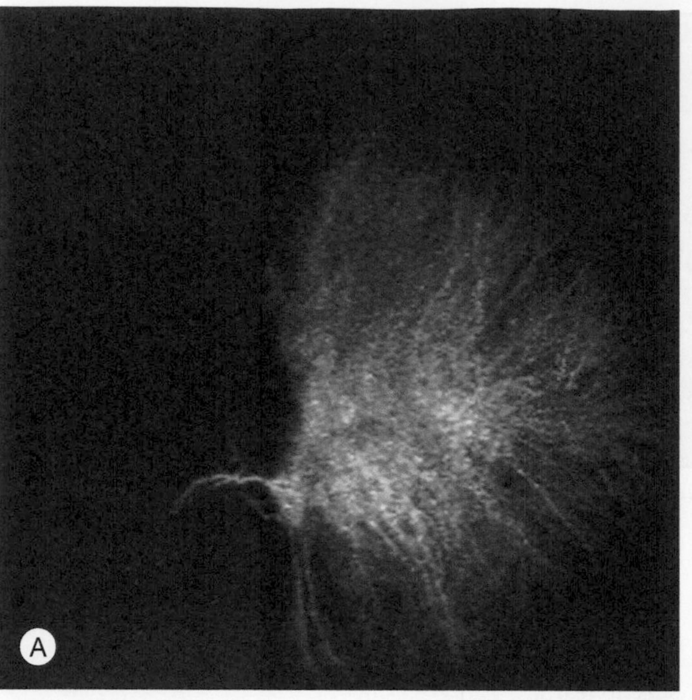

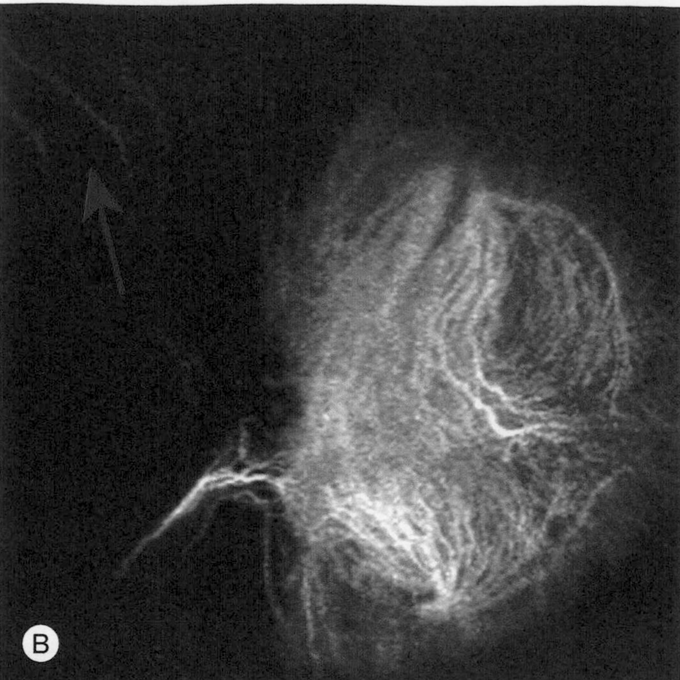

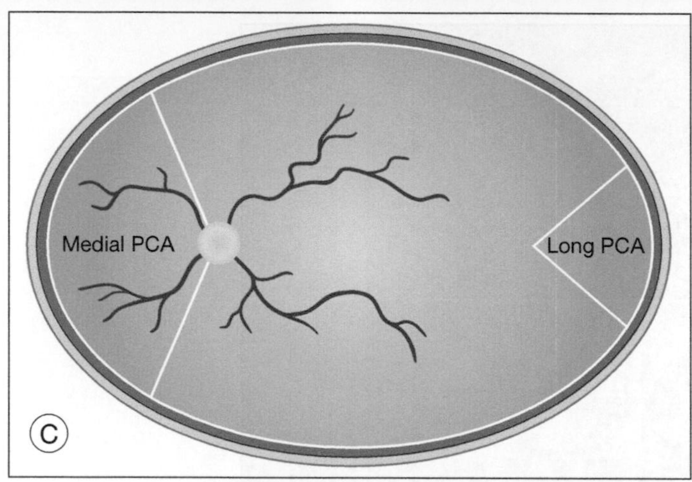

Fig. 2.4 A case of occlusion of the medial long posterior ciliary artery (PCA). (A) Indocyanine green angiography (ICGA) allows one to appreciate the different territories supplied by this artery and the lateral long PCA. (B) Venous phase of ICGA shows the filling of the lateral vortex veins. In the upper left area, the vortex vein is partially filled due to drainage from the iris (B, arrow). (C) Schematic representation of the different vascular territories of the two arteries. (Panel (C) modified with permission from Hayreh SS. Physiological anatomy of the choroidal vascular bed. Int Ophthalmol 1983;6:85–93.)

Type 2 choroidal neovascularization

In classic CNV, ICGA improves visualization of the fine structure of the neovascular network[1] (Fig. 2.9), allowing the choroidal and retinal circulation to be distinguished. This high spatial and temporal resolution permits identification of choroidal vessels that feed into the CNV.[58] In early phases, ICGA shows a dark rim which corresponds to a whitish ring on infrared imaging,[59] and a discrete neovascular network surrounded by a hypocyanescent margin which is more visible after 15 minutes.[60] Watzke et al.[54] showed that 87% of eyes with classic choroidal neovascular membranes were hypercyanescent with distinct edges.

This ability to provide a clear delineation of the neovascular network may confer an important advantage in the era of anti-VEGF therapy. It has been reported that VEGF inhibitors were more effective in controlling immature vessels, whereas a VEGF inhibitor along with a platelet-derived growth factor (PDGF) inhibitor appeared to show a synergistic effect for controlling the growth of mature vessels.[61] This is likely because pericyte recruitment is part of the maturation process in blood vessel development. Once the pericyte cell population is well established, the effectiveness of anti-VEGF agents is greatly reduced. PDGF-B is a key requirement for the recruitment of pericytes to the newly formed vessels. Mature, larger choroidal vessels may be readily differentiated from immature choroidal capillaries on ICGA (Fig. 2.10). Thus, in patients with chronic AMD or those who did not benefit from previous treatments with anti-VEGF, ICGA might better delineate a more mature stage of CNV. This has potential implications for therapeutic decision-making.

Type 3 choroidal neovascularization

During the past decade, RAP has been labeled with a number of different terms, including "retinal vascular anomalous complex,"

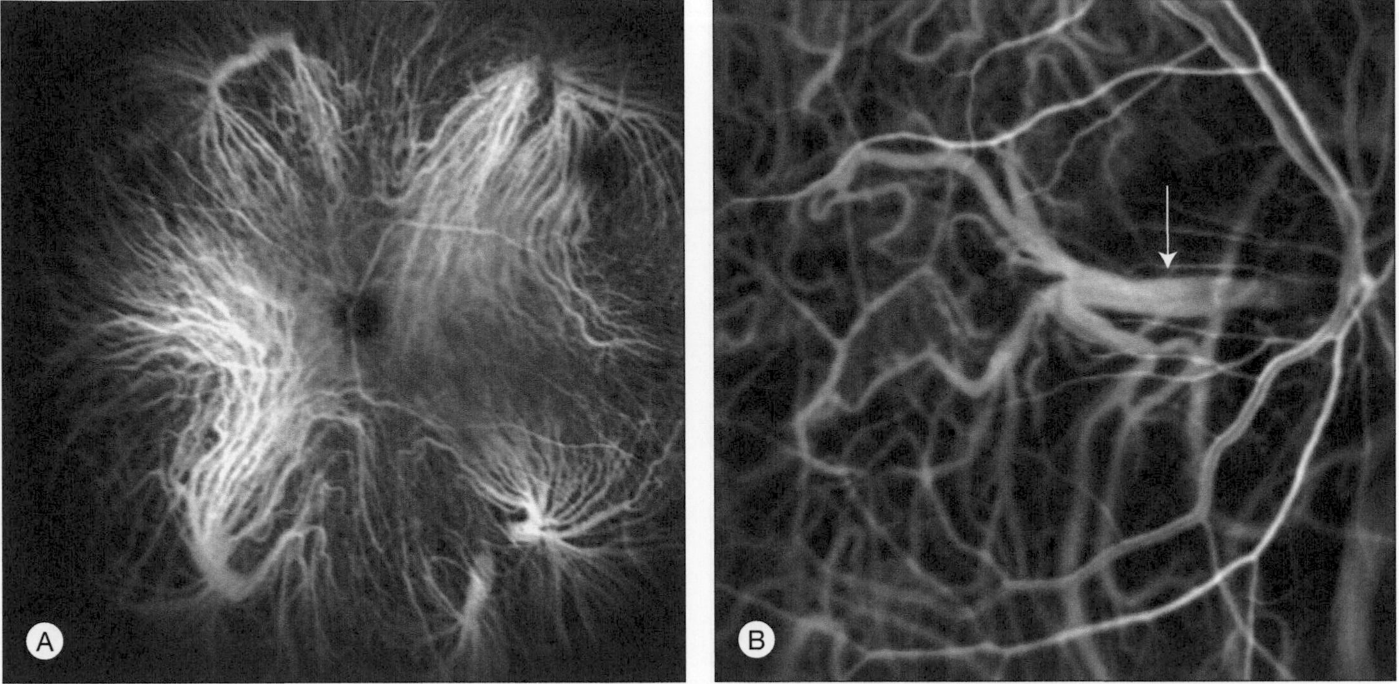

Fig. 2.5 Indocyanine green angiography allows visualization of the four vortex veins (A), and the choriovaginal vessels (B, arrow).

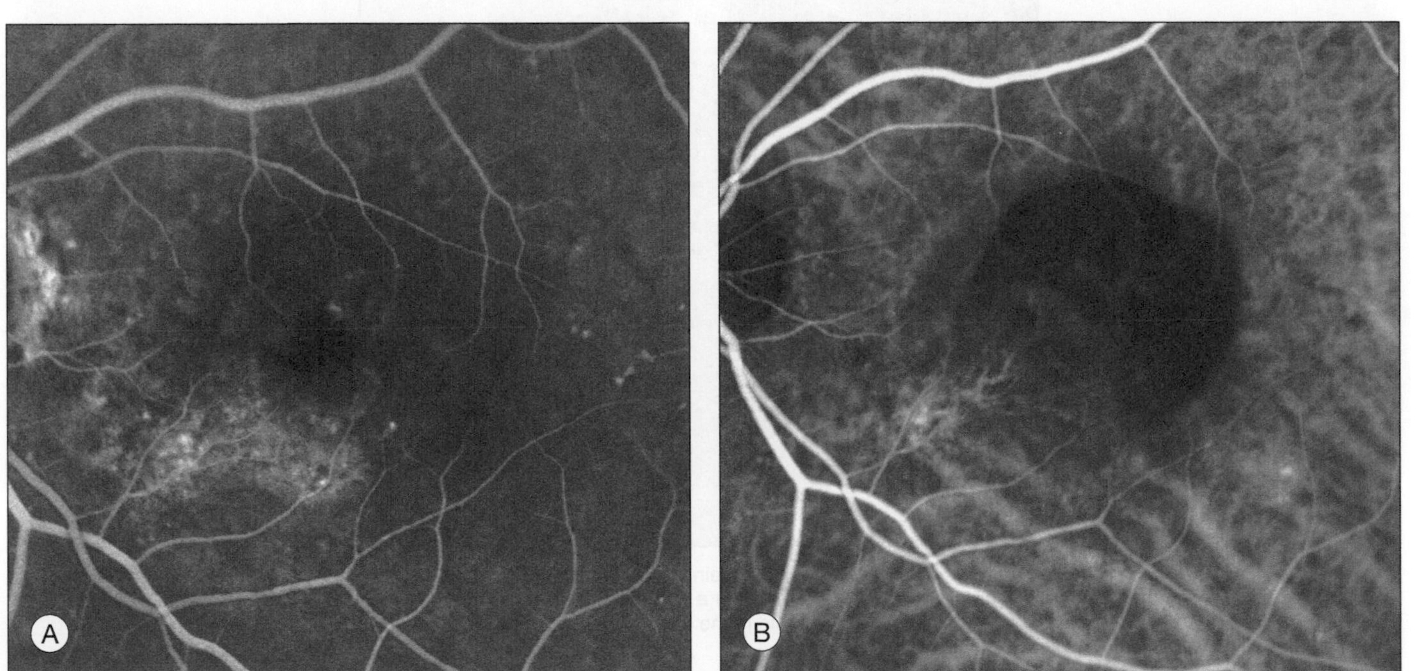

Fig. 2.6 A pigment epithelium detachment (PED) (A, fluorescein angiography) with a well-delineated neovascular network located along the edges of the PED (B, indocyanine green angiography).

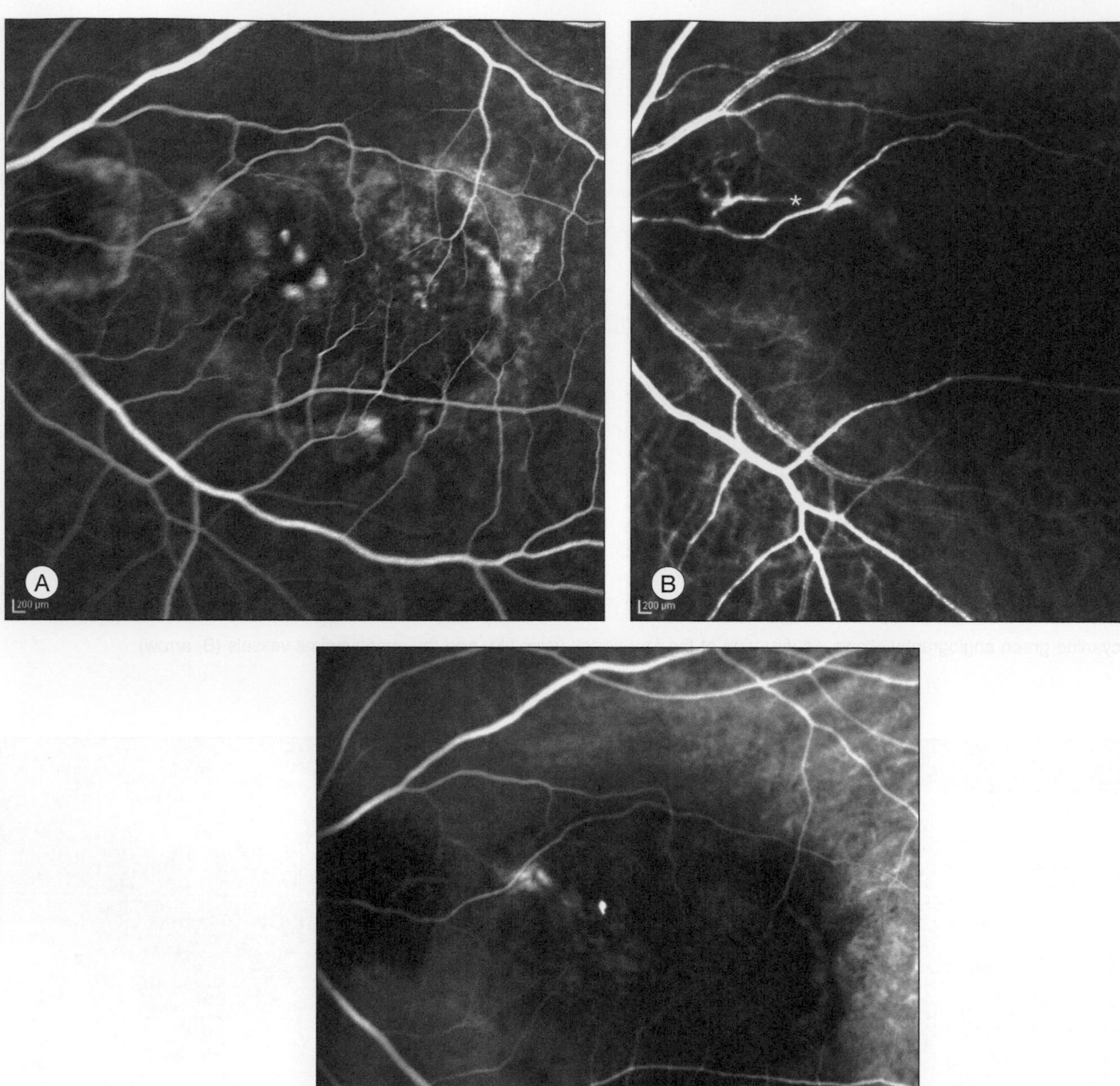

Fig. 2.7 Fibrovascular pigment epithelium detachment (PED). Fluorescein angiography demonstrates occult choroidal neovascularization with PED (A). In the early phases of indocyanine green angiography (ICGA) a feeder vessel originating in the juxtapapillary area is clearly delineated (B, asterisk). Feeder vessel and draining vein are indistinguishable in the late phases of ICGA (C).

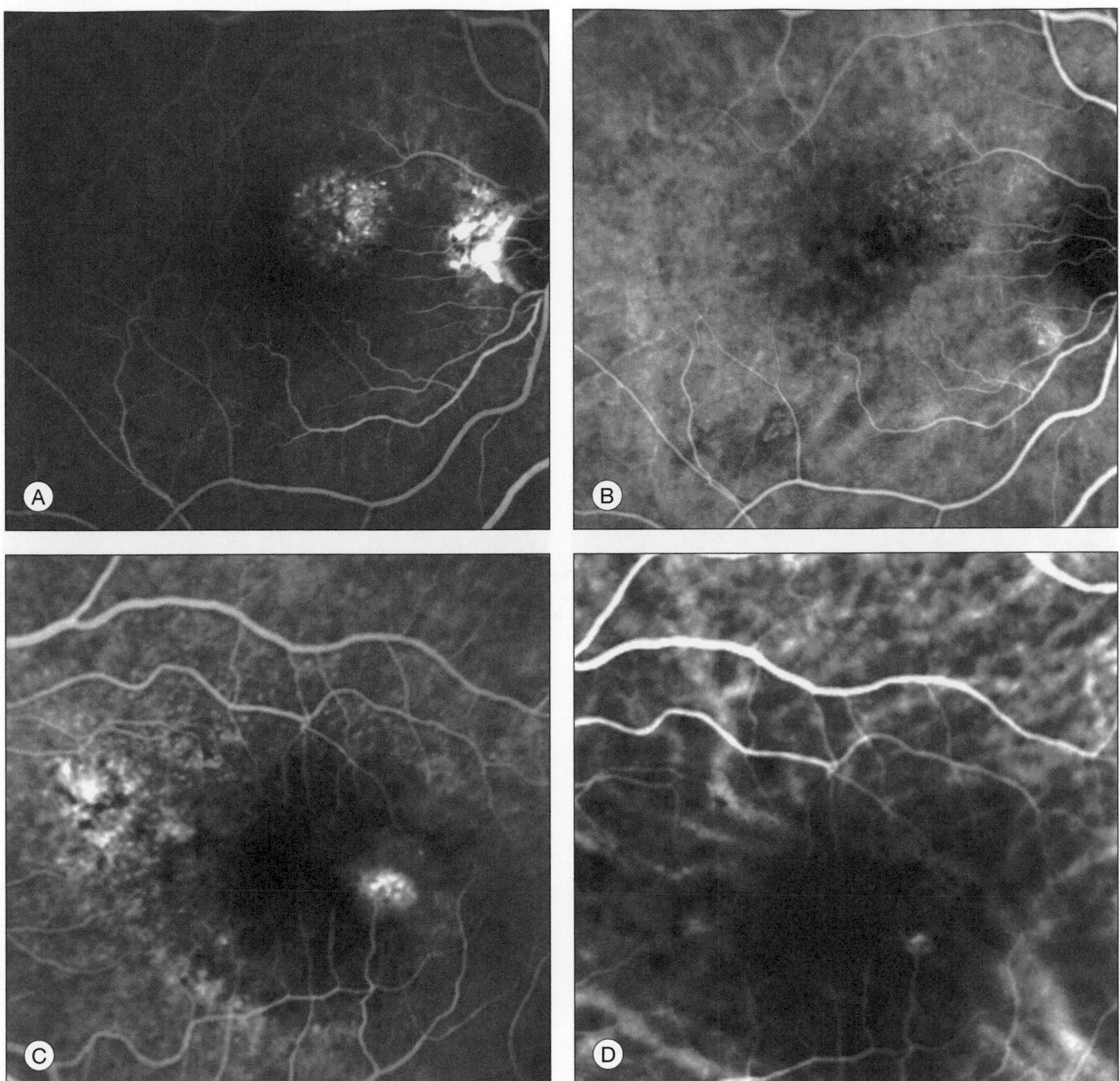

Fig. 2.8 Late leakage of undetermined source (A, C). Indocyanine green angiography may clearly differentiate a subtype of occult choroidal neovascularization (B) from retinal angiomatous proliferation (D).

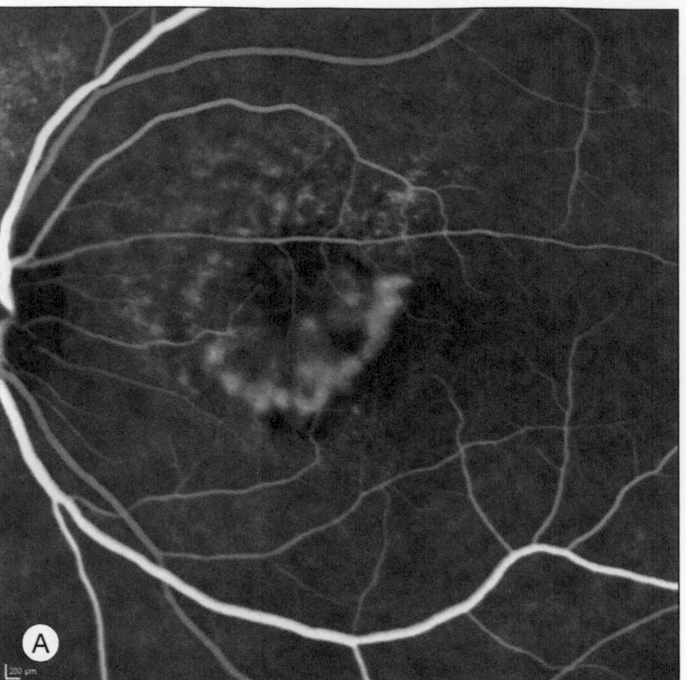

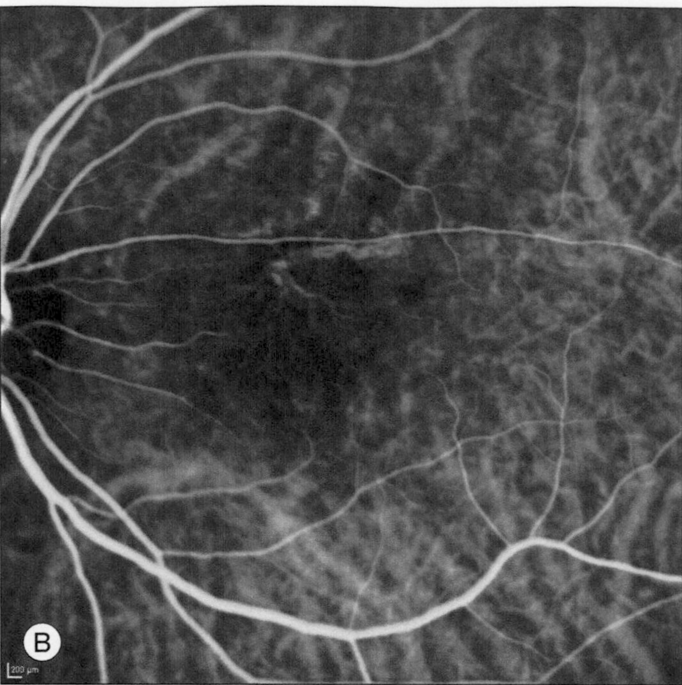

Fig. 2.9 A case of type 2 choroidal neovascularization. In fluorescein angiography image (A), the leakage of the dye from the lesion is evident, and obscures the boundaries of the neovascular network. In indocyanine green angiography (ICGA) (B), the limits of the neovascularization are much more visible. Moreover, ICGA allows the visualization of a central feeder vessel, with a surrounding net of smaller neovessels.

"retinal choroidal anastomosis," "retinal anastomosis to the lesion," and "chorioretinal anastomosis." In a comprehensive article on this entity, Yannuzzi et al.[62] provided evidence to support the original concept of capillaries arising within the inner half of the retina, or "retinal angiomatous proliferation," thus suggesting the acronym of RAP as the appropriate descriptor for the disease. Subsequently, Gass et al.[63] suggested a possible choroidal origin for these vessels, emanating from occult CNV and developing into an occult chorioretinal anastomosis. The new category, type 3 neovascularization, has been recently proposed[46] to harmonize these conflicting theories. Type 3 lesions would encompass the following disease manifestations: (1) focal neovascular proliferation arising from the deep retinal capillary plexus (the original RAP concept); (2) intraretinal neovascular extension from an underlying occult/type I CNV; and (3) de novo breaks in Bruch's membrane with neovascular infiltration into the retina.

Whatever the origin or initial location might be, our understanding of the importance of RAP as a component of neovascular AMD has been enhanced by ICGA. The fluorescein angiographic study generally shows manifestations of occult CNV, either fibrovascular PED (Fig. 2.11) or LLUS (Fig. 2.12) without a characteristic feature to identify and delineate the angiomatous process in the retina (indistinct zone of staining within and beyond the retina). By contrast, ICGA may clearly delineate the vascular structure of the lesion. When associated with PED, the RAP is usually well within the area of detachment and not at the edges, as is typically the case with CNV which vascularizes a serous PED (so-called notched PED configuration on fluorescein angiography). As previously reported, RAP may be present in up to one-fourth of eyes thought to have occult CNV with LLUS.[52] Dynamic ICGA (d-ICGA) has further expanded our capability for an early diagnosis. By definition, a diagnosis of RAP is based upon the temporal evidence of "dye filling of at least one retinal arteriole descending into the deep retinal space to a vascular communication and at least one draining retinal vein."[64] In conventional angiography, images are usually captured at 1 frame per second. This makes it virtually impossible to visualize the progression of the dye through the vascular complex, even though images are taken at very early phases. By contrast, d-ICGA takes up to 12 frames per second and captures the progressive filling of the lesion, allowing detection of very small and recent-onset cases of RAP (Fig. 2.2). The possibility of repeated viewing of the dynamic sequence of progression on ICGA may further increase our chances of an early diagnosis of RAP (Fig. 2.13). In a recent series of RAP diagnosed using d-ICGA,[52] the incidence of stage 1 RAP (64.9%) and the mean distance of the lesions from the fovea (682 ± 304 μm) were both consistent with an early-stage disease process, supporting the utility of this imaging procedure.

Early and accurate diagnosis of RAP is important for at least two reasons. First, RAP lesions are thought to be more aggressive,[65] with a treatment response that is likely to diminish with more advanced disease stages.[57] Second, recent data from the literature suggest that successful anatomic and functional results with RAP may be achieved more consistently with combined treatments (i.e., intravitreal injection of steroid or anti-VEGF + photodynamic therapy) rather than with intravitreal injection of anti-VEGF therapy alone.[66,67] Dynamic ICGA is also extremely useful for monitoring the therapeutic effect: a complete remodeling of the vascular structure may be achieved after successful closure and it is clearly highlighted in d-ICGA (Fig. 2.14).[68]

Polypoidal choroidal vasculopathy

Polypoidal choroidal vasculopathy (PCV) is a primary abnormality of the choroidal circulation characterized by an inner

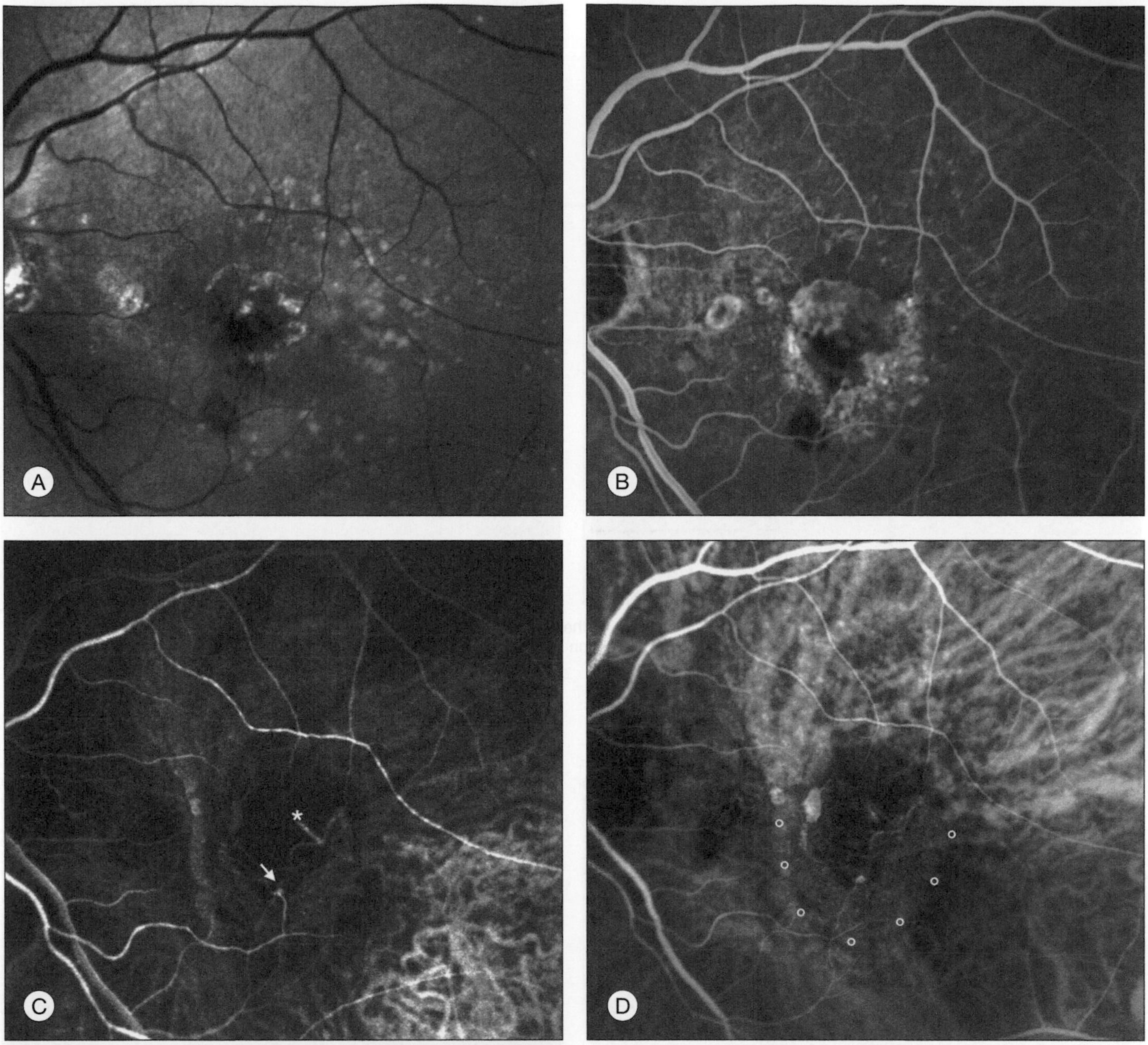

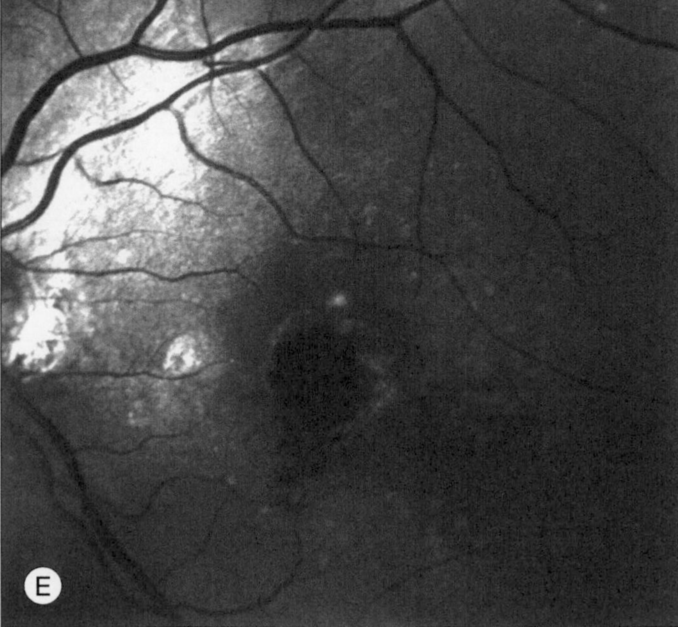

Fig. 2.10 Red-free image showing intraretinal blood within a central atrophic area. A small subretinal hemorrhage is also present inferiorly (A). Corresponding fluorescein angiogram demonstrating late leakage of undetermined source along the inferior edge of the atrophic area (B). Simultaneous early-phase indocyanine green angiography (C) reveals mature, large choroidal vessel (asterisk) feeding the large net of neovascularization along the inferior edge of the central atrophy. A real chorioretinal anastomosis (arrow) is also present. Four minutes after injection (D), the draining choroidal veins are well visualized, as is the neovascular network inferiorly (D, open circles). Red-free image after a 3-month loading phase with monthly ranibizumab (E) shows an increase in size of the central retinal hemorrhage despite anti-vascular endothelial growth factor therapy.

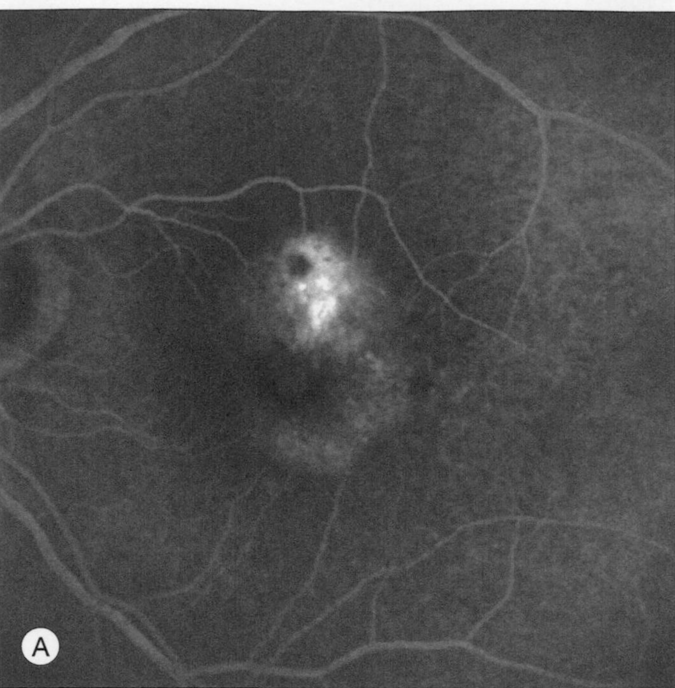

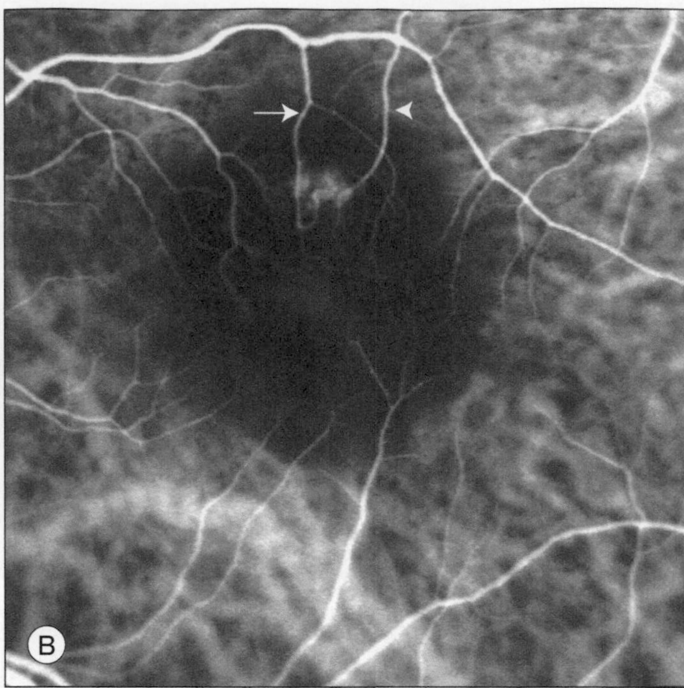

Fig. 2.11 Late-phase fluorescein angiography (A) shows a pigment epithelium detachment (PED) with a "hot spot." Indocyanine green angiography (B) reveals the presence of retinal angiomatous proliferation overlying the PED. Feeding retinal arteriole (arrow) and draining retinal venule (arrowhead) are clearly visualized.

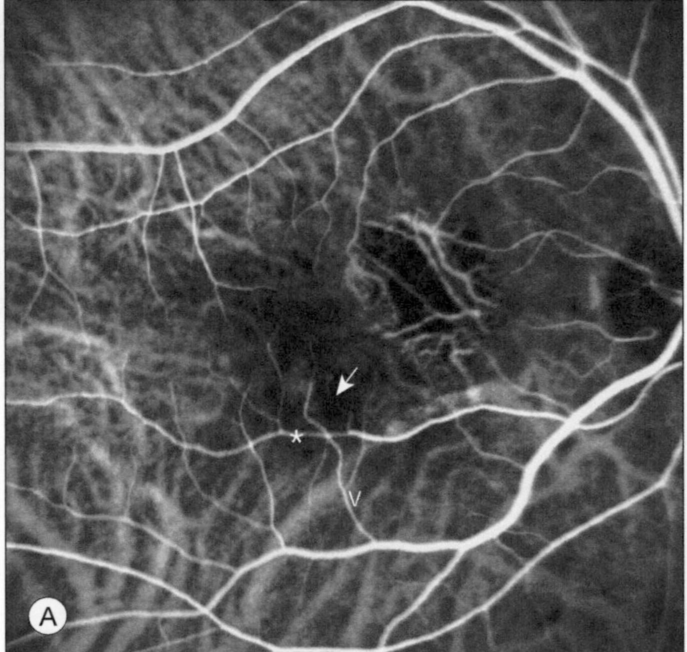

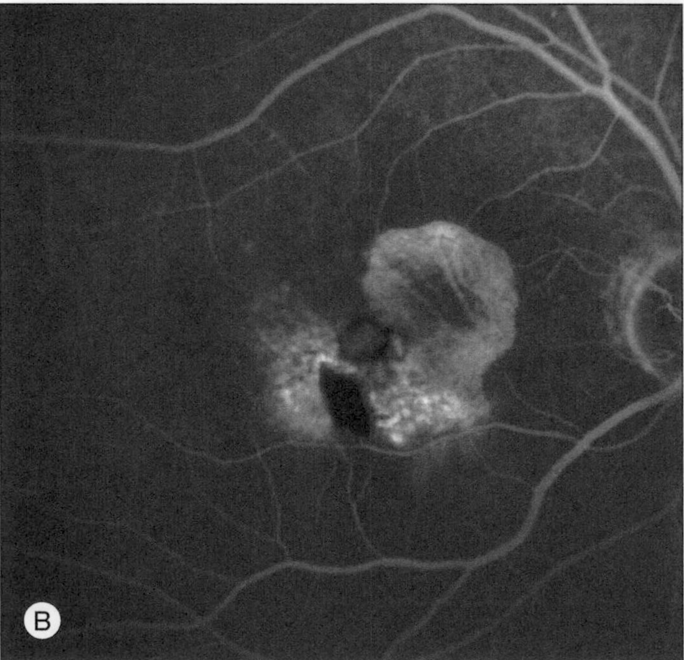

Fig. 2.12 Indocyanine green angiography (A) and fluorescein angiography (B) demonstrating an extrafoveal stage II retinal angiomatous proliferation (RAP). One feeding first-order macular arteriole (arrow) shunts blood flow from the vascular arcade (*) to the RAP and to one draining retinal vein (V). Cystoid macular edema is evident in late fluorescein phases.

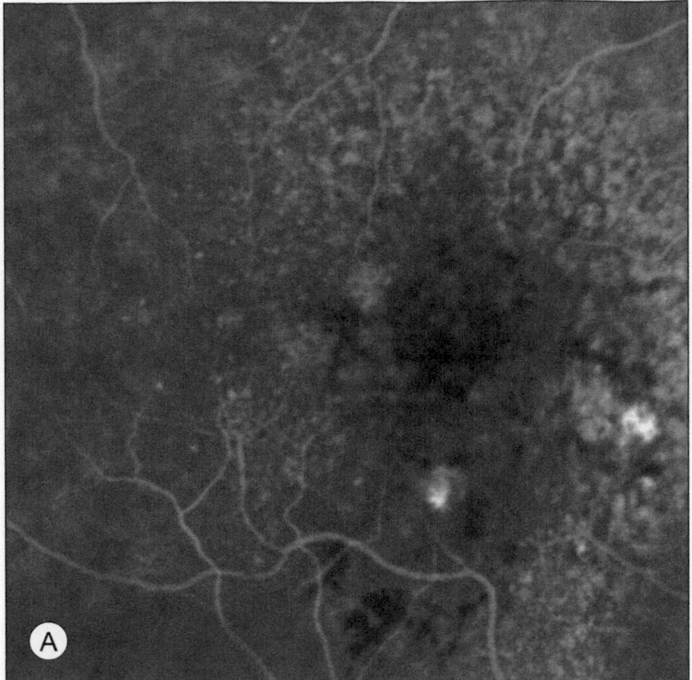

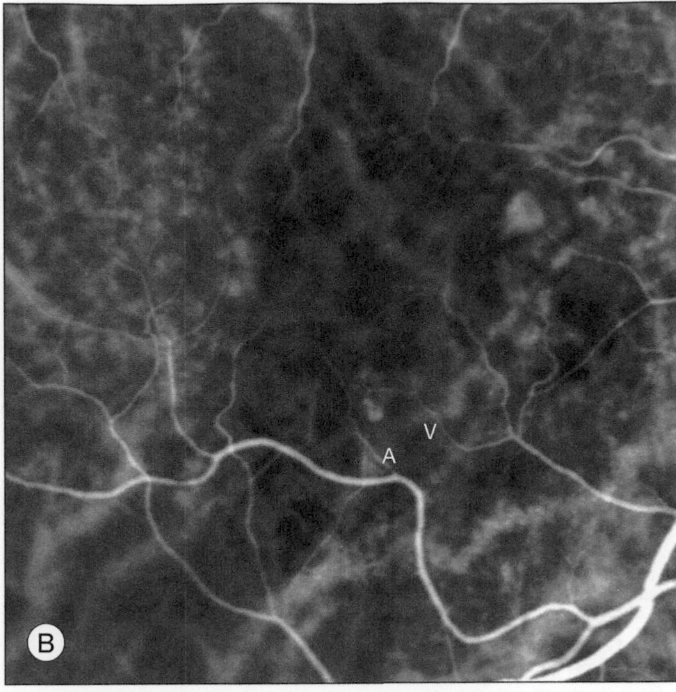

Fig. 2.13 Midphase fluorescein angiography (A) showing a small area of progressive extrafoveal staining at 6 o'clock. Dynamic indocyanine green angiography (B) reveals a well-delineated stage I retinal angiomatous proliferation with a feeding retinal arteriole (A) and a draining retinal vein (V).

choroidal vascular network of vessels ending in an aneurysmal bulge or outward projection, visible clinically as a reddish-orange, spheroid, polyp-like structure.[69] It was first described in the peripapillary area[69,70] (Fig. 2.15) but it may affect the macula[71] (Fig. 2.16), and also extramacular areas (Fig. 2.17).

The disorder is associated with multiple, recurrent, serosanguineous detachments of the RPE and neurosensory retina secondary to leakage and bleeding from the peculiar choroidal vascular abnormality. It has been reported that 85% of patients with serosanguineous detachments of the RPE have evidence of PCV.[72] ICGA has been used to detect and characterize the PCV abnormality with enhanced sensitivity and specificity.[1,71] The early phase of the ICG angiogram shows a distinct network of vessels within the choroid (Fig. 2.16B). In patients with juxtapapillary lesions, the vascular channels may follow a radial, arching pattern. In PCV limited to the macula, a vascular network often arises in the macula and follows an oval distribution pattern.[73] Larger choroidal vessels of the PCV network begin to fill before retinal vessels, and PCV network fills also at a slower rate than retinal vessels. Shortly after the network can be identified by the ICG angiogram, small hyperfluorescent "polyps" become visible (Fig. 2.16C). These polypoidal structures correspond to the reddish-orange choroidal excrescence seen clinically. They appear to leak slowly as the surrounding hypofluorescent area becomes increasingly hyperfluorescent. In the later phase of the angiogram there is uniform disappearance of dye ("washout") from the bulging polypoidal lesions.

PCV is often misdiagnosed or confused with chronic central serous chorioretinopathy (CSC)[74,75] and with exudative age-related maculopathy[71,76] and may represent a transitional condition between the two pathologies.[1] Moreover, the treatment strategies for PCV differ from exudative AMD. The use of anti-VEGF agents is controversial in PCV,[1] while verteporfin photodynamic therapy, alone or in combination with bevacizumab,[77] as well as selective laser photocoagulation have been shown to be effective treatments.[78]

Given the facts that ICGA is the most sensitive and specific tool for PCV identification and the treatment for PCV may differ from other diseases for which it is frequently confused, it would seem apparent that ICGA is an important tool in the evaluation of all cases of exudative lesions suspected of harboring PCV.

Central serous chorioretinopathy

CSC is characterized by multifocal areas of choroidal hyperpermeability on ICGA,[79-81] visible in the mid and late phases of the angiogram[82] (Fig. 2.18). These areas surround the active RPE leaks but can also be found in areas apparently unaffected by leakage or abnormal fluorescence on fluorescence angiography, even in the fellow eyes.[79] Zones of choroidal hyperpermeability tend to persist in cases of severe and chronic CSC[83] (Fig. 2.19), and are of value for distinguishing CSC from AMD in older patients with suspected occult neovascularization.[80,84]

Moreover, ICG assessment of the location of these areas of hyperpermeability may be useful when considering treatment with verteporfin photodynamic therapy, using normal[80] or half-fluence laser energy.[85] The treatment focused on these areas showed rapid reduction of fluid and improvement in visual acuity,[80] possibly by leading to hypoperfusion of choriocapillaris and vascular remodeling.[86] In these studies, verteporfin photodynamic therapy success rate seemed to be dependent on the degree of hyperpermeability, as the treatment was less effective or had more frequent recurrence of CSC in eyes without intense hyperfluorescence.[87]

Other findings in CSC using ICGA include multiple "occult" serous PED,[79] punctate hyperfluorescent spots,[88] delays in arterial filling of the choroidal arteries and choriocapillaris,[89,90] and venous congestion.[90] ICGA is also useful in differentiating CSC from PCV.[75]

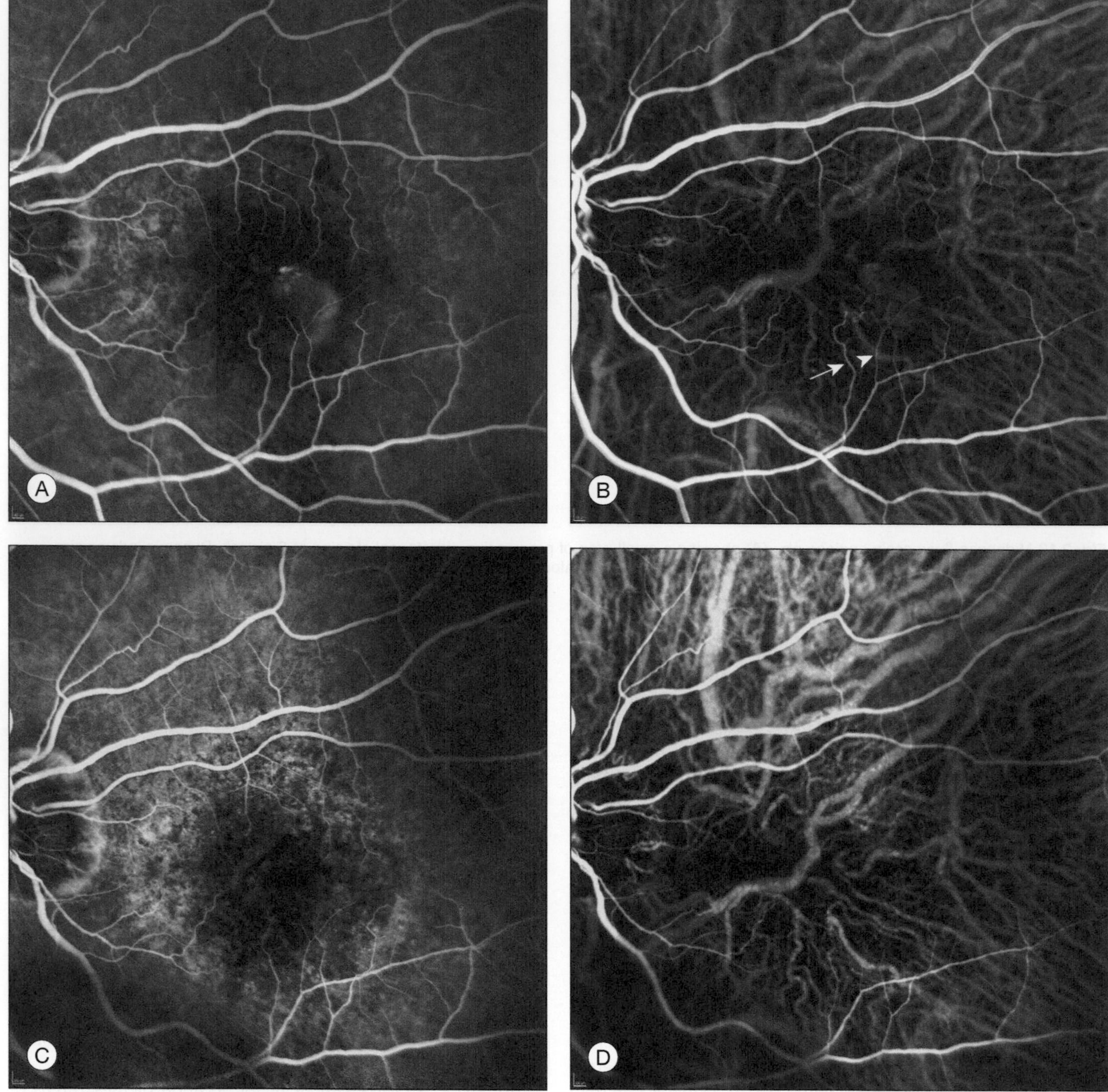

Fig. 2.14 Baseline fluorescein angiography (A) and dynamic indocyanine green angiography (ICGA) (B) shows a stage II extrafoveal retinal angiomatous proliferation (RAP) located inferotemporal to the fovea. One feeding first-order macular arteriole (arrowhead) shunts blood flow from the vascular arcade to the RAP and to the draining retinal vein (arrow). Two months after one combined treatment (intravitreal triamcinolone acetonide + photodynamic therapy), the RAP is no longer detectable by either fluorescein angiography (C) or ICGA (D). There is an evident reduction in the size of both the first-order macular arteriole and the draining retinal vein (barely visible) (C, D).

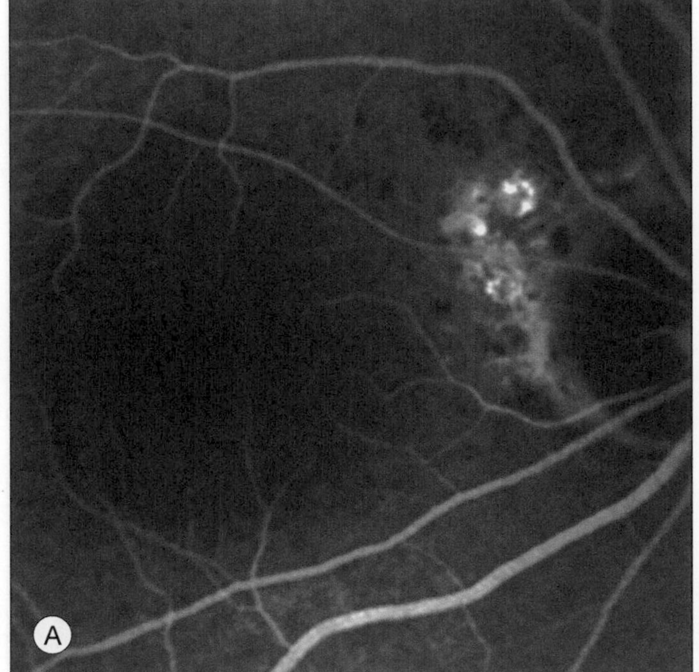

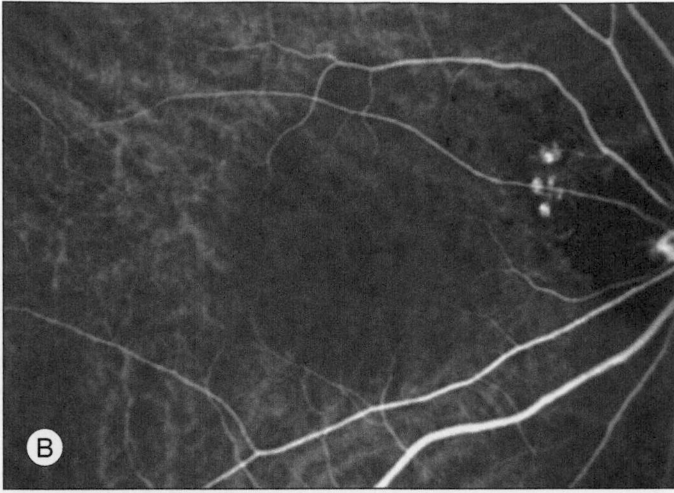

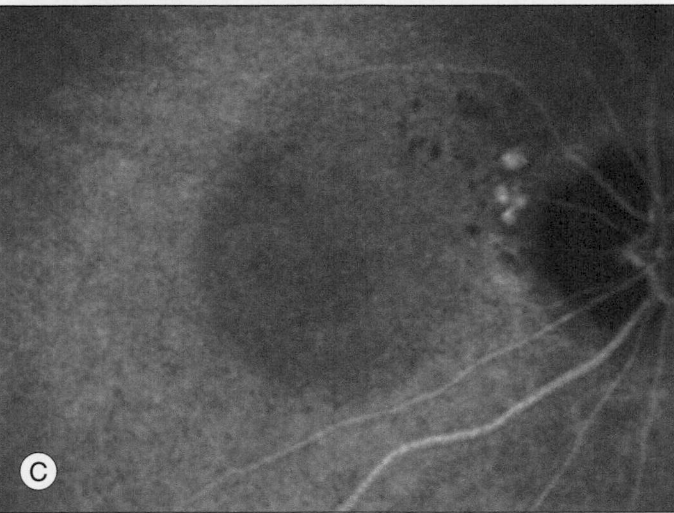

Fig. 2.15 Late-phase fluorescein angiography (A) shows a neurosensory retinal detachment with multiple juxtapapillary "hot spots." Early (B) and late (C) indocyanine green angiography reveals the presence of juxtapapillary polypoidal choroidal vasculopathy.

Choroidal tumors

Choroidal hemangioma

Unlike diffuse choroidal hemangiomas, which are usually evident at birth and typically occur as part of neuro-oculocutaneous hemangiomatosis or Sturge–Weber syndrome, circumscribed choroidal hemangioma may be more difficult to diagnose.

Circumscribed choroidal hemangiomas are benign hamartomas that typically present from the second to fourth decade of life.[91] They usually occur sporadically in the absence of systemic disease. Histopathology reveals that the tumor is composed by vascular channels lined with endothelium. It involves the full thickness of the choroid with secondary changes of the overlying RPE and the retina.[92] Although commonly asymptomatic, choroidal hemangiomas can be associated with exudative retinal detachment resulting in reduced visual function, metamorphopsia, and photopsia.

On ophthalmoscopic examination, a circumscribed choroidal hemangioma appears as an orange choroidal mass with indistinct margins that blend with the surrounding choroid. They are frequently located in the macular region of the posterior pole, and are not usually thicker than 6 mm.[93] Surrounding subretinal fluid leading to exudative retinal detachment with macular involvement is common in symptomatic cases. Retinal hard exudates are minimal or absent.

Angiographic studies such as fluorescein and ICG can be helpful in establishing the diagnosis and differentiating these benign lesions from other tumors, namely amelanotic malignant melanoma and choroidal metastases. Fluorescein angiography demonstrates a hyperfluorescent mass with a fine lacy vascular network of intrinsic vessels in the early choroidal filling phase. The hyperfluorescence increases throughout the angiogram, and there is variable leakage in late views[94] (Fig. 2.20A, B). ICGA is the most useful study for demonstrating the intrinsic vascular pattern of circumscribed choroidal hemangioma.[95] The advantage of ICG dye over sodium fluorescein dye is that it diffuses much more slowly out of fenestrated small choroidal vessels than does sodium fluorescein. Within 30 seconds of injection of the ICG dye, the tumor's intrinsic vascular pattern becomes apparent. By 1 minute, choroidal hemangiomas completely fill with the dye, showing brilliant hyperfluorescence. This 1-minute stage of intense hyperfluorescence seen with choroidal hemangiomas is brighter than any other tumor, and is very suggestive of the diagnosis. In the following phases (6–10 minutes), the hyperfluorescence can persist or begin to wane (Fig. 2.20C-E). In

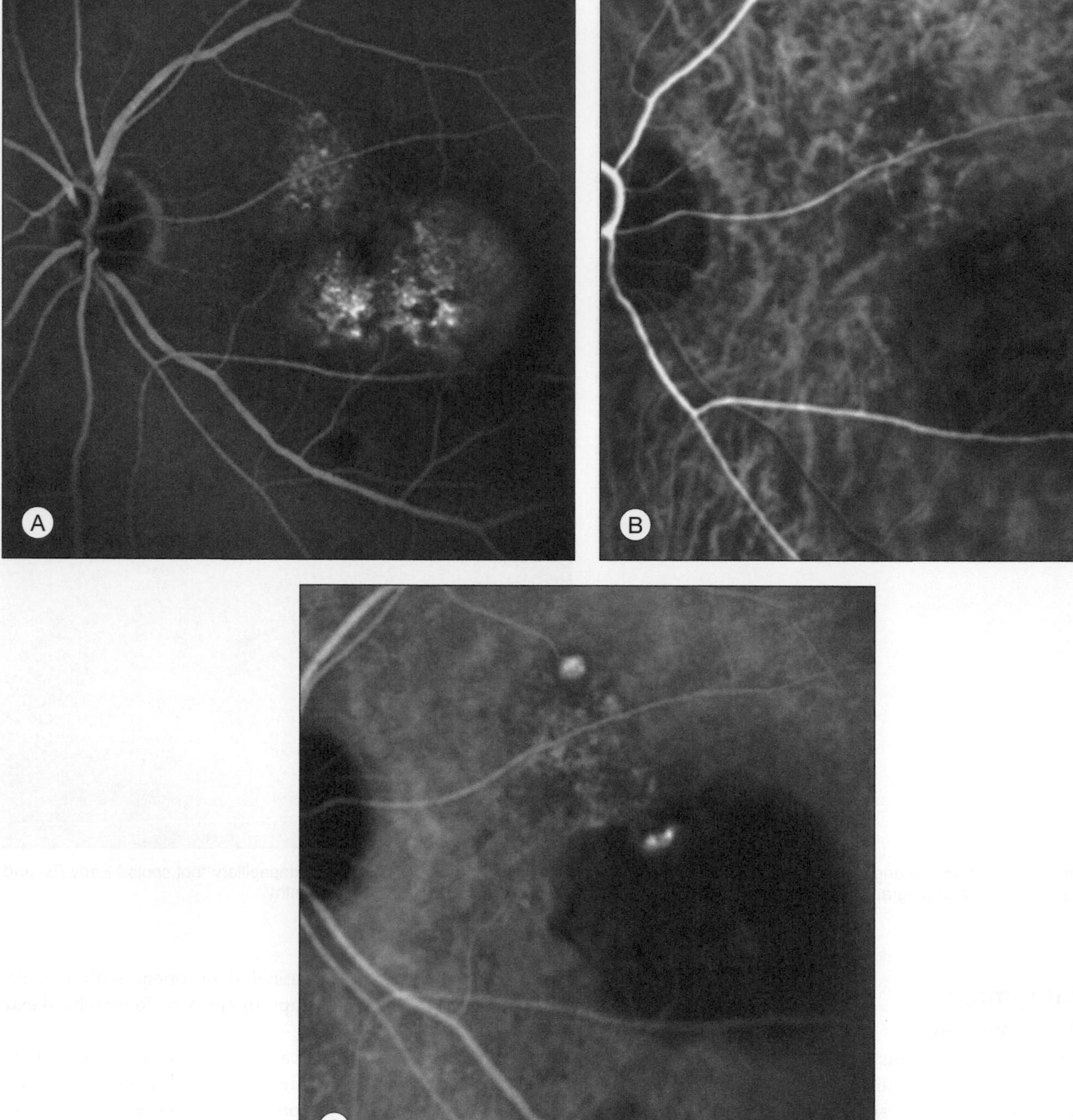

Fig. 2.16 Late-phase fluorescein angiographic image revealing type 1 occult choroidal neovascularization with a subfoveal pigment epithelium detachment (PED) (A). Early (B) and late (C) indocyanine green angiographic frames demonstrate a distinct network of vessels within the macular choroid ending with two hyperfluorescent "polyps." One of the two is located within the PED.

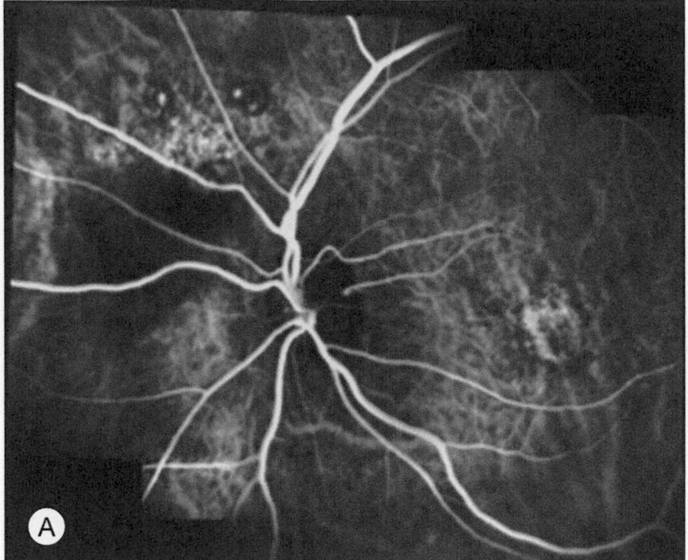

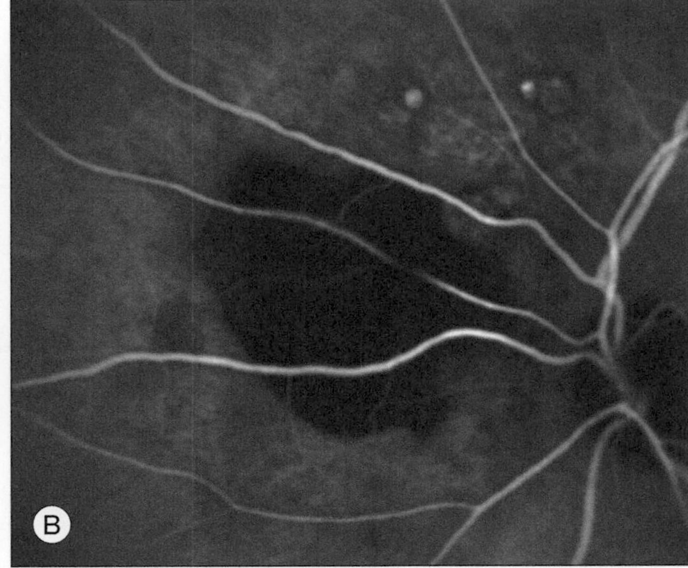

Fig. 2.17 Early (A) and late (B) indocyanine green angiography showing extramacular polypoidal choroidal vasculopathy with a pigment epithelium detachment.

the late phases of the ICG angiogram (30 minutes), a washout effect with reduction of the initial hyperfluorescence is observed secondary to the outflow of dye from the hemangioma (Fig. 2.20F).[95] The low-resistance, high-flow properties of the tumor allow rapid flow of the dye into and out of the tumor. The resulting final effect is that the tumor empties sooner than the normal surrounding choroid and thus appears hypofluorescent in comparison. This washout sign is very helpful in differentiating choroidal hemangiomas from amelanotic malignant melanoma and choroidal metastases.

Choroidal melanoma

ICGA findings in uveal melanoma are variable.[96] No study revealed any pathognomonic sign with ICGA to identify choroidal melanoma.[23,97]

Nevertheless ICGA was found to be capable of identifying tumor vessels (Fig. 2.21)[98,99] which are usually irregularly tortuous, with anarchic branching,[97] dilated with a parallel course,[98] and characterized by vasculogenic mimicry patterns.[100] ICGA was demonstrated to be superior to fluorescein angiography in detecting both tumor borders and vasculature.[97,101]

Mueller et al. found that different patterns of the microcirculation within the tumor may be useful in the prognosis of the disease.[101] The evidence of microcirculation patterns characterized by networks and a parallel course with cross-linking may be associated with a higher risk of metastatic disease.[101] Other studies reported the possible role of ICGA in evaluating the outcome of brachytherapy,[102] proton beam irradiation,[103] and transpupillary thermotherapy.[104]

Peripheral exudative hemorrhagic chorioretinopathy

Peripheral exudative hemorrhagic chorioretinopathy (PEHCR) is a bilateral peripheral exudative hemorrhagic retinal degenerative process of the eye.[105,106] The condition is characterized by blood in the subretinal or subretinal pigment epithelial space. PEHCR is most often found in older Caucasian patients and may simulate a vitreous hemorrhage with suspicion of underlying retinal detachment or break, intraocular inflammatory process, retinal artery macroaneurysm, or choroidal melanoma.[105] In fact, PEHCR often appears as a visible intraocular elevated mass with a mean basal dimension of 10 mm and a mean thickness of 3 mm, consistent with the size of a small to medium-sized melanoma.[106] The lesion is most often located temporally (77%) between the equator and the ora serrata (89%) and involves one (46%) or two (46%) quadrants.[106] In comparison, eyes with uveal melanoma show tumor location in the macula (5%), between the macula and the equator (78%), and between the equator and the ora serrata (17%).[106]

Many eyes with PEHCR have features of macular or extramacular (peripheral) degeneration such as drusen, RPE alterations, or CNV.[106] The majority of PEHCR lesions spontaneously resolve, leaving RPE atrophy, hyperplasia, and fibrosis. These features imply a bilateral generalized aging process within the eye and are consistent with the degenerative nature of the disease. Although almost half of patients may be asymptomatic, a decrease in visual acuity related to PEHCR may occur in up to 20% of cases.[106] Both for this reason and for the fact that the acute hemorrhagic form is typically mistaken for melanoma, PEHCR deserves an early and proper clinical diagnosis. Fluorescein angiography is of little help because choroidal neovascular lesions are visible in only 3% of cases.[106] This is due to the blockage of choroidal fluorescence related to subretinal hemorrhage, sub-RPE hemorrhage, or RPE hyperplasia. Diffuse peripheral changes consistent with variable degrees of RPE hyperplasia or atrophy are also common fluorescein angiographic features.

By contrast, ICGA may clearly delineate the choroidal neovascular process, which is often located at the edges of the blood pool, even in the far periphery. Photodynamic therapy or laser photocoagulation applied to the choroidal new vessels may further accelerate the reabsorption of subretinal blood with decreased risk of subsequent visual acuity loss (Figs 2.22 and 2.23).

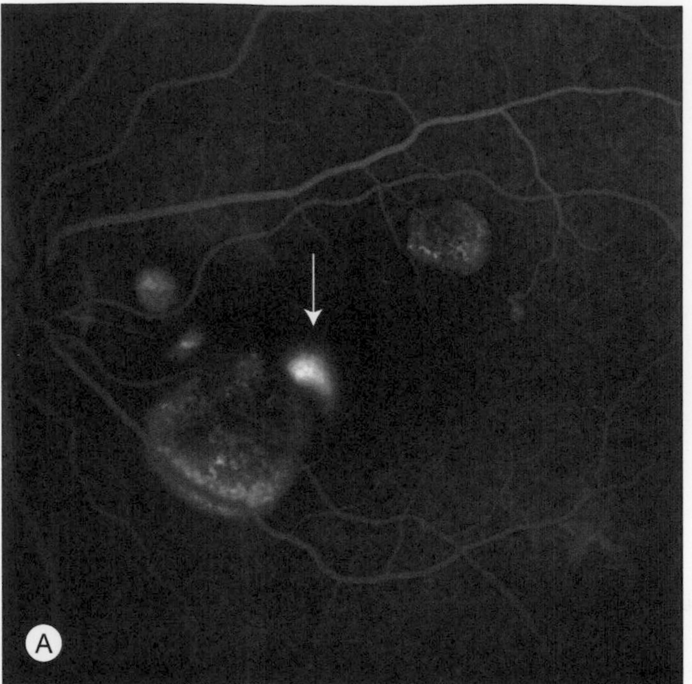

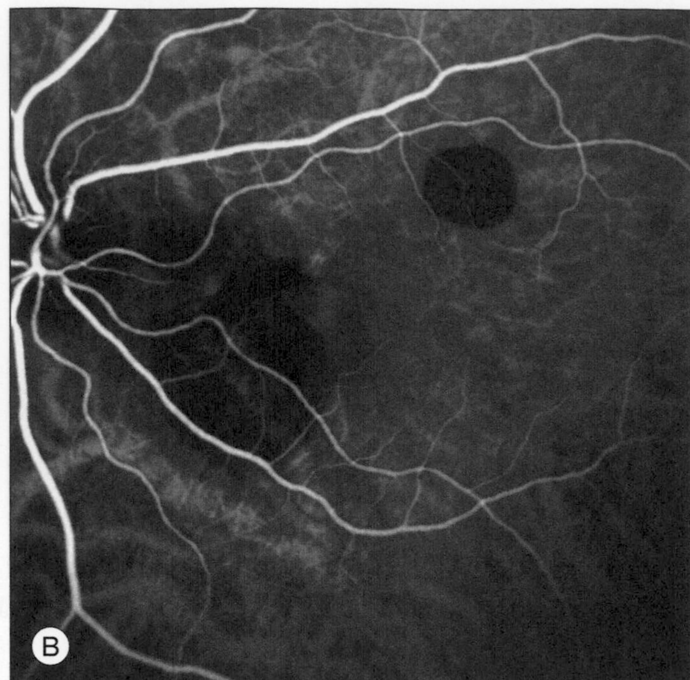

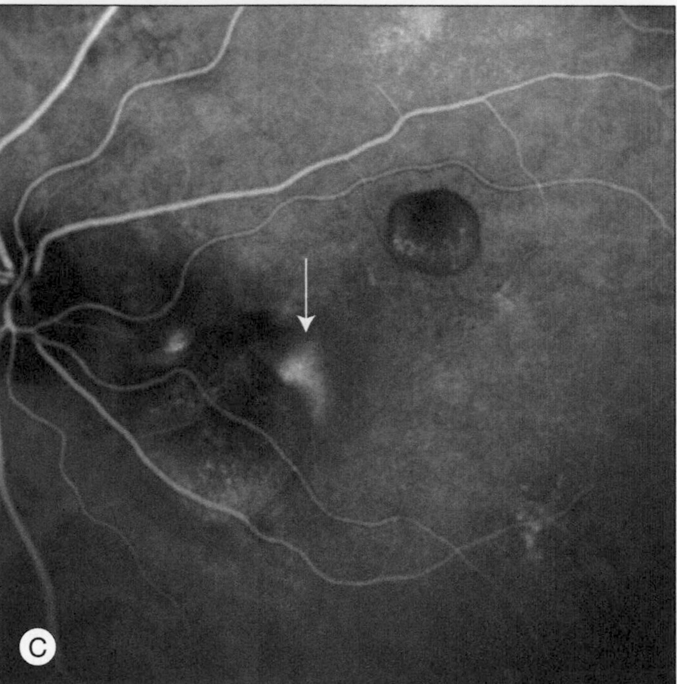

Fig. 2.18 A case of central serous chorioretinopathy. In the fluorescein angiographic image (A) it is possible to visualize three distinct serous detachments of the pigment epithelium, and one point of leakage. Another hyperfluorescent area is visible (arrow), but it is not clear if it corresponds to another point of leakage or represents an additional detachment. Indocyanine green angiographic images (B, C) allow one to distinguish clearly points of leakage as hyperfluorescent areas, with marked leakage in the late phases (C, arrow). The uncertain area noted on fluorescein angiography is another leaky point.

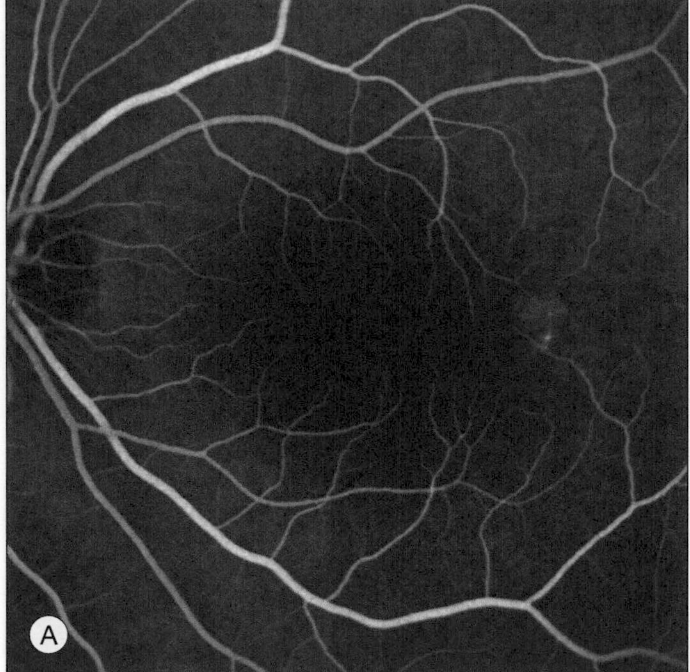

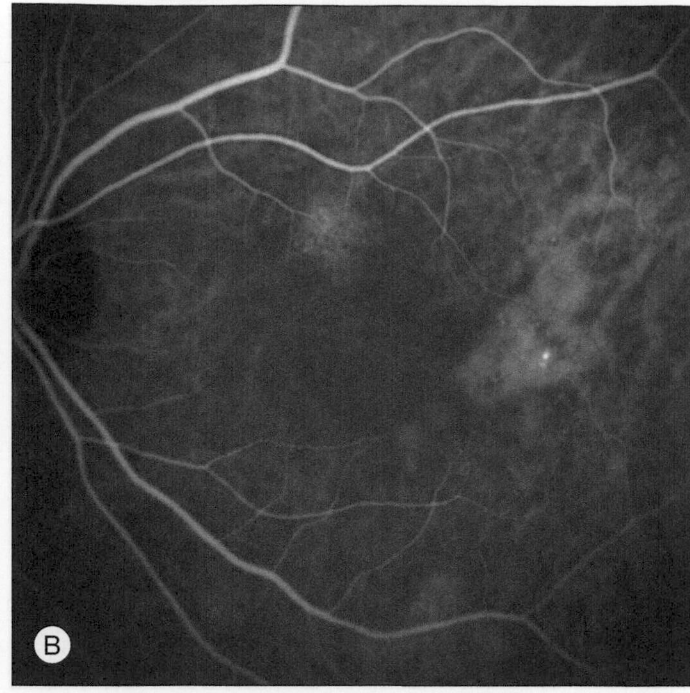

Fig. 2.19 A case of central serous chorioretinopathy. Fluorescein angiographic image (A) shows only an area of pigment epithelium disturbance. Indocyanine green angiography (B) reveals a more extensive alteration of the choriocapillaris, with multiple areas of hyperfluorescence.

Varix of the vortex vein ampulla

Varix of the vortex vein ampulla is a rare, benign, asymptomatic condition, which may be confused with a choroidal nevus or melanoma.[107] The choroidal veins drain into an average of four vortex veins, which exit the globe through scleral canals.[108] About half of the vortex veins show dilatations of varying sizes and shapes, and are referred to as vortex vein ampullae. The varix of the vortex vein ampulla is an unusually large dilatation of the vortex vein. The cause remains unclear. The gaze-dependent dynamic nature of the lesion suggested gaze-evoked kinking of the extrascleral vortex vein or narrowing of the scleral canal to be considered as the possible cause.[109] The varix may also be enlarged by factors that increase ocular venous pressure, like Valsalva maneuver, head-down positioning, and jugular vein compression.[109] Biomicroscopically, the lesion appears as a smooth red–brown elevation in the equatorial region, usually in the nasal quadrants.[107] It is usually a single lesion but may be bilateral.[109] A proper diagnosis may be achieved by pressure on the globe that readily collapses the varix (Fig. 2.24).[109] ICGA[96,107,110] is particularly useful because it demonstrates the relationship of the varix to the choroidal vasculature and also allows visualization of the pressure and gaze-dependent changes. Relatively early maximum fluorescence and a homogeneous filling pattern may further help differentiate the varix from other choroidal masses.[107]

Choroidal inflammation and white-dot syndrome

Multiple evanescent white-dot syndrome

Multiple evanescent white-dot syndrome is a unilateral acute disease that affects young women, presenting with a transient, self-limiting visual loss. The disease involves the choroid and the outer retina.[111,112] ICGA shows a pattern of multiple hypofluorescent areas at the posterior pole and peripheral retina. These spots become visible in the mid to late phases, range in size between 50 and 1000 μm,[112] and are more apparent in ICGA images than by fundus examination and fluorescein angiography[1,112] (Fig. 2.25). In addition, ICGA may show hypofluorescence surrounding the disc area.[111] The hypofluorescent spots disappear at the recovery stage of the disease, and sometimes are more persistent with ICGA.[113]

Multifocal choroiditis

In multifocal choroiditis the white lesions are visualized as hypofluorescent spots in ICGA images. These lesions may be followed up with ICGA both in the natural course of the pathology and in the response to treatment with oral prednisone.[114] A reduction in size and number of hypofluorescent spots is observed after successful treatment. Other findings visible on ICGA are hyperfluorescent spots, which usually do not correspond with the hyperfluorescent foci seen on fluorescein angiography, and a large hypofluorescent area surrounding the optic nerve.

Birdshot chorioretinopathy

This disease is characterized by deep cream-colored dots scattered diffusely throughout both fundi. The lesions appear as round-oval, hypofluorescent, symmetric dots on ICGA.[115] These lesions are typically not seen on fluorescein angiography, and therefore ICGA may detect birdshot lesions more rapidly.[116] Other findings on ICGA include diffuse ICG hyperfluorescence predominantly found in the posterior pole in the late phase of angiography, and an alteration of the vascular pattern of the choroid with choroidal vessels appearing fuzzy and indistinct in the intermediate phase of angiography.[115] In the chronic phase of the disease the hypofluorescent dots persist in the late phases of the angiogram and correspond to RPE atrophy or choroidal granulomas.[1,117]

Text continued on p. e78

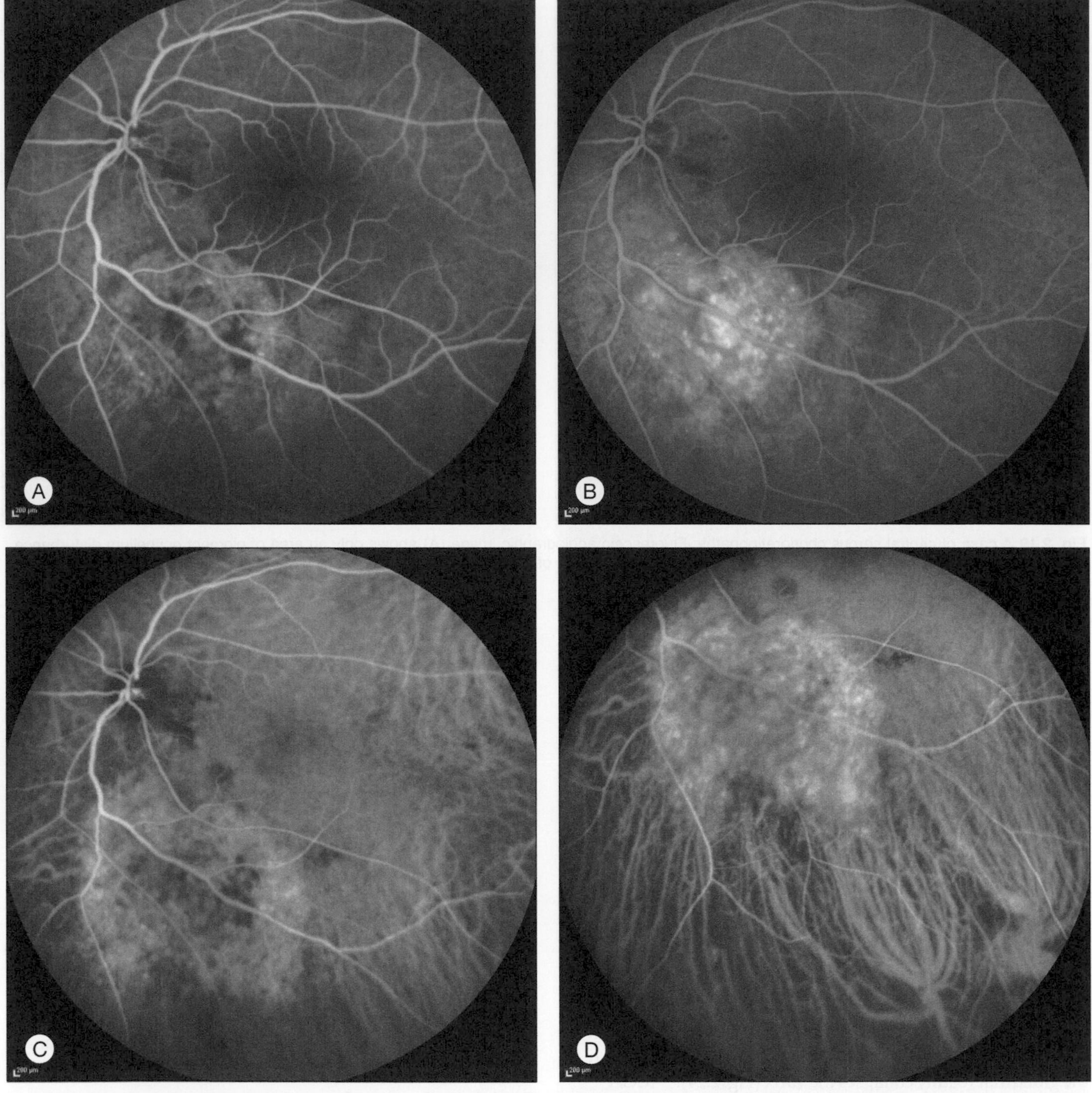

Fig. 2.20 Fluorescein angiography demonstrating a hyperfluorescent mass along the inferior vascular arcade (A). The hyperfluorescence increases progressively throughout the angiogram with variable leakage in late views (B). Early-phase indocyanine green angiography (ICGA) (49 seconds) revealing a fine lacy vascular network of intrinsic vessels (C). Increasing hyperfluorescence is detected after injection: (D) at 2 minutes.

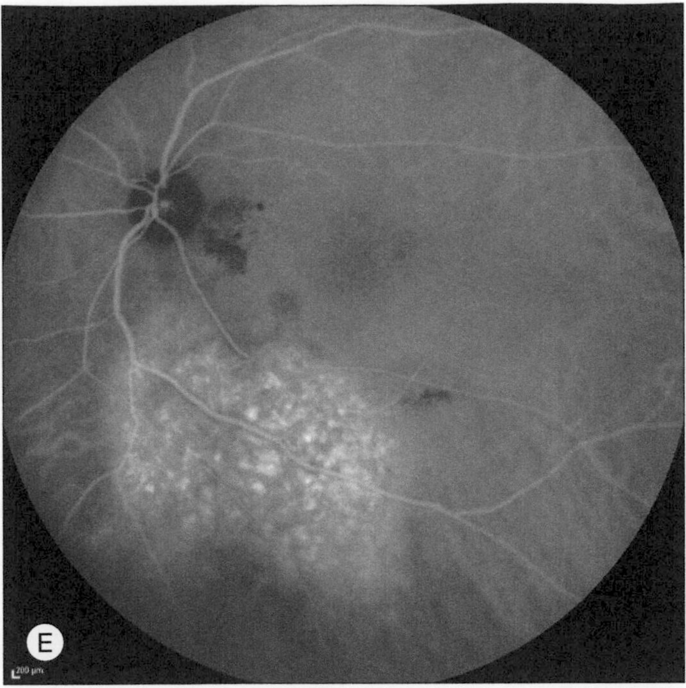

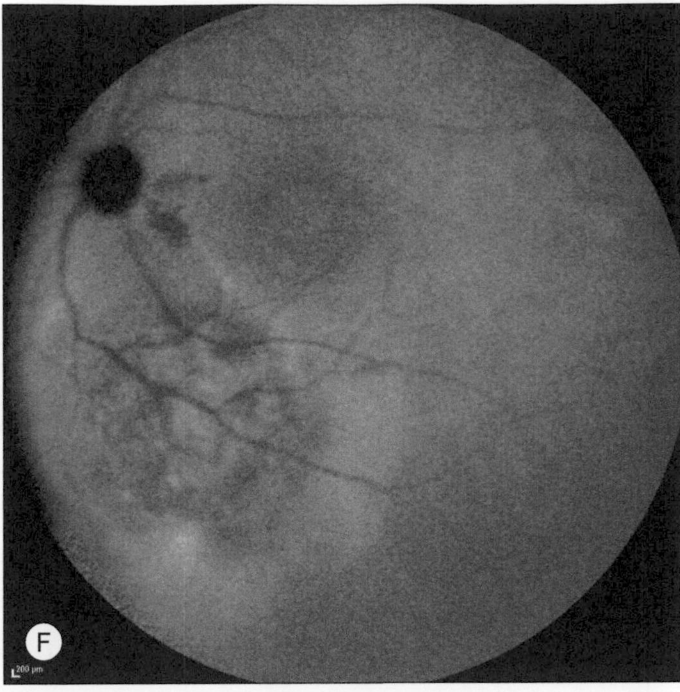

Fig. 2.20 Cont'd Increasing hyperfluorescence after injection: (E) at 5 minutes. Of note, the margins of the tumor appear scalloped. (F) Late-phase ICGA study demonstrating hypofluorescence within the tumor (washout effect). A halo of minimal hyperfluorescence surrounds the tumor. This may result from staining of the retinal pigment epithelium or leakage of indocyanine green into the subneurosensory retinal space.

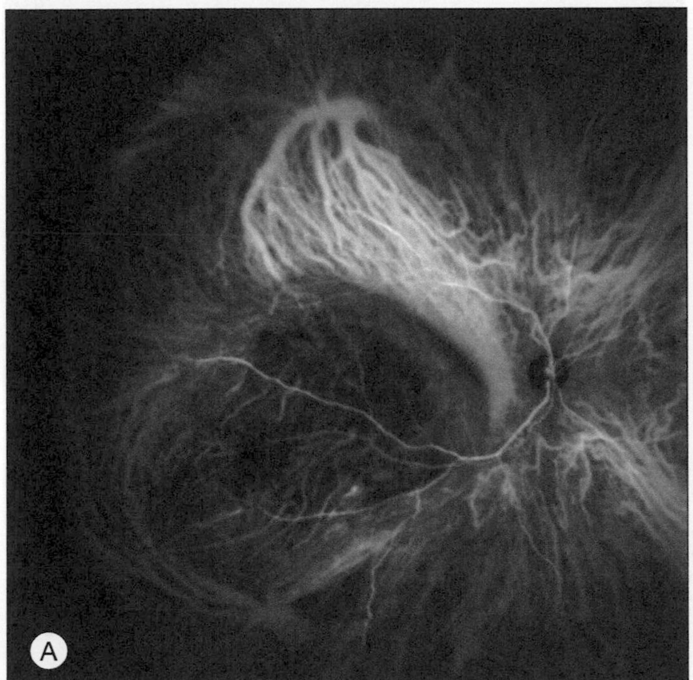

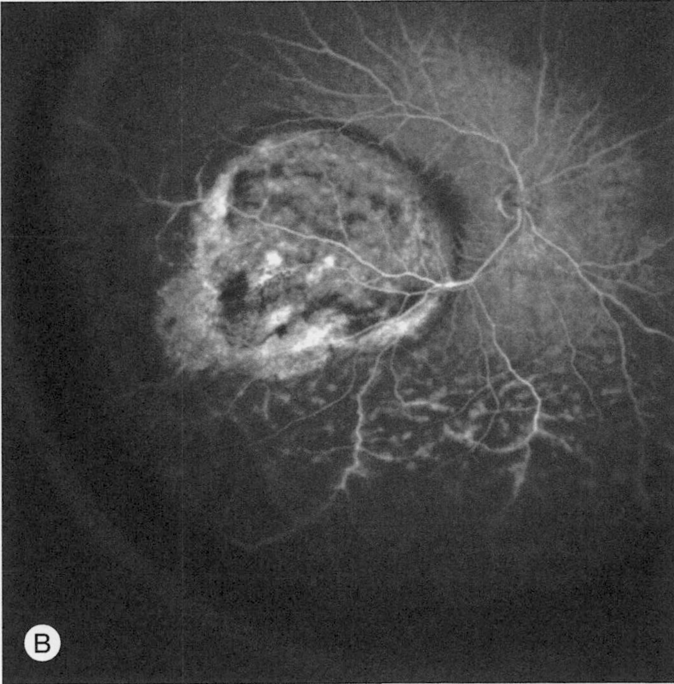

Fig. 2.21 A case of choroidal melanoma. Indocyanine green angiography (A) allows visualization of the tumor's intrinsic vasculature with irregular tortuosity and anarchic branching. Note the strong fluorescence within the large choroidal vessels around the lesion, a possible sign of increased flow due to the presence of the tumor. Melanoma-intrinsic vessels are leaky by fluorescein angiography (B), and therefore they cannot be identified with this diagnostic tool. In fluorescein angiographic images (B), in the inferior quadrant it is possible to visualize damage to retinal vessels with associated exudative detachment.

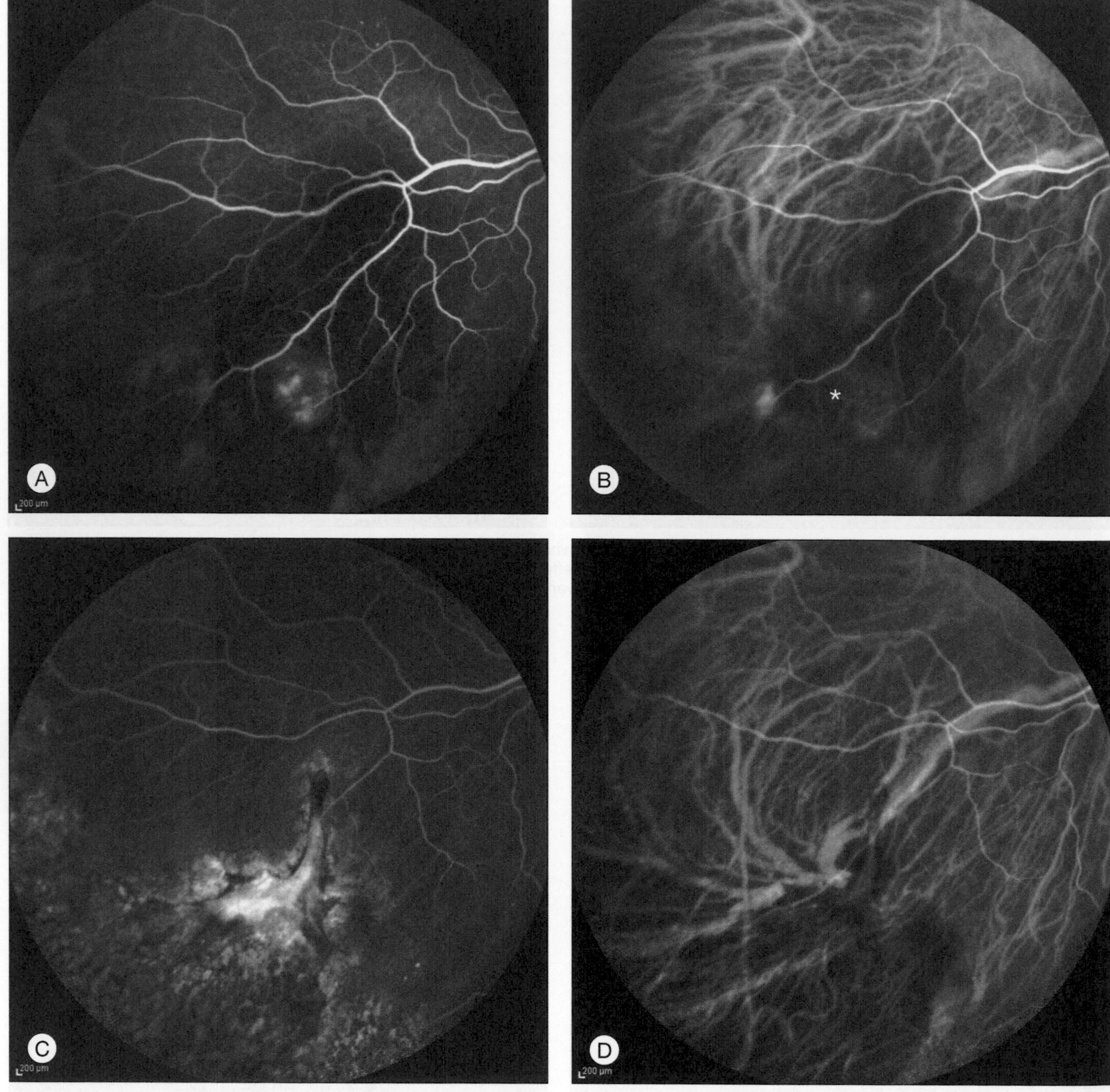

Fig. 2.22 A case of a midperipheral inferotemporal subretinal hemorrhage. Midphase fluorescein angiography showing a hyperfluorescent leaking spot within the hemorrhage (A). Note the diffuse peripheral changes consistent with variable degrees of retinal pigment epithelial hyperplasia or atrophy. Indocyanine green (ICG) angiography 31 seconds after injection (B): the choroidal neovascularization (CNV) is clearly outlined (asterisk). Six months after laser photocoagulation of the CNV: fluorescein (C) and ICG (D) angiographies reveal fibrosis of the CNV with late staining and no leakage.

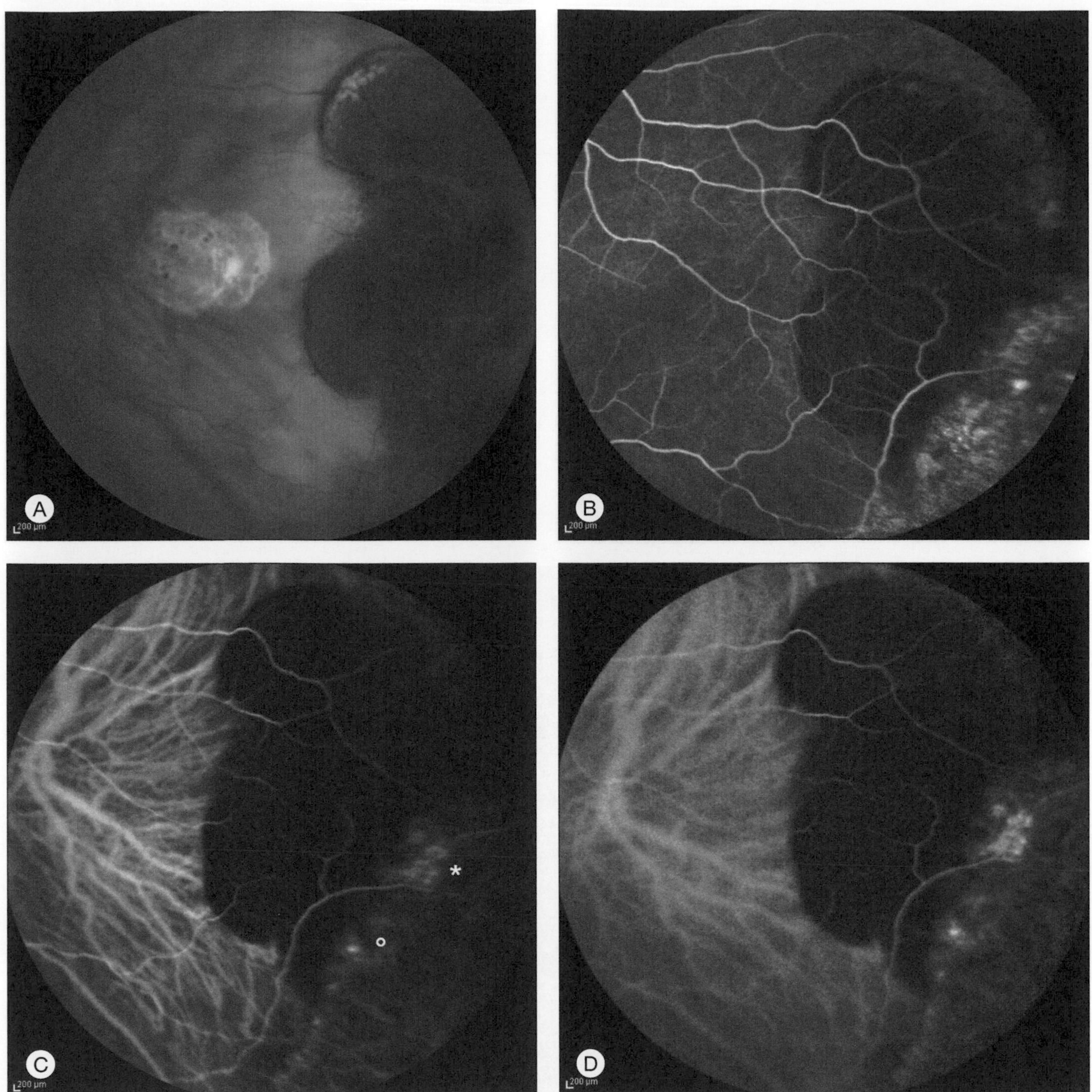

Fig. 2.23 Infrared image of a peripheral temporal subretinal hemorrhage (A). Midphase fluorescein angiography showing diffuse peripheral changes consistent with variable degrees of retinal pigment epithelium hyperplasia or atrophy. Typical features of choroidal neovascularization (CNV) are absent (B). Corresponding indocyanine green (ICG) angiography 2 minutes after injection (C): CNV is clearly visible (asterisk) while a second choroidal new vessel is suspected (circle). Six minutes after injection, ICG angiography shows progressive leakage from both areas (D).

Continued

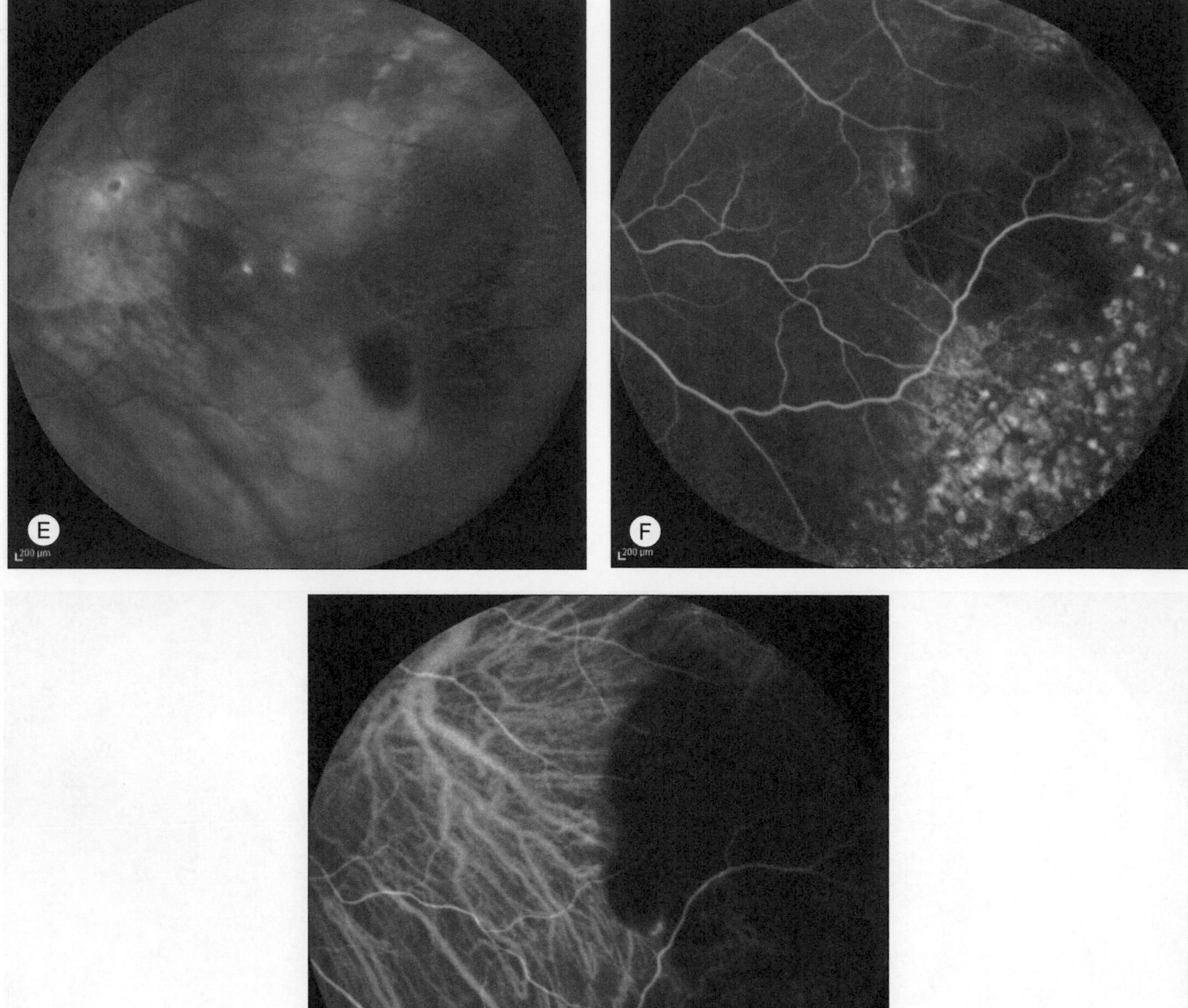

Fig. 2.23 Cont'd Infrared image 3 months after photodynamic therapy applied to the two leaking spots: the reabsorption of the subretinal hemorrhage is almost complete (E). Corresponding fluorescein (F) and ICG (G) angiograms reveal persistent obliteration of CNV with no late leakage.

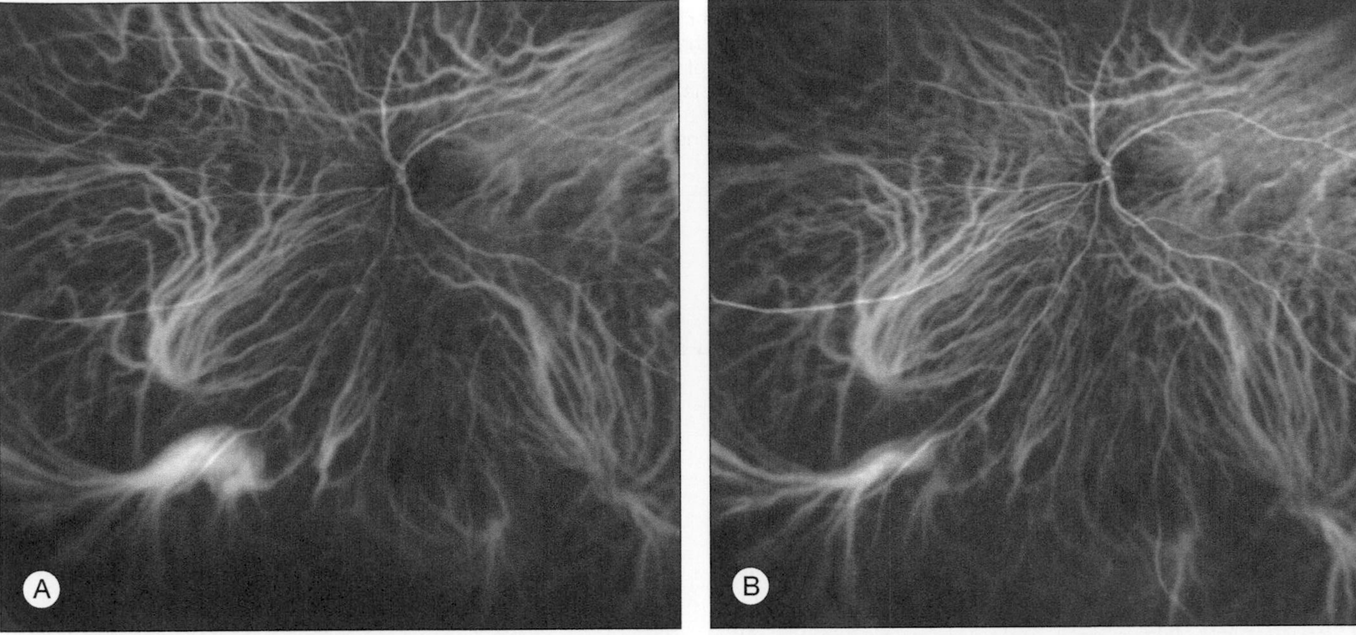

Fig. 2.24 Indocyanine green angiography in a case of varix of the vortex vein in the nasal equatorial region (A). Application of sufficient pressure on the globe readily collapses the varix (B).

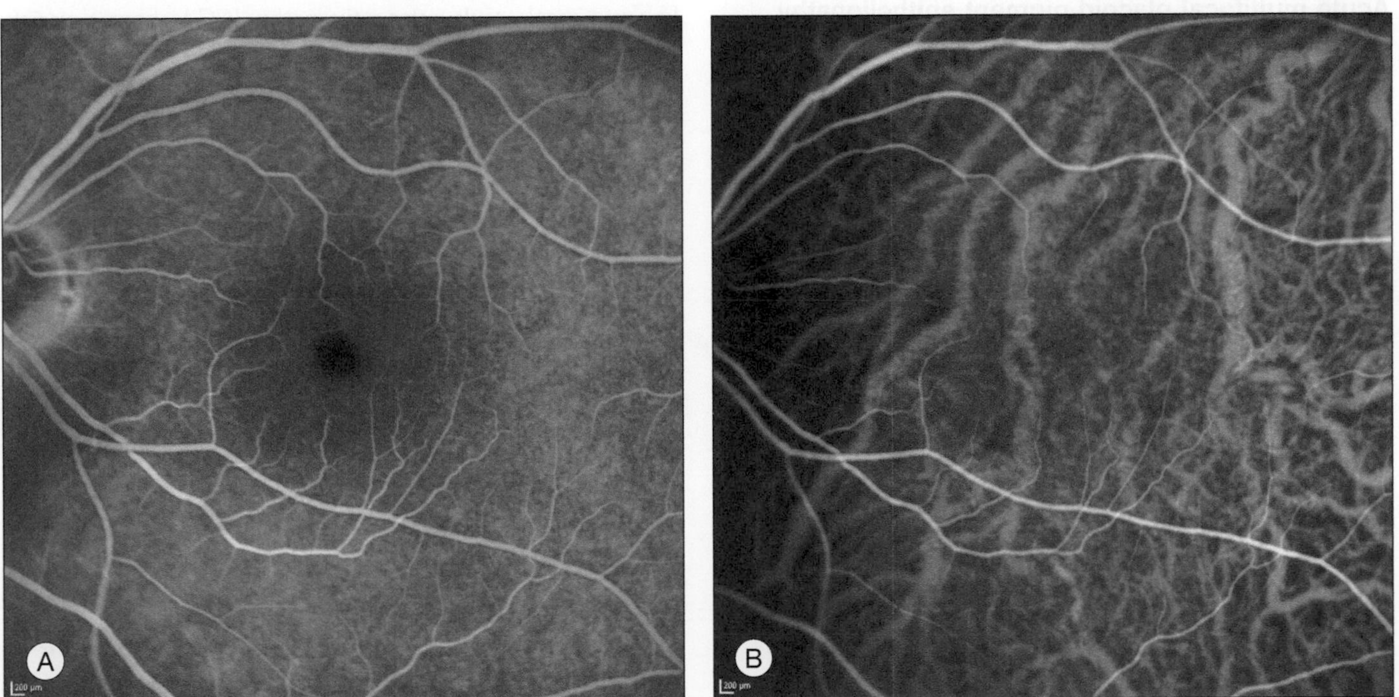

Fig. 2.25 A case of multiple evanescent white-dot syndrome. Late phases of the fluorescein angiogram reveal only mild alterations at the level of the outer retina and retinal pigment epithelium (A). Early phases of the indocyanine green angiogram (B) begin to reveal areas of hypofluorescence.

Continued

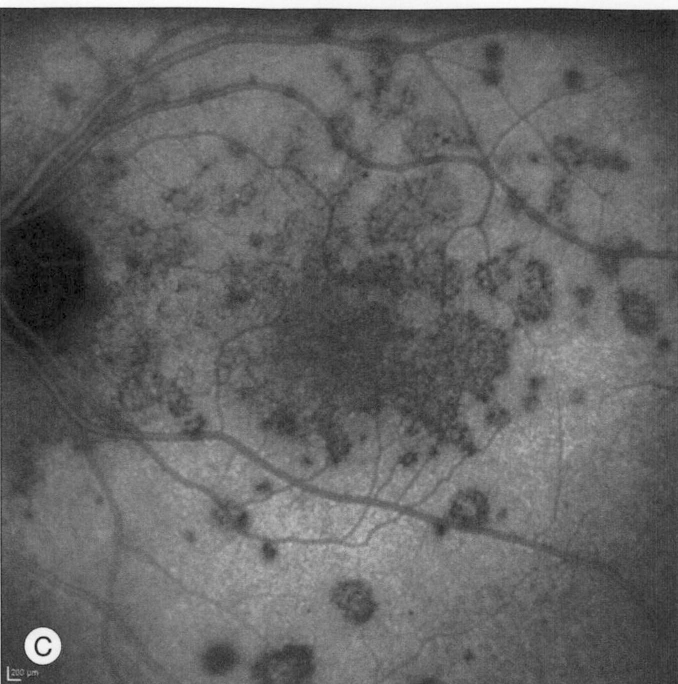

Fig. 2.25 Cont'd Areas of hypofluorescence become much more evident in the mid to late phases of the angiogram (C).

Acute multifocal placoid pigment epitheliopathy

ICG of acute posterior multifocal placoid pigment epitheliopathy (AMPPE) shows areas of hypofluorescence in both early and late phases that correlate with the placoid lesions. These lesions may be caused by choroidal hypoperfusion, secondary to occlusive vasculitis,[118] and ICGA often shows partial or complete resolution throughout the timecourse of the disease.[119] New, active and healed, inactive lesions in AMPPE can both be imaged and differentiated using ICGA.[120]

Serpiginous choroidopathy

ICG allows better staging and identification of active lesions in serpiginous chorioretinopathy.[121] The active phase of the pathology is characterized by hypofluorescent areas with poorly defined margins (Fig. 2.26). These findings can predict the active lesions observed by fluorescein angiography. The presence of late hyperfluorescence in ICG images represents a sign of choroidal hyperpermeability and may be associated with a more aggressive evolution of the disease. The healed lesions appear hypofluorescent with well-defined margins. The atrophy of the RPE and choriocapillaris allows better identification of large and medium-sized choroidal vessels.

Punctate inner chorioretinopathy

The subretinal lesions observed in punctate inner chorioretinopathy are visualized by ICG as hypofluorescent areas throughout all the phases of the angiogram.[122] These areas may correspond to localized choroidal hypoperfusion,[123] and are greater in number compared to fluorescein angiography.[124] Another finding in ICG images is the presence of hyperfluorescent points situated close to the vessel wall, representing a possible sign of vasculitis.[123]

Acute zonal occult outer retinopathy

In acute zonal occult outer retinopathy, ICGA shows a variety of patterns of presentations. Spaide reported that the peripapillary drusenoid material blocks the choroidal fluorescence in ICG and therefore the involved areas appear hypofluorescent.[125] The secondary atrophy of the choriocapillaris produces hypofluorescence as well, which does not affect the fluorescence from the underlying larger choroidal vessels.[125] In some cases, though,

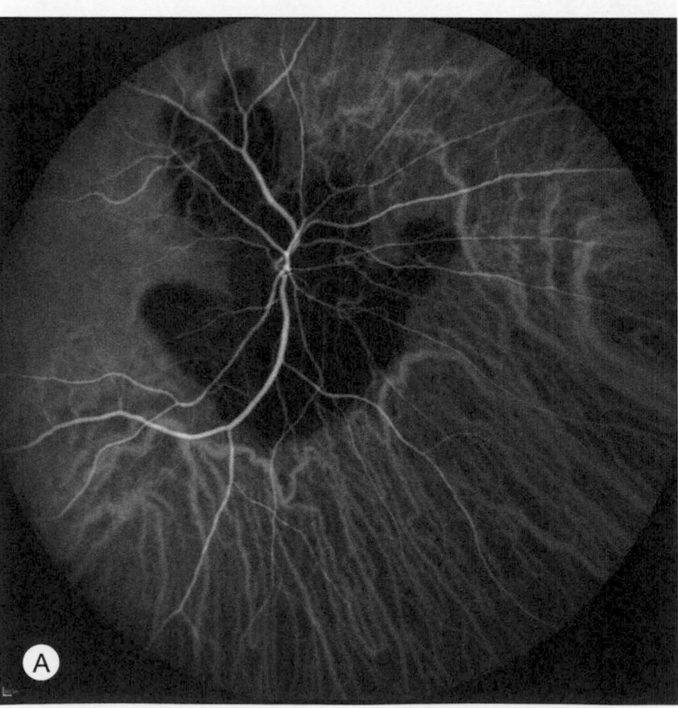

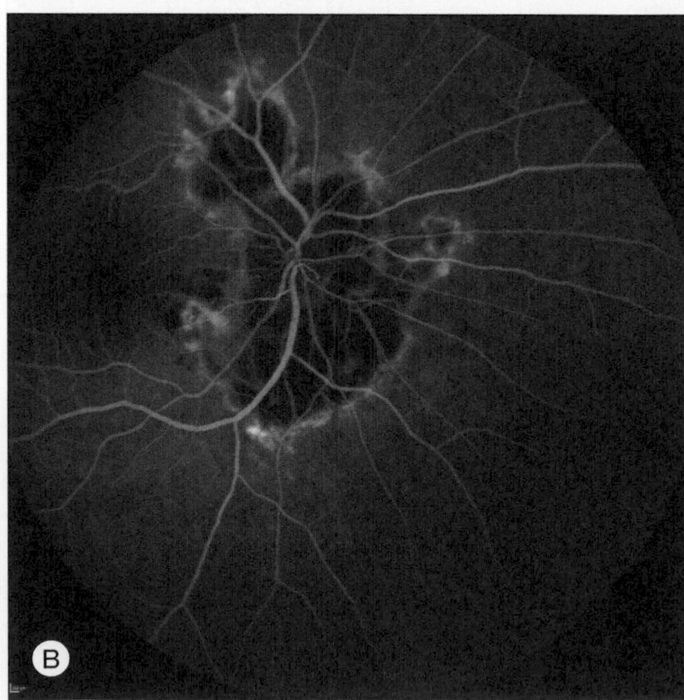

Fig. 2.26 A case of serpiginous chorioretinopathy. The lesion observed by indocyanine green angiography (A) occupies a greater extent than is evident on fluorescein angiography (B). This may indicate a progression of the pathology that can be anticipated or predicted using indocyanine green angiography.

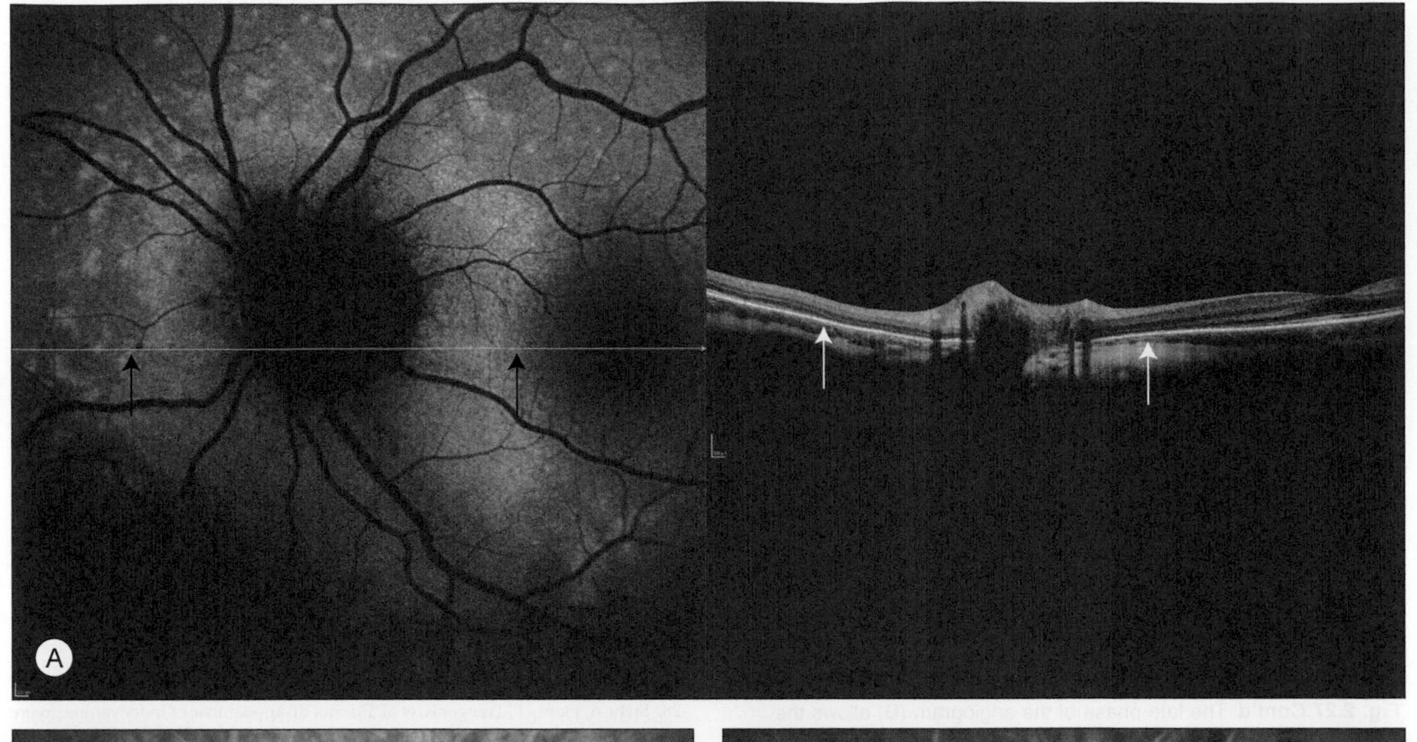

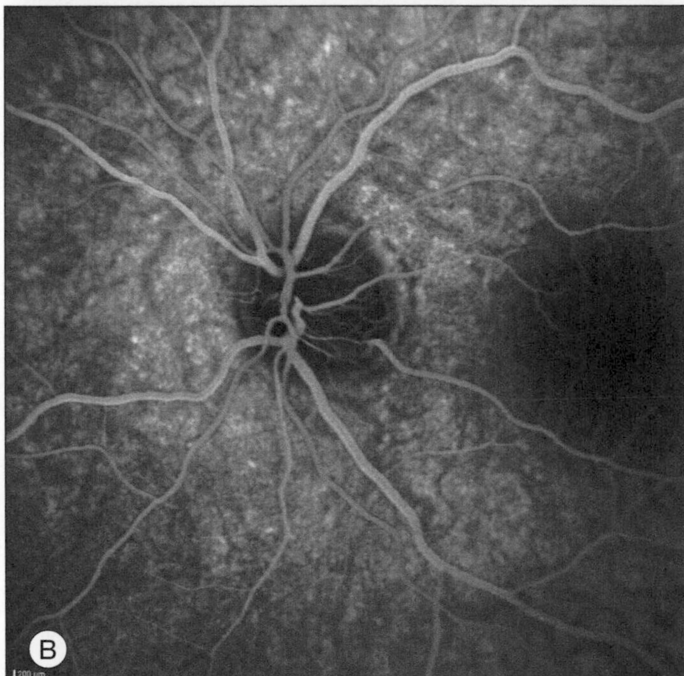

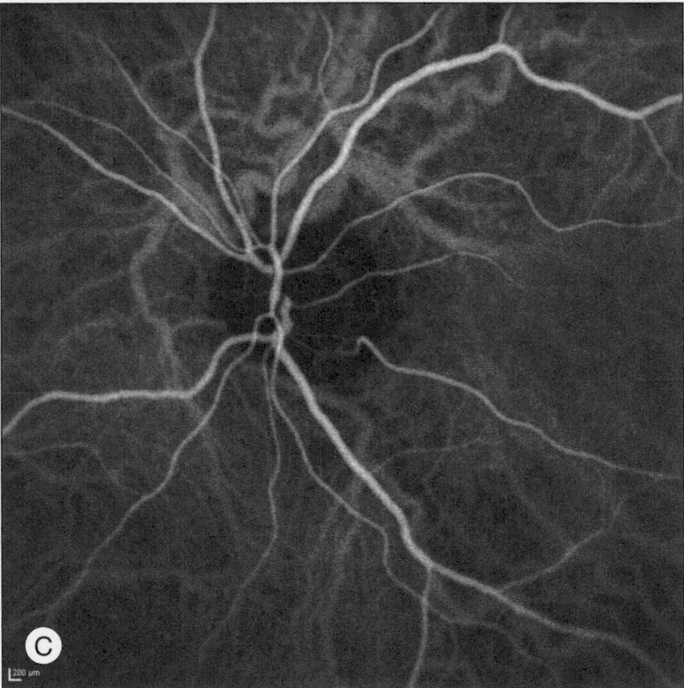

Fig. 2.27 A case of acute zonal occult outer retinopathy. Autofluorescence shows the typical features of this disorder, with hyperautofluorescent areas around the optic disc (A). Simultaneous spectral-domain optical coherence tomography suggests that these areas (black arrows) correspond to zones with loss of the outer segments of the photoreceptors (white arrows), thus resulting in less blockage of the autofluorescence originating from the retinal pigment epithelium. Fluorescein angiography shows increased fluorescence corresponding to these areas (B). Early phase of indocyanine green angiography (C) does not reveal alterations.

Continued

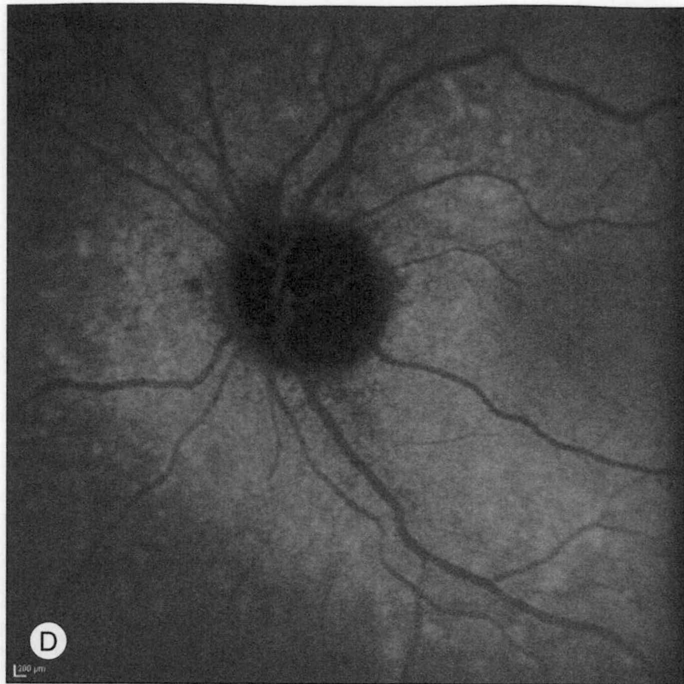

Fig. 2.27 Cont'd The late phase of the angiogram (D) allows the affected areas to be distinguished by increased fluorescence.

ICG may show an increase in fluorescence from the affected areas, due to the lack of photoreceptor outer segments and the minor blocking effect from this layer (Fig. 2.27).

CONCLUSIONS

In summary, despite the changing landscape of retinal disease therapeutics with an increased emphasis on pharmacotherapies, and the rise in prominence of noninvasive diagnostic technologies such as optical coherence tomography, ICGA remains an important tool in the diagnosis and management of a variety of retinal disorders.

REFERENCES

1. Cohen SY, Dubois L, Quentel G, et al. Is indocyanine green angiography still relevant? Retina 2011;31:209–21.
2. Ott P. Hepatic elimination of indocyanine green with special reference to distribution kinetics and the influence of plasma protein binding. Pharmacol Toxicol 1998;83(Suppl 2):1–48.
3. Fox IJ, Brooker LG, Heseltine DW, et al. A tricarbocyanine dye for continuous recording of dilution curves in whole blood independent of variations in blood oxygen saturation. Proc Staff Meet Mayo Clin 1957;32:478–84.
4. Fox IJ, Wood EH. Applications of dilution curves recorded from the right side of the heart or venous circulation with the aid of a new indicator dye. Proc Staff Meet Mayo Clin 1957;32:541–50.
5. Caesar J, Shaldon S, Chiandussi L, et al. The use of indocyanine green in the measurement of hepatic blood flow and as a test of hepatic function. Clin Sci 1961;21:43–57.
6. Hunton DB, Bollman JL, Hoffman HN. Studies of hepatic function with indocyanine green. Gastroenterology 1960;39:713–24.
7. Kogure K, Choromokos E. Infrared absorption angiography. J Appl Physiol 1969;26:154–7.
8. Kogure K, David NJ, Yamanouchi U, et al. Infrared absorption angiography of the fundus circulation. Arch Ophthalmol 1970;83:209–14.
9. Choromokos E, Kogure K, David NJ. Infrared absorption angiography. J Biol Photogr Assoc 1969;37:100–4.
10. Hochheimer BF. Angiography of the retina with indocyanine green. Arch Ophthalmol 1971;86:564–5.
11. Flower RW, Hochheimer BF. Clinical infrared absorption angiography of the choroid. Am J Ophthalmol 1972;73:458–9.
12. Hyvarinen L, Flower RW. Indocyanine green fluorescence angiography. Acta Ophthalmol (Copenh) 1980;58:528–38.
13. Hayashi K, de Laey JJ. Indocyanine green angiography of submacular choroidal vessels in the human eye. Ophthalmologica 1985;190:20–9.
14. Hayashi K, Hasegawa Y, Tokoro T. Indocyanine green angiography of central serous chorioretinopathy. Int Ophthalmol 1986;9:37–41.
15. Hasegawa Y, Hayashi K, Tokoro T, et al. [Clinical use of indocyanine green angiography in the diagnosis of choroidal neovascular diseases.] Fortschr Ophthalmol 1988;85:410–2.
16. Destro M, Puliafito CA. Indocyanine green videoangiography of choroidal neovascularization. Ophthalmology 1989;96:846–53.
17. Scheider A, Schroedel C. High resolution indocyanine green angiography with a scanning laser ophthalmoscope. Am J Ophthalmol 1989;108:458–9.
18. Guyer DR, Puliafito CA, Mones JM, et al. Digital indocyanine-green angiography in chorioretinal disorders. Ophthalmology 1992;99:287–91.
19. Yannuzzi LA, Slakter JS, Sorenson JA, et al. Digital indocyanine green videoangiography and choroidal neovascularization. Retina 1992;12:191–223.
20. Lutty GA. The acute intravenous toxicity of biological stains, dyes, and other fluorescent substances. Toxicol Appl Pharmacol 1978;44:225–49.
21. Tripp MR, Cohen GM, Gerasch DA, et al. Effect of protein and electrolyte on the spectral stabilization of concentrated solutions of indocyanine green. Proc Soc Exp Biol Med 1973;143:879–83.
22. Benya R, Quintana J, Brundage B. Adverse reactions to indocyanine green: a case report and a review of the literature. Cathet Cardiovasc Diagn 1989;17:231–3.
23. Bischoff PM, Flower RW. Ten years experience with choroidal angiography using indocyanine green dye: a new routine examination or an epilogue? Doc Ophthalmol 1985;60:235–91.
24. Flower RW, Hochheimer BF. Indocyanine green dye fluorescence and infrared absorption choroidal angiography performed simultaneously with fluorescein angiography. Johns Hopkins Med J 1976;138:33–42.
25. Geeraets WJ, Berry ER. Ocular spectral characteristics as related to hazards from lasers and other light sources. Am J Ophthalmol 1968;66:15–20.
26. Cherrick GR, Stein SW, Leevy CM, et al. Indocyanine green: observations on its physical properties, plasma decay, and hepatic extraction. J Clin Invest 1960;39:592–600.
27. Leevy CM, Bender J. Physiology of dye extraction by the liver: comparative studies of sulfobromophthalein and indocyanine green. Ann N Y Acad Sci 1963;111:161–76.
28. Stehr A, Ploner F, Traeger K, et al. Plasma disappearance of indocyanine green: a marker for excretory liver function? Intens Care Med 2005;31:1719–22.
29. Costa DL, Huang SJ, Orlock DA, et al. Retinal-choroidal indocyanine green dye clearance and liver dysfunction. Retina 2003;23:557–61.
30. Fineman MS, Maguire JI, Fineman SW, et al. Safety of indocyanine green angiography during pregnancy: a survey of the retina, macula, and vitreous societies. Arch Ophthalmol 2001;119:353–5.
31. Hope-Ross M, Yannuzzi LA, Gragoudas ES, et al. Adverse reactions due to indocyanine green. Ophthalmology 1994;101:529–33.
32. Speich R, Saesseli B, Hoffmann U, et al. Anaphylactoid reactions after indocyanine-green administration. Ann Intern Med 1988;109:345–6.
33. Michie DD, Wombolt DG, Carretta RF, et al. Adverse reactions associated with the administration of a tricarbocyanine dye (Cardio-Green) to uremic patients. J Allergy Clin Immunol 1971;48:235–9.
34. Iseki K, Onoyama K, Fujimi S, et al. Shock caused by indocyanine green dye in chronic hemodialysis patients. Clin Nephrol 1980;14:210.
35. Robson SC, Mutch E, Boys RJ, et al. Apparent liver blood flow during pregnancy: a serial study using indocyanine green clearance. Br J Obstet Gynaecol 1990;97:720–4.
36. Flower RW, Csaky KG, Murphy RP. Disparity between fundus camera and scanning laser ophthalmoscope indocyanine green imaging of retinal pigment epithelium detachments. Retina 1998;18:260–8.
37. Wolf S, Wald KJ, Elsner AE, et al. Indocyanine green choroidal videoangiography: a comparison of imaging analysis with the scanning laser ophthalmoscope and the fundus camera. Retina 1993;13:266–9.
38. Stanga PE, Lim JI, Hamilton P. Indocyanine green angiography in chorioretinal diseases: indications and interpretation: an evidence-based update. Ophthalmology 2003;110:15–21; quiz 22-3.
39. Yannuzzi LA, Flower RW, Slakter JS. Indocyanine green angiography. St Louis: Mosby Year Book; 1997. p. 46.
40. Hayreh SS. Physiological anatomy of the choroidal vascular bed. Int Ophthalmol 1983;6:85–93.
41. Mutoh T, Sakurai M, Tamai M. Indocyanine green fundus angiography of retrobulbar vasculature. Arch Ophthalmol 1995;113:631–3.
42. Ohno-Matsui K, Morishima N, Ito M, et al. Indocyanine green angiography of retrobulbar vascular structures in severe myopia. Am J Ophthalmol 1997;123:494–505.
43. Gass JD. Biomicroscopic and histopathologic considerations regarding the feasibility of surgical excision of subfoveal neovascular membranes. Am J Ophthalmol 1994;118:285–98.
44. Macular Photocoagulation Study Group. Subfoveal neovascular lesions in age-related macular degeneration. Guidelines for evaluation and treatment in the macular photocoagulation study. Arch Ophthalmol 1991;109:1242–57.
45. Sadda SR, Liakopoulos S, Keane PA, et al. Relationship between angiographic and optical coherence tomographic (OCT) parameters for quantifying choroidal neovascular lesions. Graefes Arch Clin Exp Ophthalmol 2010;248:175–84.
46. Freund KB, Ho IV, Barbazetto IA, et al. Type 3 neovascularization: the expanded spectrum of retinal angiomatous proliferation. Retina 2008;28: 201–11.
47. Olsen TW, Feng X, Kasper TJ, et al. Fluorescein angiographic lesion type frequency in neovascular age-related macular degeneration. Ophthalmology 2004;111:250–5.
48. Guyer DR, Yannuzzi LA, Slakter JS, et al. Classification of choroidal neovascularization by digital indocyanine green videoangiography. Ophthalmology 1996;103:2054–60.

49. Yannuzzi LA, Hope-Ross M, Slakter JS, et al. Analysis of vascularized pigment epithelial detachments using indocyanine green videoangiography. Retina 1994;14:99–113.
50. Brown DM, Kaiser PK, Michels M, et al. Ranibizumab versus verteporfin for neovascular age-related macular degeneration. N Engl J Med 2006;355:1432–44.
51. Rosenfeld PJ, Brown DM, Heier JS, et al. Ranibizumab for neovascular age-related macular degeneration. N Engl J Med 2006;355:1419–31.
52. Massacesi AL, Sacchi L, Bergamini F, et al. The prevalence of retinal angiomatous proliferation in age-related macular degeneration with occult choroidal neovascularization. Graefes Arch Clin Exp Ophthalmol 2008;246:89–92.
53. Lim JI, Aaberg TM, Capone AJ, et al. Indocyanine green angiography-guided photocoagulation of choroidal neovascularization associated with retinal pigment epithelial detachment. Am J Ophthalmol 1997;123:524–32.
54. Watzke RC, Klein ML, Hiner CJ, et al. A comparison of stereoscopic fluorescein angiography with indocyanine green videoangiography in age-related macular degeneration. Ophthalmology 2000;107:1601–6.
55. Shiraga F, Ojima Y, Matsuo T, et al. Feeder vessel photocoagulation of subfoveal choroidal neovascularization secondary to age-related macular degeneration. Ophthalmology 1998;105:662–9.
56. Staurenghi G, Orzalesi N, La Capria A, et al. Laser treatment of feeder vessels in subfoveal choroidal neovascular membranes: a revisitation using dynamic indocyanine green angiography. Ophthalmology 1998;105:2297–305.
57. Bottoni F, Massacesi A, Cigada M, et al. Treatment of retinal angiomatous proliferation in age-related macular degeneration: a series of 104 cases of retinal angiomatous proliferation. Arch Ophthalmol 2005;123:1644–50.
58. Flower RW. Optimizing treatment of choroidal neovascularization feeder vessels associated with age-related macular degeneration. Am J Ophthalmol 2002;134:228–39.
59. Semoun O, Guigui B, Tick S, et al. Infrared features of classic choroidal neovascularisation in exudative age-related macular degeneration. Br J Ophthalmol 2009;93:182–5.
60. Schmidt-Erfurth U, Kriechbaum K, Oldag A. Three-dimensional angiography of classic and occult lesion types in choroidal neovascularization. Invest Ophthalmol Vis Sci 2007;48:1751–60.
61. Hlushchuk R, Baum O, Gruber G, et al. The synergistic action of a VEGF-receptor tyrosine-kinase inhibitor and a sensitizing PDGF-receptor blocker depends upon the stage of vascular maturation. Microcirculation 2007;14:813–25.
62. Yannuzzi LA, Negrao S, Iida T, et al. Retinal angiomatous proliferation in age-related macular degeneration. Retina 2001;21:416–34.
63. Gass JD, Agarwal A, Lavina AM, et al. Focal inner retinal hemorrhages in patients with drusen: an early sign of occult choroidal neovascularization and chorioretinal anastomosis. Retina 2003;23:741–51.
64. Hartnett ME, Weiter JJ, Staurenghi G, et al. Deep retinal vascular anomalous complexes in advanced age-related macular degeneration. Ophthalmology 1996;103:2042–53.
65. Viola F, Massacesi A, Orzalesi N, et al. Retinal angiomatous proliferation: natural history and progression of visual loss. Retina 2009;29:732–9.
66. Rouvas AA, Papakostas TD, Vavvas D, et al. Intravitreal ranibizumab, intravitreal ranibizumab with PDT, and intravitreal triamcinolone with PDT for the treatment of retinal angiomatous proliferation: a prospective study. Retina 2009;29:536–44.
67. Saito M, Shiragami C, Shiraga F, et al. Comparison of intravitreal triamcinolone acetonide with photodynamic therapy and intravitreal bevacizumab with photodynamic therapy for retinal angiomatous proliferation. Am J Ophthalmol 2010;149:472–81.e1.
68. Bottoni F, Romano M, Massacesi A, et al. Remodeling of the vascular channels in retinal angiomatous proliferations treated with intravitreal triamcinolone acetonide and photodynamic therapy. Graefes Arch Clin Exp Ophthalmol 2006;244:1528–33.
69. Yannuzzi LA, Sorenson J, Spaide RF, et al. Idiopathic polypoidal choroidal vasculopathy (IPCV). Retina 1990;10:1–8.
70. Spaide RF, Yannuzzi LA, Slakter JS, et al. Indocyanine green videoangiography of idiopathic polypoidal choroidal vasculopathy. Retina 1995;15:100–10.
71. Yannuzzi LA, Wong DW, Sforzolini BS, et al. Polypoidal choroidal vasculopathy and neovascularized age-related macular degeneration. Arch Ophthalmol 1999;117:1503–10.
72. Ahuja RM, Stanga PE, Vingerling JR, et al. Polypoidal choroidal vasculopathy in exudative and haemorrhagic pigment epithelial detachments. Br J Ophthalmol 2000;84:479–84.
73. Ciardella AP, Donsoff IM, Huang SJ, et al. Polypoidal choroidal vasculopathy. Surv Ophthalmol 2004;49:25–37.
74. Ahuja RM, Downes SM, Stanga PE, et al. Polypoidal choroidal vasculopathy and central serous chorioretinopathy. Ophthalmology 2001;108:1009–10.
75. Yannuzzi LA, Freund KB, Goldbaum M, et al. Polypoidal choroidal vasculopathy masquerading as central serous chorioretinopathy. Ophthalmology 2000;107:767–77.
76. Maruko I, Iida T, Saito M, et al. Combined cases of polypoidal choroidal vasculopathy and typical age-related macular degeneration. Graefes Arch Clin Exp Ophthalmol 2010;248:361–8.
77. Lai TY, Chan WM, Liu DT, et al. Intravitreal bevacizumab (Avastin) with or without photodynamic therapy for the treatment of polypoidal choroidal vasculopathy. Br J Ophthalmol 2008;92:661–6.
78. Eandi CM, Ober MD, Freund KB, et al. Selective photodynamic therapy for neovascular age-related macular degeneration with polypoidal choroidal neovascularization. Retina 2007;27:825–31.
79. Guyer DR, Yannuzzi LA, Slakter JS, et al. Digital indocyanine green videoangiography of central serous chorioretinopathy. Arch Ophthalmol 1994;112:1057–62.
80. Yannuzzi LA, Slakter JS, Gross NE, et al. Indocyanine green angiography-guided photodynamic therapy for treatment of chronic central serous chorioretinopathy: a pilot study. Retina 2003;23:288–98.
81. Piccolino FC, Borgia L. Central serous chorioretinopathy and indocyanine green angiography. Retina 1994;14:231–42.
82. Spaide RF, Hall L, Haas A, et al. Indocyanine green videoangiography of older patients with central serous chorioretinopathy. Retina 1996;16:203–13.
83. Shiraki K, Moriwaki M, Matsumoto M, et al. Long-term follow-up of severe central serous chorioretinopathy using indocyanine green angiography. Int Ophthalmol 1997;21:245–53.
84. Lafaut BA, Salati C, Priem H, et al. Indocyanine green angiography is of value for the diagnosis of chronic central serous chorioretinopathy in elderly patients. Graefes Arch Clin Exp Ophthalmol 1998;236:513–21.
85. Reibaldi M, Cardascia N, Longo A, et al. Standard-fluence versus low-fluence photodynamic therapy in chronic central serous chorioretinopathy: a nonrandomized clinical trial. Am J Ophthalmol 2010;149:307–15.e2.
86. Chan WM, Lam DS, Lai TY, et al. Choroidal vascular remodelling in central serous chorioretinopathy after indocyanine green guided photodynamic therapy with verteporfin: a novel treatment at the primary disease level. Br J Ophthalmol 2003;87:1453–8.
87. Inoue R, Sawa M, Tsujikawa M, et al. Association between the efficacy of photodynamic therapy and indocyanine green angiography findings for central serous chorioretinopathy. Am J Ophthalmol 2010;149:441–6.e1-2.
88. Tsujikawa A, Ojima Y, Yamashiro K, et al. Punctate hyperfluorescent spots associated with central serous chorioretinopathy as seen on indocyanine green angiography. Retina 2010;30:801–9.
89. Kitaya N, Nagaoka T, Hikichi T, et al. Features of abnormal choroidal circulation in central serous chorioretinopathy. Br J Ophthalmol 2003;87:709–12.
90. Prunte C, Flammer J. Choroidal capillary and venous congestion in central serous chorioretinopathy. Am J Ophthalmol 1996;121:26–34.
91. Anand R, Augsburger JJ, Shields JA. Circumscribed choroidal hemangiomas. Arch Ophthalmol 1989;107:1338–42.
92. Shields CL, Honavar SG, Shields JA, et al. Circumscribed choroidal hemangioma: clinical manifestations and factors predictive of visual outcome in 200 consecutive cases. Ophthalmology 2001;108:2237–48.
93. Witschel H, Font RL. Hemangioma of the choroid. A clinicopathologic study of 71 cases and a review of the literature. Surv Ophthalmol 1976;20:415–31.
94. Singh AD, Kaiser PK, Sears JE. Choroidal hemangioma. Ophthalmol Clin North Am 2005;18:151–61. ix.
95. Arevalo JF, Shields CL, Shields JA, et al. Circumscribed choroidal hemangioma: characteristic features with indocyanine green videoangiography. Ophthalmology 2000;107:344–50.
96. Shields CL, Shields JA, De Potter P. Patterns of indocyanine green videoangiography of choroidal tumours. Br J Ophthalmol 1995;79:237–45.
97. Sallet G, Amoaku WM, Lafaut BA, et al. Indocyanine green angiography of choroidal tumors. Graefes Arch Clin Exp Ophthalmol 1995;233:677–89.
98. Andersen MV, Scherfig E, Prause JU. Differential diagnosis of choroidal melanomas and nevi using scanning laser ophthalmoscopical indocyanine green angiography. Acta Ophthalmol Scand 1995;73:453–6.
99. Mueller AJ, Bartsch DU, Folberg R, et al. Imaging the microvasculature of choroidal melanomas with confocal indocyanine green scanning laser ophthalmoscopy. Arch Ophthalmol 1998;116:31–9.
100. Frenkel S, Barzel I, Levy J, et al. Demonstrating circulation in vasculogenic mimicry patterns of uveal melanoma by confocal indocyanine green angiography. Eye (Lond) 2008;22:948–52.
101. Mueller AJ, Freeman WR, Schaller UC, et al. Complex microcirculation patterns detected by confocal indocyanine green angiography predict time to growth of small choroidal melanocytic tumors: MuSIC Report II. Ophthalmology 2002;109:2207–14.
102. Schaller UC, Mueller AJ, Bartsch DU, et al. Choroidal melanoma microcirculation with confocal indocyanine green angiography before and 1 year after radiation brachytherapy. Retina 2000;20:627–32.
103. Krause L, Bechrakis NE, Heinrich S, et al. Indocyanine green angiography and fluorescein angiography of malignant choroidal melanomas following proton beam irradiation. Graefes Arch Clin Exp Ophthalmol 2005;243:545–50.
104. Midena E, Pilotto E, de Belvis V et al. Choroidal vascular changes after transpupillary thermotherapy for choroidal melanoma. Ophthalmology 2003;110:2216–22.
105. Annesley WHJ. Peripheral exudative hemorrhagic chorioretinopathy. Trans Am Ophthalmol Soc 1980;78:321–64.
106. Shields CL, Salazar PF, Mashayekhi A, et al. Peripheral exudative hemorrhagic chorioretinopathy simulating choroidal melanoma in 173 eyes. Ophthalmology 2009;116:529–35.
107. Gunduz K, Shields CL, Shields JA. Varix of the vortex vein ampulla simulating choroidal melanoma: report of four cases. Retina 1998;18:343–7.
108. Rutnin U. Fundus appearance in normal eyes. I. The choroid. Am J Ophthalmol 1967;64:821–39.
109. Osher RH, Abrams GW, Yarian D, et al. Varix of the vortex ampulla. Am J Ophthalmol 1981;92:653–60.
110. Singh AD, De Potter P, Shields CL, et al. Indocyanine green angiography and ultrasonography of a varix of vortex vein. Arch Ophthalmol 1993;111:1283–4.
111. Gross NE, Yannuzzi LA, Freund KB, et al. Multiple evanescent white dot syndrome. Arch Ophthalmol 2006;124:493–500.

112. Dell'omo R, Wong R, Marino M, et al. Relationship between different fluorescein and indocyanine green angiography features in multiple evanescent white dot syndrome. Br J Ophthalmol 2010;94:59–63.
113. Tsukamoto E, Yamada T, Kadoi C, et al. Hypofluorescent spots on indocyanine green angiography at the recovery stage in multiple evanescent white dot syndrome. Ophthalmologica 1999;213:336–8.
114. Slakter JS, Giovannini A, Yannuzzi LA, et al. Indocyanine green angiography of multifocal choroiditis. Ophthalmology 1997;104:1813–9.
115. Fardeau C, Herbort CP, Kullmann N, et al. Indocyanine green angiography in birdshot chorioretinopathy. Ophthalmology 1999;106:1928–34.
116. Howe LJ, Stanford MR, Graham EM, et al. Choroidal abnormalities in birdshot chorioretinopathy: an indocyanine green angiography study. Eye (Lond) 1997;11:554–9.
117. Trinh L, Bodaghi B, Fardeau C, et al. Clinical features, treatment methods, and evolution of birdshot chorioretinopathy in 5 different families. Am J Ophthalmol 2009;147:1042–7. 1047.e1.
118. Park D, Schatz H, McDonald HR, et al. Indocyanine green angiography of acute multifocal posterior placoid pigment epitheliopathy. Ophthalmology 1995;102:1877–83.
119. Howe LJ, Woon H, Graham EM, et al. Choroidal hypoperfusion in acute posterior multifocal placoid pigment epitheliopathy. An indocyanine green angiography study. Ophthalmology 1995;102:790–8.
120. Schneider U, Inhoffen W, Gelisken F. Indocyanine green angiography in a case of unilateral recurrent posterior acute multifocal placoid pigment epitheliopathy. Acta Ophthalmol Scand 2003;81:72–5.
121. Giovannini A, Mariotti C, Ripa E, et al. Indocyanine green angiographic findings in serpiginous choroidopathy. Br J Ophthalmol 1996;80:536–40.
122. Amer R, Lois N. Punctate inner choroidopathy. Surv Ophthalmol 2011;56:36–53.
123. Tiffin PA, Maini R, Roxburgh ST, et al. Indocyanine green angiography in a case of punctate inner choroidopathy. Br J Ophthalmol 1996;80:90–1.
124. Levy J, Shneck M, Klemperer I, et al. Punctate inner choroidopathy: resolution after oral steroid treatment and review of the literature. Can J Ophthalmol 2005;40:605–8.
125. Spaide RF. Collateral damage in acute zonal occult outer retinopathy. Am J Ophthalmol 2004;138:887–9.

Chapter 3

Optical Coherence Tomography

Carlos Alexandre de Amorim Garcia Filho, Zohar Yehoshua, Giovanni Gregori, Carmen A. Puliafito, Philip J. Rosenfeld

PHYSICAL PRINCIPLES OF OPTICAL COHERENCE TOMOGRAPHY

During the past two decades, optical coherence tomography (OCT) has become an essential tool in ophthalmology. Its ability to image detailed ocular structures noninvasively in vivo with high resolution has revolutionized patient care.[1,2] OCT technology is based on the principle of low-coherence interferometry, where a low-coherence (high-bandwidth) light beam is directed on to the target tissue and the scattered back-reflected light is combined with a second beam (reference beam), which was split off from the original light beam. The resulting interference patterns are used to reconstruct an axial A-scan, which represents the scattering properties of the tissue along the beam path. Moving the beam of light along the tissue in a line results in a compilation of A-scans with each A-scan having a different incidence point. From all these A-scans, a two-dimensional cross-sectional image of the target tissue can be reconstructed and this is known as a B-scan.

Typically OCT instruments use an infrared light source centered at a wavelength of about 840 nm. For a given wavelength, the axial resolution is dictated by the bandwidth of the light source. The latest commercial instruments typically have an axial resolution of approximately 5 μm, while research instruments have been built with a resolution as high as approximately 2 μm.[1] The lateral resolution is limited by the diffraction caused by the pupil and it is normally about 20 μm. For clinical purposes, the image acquisition time is limited by the patient's ability to avoid eye movements, i.e., less than 2 seconds in the typical patient. The instrument's scanning speed (number of A-scans acquired per second) is then the crucial parameter determining the amount of data available for a single OCT dataset.

The early OCT instruments, known as time domain OCT (TD-OCT), used a single photo detector, and an A-scan was created by moving a mirror to change the optical path of the reference beam in order to match different axial depths in the target tissue. This setup limited the scanning speed to a few thousand A-scans per second. A newer technique, known as spectral domain OCT (SD-OCT), Fourier domain OCT (FD-OCT), or high-definition OCT (HD-OCT), is able to acquire an entire A-scan by using an array of detectors instead of using multiple reference beams from a moving mirror. Scanning speeds with SD-OCT instruments can exceed 100000 A-scans per second, about 200 times faster than TD-OCT. Currently available SD-OCT commercial systems operate at a scanning rate of approximately 27000 A-scans per second.[1]

The scanning pattern with the commercial TD-OCT instrument (Stratus OCT, Carl Zeiss Meditec, Dublin, CA) incorporated six radial, concentric, 6-mm-long B-scans centered on the fovea. With the recent development of high-speed SD-OCT systems, several novel and important imaging strategies have been introduced based on acquiring three-dimensional datasets and B-scan averaging (Fig. 3.1).

Three-dimensional datasets are obtained using a dense two-dimensional raster array over a relatively large retinal region. The resulting datasets can be rendered as a volume image in three dimensions and can be analyzed by showing two-dimensional slices (i.e., sequences of parallel B-scans). Three-dimensional datasets give detailed information about the retinal structure over large areas. In addition, it is possible to generate en face fundus-like images directly from the OCT datasets. These OCT fundus images (OFIs) provide an accurate spatial colocalization of retinal features observed on the en face and cross-sectional images. Therefore, exact correlations can be achieved between the retinal cross-sectional geometry seen on the OCT B-scans and the retinal landmarks seen on en face images, known as the OFI. The potential exists for registration between several SD-OCT datasets of the same eye and images obtained using other imaging modalities, such as color fundus photography, fluorescein angiography, and fundus autofluorescence imaging. This holds the promise for an unprecedented ability

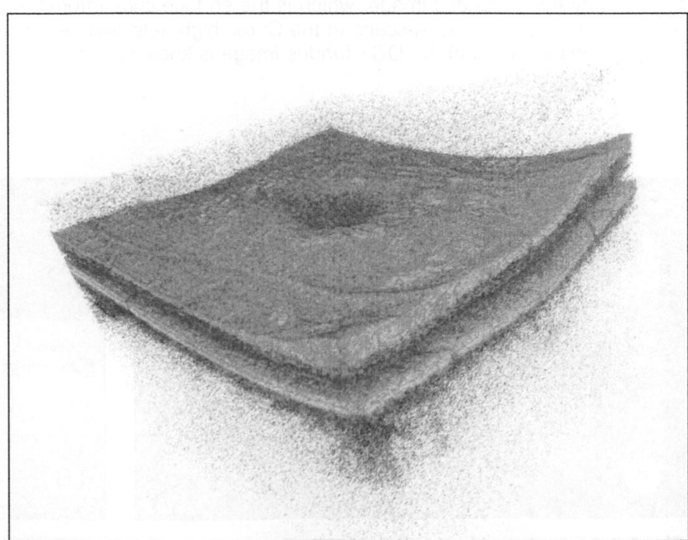

Fig. 3.1 Three-dimensional dataset. (Courtesy of Cirrus HD-OCT, Carl Zeiss Meditec, Dublin, CA.)

to describe and monitor changes in the local geometry of the retina.[3] In addition to the OFI generated by a full OCT dataset, partial OFIs (or slabs) can be generated to produce en face renderings that correspond to particular retinal layers or features.[4] These slabs can be very useful to visualize and quantify specific pathologies (Fig. 3.2).

The scanning speed of SD-OCT can also be used to produce very high-quality individual B-scan images through a combination of high sampling density and image averaging. One of the main factors affecting the perceived quality of OCT images is noise, in particular the speckle noise which is responsible for the characteristic "granular" appearance of OCT. Noise can be reduced through the acquisition, registration, and averaging of a number of B-scans at approximately the same retinal position (Fig. 3.3).

Although en face registration and B-scan averaging strategies can be implemented in many ways, a particularly powerful and flexible solution is the use of a built-in laser eye-tracking system. The main limitation of this approach is that the necessary acquisition times can become very long and sometimes unmanageable, particularly for large raster scans and for subjects with poor fixation.

Recently, different companies have invested in research in the field of retinal imaging, especially in the development and improvement of SD-OCT. It is not an objective of this section to discuss the differences between each of the currently available instruments since these instruments are continuously evolving. Table 3.1 lists currently available instruments.

QUANTITATIVE ANALYSIS OF OCT DATASETS

A crucial step towards a clinically useful, quantitative understanding of the retinal anatomy is the development of accurate, robust, reproducible segmentation algorithms that can automatically identify the boundaries between specific retinal layers and/or other retinal features. The currently available SD-OCT instruments have several advantages over the previous generation of TD-OCT instruments. SD-OCT instruments generally have a higher axial resolution and can produce B-scans with better image quality by increasing the A-scan density and through averaging techniques. Much more importantly, the higher scanning speed made possible by the SD-OCT technology reduces the effect of artifacts associated with eye motion and produces images that provide a true picture of the retinal geometry. The large, dense raster scans make it possible to obtain detailed surfaces of individual retina layers over large areas, resulting in segmentation maps. These maps allow for an

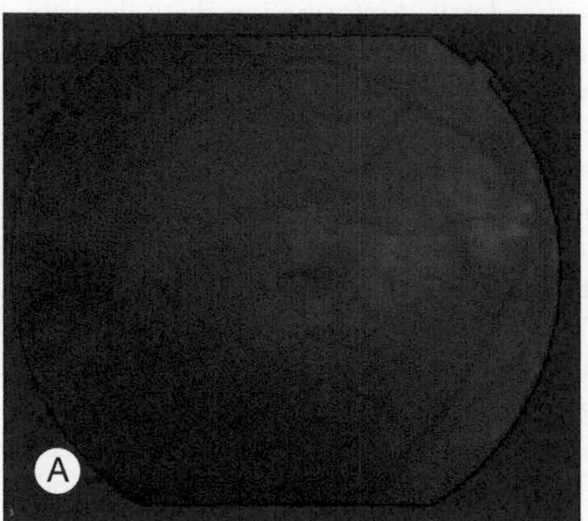

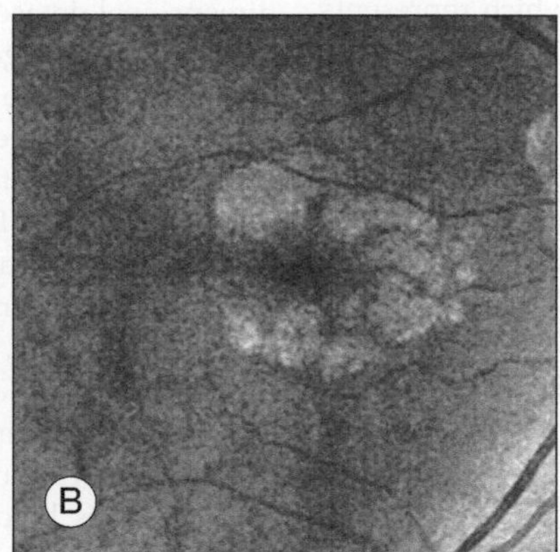

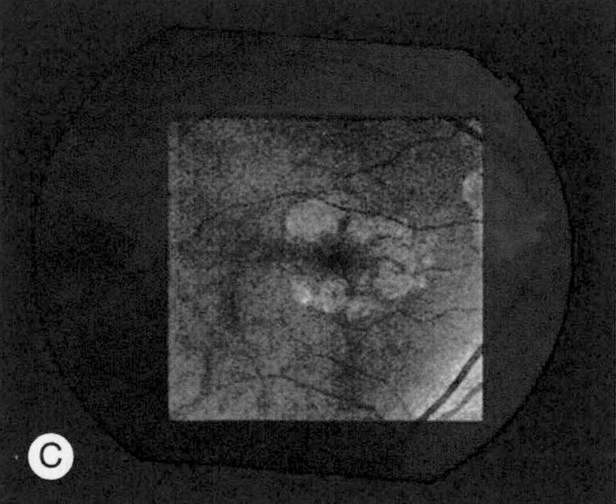

Fig. 3.2 (A) Color fundus image of a patient with geographic atrophy secondary to age-related macular degeneration. (B) Optical coherence tomography (OCT) fundus image, which is the en face image from the reflected light from each A-scan, of the same patient obtained with a scan pattern of 200 × 200 A-scans in the Cirrus high-definition OCT instrument. (C) Registration of the color fundus image with the OCT fundus image. Since the area of the OCT fundus image is known to be 6 × 6 mm, it is possible to quantify lesion area and calibrate the fundus camera to use this technique.

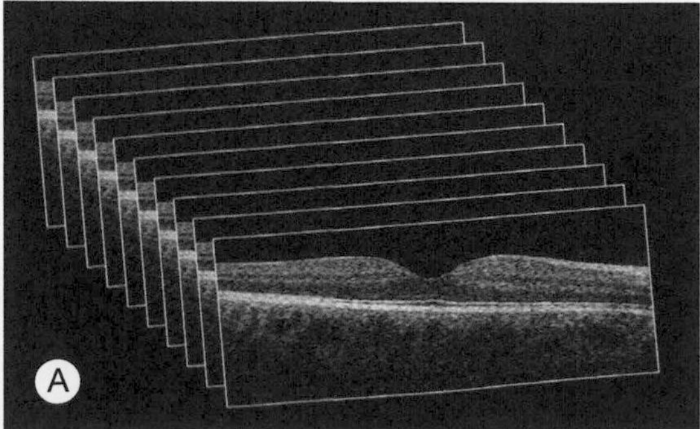

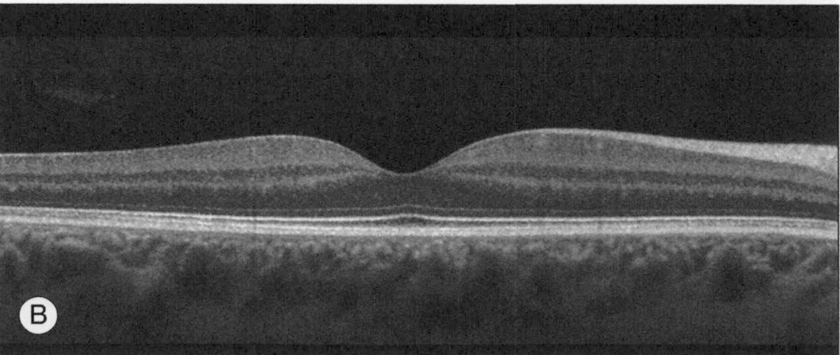

Fig. 3.3 Averaging process. (A) Multiple B-scans acquired through the foveal center of a normal patient. (B) The registration and averaging of these B-scans can reduce the speckled noise and improve the image quality. In these examples the image was averaged 20 times using the Cirrus high-definition optical coherence tomograph.

Table 3.1 Commercially available spectral domain optical coherence tomography (OCT) instruments

Device (manufacturer)	Axial resolution; scanning rate	Special characteristics
3D-OCT 2000 (Topcon, Tokyo, Japan)	5 μm; 27 kHz	Fundus camera
Bioptigen SD-OCT (Bioptigen, Research Triangle Park, NC)	4 μm; 20 kHz	Designed for research applications
Cirrus HD-OCT (Carl Zeiss Meditec, Dublin, CA)	5 μm; 27 kHz	
RTVue-100 (Optovue, Fremont, CA)	5 μm; 26 kHz	
SOCT Copernicus (Optopol, Zawiercie, Poland)	6 μm; 27 kHz	
Spectral OCT SLO (Opko, Miami, FL)	6 μm; 27 kHz	Microperimetry
Spectralis OCT (Heidelberg Engineering, Heidelberg, Germany)	8 μm; 40 kHz	Eye-tracking, fluorescein angiography, ICG angiography, autofluorescence

3D, three-dimensional; SD, spectral domain; HD, high-definition; SOCT, spectral optical coherence tomography; SLO, scanning laser ophthalmoscope; ICG, indocyanine green.

unprecedented visualization and quantitative evaluation of the corresponding retinal structures.

Several commercially available SD-OCT instruments offer some level of quantitative analysis using different, proprietary segmentation algorithms. The various segmentation algorithms make different design choices and have been shown to have very different performance profiles in terms of accuracy, reproducibility, and robustness.[5–8] Care should be exercised when comparing measurements obtained from different OCT instruments.

The most commonly used quantitative parameter derived from OCT datasets is retinal thickness, obtained by segmenting the internal limiting membrane (ILM) and a boundary representing the retinal pigment epithelium (RPE). This information can be used to generate surface maps of the ILM and the RPE as well as two-dimensional and three-dimensional retinal thickness maps. These maps can be very useful in identifying and describing deviations from the normal anatomy and changes over time. Registering OCT datasets acquired over time can give very precise information about the dynamics of disease progression and response to treatment based on changes in retinal anatomy (Fig. 3.4).

It is important to keep in mind that there is some confusion in the definition of the outer retinal boundary. In a normal eye, the bright reflective band at the external aspect of the retina, often referred to as the RPE complex, can be resolved in ultrahigh-resolution images, and occasionally in images acquired with a commercially available SD-OCT instrument, consisting of three individual layers.[9] Different segmentation algorithms from different instruments tend to follow

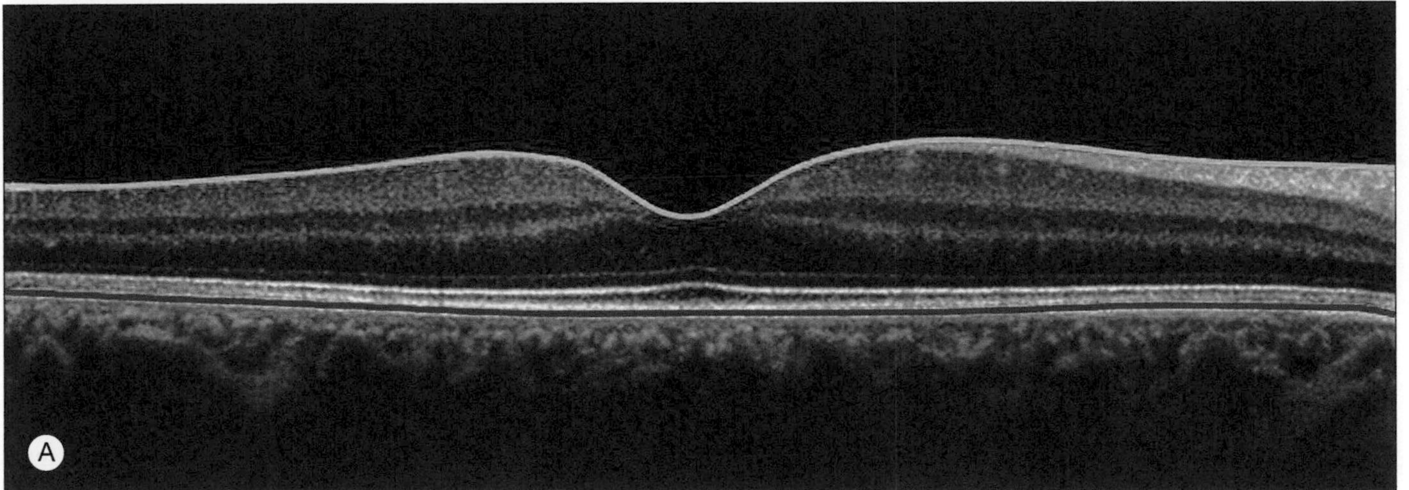

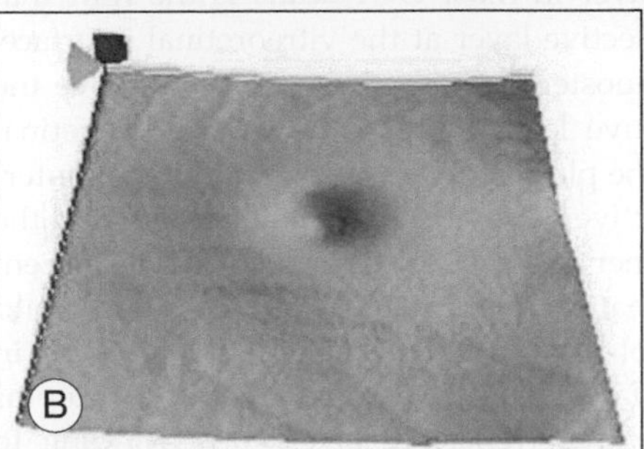

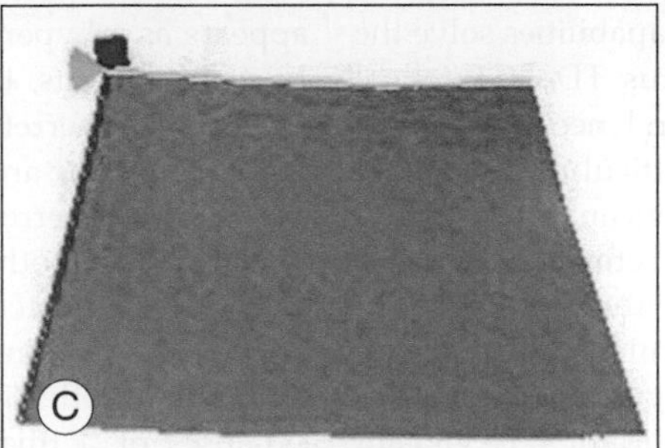

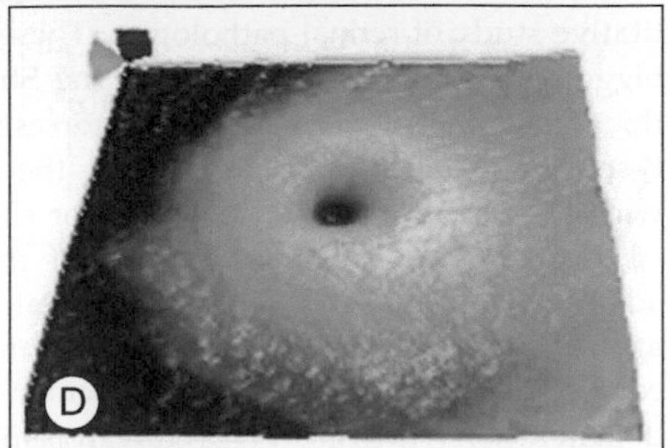

Fig. 3.4 Segmentation process. (A) B-scan through the foveal center of a normal patient with a yellow line identifying the internal limiting membrane (ILM) and a red line corresponding to the retinal pigment epithelium (RPE). Three-dimensional map of the ILM (B), RPE (C), and the retinal thickness map (D) acquired with a 200 × 200 scan pattern with the Cirrus high-definition optical coherence tomography instrument.

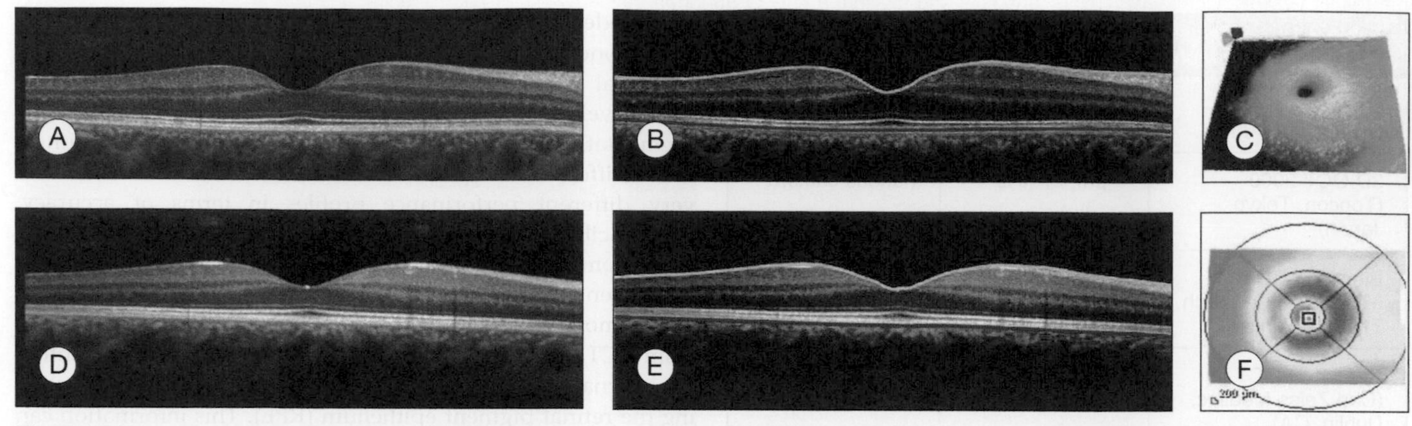

Fig. 3.5 Differences in segmentation and retinal thickness maps between instruments. The B-scan, the B-scan identifying the internal limiting membrane (yellow line), and the retinal pigment epithelium (red line), and the retinal thickness map acquired with the Cirrus high-definition optical coherence tomograph (A–C) and the Spectralis (D–F). Note that, using the Cirrus instrument, the segmentation algorithm identifies the actual retinal pigment epithelium (B) and using the Spectralis the segmentation algorithm identifies Bruch's membrane. This subtle difference in the segmentation algorithm between each instrument can be responsible for different retinal thickness measurements.

different edges and therefore result in different measurements. For example, the Spectralis SD-OCT instrument typically follows the posterior edge of the RPE complex, the Stratus TD-OCT instrument typically follows the inner segment–outer segment (IS/OS) junction, which is anterior to the RPE complex, and the Cirrus SD-OCT instrument typically follows the anterior edge of the RPE layer (Fig. 3.5). This situation becomes even more complicated and sometimes inconsistent when the normal retinal structure is deformed by the presence of pathology.[10]

In addition to total retinal thickness, a number of other quantitative parameters have been proposed. For example, it is possible to obtain measurements of particular retinal layers, such as the thickness of the ganglion cell layer or the thickness of the photoreceptors' outer segments, as well as measurements of retinal lesions, like the area of geographic atrophy (GA).[9,11,12]

An area of particular promise is the measurement of RPE deformations associated with drusen.[13,14] These measurements are obtained by comparing the actual RPE geometry with the geometry of a virtual RPE free of deformations. Parameters like drusen area and volume can be generated in a fully automated manner and have been shown to be quite robust and reproducible (Fig. 3.6).

The amount of information provided by each dataset, together with the possibility for image registration and longitudinal studies, makes SD-OCT a very promising new tool for the quantitative study of retinal pathologies. These capabilities solve the biggest problems associated with the Stratus TD-OCT retinal thickness maps: the lack of precise correspondence between the B-scans and the retinal topography, the difficulties associated with eye movements, and the need for significant interpolation of the data due to undersampling of the retina. Despite the advantages of SD-OCT, segmentation algorithms can produce artifacts, particularly in the presence of macular disorders with complex morphology like neovascular age-related macular degeneration (AMD).[15–19] Therefore, it is important to be vigilant and monitor the quality of the segmentation in order to eliminate artifacts arising from flawed segmentation and associated measurements.

NORMAL MACULAR ANATOMY

The OCT image closely approximates the histological appearance of the macula and, for this reason, it has been referred to as an in vivo optical biopsy. With the increase in the axial resolution of the new SD-OCT instruments (5–8 μm) and the ultrahigh-resolution OCT (2 μm), it has become possible to correlate OCT images accurately with histological features of the retina.[20] However, care must be taken when making assumptions about these correlations because histological sections require fixation and exogenous staining to produce contrast within tissue, and this can introduce artifacts, while OCT relies on intrinsic differences in tissue optical properties to produce image contrast.[21] When light travels through the retinal tissue it can be reflected, scattered, or absorbed, and this creates the multilayered pattern of the retina. The angle of incidence of the light, motion artifacts, speckled noise, and image contrast can affect the axial resolution of retinal imaging. Therefore, one-to-one correspondence of histology with OCT images cannot be expected.[2,21]

Although the interpretation of features of the inner retina, which can be defined for our purpose to span from the ILM to the junction of the inner and outer segments of the photoreceptors, appears to correlate well with histology, the OCT features of the outer retina are less well understood and remain a topic of discussion (Fig. 3.7).[9,22,23]

The first detected layer in most OCT scans is the ILM that appears as a hyperreflective layer at the vitreoretinal interface. In some patients, the posterior hyaloid can be seen above the ILM as a hyperreflective layer. Within the retina, the retinal nerve fiber layer and the plexiform layers (both inner and outer) are seen as hyperreflective while the ganglion cell layer and the nuclear layers (both inner and outer) are hyporeflective. A recent study demonstrated that the incidence of the light beam could affect the appearance of Henle's fiber layer by OCT, resulting in a thin hyperreflective layer corresponding to the photoreceptor synapses or a thicker hyperreflective layer corresponding to photoreceptor axonal extensions enveloped by the outer cytoplasm of Müller cells (Fig. 3.8).[24] The retinal vessels may sometimes be seen on OCT images as circular hyperreflective

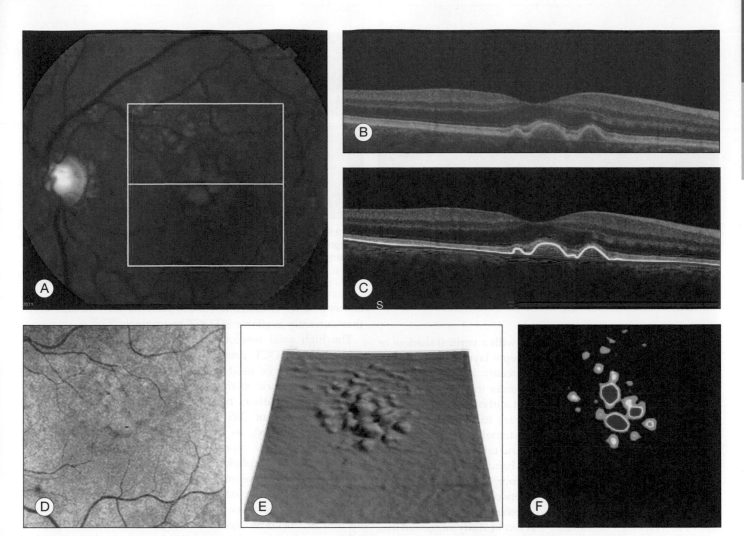

Fig. 3.6 Retinal pigment epithelium (RPE) deformation algorithm. (A) Color fundus image of a patient with drusen. A 6 × 6 mm white box was superimposed on the image to represent the scan area. (B) B-scan from the spectral domain optical coherence tomography dataset that corresponds to the central line on the color fundus image. (C) B-scan with a yellow line representing the RPE segmentation and a red line showing the RPE floor (virtual map of the RPE free of deformations). (D) En face image of the 6 × 6 mm scan pattern (optical coherence tomography fundus image). (E) Three-dimensional RPE map delineating the drusen conformation. (F) RPE elevation map with drusen area (1.41 mm^2) and volume (0.08 mm^3).

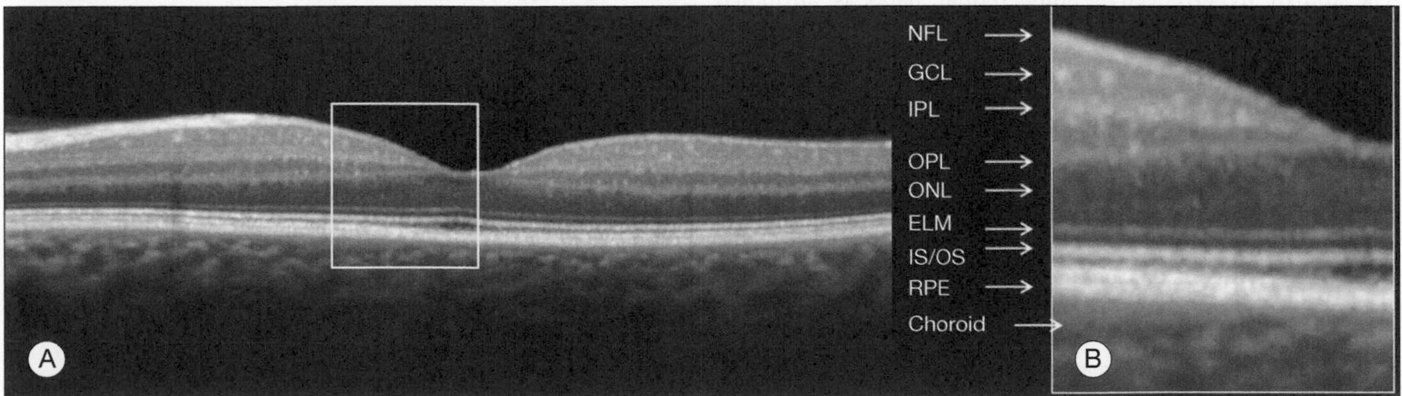

Fig. 3.7 Spectral domain optical coherence tomography (Spectralis, Heidelberg) image of a normal individual. The multilayered retinal architecture can be observed and each retinal layer can be identified. NFL, nerve fiber layer; GCL, ganglion cell layer; IPL, inner plexiform layer; OPL, outer plexiform layer; ONL, outer nuclear layer; ELM, external limiting membrane; IS/OS, junction of the inner and outer segments of the photoreceptors; RPE, retinal pigment epithelium.

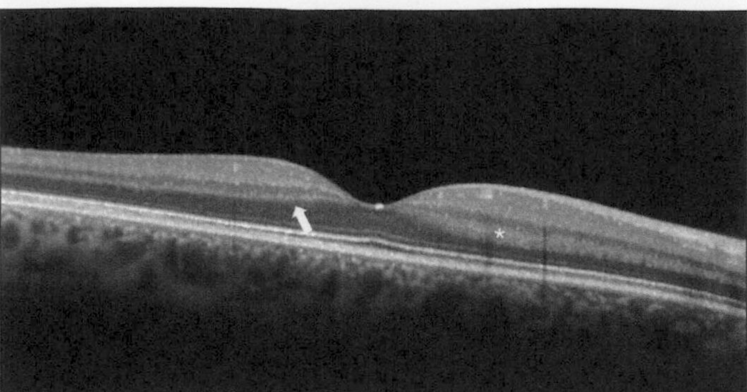

Fig. 3.8 Spectral domain optical coherence tomography of the same patient using a different light incidence. This results in a thin hyperreflective layer that corresponds to the photoreceptor synapses (white arrow) or a thicker hyperreflective layer corresponding to photoreceptor axonal extensions enveloped by the outer cytoplasm of Müller cells (white asterisk).

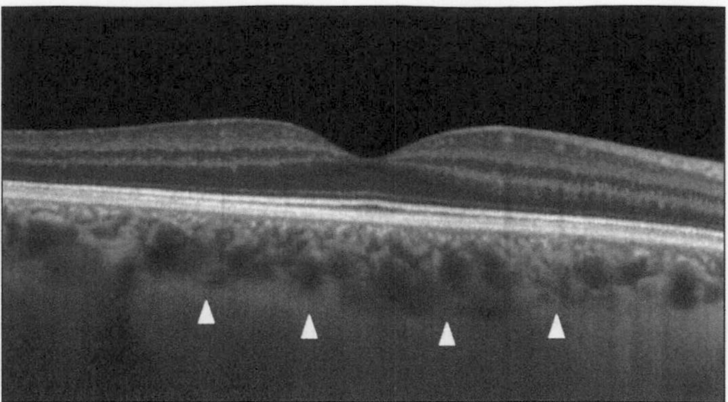

Fig. 3.9 Enhanced-depth spectral domain optical coherence tomography image (Spectralis, Heidelberg) of a normal subject showing the boundaries of the choroid (arrowheads).

structures located in the inner retina, with a vertical shadow or reduced reflectivity extending into deeper layers.

Outside the central fovea, commercially available SD-OCT instruments typically resolve four bands in the outer retina. There is discordance between different authors regarding which anatomical structure correlates with each band.[20,21,25] The innermost band has been attributed to the external limiting membrane (ELM). This band is typically thinner and fainter than the others. The nomenclature for the middle two bands has much less supportive evidence. The second of the four bands has been commonly ascribed to the boundary between the IS/OS of the photoreceptors and the third band is referred to as either the OS tips or as Verhoeff's membrane.[9,26] A recent study suggested that the second band was the ellipsoid section of the photoreceptors (inner segment) instead of the IS/OS junction and that the third band appears to correspond to the contact cylinder between the RPE apical process and the external portion of the cone outer segment. This band typically merges with the fourth band in the central fovea and this is explained by a greater height of the contact cylinder of the cones and RPE outside the fovea.[25] The fourth hyperreflective outer retinal band is attributed to the RPE, with potential contribution from Bruch's membrane and choriocapillaris, with abundant experimental and clinical evidence supporting this designation.[9,22,27]

Although the current SD-OCT uses a short wavelength of approximately 840 nm, which results in light scattering at the level of the RPE and a lower signal from the deep choroidal tissue, it is also possible to image the choroid and extract quantitative information (Fig. 3.9).[28–31] Choroidal thickness may be influenced by age, axial length, and perhaps refractive abnormalities. It also varies in different retinal regions within the same normal subject, being thickest beneath the fovea,[31] or in the superior outer macula (Early Treatment Diabetic Retinopathy Study (ETDRS) subfield), with the thinnest choroid being located in the nasal outer ETDRS subfield.[32] When centering the optic nerve head as a reference point, the choroid appears thin in the peripapillary region and increases in thickness with eccentricity in all directions, up to a certain point, except inferiorly.[32] This is the embryonic location of the optic fissure closure and thus may be responsible for the localized thinning.[32,33] High-penetration OCT uses a light source with a wavelength around 1050 nm that allows a better visualization of the posterior choroid and sclera than currently available SD-OCT instruments.[30,33,34]

The high axial resolution and the different scan patterns offered by SD-OCT provide comprehensive structural information that can be used to map retinal layer thicknesses and perform volumetric analyses. Using different SD-OCT instruments, several authors have reported an approximate central retinal thickness of 265 μm in normal subjects.[35] However, caution is required, as errors in automated measurements may occur and are more often found in macular disorders with complex morphology like neovascular AMD, which alters the ability of segmentation algorithms to detect normal boundaries.[15–19] Therefore, care must be taken that high-quality and artifact-free scans are obtained before running the retinal thickness algorithm.

It is essential to consider the following points when analyzing OCT images: location, shape, and reflectivity of the structure, along with its histological correlation. It is also important to remember that the alignment of the instrument with the pupil can generate signals that may lead to a misinterpretation of the exam.

Characteristic OCT findings in several common retinal disorders which are frequently studied using OCT are discussed below. For OCT findings, in other disorders, such as retinal degenerations, the reader is directed to the specific chapters describing these diseases.

SD-OCT IN RETINAL DISORDERS

Vitreoretinal interface disorders

Abnormalities of the vitreoretinal interface are involved in the pathogenesis of several macular conditions. In idiopathic epiretinal membranes (ERMs), a layer of fibrotic tissue develops on the surface of the retina, usually after a posterior vitreous detachment. Contraction of this membrane can result in retinal distortion, leading to vision loss. In other conditions, such as vitreomacular traction (VMT) syndrome or idiopathic macular hole, there are abnormal attachments between the vitreous and the retina. The resulting traction exerted on the retina causes anatomical alteration and subsequent visual loss.

Vitreomacular traction

VMT syndrome results from persistent vitreoretinal adhesions in the setting of a partial posterior vitreous detachment.[36] In normal eyes, as the vitreous liquefies due to age, it detaches from the macula. This natural progression has been demonstrated using OCT.[37] In some people, an unusually strong adhesion is present between the vitreous and macula, and as the vitreous detaches peripherally, it continues to pull on areas of the macula. The vitreoretinal adhesions transmit tractional forces to the retina from the vitreous body, having the potential to cause tensile deformation, foveal cavitations, cystoid macular edema (CME), limited macular detachment, or a macular hole.[38,39] Patients can present with visual loss and metamorphopsia.

Diagnosis of VMT by biomicroscopy may be challenging, particularly when the area of vitreoretinal attachment is broad. OCT better defines the vitreoretinal relationships in eyes with VMT and also documents concomitant ERM and macular edema.[40–44] With OCT imaging, the abnormal VMT bands from the prominent posterior hyaloid are well delineated as reflective lines from the perifoveal area into the vitreous cavity, distorting the macular contour with or without accumulation of intraretinal or subretinal fluid (Fig. 3.10).

In recent years OCT has been most beneficial in diagnosing VMT and subsequently directing treatment of this condition. In some cases, spontaneous resolution can occur with separation of the vitreous from the macula, leading to subsequent resolution of the intraretinal and subretinal fluid and restoration of normal vision.[45,46] However, in most eyes, VMT persists and vitrectomy may be an effective treatment option for patients with symptomatic VMT.[40,47,48] Consequently, OCT is useful in monitoring subtle changes in vitreoretinal adhesions and retinal architecture and assisting the treatment decision-making process.

Epiretinal membrane

ERM occurs in approximately 6% of patients over the age of 60, with incidence increasing with age.[49,50] ERMs can be classified as idiopathic or secondary to an initiating event. Most idiopathic ERMs are thought to result from fibroglial proliferation on the inner surface of the retina secondary to a break in ILM occurring during posterior vitreous detachment.[51,52] Secondary ERMs result from an already-existing ocular pathology such as central or branch retinal vein occlusion, diabetic retinopathy, uveitis, and retinal breaks with or without detachment.[53] Glial cells, RPE cells, and myofibroblasts are shown to be mostly involved in ERM formation.[51,52] ERM may lead to loss of normal retinal anatomy, with the patient experiencing metamorphopsia, micropsia, monocular diplopia, and decreased visual acuity. These symptoms vary in severity depending on the location, density, and contraction of the membrane.

On slit-lamp biomicroscopy, a mild ERM appears as a glistening layer on the retinal surface. Denser membranes may be seen as a gray sheet overlying the retina and causing distortion in the macular vascular architecture. Occasionally, ERMs can evolve into macular pseudoholes and ERMs are often seen in conjunction with idiopathic full-thickness macular holes.[38] Fluorescein angiography may demonstrate macular leakage, which can be variable from case to case.

OCT provides qualitative and quantitative information about the retinal anatomy, which can identify factors contributing to vision loss in patients with ERM. On OCT, ERMs are seen as a highly reflective layer on the inner retinal surface (Fig. 3.11). In most eyes, the membrane is globally adherent to the retina but, in some cases, it can be separated from the inner aspect of the retina, which enhances its visibility by OCT. In this situation, it

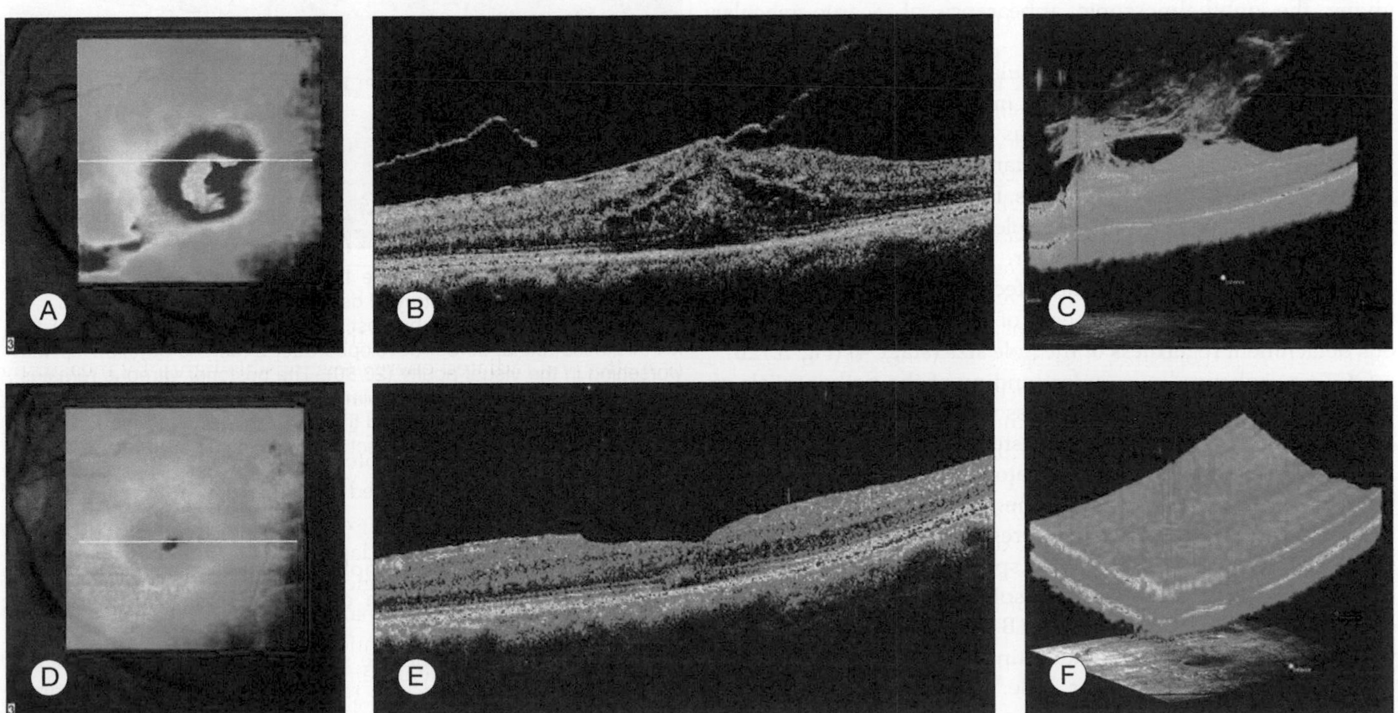

Fig. 3.10 Vitreomacular traction syndrome: color fundus image of the left eye of a 71-year-old woman superimposed with the retinal thickness map (A) showing an increase in the retinal thickness (red areas). The B-scan of the macular region shows an increase in the retinal thickness and the presence of subretinal fluid and intraretinal cysts due to vitreomacular traction and an epiretinal membrane (B). A three-dimensional spectral domain optical coherence tomography (courtesy of Cirrus, Carl Zeiss Meditec) is presented (C). The patient underwent surgery and, 2 months after pars plana vitrectomy, the retinal thickness decreased, with resolution of the intraretinal cysts (D–F).

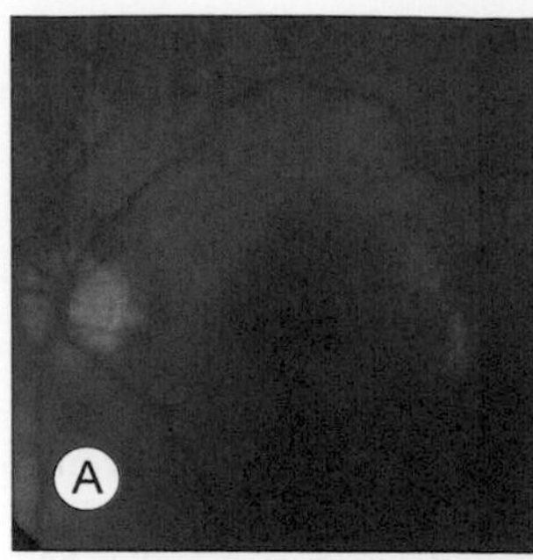

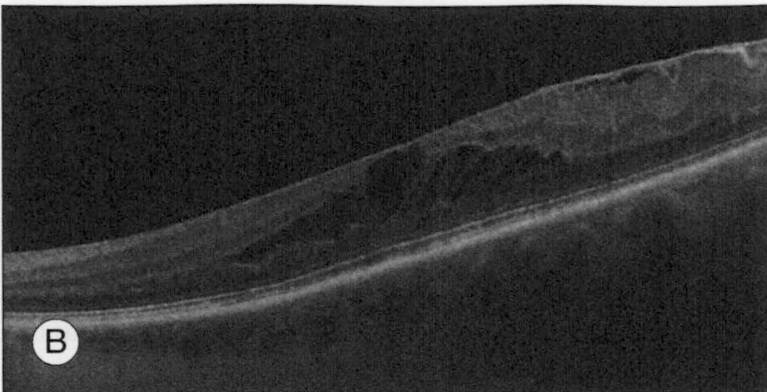

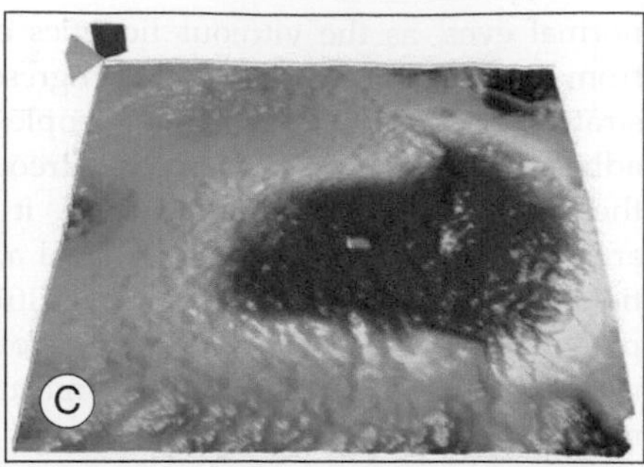

Fig. 3.11 Epiretinal membrane – color fundus image of the left eye of a 65-year-old man with grayish tissue over the retina (A). Cross-sectional optical coherence tomography image showing a hyperreflective tissue overlying the retina, resulting in increased retinal thickness and cysts in the retina (B and C).

is usually distinguishable from a detached posterior hyaloid. Secondary effects of the membrane include loss of the normal foveal contour, increased retinal thickness, and the presence of cystoid changes, and these features may be observed in more advanced membranes. OCT is useful for monitoring changes in cases that are being observed and for documenting the response to treatment in patients undergoing pars plana vitrectomy with membrane peeling.

Macular hole

Idiopathic macular holes typically occur in the sixth to seventh decade of life with a 2:1 female preponderance. Symptoms include decreased visual acuity, metamorphopsia, and central scotoma. Bilateral involvement occurs in 15–20% of patients.[21]

A full-thickness defect in the neural retina as seen with OCT can differentiate a true macular hole from a pseudohole seen clinically. Pseudoholes are seen in the presence of a dense sheet of ERM with a central defect that overlies the foveal center, giving the ophthalmoscopic appearance of a true macular hole.[21,54]

Gass described the stages of macular hole formation based on biomicroscopic findings.[55] A stage 1 impending hole is characterized by a foveal detachment seen as a yellow spot (1A) or ring (1B) in the fovea (Fig. 3.12A). Spontaneous resolution will occur in approximately 50% of these cases. In stages 2–4, there is a full-thickness retinal defect, with a complete absence of neural retinal tissue overlying the foveal center. What differentiates these stages is the size of the retinal defect (<400 μm in stage 2 and >400 μm in stage 3) or the presence of a complete posterior vitreous detachment regardless of the hole size (stage 4) (Fig. 3.12B).

OCT has enhanced our understanding of the pathogenesis of macular holes, the healing process after surgical repair, and helped in identifying pre- and postoperative features that are related to visual outcome. The anatomic changes identified on OCT have been correlated with the various stages of macular hole. In stage 1A, patients usually present with a localized foveolar detachment, which can resolve spontaneously after the posterior vitreous detachment with resolution of the yellow foveal spot, or it can progress to stage 1B with a development of a pseudocyst with loss of the outer retinal layers, and later develop into a full-thickness macular hole.[56,57] Generally, the retinal defect is accompanied by a variable amount of intraretinal fluid appearing as cysts and a variable amount of subretinal fluid at the edge of the hole. The edge of the hole can appear elevated, as a result of the significant intraretinal fluid accumulation or due to persistent vitreofoveal traction. In a stage 4 macular hole,

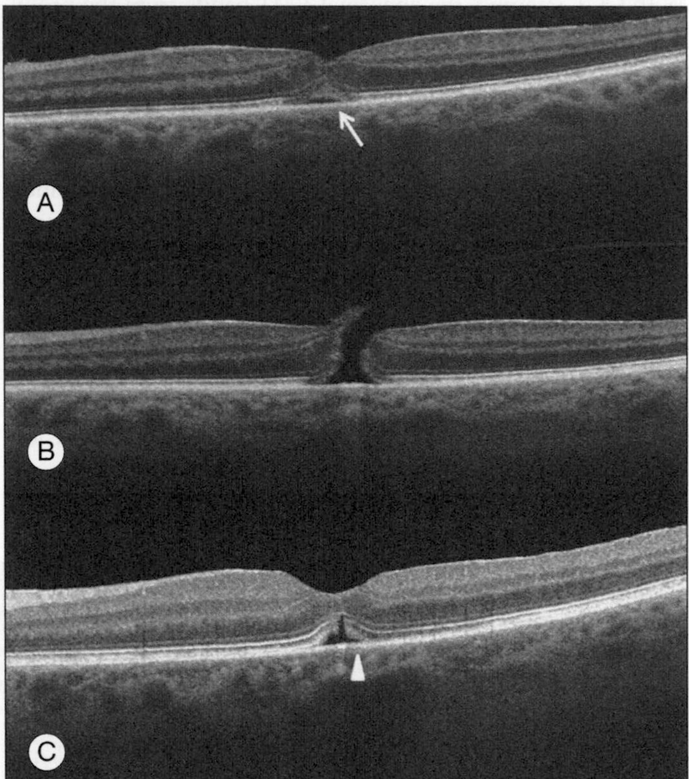

Fig. 3.12 Macular hole. (A) Stage 1 macular hole in a 63-year-old woman with a 3-month history of decreased visual acuity (20/60). An outer retinal defect can be observed in the B-scan (arrow). (B) A full-thickness retinal defect developed after 2 months of follow-up with worsening in the visual acuity (20/80). The posterior vitreous remains adhered to the edge of the macular hole. (C) One month after surgery, the macular hole was closed and the visual acuity improved to 20/50, but a persistent foveal outer defect could be observed (arrowhead).

OCT can demonstrate the complete hyaloid separation and occasionally a retinal operculum can be seen floating above the foveal center.

Vitrectomy has become the standard treatment for macular hole with anatomical success rates of 85–100%.[58,59] OCT can be used to confirm complete macular hole closure and restoration of the normal foveal contour.[60–63] In cases with suboptimal postoperative visual outcomes, OCT can visualize persistent retinal abnormalities despite anatomically successful macular hole surgery (Fig. 3.12C). Restoration of the ELM and the so-called junction of the inner and outer segment of photoreceptors may reflect the morphologic and functional recovery of the photoreceptors in surgically closed macular holes.[62–65] A residual small defect in the ELM is often still evident in closed holes, particularly in those that are spontaneously healed. The ability to perform OCT imaging in eyes filled with gas or silicone oil has also been useful as an adjunct to determine the extension of the face-down position in patients following vitrectomy for macular hole.[66–68]

Age-related macular degeneration

AMD is a common cause of irreversible vision loss among the elderly worldwide. It is estimated that approximately 30% of adults older than 75 years have some sign of AMD and that approximately 10% of these patients have advanced stages of the disease.[69–72] AMD can be classified in two forms: non-neovascular (dry) and neovascular (wet or exudative). The non-neovascular form accounts for 80–90% of cases while the neovascular form accounts for 10–20% of cases, but was responsible for the majority of severe vision loss (80–90%) prior to the widespread use of vascular endothelial growth factor (VEGF) inhibitors.[71,73]

Non-neovascular AMD

Non-neovascular (dry) AMD is characterized by abnormalities of the RPE, Bruch's membrane, and choriocapillaris. These abnormalities may be asymptomatic or accompanied by compromised vision, and are considered to be the precursors of GA and choroidal neovascularization (CNV).[74,75]

Early non-neovascular AMD: drusen and pigmentary changes

Drusen appear clinically as focal white-yellow excrescences deep to the retina. They vary in number, size, shape, and distribution. Several grading strategies have been developed to image drusen using color fundus imaging.[76,77] Although color fundus imaging is useful for assessing the appearance of drusen, these images only provide two-dimensional area information on the geometry of the drusen and cannot be used to measure quantitative properties such as drusen volume. Until the advent of high-speed spectral domain technology, evaluation of drusen with OCT was often difficult as motion artifacts commonly resulted in apparent undulation of the RPE, mimicking the appearance of drusen.[78,79] SD-OCT can provide a three-dimensional, geometric assessment of drusen.

The high-definition B-scans obtained with SD-OCT are useful to assess the ultrastructure of drusen and to evaluate for evidence of disruption of adjacent retinal layers. Drusen are seen as discrete areas of RPE elevation with variable reflectivity, which is consistent with the variable composition of the underlying material (Fig. 3.13).[80,81] In larger drusen or drusenoid retinal pigment epithelial detachments (PEDs), the RPE has a greater elevation with a dome-shaped configuration.[82] Larger drusen may often become confluent and can sometimes be accompanied

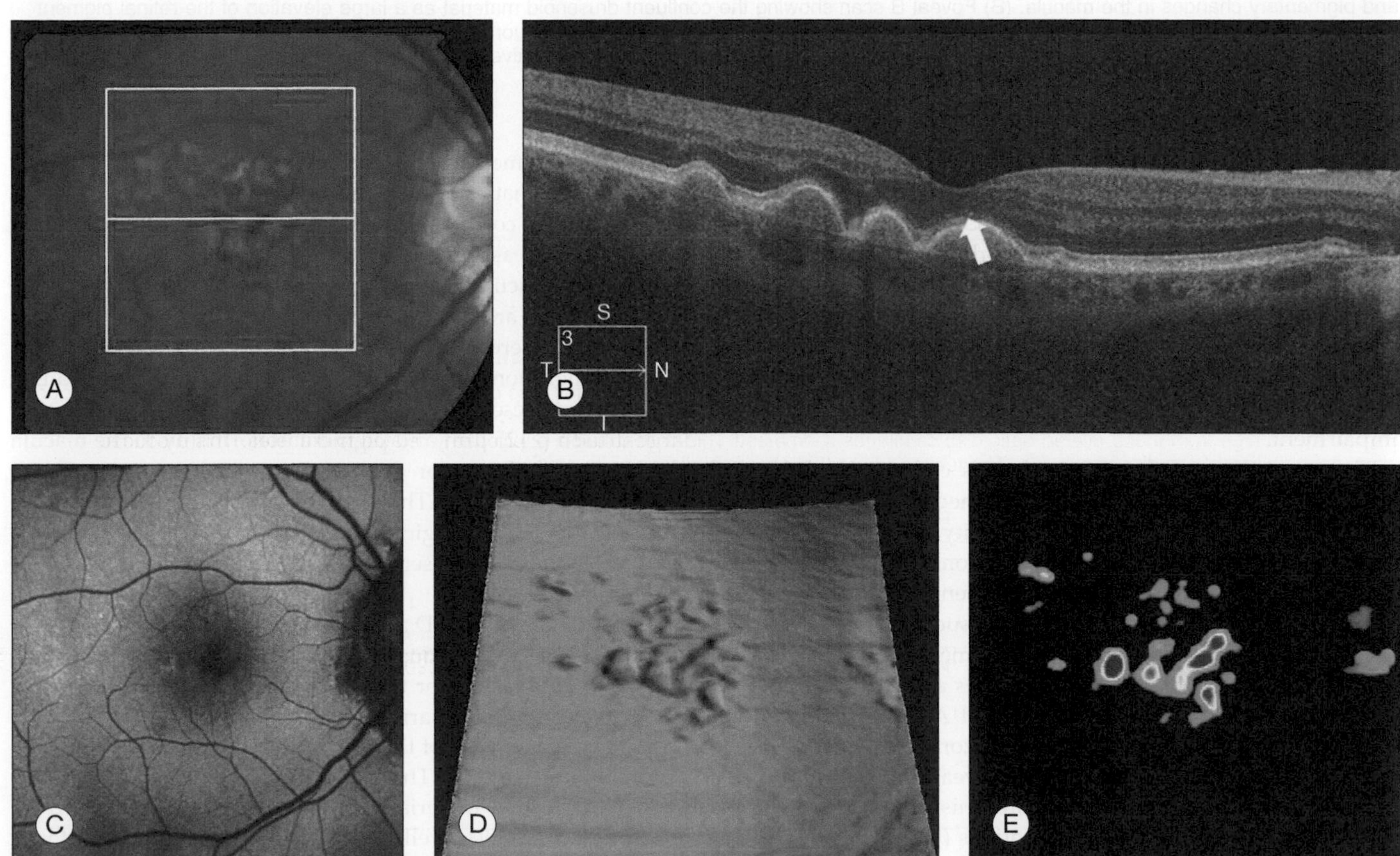

Fig. 3.13 Early non-neovascular age-related macular degeneration. (A) Color fundus image of the right eye of a 61-year-old man with drusen and pigmentary changes in the macula. (B) Foveal B-scan showing the drusen as elevations of the retinal pigment epithelium (RPE). The inner and outer segment junction of the photoreceptors adjacent to the drusen appears disrupted (arrow). (C) Fundus autofluorescence illustrating that drusen cannot be reliably identified by this imaging modality. (D) RPE segmentation map showing drusen in a unique three-dimensional perspective. (E) RPE elevation map providing the drusen area (1.37 mm^2) and volume (0.063 mm^3).

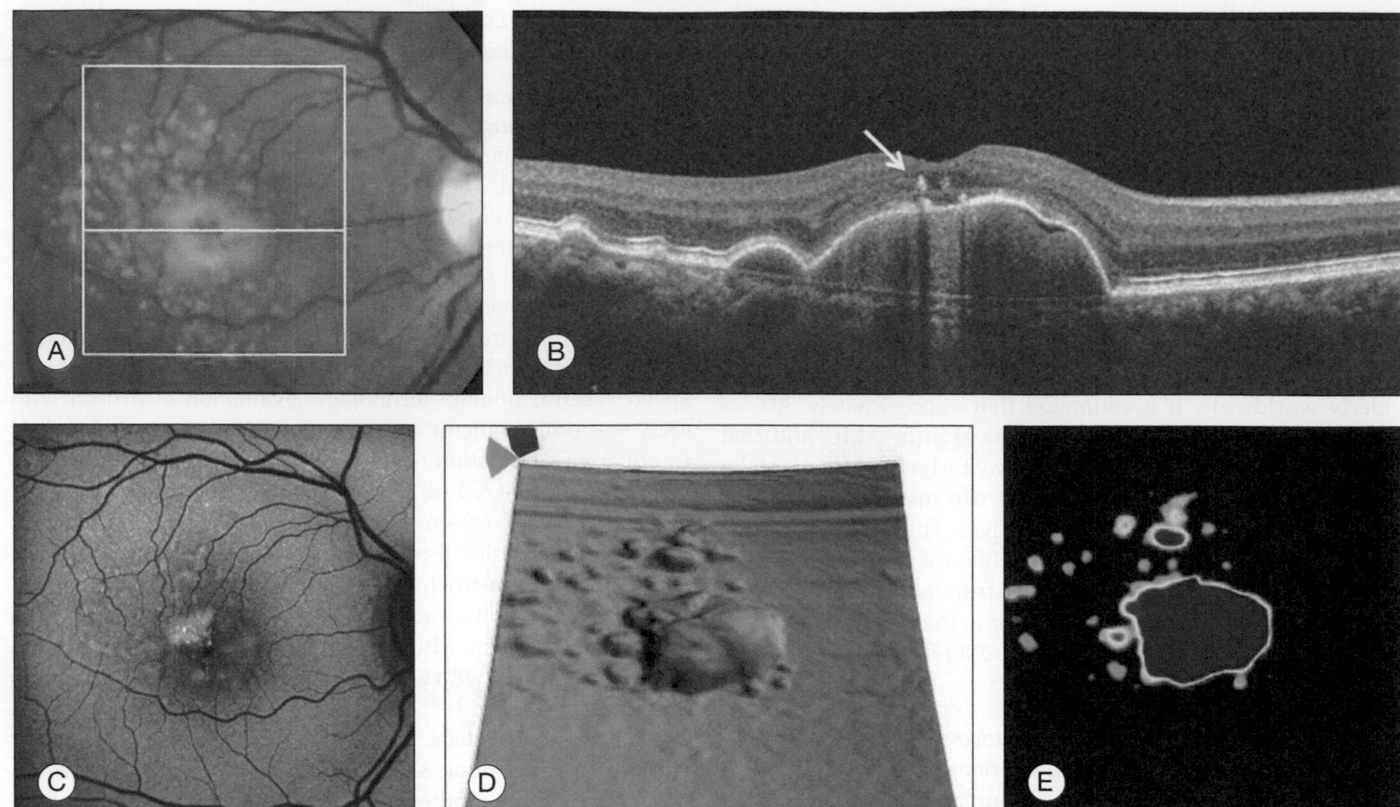

Fig. 3.14 Drusenoid retinal pigment epithelium detachment (DPED). (A) Color fundus image of the right eye of a 66-year-old man with a DPED and pigmentary changes in the macula. (B) Foveal B-scan showing the confluent drusenoid material as a large elevation of the retinal pigment epithelium (RPE). Intraretinal pigment migration can be observed (arrow). (C) Fundus autofluorescence image (Heidelberg retina angiograph, Heidelberg). (D) RPE segmentation map showing the DPED in a three-dimensional perspective. (E) RPE elevation map providing the DPED area (3.87 mm^2) and volume (0.508 mm^3).

by fluid accumulation under the retina in the absence of CNV (Fig. 3.14).[80] Recognition of this feature may avoid unnecessary treatment with anti-VEGF drugs. SD-OCT imaging has the resolution to evaluate the retinal layers overlying drusen. A thinning in the photoreceptor layer can be observed in up to 97% of cases, with average photoreceptor layer thickness reduced by 27% compared to age-matched control eyes. The inner retinal layers usually remain unchanged. These findings demonstrate a degenerative process with photoreceptor loss leading to visual impairment.[83]

The acquisition of dense raster scans comprised of a large number of lower-density B-scans combined with the use of segmentation algorithms results in the ability to generate maps of the RPE, which provides information on RPE geometry and therefore a unique perspective of drusen. A novel algorithm developed to identify RPE deformations such as drusen has been shown to be highly reproducible in the measurement of drusen area and volume.[13] The algorithm creates a drusen map from a scan pattern of 40000 uniformly spaced A-scans organized as 200 A-scans in each B-scan and 200 horizontal B-scans, covering an area of 6 × 6 mm centered in the fovea. The algorithm uses the actual RPE geometry and compares this RPE map to a virtual map of the RPE free of any deformations (RPE floor). The algorithm creates a difference map from these two maps, which permits reproducible measurements of drusen area and volume (Fig. 3.6). This algorithm was used to study the natural history of drusen in AMD.[14] Drusen were shown to undergo three different growth patterns. In most eyes, drusen were found to increase in volume and area. Drusen could also remain stable or they could dramatically decrease over time. When these drusen decreased, they could evolve into GA or neovascular AMD, or they could decrease, resulting in no apparent residual anatomic defect in the macula.

The RPE cells are capable of hypertrophy and proliferation in response to different stimuli and in many cases an intraretinal pigment migration may occur (Fig. 3.14B). The Age-Related Eye Disease Study research group reported a severity scale defining large drusen (≥125 μm) and pigment abnormality in the macula as being a risk factor for disease progression in patients with intermediate AMD.[84,85] This pigmentary abnormality can be observed on OCT imaging as small discrete hyperreflective lesions within the neurosensory retina, usually within the outer nuclear layer.[86]

Typical drusen in AMD are seen as deposits between the RPE and the inner collagenous layer of Bruch's membrane. OCT imaging is also useful for the assessment of a variety of conditions characterized by variant forms of drusen. These deposits can also be seen on top of the RPE and are known as "subretinal drusenoid deposits."[87,88] They appear on OCT imaging as granular hyperreflective material between the RPE and the IS/OS junction and are also well visualized on blue-light reflectance imaging and autofluorescence imaging (Fig. 3.15).

Another form of drusen, known as "cuticular drusen," appears as numerous, uniform, round, yellow-white punctuate accumulations under the RPE. Cuticular drusen are usually seen on OCT imaging as elevations of the RPE with occasional disruption of

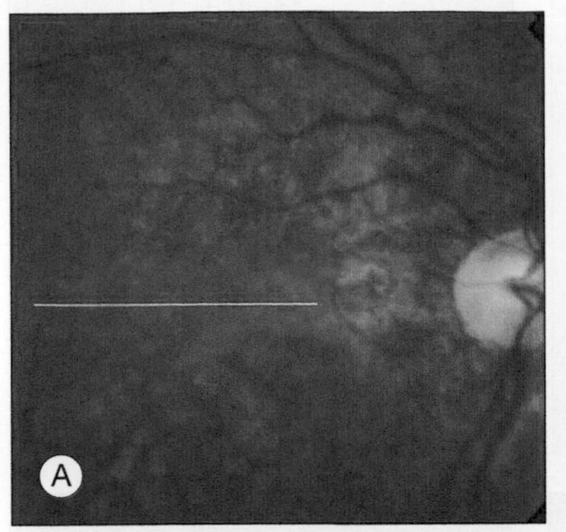

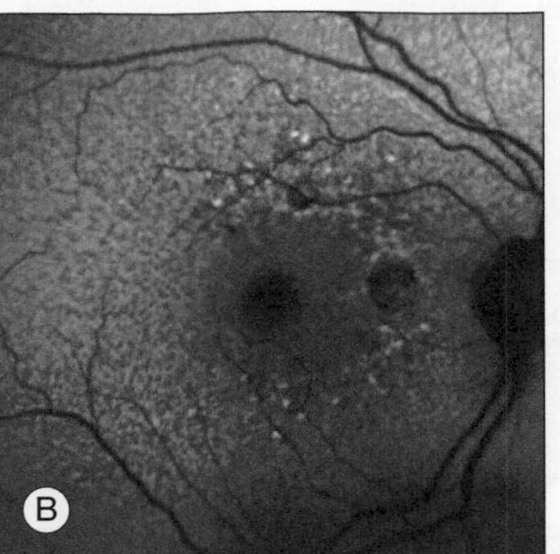

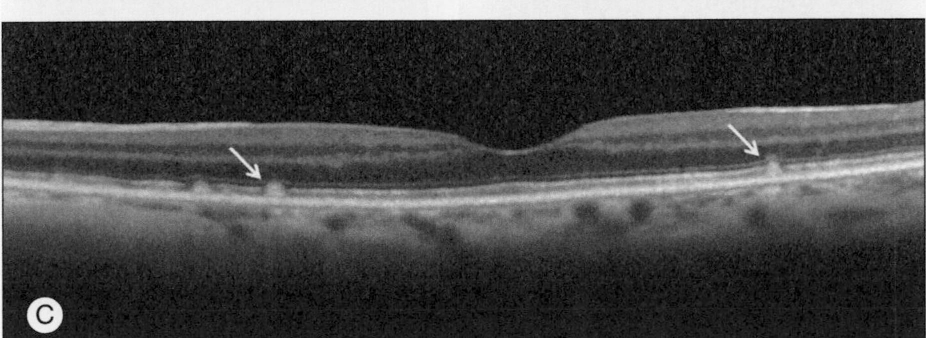

Fig. 3.15 Subretinal drusenoid deposits. (A) Color fundus image of a 76-year-old woman shows multiple yellowish, small, and round lesions. (B) Fundus autofluorescence clearly shows these deposits as small and multiple hyperautofluorescent spots. (C) On optical coherence tomography, these lesions appear as multiple areas of granular hyperreflectivity between the retinal pigment epithelium and the inner segment–outer segment junction (arrows).

the overlying IS/OS junction and ELM.[81] Although cuticular drusen, subretinal drusenoid deposits, and soft drusen are composed of common components, they are distinguishable by multimodal imaging because of differences in location, morphology, and the optical properties of the drusenoid material and the RPE.

Late non-neovascular AMD: geographic atrophy

The natural history of GA has been described as a progressive condition that evolves through stages with loss of vision occurring over many years.[89–91] Multiple imaging modalities have been used to document and quantify the area of GA. Until recently, color fundus photography was used as the standard method to image GA; however, the use of color photos can be challenging due to the reported difficulty in detecting and accurately delineating GA.[91,92] Other imaging modalities such as fluorescein angiography, fundus autofluorescence, and SD-OCT imaging are now used to evaluate and quantify GA (Fig. 3.16). Although these imaging modalities provide different information, none has been shown to be superior to the other.

GA is seen clinically as one or more well-demarcated areas of hypopigmentation or depigmentation due to the absence or severe attenuation of the underlying RPE. The larger, deeper choroidal vessels are more readily visualized through the atrophic areas, and are accompanied by varying degrees of photoreceptor and choriocapillaris loss. Associated retinal atrophy is seen as thinning or loss of the outer nuclear layer and the absence of ELM and IS/OS junctions.[93,94] The loss of photoreceptors often extends beyond the margins of GA, with the ELM and IS/OS junctions disappearing while bridging across the GA margin.[95] Evaluation of these junctional zones may provide information about the pathogenesis of GA, and the role of RPE, photoreceptor, and choriocapillaris loss in the initiation and propagation of this condition.[95] SD-OCT has been shown to be useful in detecting some of these morphologic alterations (Fig. 3.16D).

With the use of SD-OCT enhanced depth imaging (EDI) protocols, it is now possible to visualize the structure of the choroid in greater detail.[29] EDI demonstrated that subfoveal choroidal thickness decreases with age and axial length.[31] In a subset of elderly patients complaining of unexplained vision loss, abnormal choroidal thinning was identified, and this condition was named "age-related choroidal atrophy."[96] Future studies are necessary to confirm if this represents a new clinical entity or a subtype of AMD. In contrast, the choroidal thickness appears to be unaffected in early non-neovascular AMD patients.[97]

SDOCT can also be used to quantify the areas of GA and monitor the progression of the disease. GA is currently imaged with SDOCT by using the OFI, which represents a virtual fundus image resulting from the en face summation of the reflected light from each A-scan. This en face OCT fundus image identifies GA as a bright area due to the increased penetration of light into the choroid where atrophy has occurred in the macula. The absence of the RPE and choriocapillaris is responsible for this increased penetration of light associated with GA. The OFI was shown to correlate well with the GA seen on clinical examination, color fundus imaging, and autofluorescence imaging (Fig. 3.16E).[12,98,99] More recently, a newer algorithm provides an enhanced (partial) OFI, which is the summation of the reflected light from beneath the RPE (Fig. 3.17). In addition, this new algorithm is able to quantify the area of GA automatically. The enhanced OFI has advantages over the conventional OFI because the area of GA appears brighter than in the conventional OFI due to a better contrast at the boundaries of the lesions and there is less interference from other macular pathologies such as ERMs.

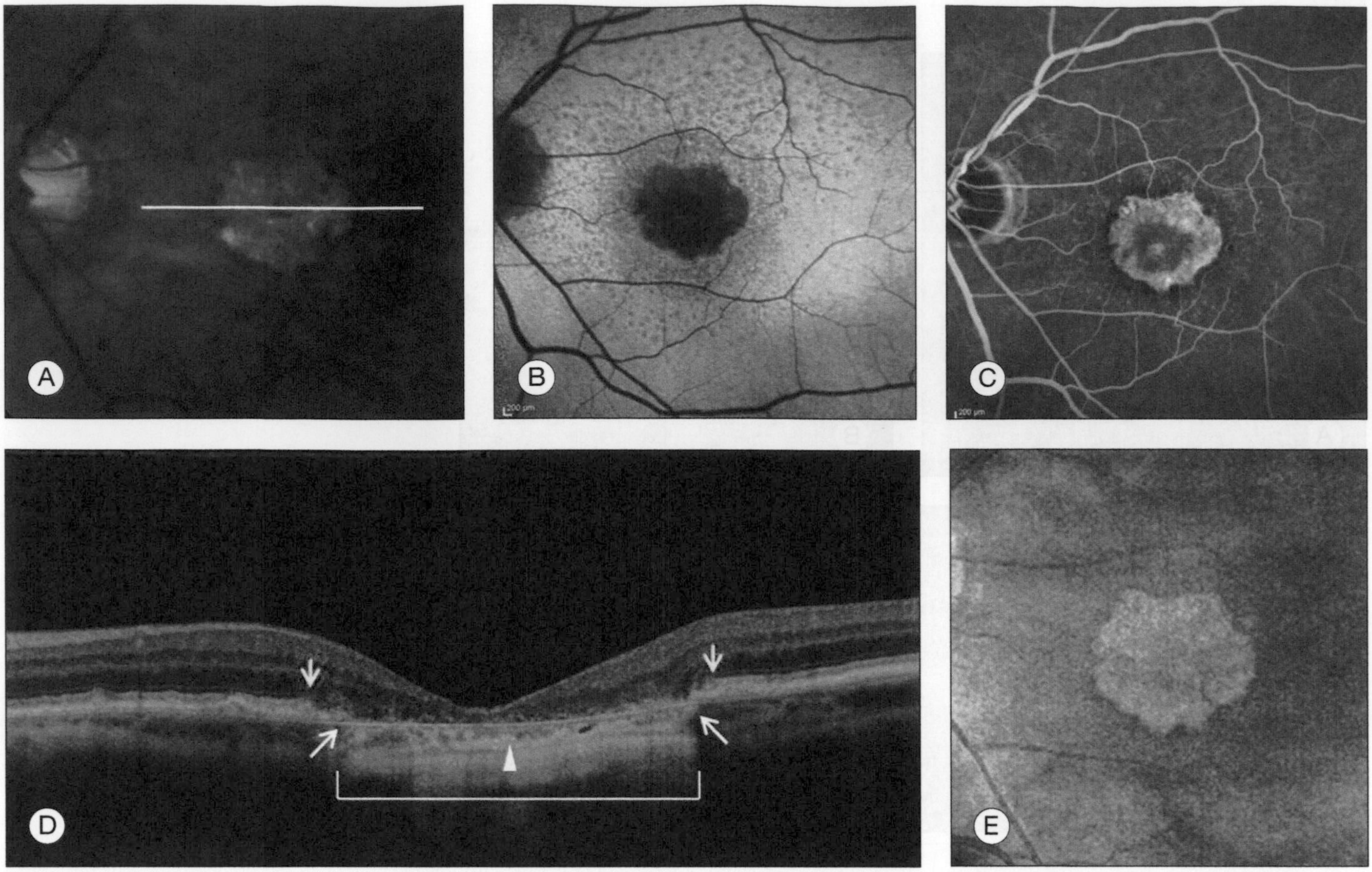

Fig. 3.16 Geographic atrophy (GA). (A) Color fundus image of the left eye of a 74-year-old male with central GA secondary to age-related macular degeneration. (B) Fundus autofluorescence (Spectralis, Heidelberg) showing a central area of hypoautofluorescence corresponding to the GA seen on the color image. (C) Late-phase fluorescein angiography showing a central window defect corresponding to the GA. (D) Horizontal B-scan through the foveal center demonstrating retinal thinning, loss of the retinal pigment epithelium (RPE), and photoreceptors. The loss of photoreceptors (yellow arrows) often extends beyond the margins of the RPE loss (white arrows). Observe the increased light penetration in the areas where the RPE is absent (bracket) and thin choroid (arrowhead). (E) Optical coherence tomography fundus image (courtesy of Cirrus, Carl Zeiss Meditec), showing the GA as a bright area.

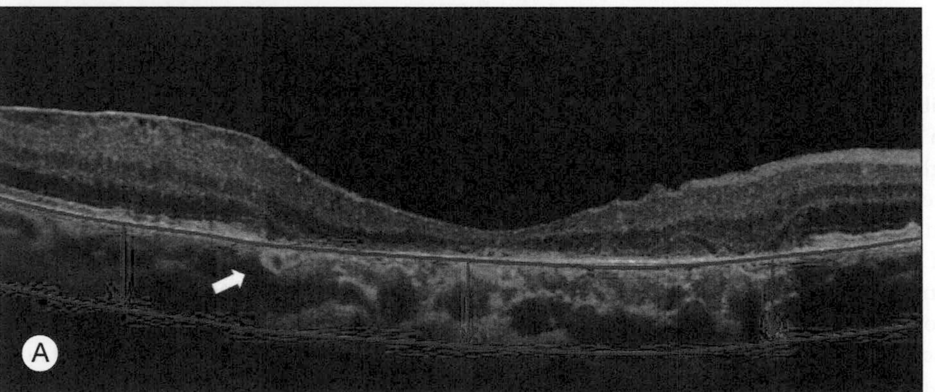

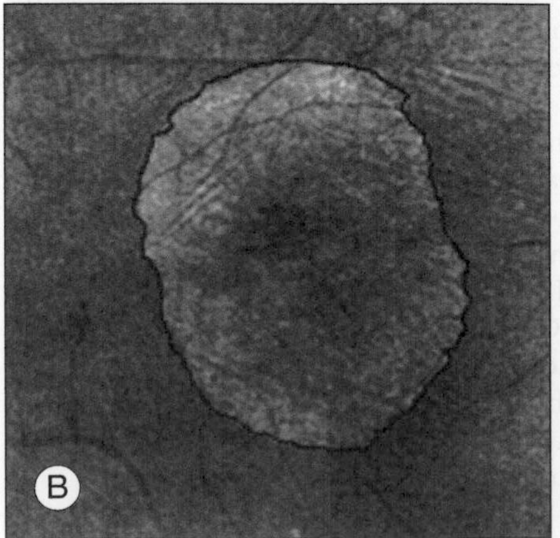

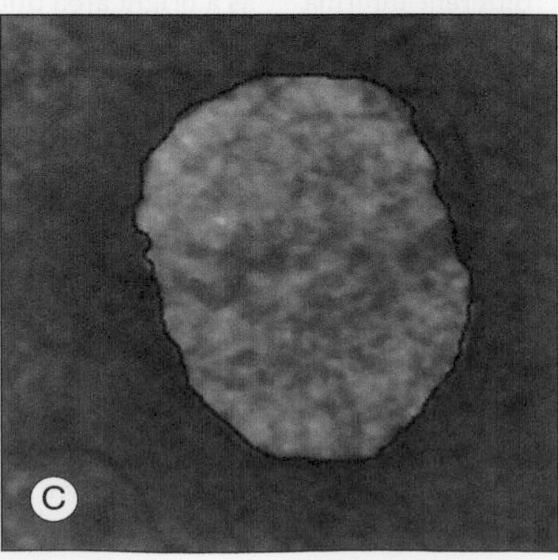

Fig. 3.17 Geographic atrophy (GA). (A) Horizontal B-scan through the foveal center of a 73-year-old man with GA showing increased light penetration in the areas where the retinal pigment epithelium (RPE) is absent. The white arrow shows the junction where the RPE is present and absent. (B) Optical coherence tomography (OCT) fundus image (OFI) represents a virtual fundus image resulting from the en face summation of the reflected light from each A-scan. GA lesions are identified as a bright area due to the increased penetration of light into the choroid where atrophy has occurred. (C) Enhanced OCT fundus image (courtesy of Cirrus, Carl Zeiss Meditec), which represents the summation of the reflected light from beneath the RPE (red lines and arrows on (A)).

Neovascular AMD

The neovascular (wet) form of AMD is characterized by the overproduction of VEGF and the growth of abnormal vessels in the macular region. These vessels may arise from the choroidal circulation and penetrate Bruch's membrane to form a fibrovascular tissue beneath or above the RPE, or these vessels may arise primarily from the retinal circulation. In either case, the presence of VEGF and abnormal vessels leads to structural changes in the retina and choroid with the accumulation of fluid within the retina, in the subretinal space, or under the RPE. Furthermore, this neovascular invasion may lead to significant disorganization and remodeling of the retina, resulting in the loss of the RPE and photoreceptors with the formation of a disciform scar.[100,101]

Intraretinal and subretinal fluid

In cases suspicious for exudative changes, OCT imaging can be extremely useful in detecting intraretinal, subretinal, or sub-RPE fluid. In cases with active neovascular AMD, OCT imaging can be used to establish baseline retinal thickness and volume, and determine the extent of neovascularization, fluid involvement, and other lesion components (blood, fluid, pigment, and fibrosis).

The growth of neovascularization is often accompanied by VEGF-dependent leakage from both the mature vessels and the growing immature vessels. Intraretinal edema can range from mild retinal thickening of the outer nuclear layer to large and diffuse cystoid edema, seen as round or oval hyporeflective areas (Fig. 3.18).[21] Lipid exudation can also be present in patients with profuse intraretinal edema and appear as small hyperreflective dots in the outer retina. The fluid may also accumulate in the space between the RPE and the neurosensory retina. The subretinal fluid appears on OCT imaging as homogeneous hyporeflective spaces when the fluid exudation is serous, or may be separated by fibrinous membranes when profuse proteinaceous exudation is present.[102] Usually neovascular lesions growing in the subretinal space are associated with a larger volume of subretinal fluid compared with sub-RPE lesions.[103]

Retinal pigment epithelium detachment

In wet AMD, a retinal PED is formed by the separation of the RPE from Bruch's membrane due to the presence of sub-RPE fluid, blood, or fibrovascular tissue. A serous PED is defined as an area of smooth, sharply demarcated dome-shaped elevation of the RPE, often yellow–orange in color with a reddish halo of subretinal fluid. On fluorescein angiography, serous PEDs are associated with early hyperfluorescence with a well-defined border, which increases gradually throughout the study and classically demonstrates a pooling of dye rather than leakage.[104,105] Serous PEDs can be categorized as vascular or avascular.[106] On OCT imaging, serous PEDs appear as a dome-shaped elevation of the RPE typically seen overlying a homogeneously hyporeflective space, bound inferiorly by a visible Bruch's membrane, which is seen as a thin hyperreflective line at the outer aspect of the PED (Fig. 3.19).[107,108] The appearance of vascularized serous PEDs is similar. However, in some cases, the apparent fibrovascular proliferation can be seen adjacent to the PED and even adherent to the outer surface of the RPE.

The fibrovascular PED usually produces an irregularly elevated lesion visible on clinical examination and can be associated with RPE hyperpigmentation, subretinal hemorrhage, subretinal lipid exudation, and intra- or subretinal fluid collection.[109] The elevation is often low and the borders are ill defined. The detailed structural characteristics and precise mechanism of PED formation have not been completely resolved. Recent studies using SD-OCT imaging revealed that many of the fibrovascular PEDs appear to be filled with solid layers of material of medium reflectivity, separated by hyporeflective clefts (Fig. 3.20).[110]

Hemorrhagic PEDs occur when a CNV membrane bleeds into the sub-RPE space or as a result of an RPE tear. The hemorrhage can invade the subretinal space, with the sub-RPE blood having a typically darker appearance than subretinal blood. OCT

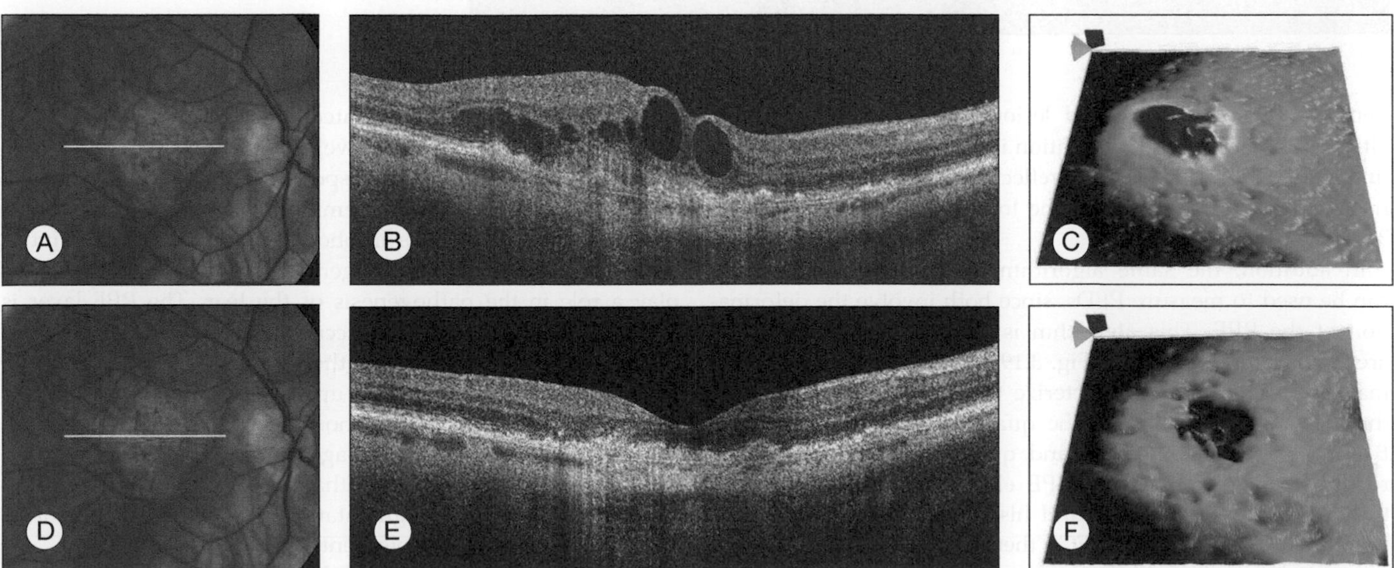

Fig. 3.18 Neovascular age-related macular degeneration. (A) Color fundus image of the right eye of an 81-year-old man with a 1-month history of vision loss. Visual acuity was 20/100. (B) Horizontal B-scan through the foveal center showing retinal thickening and the presence of intraretinal fluid with large cysts. (C) Retinal thickness map (courtesy of Cirrus, Carl Zeiss Meditec) showing the increase in retinal thickness (red areas). After three intravitreal injections of antivascular endothelial growth factor, the intraretinal fluid was reabsorbed (D). This is better observed in the B-scan and retinal thickness map (E, F).

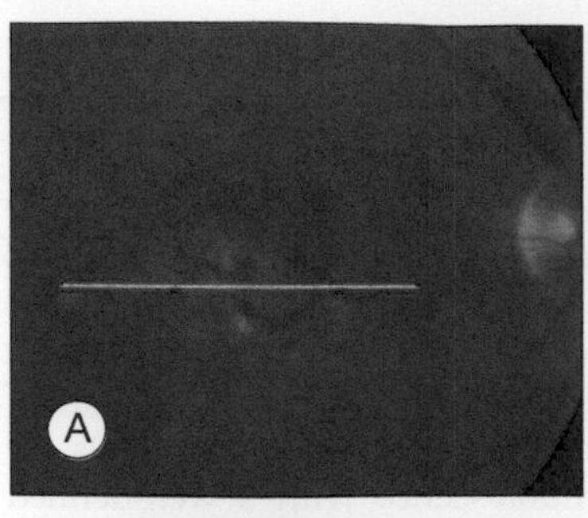

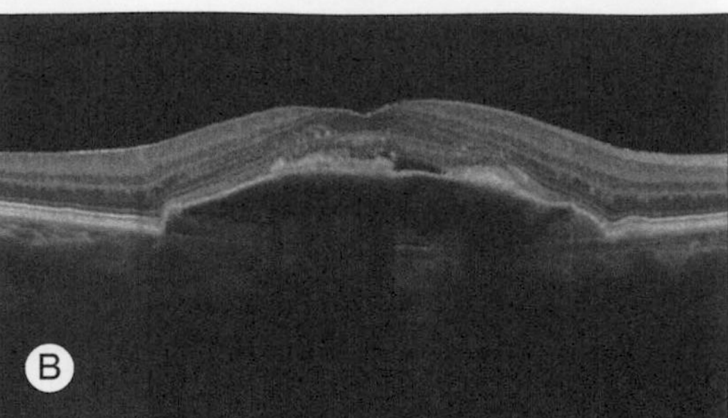

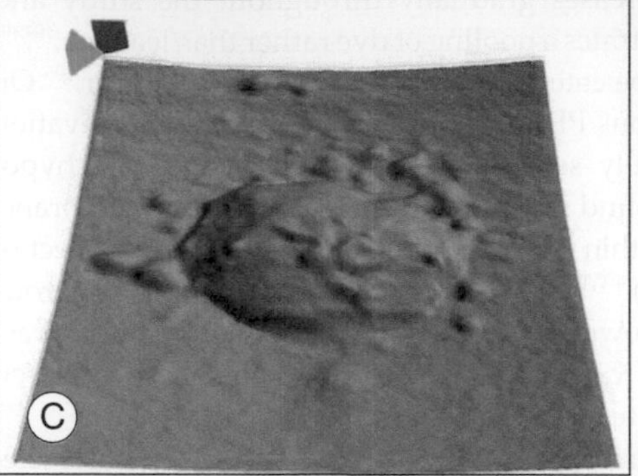

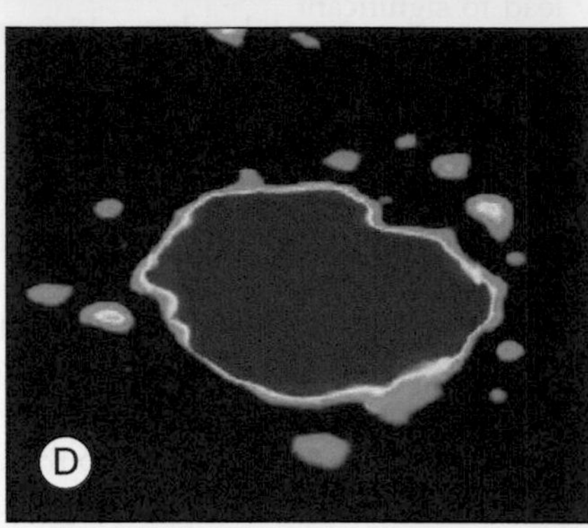

Fig. 3.19 Vascularized serous retinal pigmented epithelium detachment (PED). (A) Color fundus image of the left eye of a 77-year-old woman with pigmentary changes in the macula associated with an elevation of the macula. (B) Horizontal B-scan through the fovea showing a dome-shaped retinal pigment epithelium (RPE) elevation overlying a homogeneous hyporeflective space. Observe the presence of subretinal fluid above the PED. (C) RPE segmentation map showing a three-dimensional perspective of the PED. (D) RPE elevation map showing the area (5.84 mm^2) and volume (0.83 mm^3) measurements of the PED.

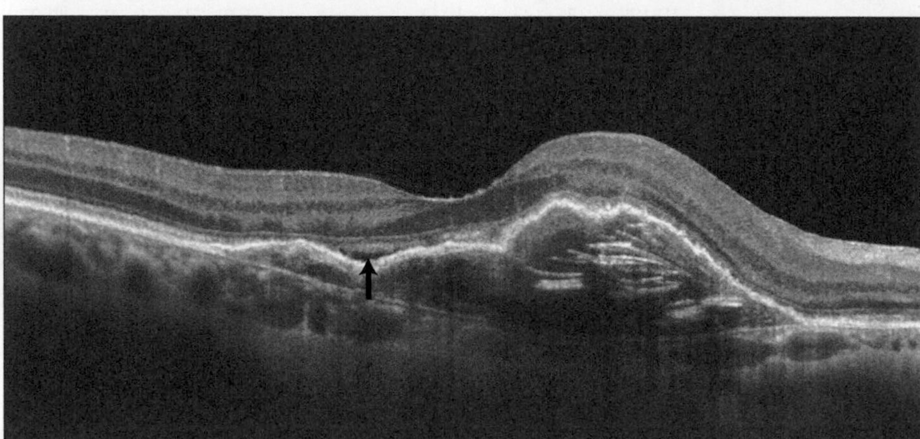

Fig. 3.20 Fibrovascular retinal pigmented epithelium detachment (PED). Cross-sectional B-scan of the right eye of an 87-year-old woman with a fibrovascular PED. The space below the retinal pigment epithelium is filled with solid layers of medium reflectivity separated by hyporeflective clefts. A small amount of subretinal fluid can be identified over the PED (arrow).

demonstrates a dome-shaped lesion, similar to serous PEDs, although the slope of the elevation is more acute and the blood under the RPE appears hyperreflective, attenuating the signal from deeper structures, with the loss of choroidal detail (Fig. 3.21).[107,109,111]

In addition, the same algorithm used to measure drusen can be used to measure PEDs, since both involve the deformation of the RPE. This algorithm is able to measure both the area and volume of PEDs (Fig. 3.19D). In addition, algorithms may be developed to characterize the internal architecture of the PEDs automatically.[112] The qualitative appearance of the B-scans and the qualitative and quantitative changes in the retinal thickness maps and RPE elevation map can be used to appreciate better the natural history of the disease and to monitor the effect of anti-VEGF therapy in patients with PEDs associated with wet AMD.

Tear of the retinal pigment epithelium

RPE tears are most commonly seen in association with CNV secondary to AMD, especially when a PED is present.[113,114] RPE tears may also be associated with central serous chorioretinopathy (CSC), trauma, as well as other causes of CNV.[115,116] Although RPE tears can occur spontaneously in AMD patients, they have also been related temporally to various treatments for AMD, such as verteporfin photodynamic therapy and intravitreal injection of anti-VEGF agents.[117-121] Hemodynamic factors play a role in the pathogenesis of the tear. The RPE layer is put on stretch as a result of accumulating sub-RPE fluid and this stress leads to a tear in the RPE. A sheet of RPE cells then contracts and scrolls up upon itself in a radial fashion, leaving an area of retina without underlying RPE.[114,122] Subretinal and sub-RPE hemorrhages frequently accompany an RPE tear, which appears ophthalmoscopically as an area of well-demarcated hyperpigmentation immediately adjacent to an area of relative hypopigmentation.

On OCT imaging, an area of discontinuity in a large PED is often seen, with the free edge of the RPE often curled under the PED. Adjacent to the tear, there is increased reflectivity from the choroid vessels, due to the absence of the RPE. The overlying retina is typically intact, but may be separated from the area of atrophy by subretinal fluid.[114] The tear tends to occur at the base of the PED, near or at the intersection of attached and detached retina (Fig. 3.22).[113] During anti-VEGF therapy, the height of the PED and the irregular surface contour may help in predicting the risk for RPE tear, which may also occur without treatment as part of normal disease progression.[123,124] The visual outcome in patients with RPE tears is generally poor when the fovea is involved.

Disciform scarring

Disciform scarring and subretinal fibrosis mark the endstage of CNV. The vascular components of CNV typically regress as the lesion becomes less active, and the fibrous components typically increase, resulting in disciform scar formation. Clinically the scar appears as smooth, elevated white or gray tissue in the subretinal space and on OCT imaging the scar corresponds to a highly reflective outer retinal or subretinal lesion (Fig. 3.23).[21] Scar formation may be associated with loss of the overlying photoreceptor layer and irreversible reduction in visual acuity. This may be observed on OCT imaging as a disruption of the IS/OS junction and ELM.[125,126] In this stage of the disease, the OCT is very helpful in identifying the presence of subretinal fluid or intraretinal cysts that are associated with the neovascular activity of the lesion, and may help in making the retreatment decision.

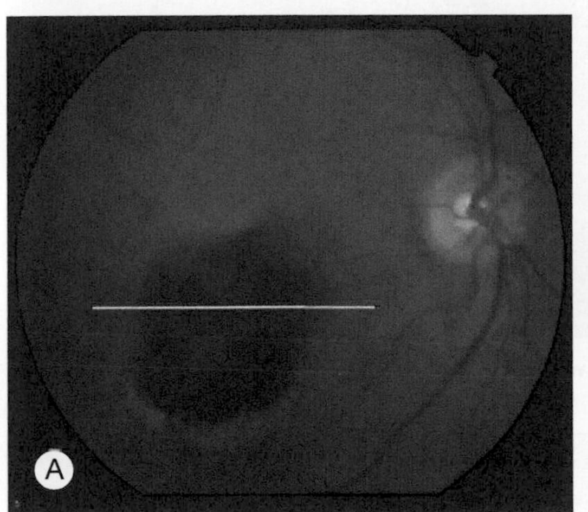

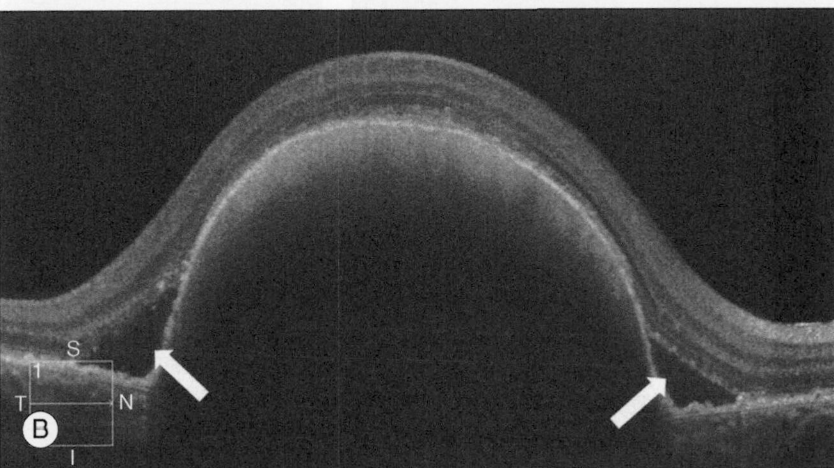

Fig. 3.21 Hemorrhagic retinal pigmented epithelium detachment (PED). (A) Color fundus image of the right eye of a 65-year-old woman with a large subretinal pigment epithelium (RPE) hemorrhage secondary to neovascular age-related macular degeneration. (B) Optical coherence tomography demonstrates a dome-shaped lesion, similar to serous PEDs. The blood under the RPE appears hyperreflective, attenuating the signal from deeper structures. Subretinal fluid can be observed as hyporeflective spaces above the RPE (arrows).

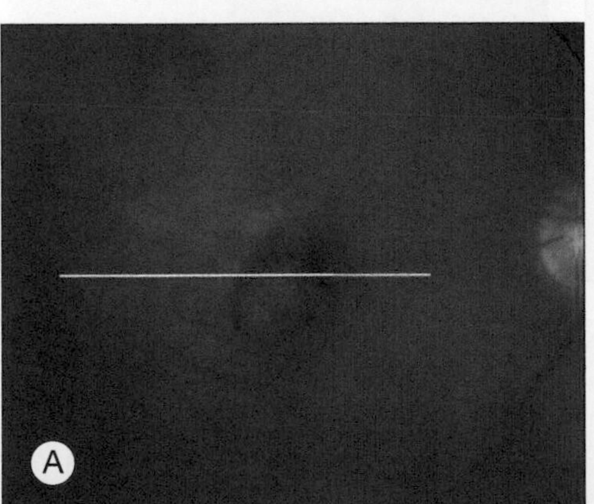

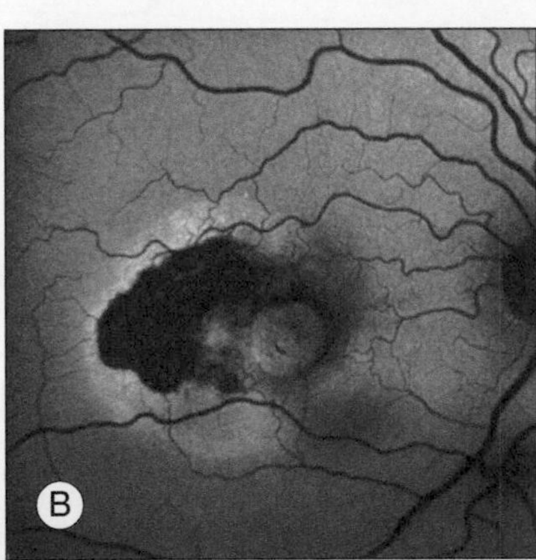

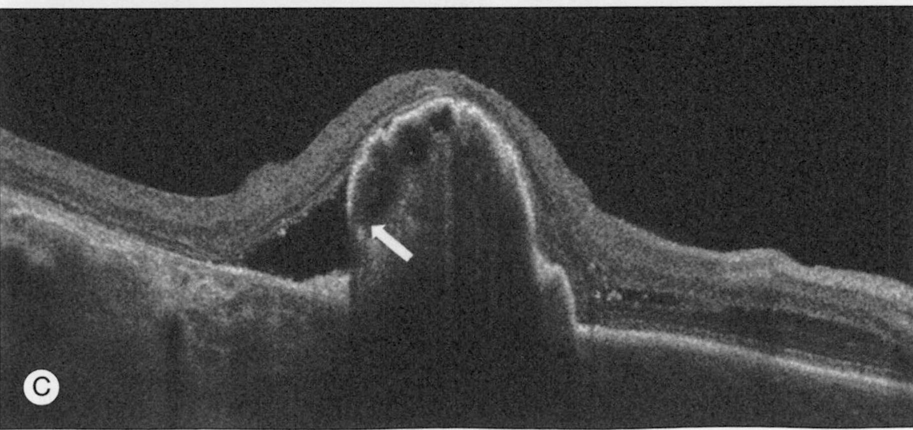

Fig. 3.22 Retinal pigment epithelium (RPE) tear. (A) Color image of the right eye of an 81-year-old man with an area of relative hypopigmentation that corresponds to the RPE tear. (B) Heidelberg fundus autofluorescence showing hypoautofluorescence in the area where the RPE is absent. (C) On the B-scan there is an area of discontinuity of the RPE near the base of the pigmented epithelium detachment with the free edge of the RPE curled under the pigmented epithelium detachment (arrow).

Retinal angiomatous proliferation

The term "retinal angiomatous proliferation" was introduced by Yannuzzi and coworkers to describe a form of neovascularization in AMD patients, which arises from within the retina with possible formation of a retinochoroidal anastomosis as the disease progresses.[127] Whether the development of the retinochoroidal anastomosis is a result of a primary intraretinal neovascularization or a sub-RPE lesion remains controversial.[127,128] Recently, studies with SD-OCT imaging concluded that the initial neovascular process could originate from either the retinal or choroidal circulation; however, histopathological studies suggest that all the neovascularization is within the retina.[129,130] On OCT imaging, the most common feature is the presence of a serous PED with CME overlying the PED (Fig. 3.24).[129,131,132] An intraretinal hyperreflective angiomatous complex consistent with the intraretinal neovascularization and subretinal fluid may also be seen.[127]

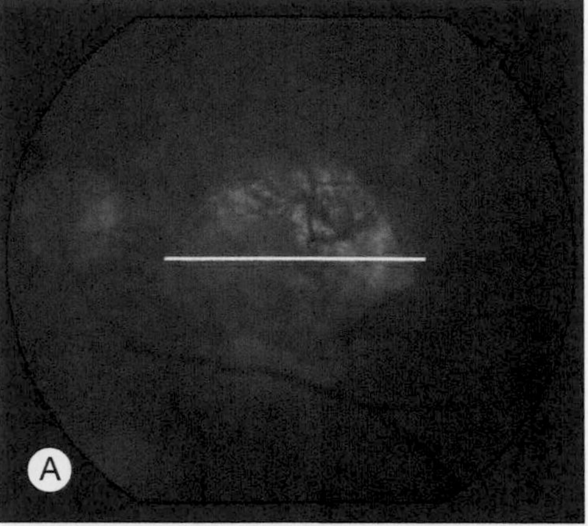

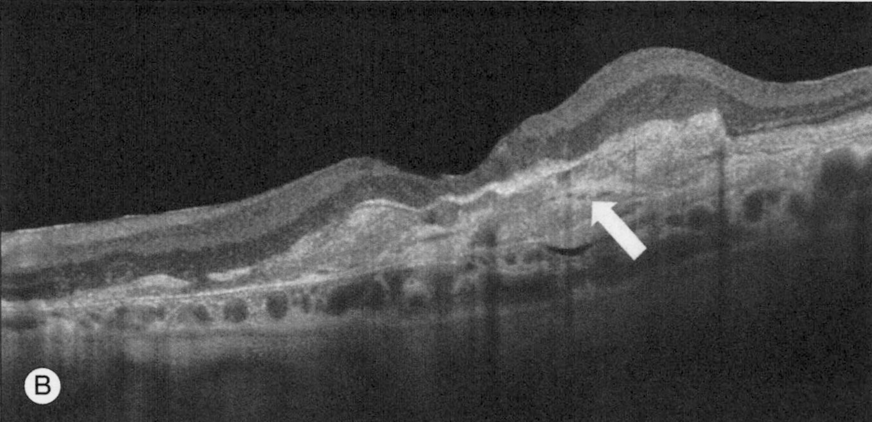

Fig. 3.23 Disciform scar. (A) Color fundus image of the left eye of an 80-year-old woman with a white-grayish tissue involving the macula. (B) Horizontal B-scan with a large hyperreflective lesion under the retina (arrow).

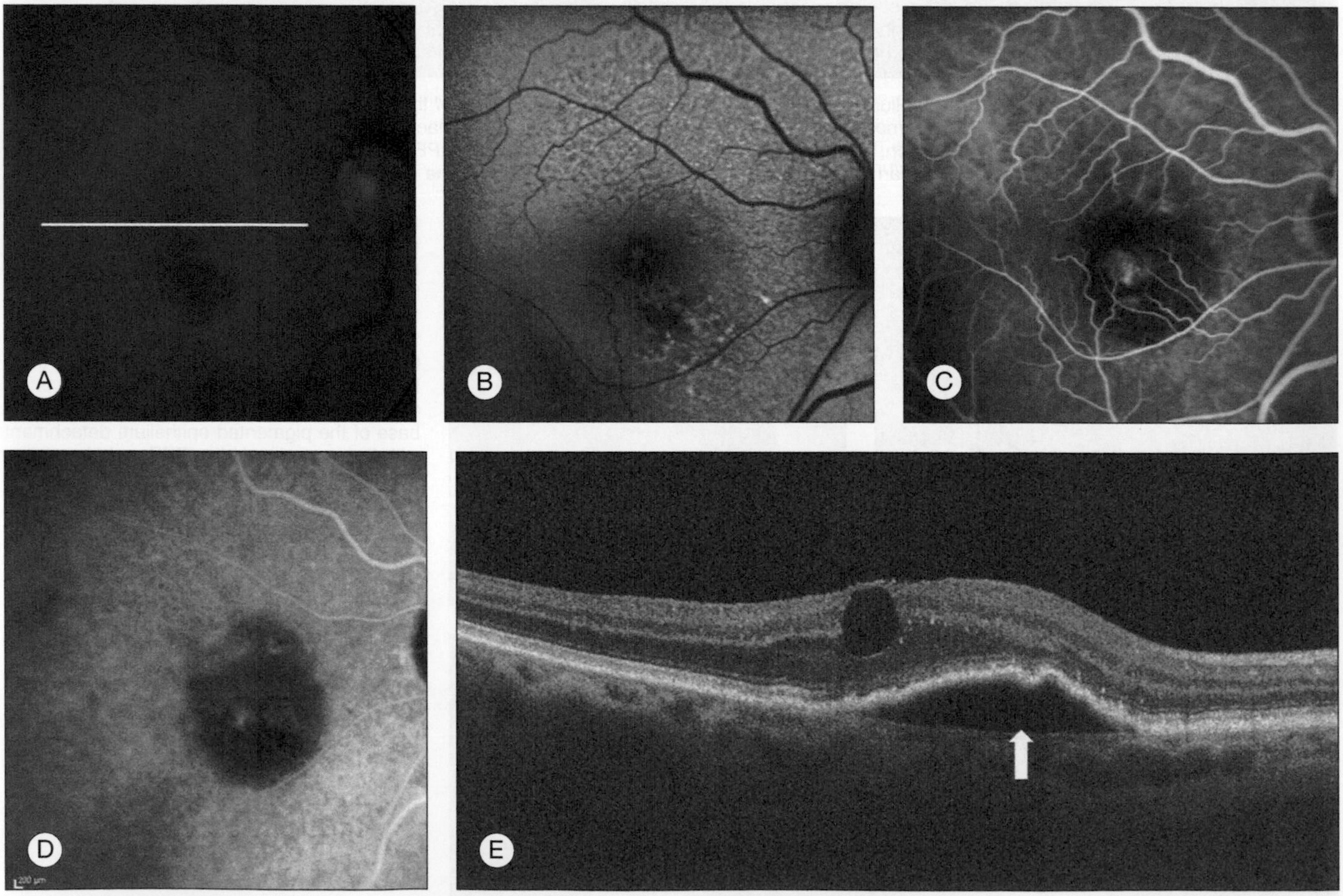

Fig. 3.24 Retinal angiomatous proliferation. (A) Color fundus image of the right eye of a 90-year-old woman with a history of blurred vision and metamorphopsia for 2 weeks. Visual acuity was 20/40. Fundus examination revealed multiple drusen, pigmentary changes, and hemorrhage inferior to the fovea with a subtle elevation of the retina. (B) Fundus autofluorescence demonstrates hypoautofluorescence in the area corresponding to the hemorrhage. (C) Fluorescein angiography demonstrates a focal area of leakage inferior to the fovea. (D) Late-phase indocyanine green angiography reveals a hot spot. (E) B-scan through the lesion reveals a retinal pigment epithelium detachment (arrow) with cystoid macular edema overlying the pigmented epithelium detachment.

Polypoidal choroidal vasculopathy

Polypoidal choroidal vasculopathy is considered a variant form of CNV characterized by the presence of multiple vascular sacular dilations (polyps) in the choroidal circulation that manifests clinically with variably sized serous and serosanguineous detachments of the neurosensory retina and RPE, usually around the optic nerve or in the central macula.[133] Indocyanine green (ICG) angiography is particularly useful in imaging the polypoidal abnormalities seen in polypoidal choroidal vasculopathy, with a branching vascular network of vessels ending in polyp-like structures.[134] SD-OCT images can demonstrate the polypoidal structure beneath the RPE, which remains adherent to the RPE, even with increased exudation. It is especially useful to detect the abnormalities surrounding the polypoidal lesions such as intraretinal, subretinal, and sub-RPE fluid.[135,136]

Choroidal neovascularization: response to treatment

The combination of clinical examination, fluorescein angiography, OCT images, and, less frequently, ICG angiography is usually required to diagnose neovascular AMD and exclude other macular conditions that can mimic the features of neovascular AMD.[137] With the use of anti-VEGF drugs, the ideal strategy for following eyes with wet AMD has evolved from monthly injections to OCT imaging to determine whether the treatment is effective in resolving the macular fluid.[138,139] Many alternative treatment regimens have used OCT-guided strategies, with good visual and anatomical results with fewer intravitreal injections compared with monthly dosing.[140–144] The macular fluid can be identified by examining the B-scans and reviewing the retinal thickness maps, which calculate the retinal thickness between the ILM and the RPE segmentation maps. The effect of anti-VEGF therapy can then be assessed based on the qualitative appearance of the B-scans and the qualitative, as well as quantitative, changes in the retinal thickness maps (Figs 3.18 and 3.25). The presence or recurrence of intraretinal or subretinal fluid has to be differentiated from the appearance of "outer retinal tubulation", since the latter represents a rearrangement of photoreceptors in response to injury and RPE loss and is usually present in patients with chronic and advanced neovascular AMD (Fig. 3.26). Importantly, this tubulation does not respond to anti-VEGF therapy.[145] In patients with PEDs, the area and volume of the lesion can be assessed and used to monitor the effect of anti-VEGF therapy in patients with wet AMD associated with PEDs, and an increase in the area and volume of PEDs could be used to indicate when retreatment is necessary.

Central serous chorioretinopathy

CSC is an idiopathic syndrome that typically affects young to middle-aged males and is characterized by serous detachment of the neurosensory retina. Focal and multifocal areas of leakage secondary to increased permeability of the choroidal vessels and a barrier defect at the level of the RPE have been described in the pathogenesis of this disorder.[146–148]

Presenting symptoms include central vision loss, a decrease in vision that can be corrected with an increased hyperopic correction, metamorphopsia, central scotoma, and decreased color saturation. The symptoms are usually self-limited but can recur in the same or the opposite eye. In most cases, CSC resolves spontaneously within 6 months, with a good visual prognosis. However, prolonged and recurrent macular detachment in some cases may cause degenerative changes in the subfoveal RPE and neurosensory retina with poor visual outcome.[149,150]

The primary pathology of acute CSC is thought to begin with disruption of the choroidal circulation. The RPE then decompensates and exudation from the choroidal vasculature passes into the subretinal space. These hypotheses were based on fluorescein angiography and ICG angiography findings.[147,151–154] The development of OCT imaging has provided a better understanding of CSC, especially the abnormalities in the RPE layer.[155–159]

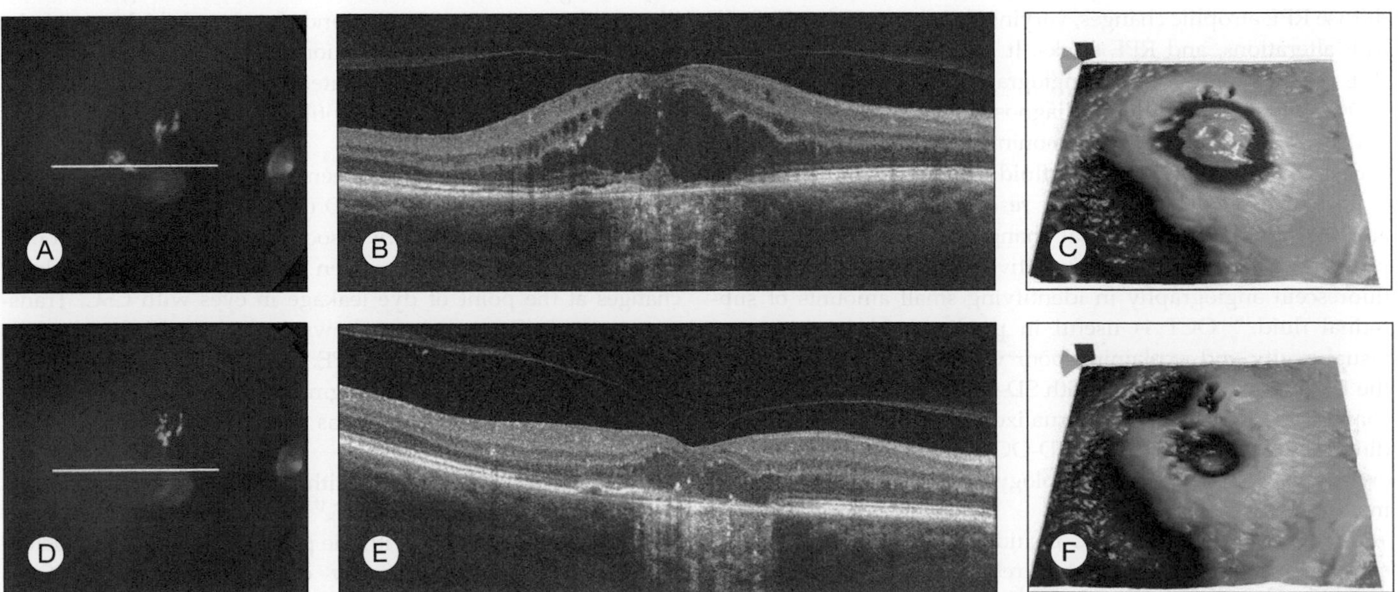

Fig. 3.25 Neovascular age-related macular degeneration (response to treatment). Color fundus image, horizontal B-scan, and retinal thickness map of the right eye of a 65-year-old man with wet age-related macular degeneration before (A–C) and after (D–F) a single treatment with intravitreal anti-vascular endothelial growth factor. Observe the improvement of the intraretinal fluid and cysts in the B-scans (B, E) and the decrease in retinal thickness (C, F).

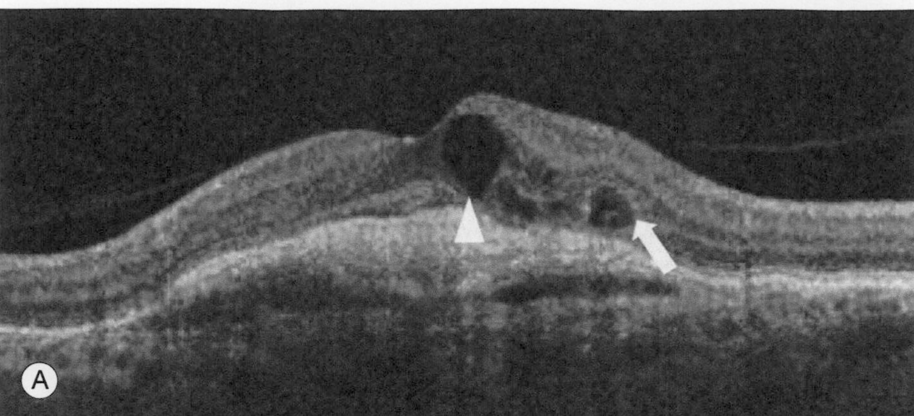

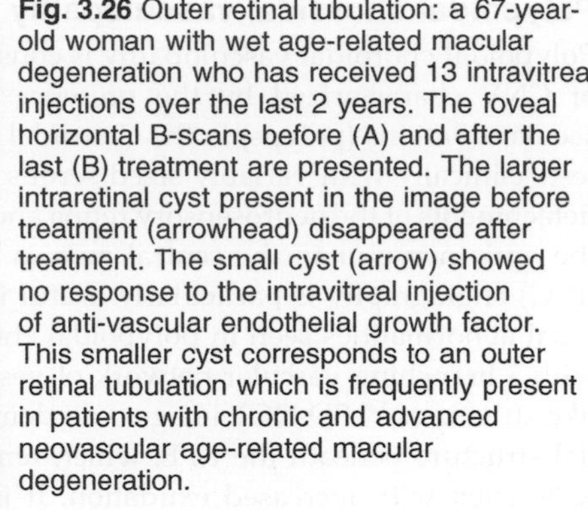

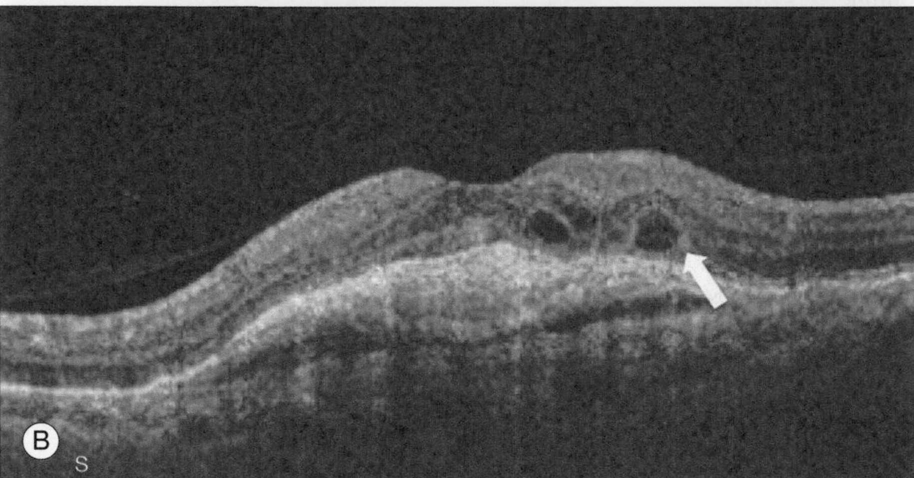

Fig. 3.26 Outer retinal tubulation: a 67-year-old woman with wet age-related macular degeneration who has received 13 intravitreal injections over the last 2 years. The foveal horizontal B-scans before (A) and after the last (B) treatment are presented. The larger intraretinal cyst present in the image before treatment (arrowhead) disappeared after treatment. The small cyst (arrow) showed no response to the intravitreal injection of anti-vascular endothelial growth factor. This smaller cyst corresponds to an outer retinal tubulation which is frequently present in patients with chronic and advanced neovascular age-related macular degeneration.

There are two forms of the disease, acute and chronic. Acute CSC (Fig. 3.27) is classically unilateral and characterized by one or more focal leaks at the level of the RPE on fluorescein angiography. The chronic form (Fig. 3.28) is believed to be due to diffuse RPE disease and is usually bilateral. It presents with diffuse RPE atrophic changes, varying degree of subretinal fluid, RPE alterations, and RPE tracks. It is characterized by diffuse RPE leakage on fluorescein angiography.

OCT imaging is helpful in diagnosing and managing patients with CSC. OCT imaging can noninvasively identify the presence and extent of subretinal fluid and PEDs. OCT imaging is also useful for assessing the resolution of subretinal fluid and the morphological retinal changes during normal disease progression. OCT is more sensitive than clinical exam and fluorescein angiography in identifying small amounts of subretinal fluid.[160] OCT is useful in predicting the recovery of visual acuity and explaining poor visual outcomes even after the resolution of the fluid. With SD-OCT imaging, topographic changes in CSC can be visualized with two- and three-dimensional reconstructions. SD-OCT also offers the ability of exact localization of the pathology and accurate volumetric measurements.[161]

OCT features of acute CSC include thickening of the neurosensory retina within the area of retinal detachment, PED, the presence of fibrinous exudates in the subretinal space, and the shaggy outer segments of the neurosensory retina above the leakage site. OCT features of the chronic form include foveal atrophy, retinal thinning, and cystoid degenerative changes.[156,157,162–166] OCT can also visualize the subretinal yellow deposits as highly reflective material. Precipitates are not only on the posterior surface of the detached retina but also in the detached neurosensory retina. Photoreceptor segment morphologic changes along the detached retina show elongation of the photoreceptor outer segments and decreased thickness of the outer nuclear layer.[167] Accumulation of abnormal outer segments in the neurosensory retina is related to clinical manifestation on OCT as a granulated shaggy profile of the outer surface of the detached retina.[168]

En face OCT imaging has been found to detect alterations of the RPE in the form of a PED or a small defect in the RPE. Most alterations of RPE are associated with choroidal abnormalities.[159] OCT imaging has been found to detect morphologic changes at the point of dye leakage in eyes with CSC. Transverse images (C-scans) have shown serous retinal detachments and irregular lesions of the RPE. These findings, along with other findings on B-scans and segmentation maps, are consistent with location of lesions in areas of fluorescein angiographic leakage.[169,170]

Visual prognosis in patients with CSC can be linked to retinal morphological changes by OCT.[171,172] Mastsumoto et al. correlated the visual outcome with the preservation of outer nuclear layer thickness and continuity of photoreceptor IS/OS in resolved CSC. The outer nuclear layer thickness was positively correlated with visual acuity. Discontinuity of the IS/OS line was prevalent in eyes with thinner outer nuclear layer and lower visual acuity.[172] Ojima et al.[171] reported that microstructural

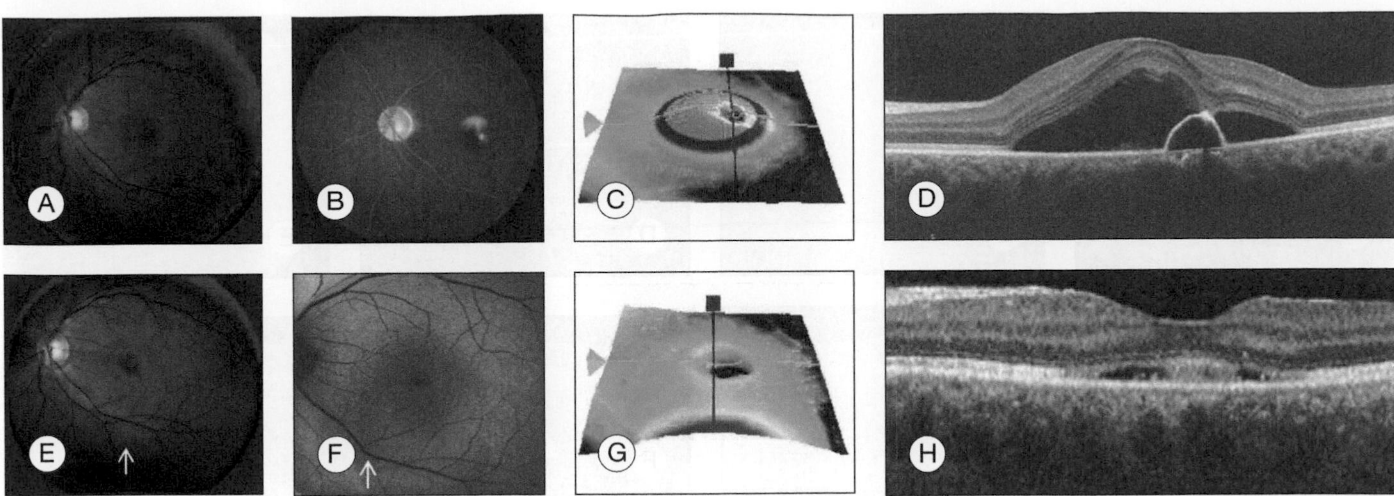

Fig. 3.27 Acute central serous chorioretinopathy. (A) Color photo shows a well-defined, circular area of retinal elevation. (B) Fluorescein angiography shows an area of hyperfluorescence with "smokestack" leakage. (C) Retinal thickness map shows elevation of the retina. (D) Spectral domain optical coherence tomography (OCT), horizontal, acquired through the fovea, shows serous detachment of the neurosensory retina above an optically clear, fluid-filled cavity, associated with a pigment epithelial detachment. The retinal pigment epithelium detachment corresponds to the area of hyperfluorescence seen on the angiogram. (E–H) Follow-up visit 1 month later. (E) Color photo shows resolution of the retinal elevation in the area of the fovea but illustrates a well-defined, circular area of retinal elevation inferior to the fovea (small arrow). (F) Fundus autofluorescence shows a well-defined, circular area of retinal elevation inferior to the fovea involving the inferior arcade (small arrow). (G) Retinal thickness map shows decrease in the thickness of the retina in the fovea. (H) Spectral domain OCT, horizontal B-scan acquired through the fovea, shows decrease in the amount of subretinal fluid.

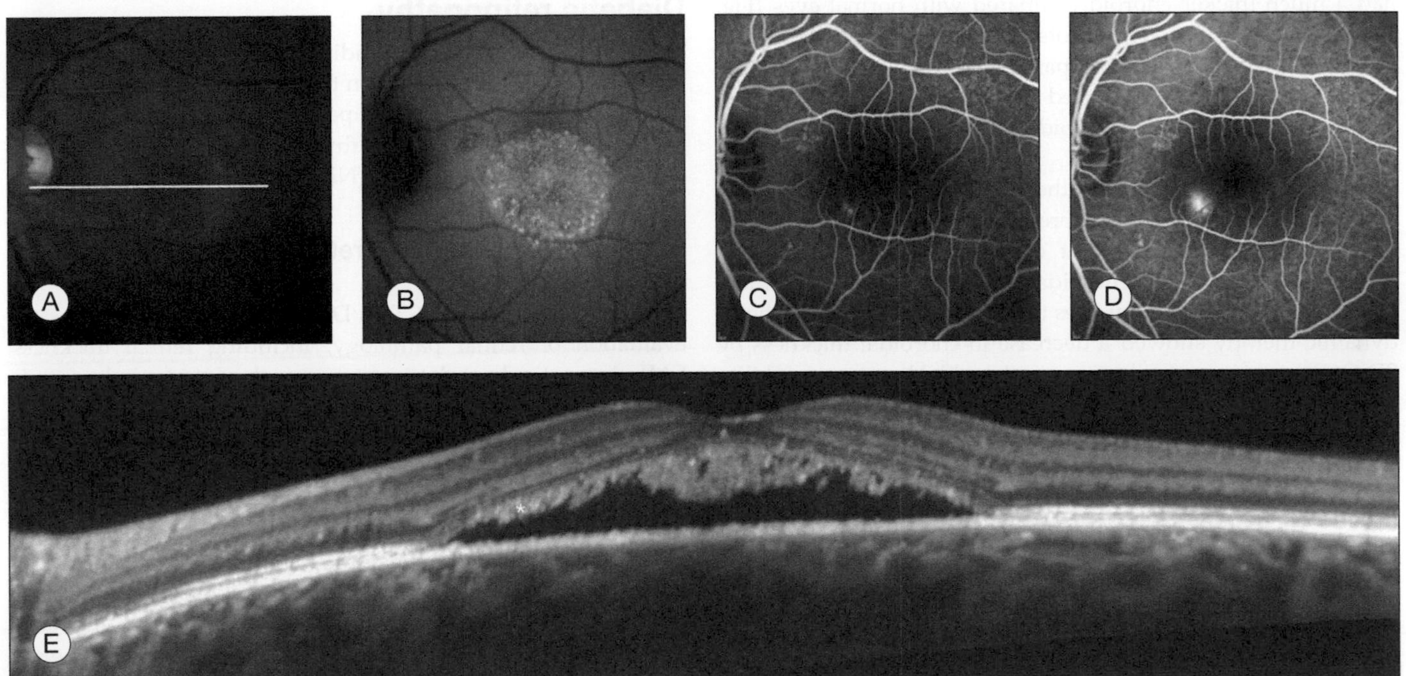

Fig. 3.28 Central serous chorioretinopathy. (A) Color photo shows a well-defined, circular area of retinal elevation; white line represents the location of the B-scan. (B) Fundus autofluorescence shows an area of hyperfluorescence. (C, D) Fluorescein angiography shows an inkblot appearance that leaks later. (E) Spectral domain optical coherence tomography shows serous detachment of the neurosensory retina associated with an irregular, granulated retinal pigment epithelial layer and sagging/dipping of the posterior layer of the neurosensory retina (asterisk).

changes occur in the photoreceptor layer of the detached retina and the visualization of the ELM and the photoreceptor layer correlates with visual function. Foveal thickness can be a predictor of visual outcome in patients with CSC.[163] Both foveal thickness and visual acuity have been observed to be proportional to the duration of symptoms, Foveal attenuation, and atrophy, which may be a consequence of prolonged absence of contact between photoreceptor and RPE cells.[160]

Enhanced depth imaging OCT IN CSC

Conventional SD-OCT has a limited ability to image the choroid because of scattering by the pigment granules within the RPE and by the pigment and blood within the choroid, and because of a depth-dependent roll-off in sensitivity of SD-OCT instruments in general.[29] A method to improve imaging of the choroid, known as EDI OCT, showed that eyes with CSC

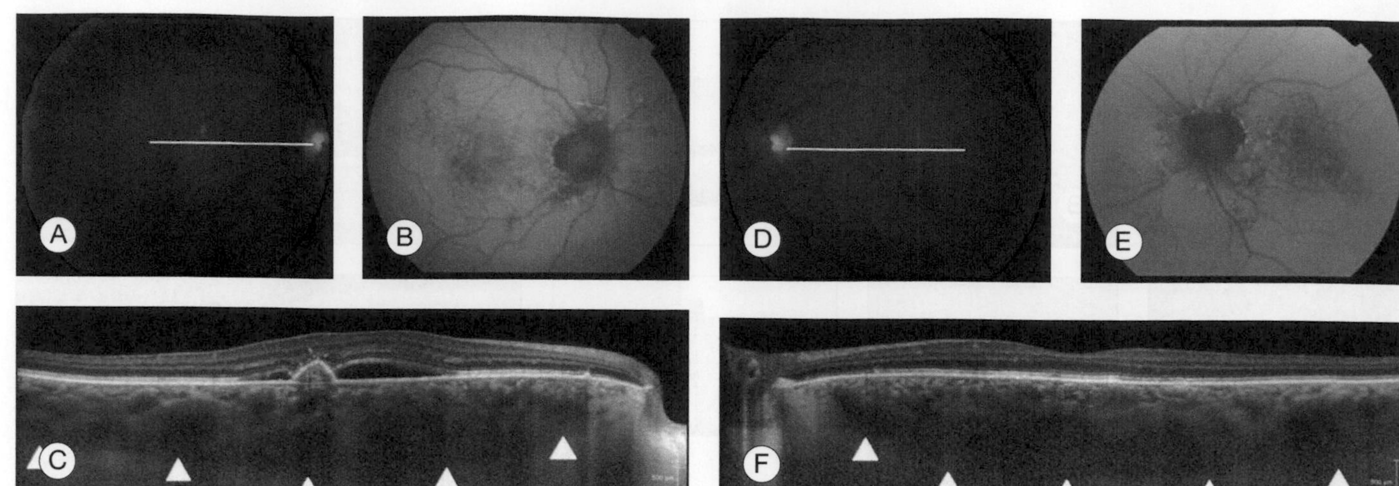

Fig. 3.29 Central serous chorioretinopathy. (A) Color photo of the right eye shows area of retinal elevation with pigmentary changes; white line represents the position of B-scan. (B) Fundus autofluorescence shows an area of hyperfluorescence and hypofluorescence. (C) Spectral domain optical coherence tomography (OCT), enhanced depth imaging, shows serous detachment of the neurosensory retina along with pigmented epithelium detachment, retinal pigment epithelial alterations, granulated posterior detached retina, and thick choroid (arrowheads represent the outer boundary of the choroid). (D) Color photo of the left eye shows pigmentary changes without retinal elevation; white line represents location of B-scan. (E) Fundus autofluorescence shows an area of hyperfluorescence and hypofluorescence. (F) Spectral domain OCT, enhanced depth imaging, demonstrates a thick choroid (arrowheads represent the boundary of the choroid) without serous detachment of the neurosensory retina.

had a much thicker choroid compared with normal eyes (Fig. 3.29).[173] Fellow eyes of patients with CSC were also found to have thicker choroids compared with age-matched normal eyes.[174] Maruko et al. reported a thickened choroid in CSC and the association with choroidal vascular hyperpermeability on ICG angiography.[175]

Verteporfin photodynamic therapy is one of the therapies used to treat leakage and subretinal fluid in eyes with CSC. Maruko et al.[175] reported that eyes treated with focal laser showed no alteration in choroidal thickness even though there was fluid reabsorption, but eyes treated with verteporfin photodynamic therapy showed a decrease in choroidal thickness by SD-OCT imaging and a decrease in choroidal hyperpermeability seen during ICG angiography. The changes occurring in the choroid after photodynamic therapy may reflect a more normalized choroidal permeability.

Cystoid macular edema

CME is an important cause of reduced visual acuity in a wide variety of retinal diseases such as diabetic retinopathy, retinal vein occlusion, CNV, retinal dystrophies, uveitis, and following intraocular surgery. Regardless of the underlying etiology, CME appears as retinal thickening with intraretinal cavities of reduced reflectivity on OCT (Fig. 3.30).

Clinically significant pseudophakic CME is estimated to occur in 1–2% of patients undergoing cataract extraction.[176,177] Inflammatory components induced by surgery along with mechanical forces induced by a modified vitreous are responsible for the macular changes in these patients.[178,179] The diagnosis based only on fundus examination can be challenging and usually fluorescein angiographic imaging, which shows a classic petaloid pattern of leakage, or OCT imaging is needed for confirmation. OCT has the advantage of being a faster and noninvasive imaging technique which can also provide quantitative assessment of the macular thickness that can be used to monitor the clinical course and to make therapeutic decisions.

Diabetic retinopathy

Diabetic retinopathy is the leading cause of blindness in individuals under 65 years of age in the USA, with diabetic macular edema (DME) being the principal cause of vision loss in these patients.[180,181] Diabetic retinopathy can be classified into nonproliferative diabetic retinopathy (NPDR) and proliferative diabetic retinopathy (PDR).

Nonproliferative diabetic retinopathy and diabetic macular edema

The important role of OCT in DME management involves the evaluation of retinal pathology, including retinal thickness, CME, intraretinal exudates, vitreomacular interface abnormalities, subretinal fluid, and photoreceptor IS/OS junction abnormalities. OCT is also important in monitoring the response to treatment of DME by laser, intravitreal pharmacotherapies, and vitreoretinal surgery.

Determination of macular edema can be difficult with biomicroscopy or color fundus imaging, especially when the edema is mild.[182–184] It has been suggested that OCT measurements may be a more sensitive and reproducible indicator of true change in retinal thickness than color fundus imaging, supporting the use of OCT as the principal method for documenting retinal thickness. However, OCT is less suitable than fundus imaging for documenting the location and severity of other morphologic features of diabetic retinopathy, such as hard exudates, retinal hemorrhages, microaneurysms, and vascular abnormalities. Furthermore, OCT cannot provide information on overall retinopathy severity, for which color photographs remain the gold standard.[185–188]

OCT can be used to distinguish patients with normal retinal contour and thickness despite extensive angiopathy from those with early retinal edema. In general, the DME can be classified into several categories: diffuse retinal thickening, CME, serous retinal detachment or subretinal fluid, and vitreomacular interface abnormality.[189–191] Diffuse retinal thickening is usually

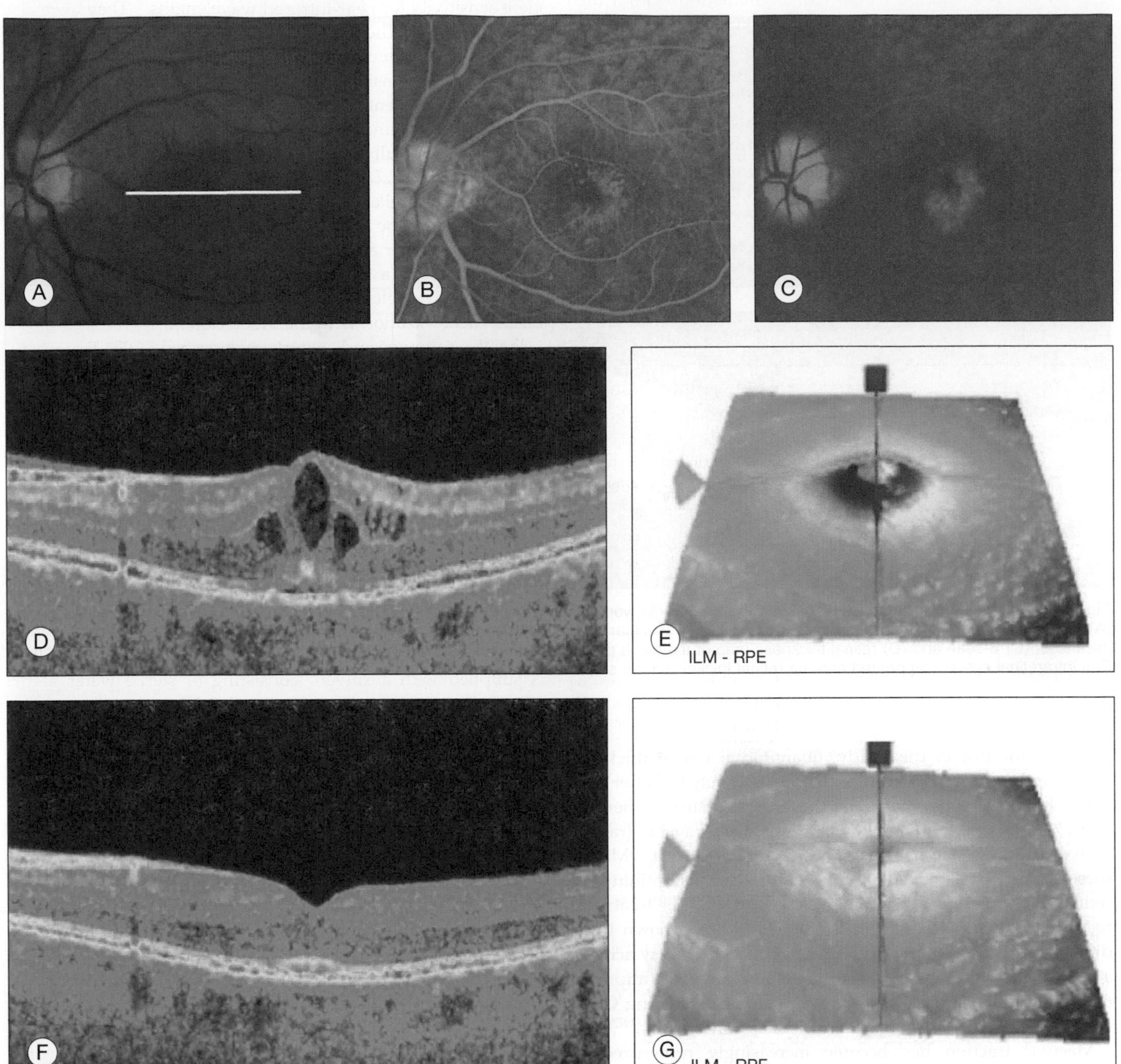

Fig. 3.30 Cystoid macular edema. Left eye of a 64-year-old man 30 days after phacoemulsification. The visual acuity was 20/50. (A) Color fundus image with some cystic changes; white line represents where the B-scan was acquired. (B, C) Fluorescein angiography showing the classic petaloid leakage pattern. (D) B-scan showing the intraretinal cysts as hyporeflective spaces within the retina. (E) Retinal thickness map showing increased retinal thickness due to the presence of cysts. (F, G) Same patient after 45 days of treatment with topical nonsteroid anti-inflammatory medication. The retinal thickness decreased and the intraretinal cysts disappeared. ILM, internal limiting membrane; RPE, retinal pigment epithelium.

defined as a sponge-like swelling of the retina with a generalized, heterogeneous, mild hyporeflectivity compared with normal retina. CME is characterized by the presence of intraretinal cystoid areas of low reflectivity, which are typically separated by highly reflective septa (Fig. 3.31). Serous retinal detachment is defined on OCT as a focal elevation of neurosensory retina overlying a hyporeflective, dome-shaped space. The posterior border of the detached retina is usually highly reflective, which helps to differentiate subretinal from intraretinal fluid. Vitreomacular interface abnormalities include the presence of ERMs, VMT, or both. Intraretinal focal hyperreflections that correspond clinically to retinal exudates are a frequent finding in all the patterns described above.

OCT has become widely accepted in monitoring progression and treatment response in patients with DME. Prior to OCT imaging, precision in central retinal thickness monitoring was not possible. The ETDRS provided guidelines for laser management of patients with DME.[192-194] Although OCT was not

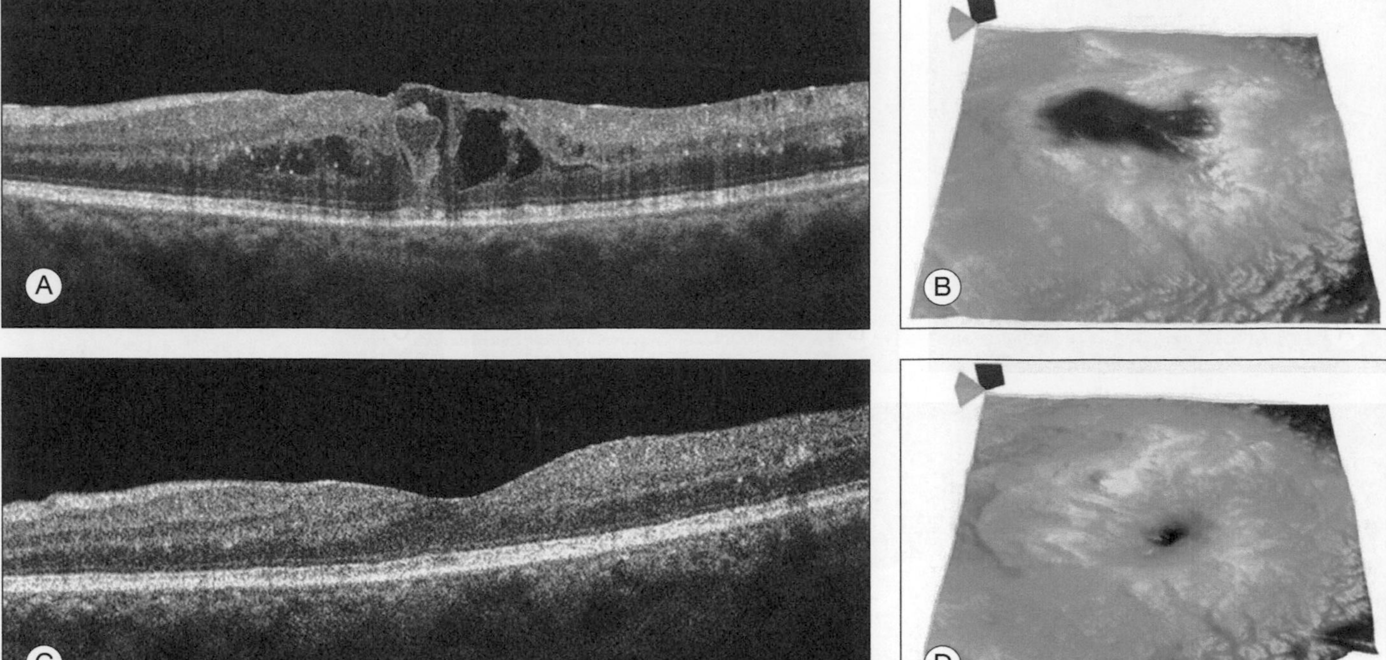

Fig. 3.31 Diabetic macular edema. Right eye of a 43-year-old woman with type 2 diabetes and moderate nonproliferative diabetic retinopathy. (A) B-scan and (B) retinal thickness map showing diffuse macular edema and the presence of intraretinal cysts with an increased retinal thickness. (C) B-scan and (D) retinal thickness map of the same patient after 3 months of intensive blood sugar control and focal laser therapy. The intraretinal cysts disappeared and the retinal thickness map shows an important decrease in the retinal thickness.

available for use in this study, quantitative retinal thickness maps can be used to direct laser therapy and may be better than using biomicroscopy alone. In the era of pharmacotherapy, many agents like triamcinolone and anti-VEGF agents (ranibizumab and bevacizumab) have been studied to treat DME. In these studies, OCT played an important role in determining the retinal thickness and the treatment response.[195,196] The treatment response of each OCT pattern of DME has been shown to be different.[197] Patients with diffuse retinal thickening may achieve a greater reduction in retinal thickness and a greater improvement in visual acuity compared with patients exhibiting CME, subretinal fluid, or vitreomacular interface abnormality.[197,198]

Macular traction has become increasingly recognized in patients with DME, especially in eyes with persistent edema after focal laser or pharmacological treatment. These patients often show the clinical appearance of a thick posterior hyaloid with diffuse fluorescein leakage. Recognition of this condition can be difficult using the clinical exam alone. This is readily recognized on OCT imaging as diffuse cystoid retinal thickening, a flat-appearing foveal contour, and a thickened hyperreflective linear vitreoretinal interface. Focal vitreoretinal adhesions that cannot be identified on clinical exam are also often evident on OCT.[199,200] These findings can direct the decision as to whether to proceed with pars plana vitrectomy and membrane peeling.[201]

Furthermore, the improvement in axial resolution with SD-OCT has enhanced the ability to evaluate foveal microstructural abnormalities, including the photoreceptor IS/OS junction, which may reveal damage to macular photoreceptors. Several studies have demonstrated that an intact IS/OS junction is predictive of a better visual acuity in patients after treatment for DME.[202–204]

Proliferative diabetic retinopathy

PDR can be visualized with OCT imaging as highly reflective preretinal bands anterior to the retinal surface, consistent with preretinal fibrovascular or fibroglial proliferation. Diffuse retinal thickening, distortion, and irregularity of the retinal contour can also occur as a result of the contraction of these preretinal membranes. An associated traction retinal detachment may be observed as well. OCT imaging is valuable in determining the extent of the tractional component as well as the presence of foveal involvement, assisting in the decision to intervene surgically (Fig. 3.32).[21] The decision for surgery typically hinges on the progressive nature of the traction and the degree to which the macula is affected by the traction.

Retinal vein occlusion

Retinal vein occlusions have been defined as retinal vascular disorders characterized by engorgement and dilatation of the retinal veins with secondary, mostly intraretinal, hemorrhages and mostly intraretinal (and partially subretinal) fluid, retinal ischemia, including cotton-wool spots, and retinal exudates.[205] Retinal vein occlusions are commonly divided into central retinal vein occlusion and branch retinal vein occlusion, and as soon as the foveal region is involved with macular edema, central visual acuity may be affected.

In retinal vein occlusions, OCT can display intraretinal cysts responsible for the increase in retinal thickness often associated with serous detachment of the neurosensory retina. Retinal cysts can be numerous and confluent, forming large central cystoid spaces. Associated findings can be observed, such as vitreous macular adherence, ERM, and hyperreflectivity of the posterior layer corresponding to atrophy or fibrosis of the RPE, subretinal

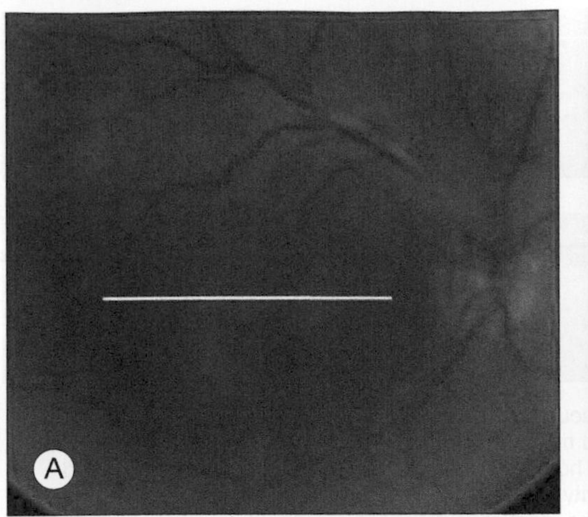

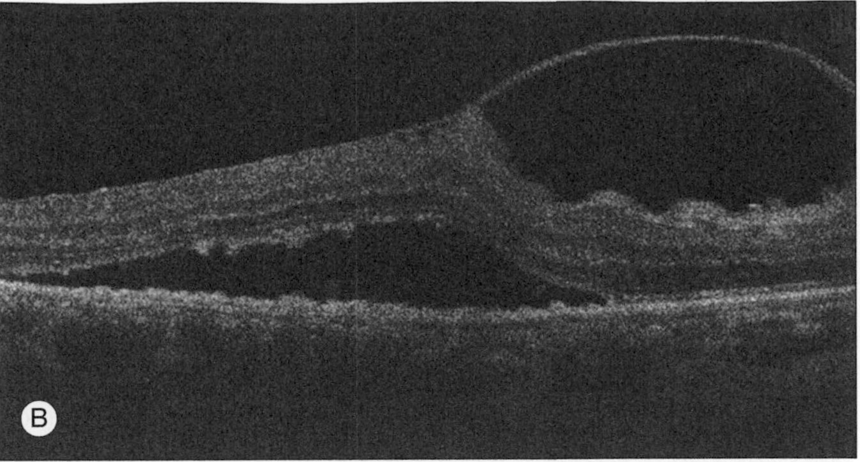

Fig. 3.32 Diabetic retinal tractional detachment. (A) Color fundus image of the right eye of a 72-year-old woman with proliferative diabetic retinopathy. (B) Foveal B-scan of the same patient showing a thick posterior hyaloid distorting the retinal architecture with traction and accumulation of fluid under the retina.

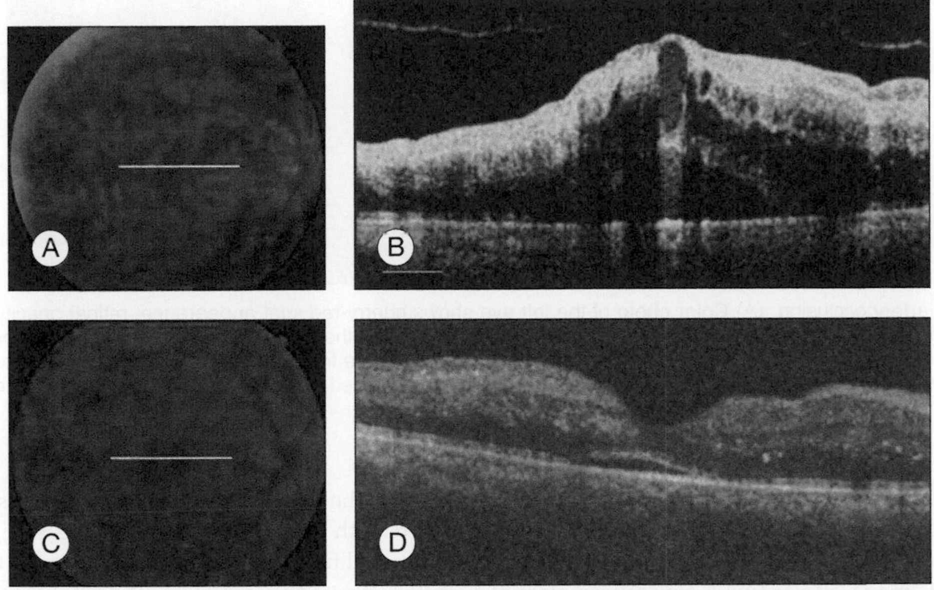

Fig. 3.33 Central retinal vein occlusion. (A) Color photo of the right eye shows optic nerve head edema, dilated tortuous retinal veins, scattered intraretinal hemorrhages in all quadrants, and macular edema; white line represents the location of the B-scan. (B) Spectral domain optical coherence tomography (OCT) obtained through the fovea illustrates loss of normal foveal contour and marked and diffuse retinal thickening. Large areas of low intraretinal reflectivity consistent with cystic fluid accumulation and edema were seen. A detachment of the neurosensory retina with subretinal fluid was observed below the fovea. (C) Color photo of the right eye 1 month after bevacizumab injection shows dilated tortuous retinal veins and scattered intraretinal hemorrhages in all quadrants; white line represents area of B-scan. (D) Spectral domain OCT, 1 month after bevacizumab injection obtained through the fovea, shows that macular edema almost completely disappeared with a small amount of residual subretinal fluid. Improvement in the normal foveal contour and decrease in the retinal thickening and edema. Areas of high intraretinal reflectivity consistent with the hemorrhages.

accumulation of material, subretinal fibrosis, lamellar macular hole formation, intraretinal lipid exudates, and intraretinal hemorrhage (Fig. 3.33).

Ota et al. reported that, in branch retinal vein occlusion, visual function and recovery of vision are correlated with thickness of the central macula, and that is correlated with the integrity of the inner and outer segments of the photoreceptors in the fovea.[206] SD-OCT imaging helps to quantify the amount of CME. The accumulation of fluid can be located mostly within the retinal layers or additionally in the subretinal space.[207] Anti-VEGF therapy is increasingly used to treat macular edema in patients with retinal vein occlusions. Nevertheless, a significant proportion of eyes retain poor visual acuity despite treatment. Several studies have shown that low visual acuity has been associated with a poor functional outcome after treatment or during the natural course (Fig. 3.34). SD-OCT can help predict visual acuity based on the integrity of the neurosensory retina.

Central retinal artery occlusion

Central retinal artery occlusion shows a distinct pattern on OCT images. In the acute phase, OCT images demonstrate the increased reflectivity and thickness of the inner retina and a corresponding decrease of reflectivity in the outer layer of the retina and RPE/choriocapillaris layer. Follow-up OCT images

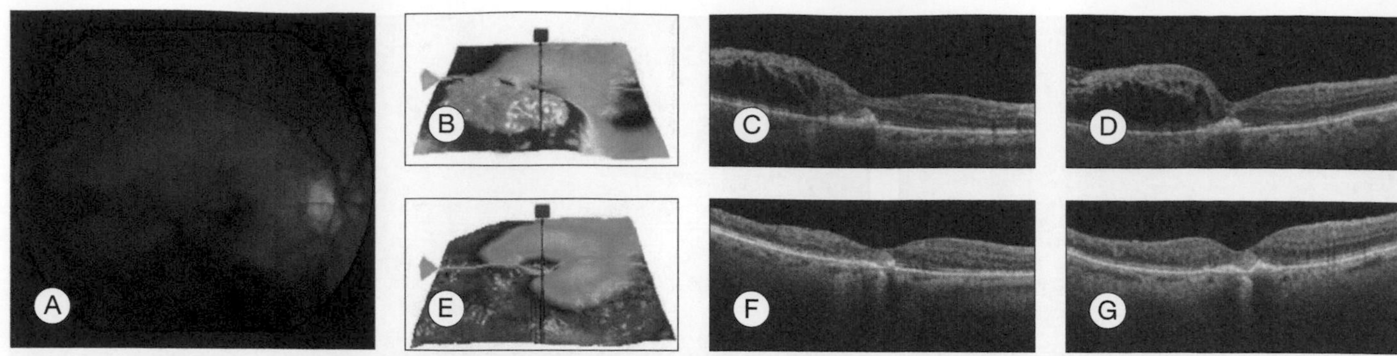

Fig. 3.34 Branch retinal vein occlusion. (A) Color photo of the right eye shows dilated tortuous retinal veins, flame-shaped hemorrhages in an arcuate configuration in the distribution of inferotemporal branch retinal vein occlusion, and macular edema. (B) Retinal thickness map showing increase in retinal thickness. (C, D) Spectral domain optical coherence tomography (OCT) horizontal and vertical scan respectively obtained through the fovea revealed that marked retinal thickening, areas of low intraretinal reflectivity consistent with cystic fluid accumulation, and edema were identified, especially in the outer plexiform layer. High reflectivity is noted in the inner layers from intraretinal hemorrhage. (E) Retinal thickness map 1 month after bevacizumab injection, showing decrease in retinal thickness. (F, G) Spectral domain OCT horizontal and vertical scan respectively, 1 month after bevacizumab injection, obtained through the fovea showed complete resolution of macular edema, improvement in foveal contour, and decrease in retinal thickening.

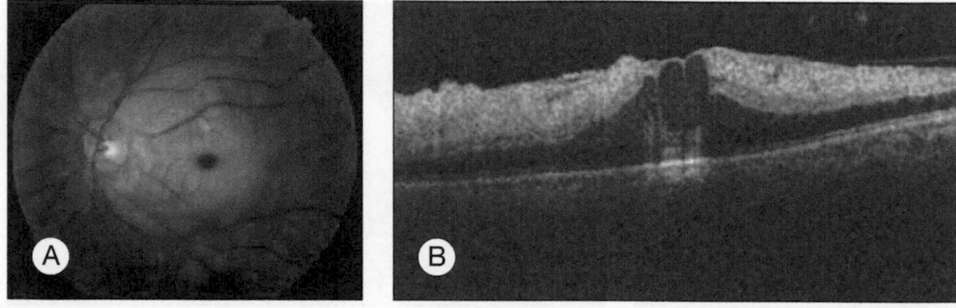

Fig. 3.35 Central retinal artery occlusion. (A) Color photo of the left eye shows cherry-red spot appearance, retinal opacity of posterior fundus, most marked in the parafoveal region, and a small area of normal retina temporal to the optic disc corresponding to the patent cilioretinal retinal artery. (B) Spectral domain optical coherence tomography horizontal scan through the fovea illustrates increased thickness and hyperreflectivity of the inner retinal layers, denoting the presence of intracellular edema, with decreased reflectivity of photoreceptor and retinal pigment epithelial layers because of the shadowing effect.

demonstrate a decrease in the reflectivity and thickness of the inner retinal layers and a corresponding increase of reflectivity in the outer retina and RPE/choriocapillaris layer compared with the baseline OCT image, suggesting a generalized atrophy of the neurosensory retina as a late finding. Therefore, the use of OCT may help facilitate prompt recognition of acute and chronic central retinal artery occlusion. In patients with central retinal artery occlusion, OCT images closely correspond with known histopathologic changes. Histology following acute central retinal artery occlusion shows retinal changes limited to the nerve fiber and ganglion cell layers. There are profound losses of ganglion cells and diffuse edema of the inner retinal layers with little change seen in the deeper retinal layers supplied by choroidal vessels. OCT images provide an in vivo view of the retinal structure following central retinal artery occlusion. Increased reflectivity of the inner retina, presumably because of opacification of the ganglion cell and nerve fiber layers, corresponds to previously described histologic findings of "cloudy swelling" of these layers. Attenuation of reflectivity in the outer layer of the retina and the RPE/choriocapillaris layer is due to the ganglion cell and nerve fiber changes allowing less light reflected back from the outer portions of the retina. Further evidence of this phenomenon is at the foveal depression where the ganglion cell layer is absent. As more light is allowed through the fovea, the RPE/choriocapillaris layer directly beneath the fovea shows a relative increase in reflectivity compared with the other regions of the RPE/choriocapillaris. An additional finding on OCT imaging is the thinning and atrophy in the affected area of the retina, which occurs after a period of time (Fig. 3.35).[208]

Branch retinal artery occlusion

Branch retinal artery occlusions are usually embolic in nature. The embolic source is either a carotid artery atheroma or myocardial thrombus. The embolus usually lodges at the bifurcation of the central retinal artery into the branch retinal artery. Histopathologically, acute branch retinal artery occlusions reveal ischemia in the corresponding retinal quadrant marked by inner retinal edema at the initial stage followed by atrophy in longstanding cases. SD-OCT imaging shows the edematous inner retina, comprising the inner nuclear layer, inner plexiform layer, and ganglion cell layer, as a hyperintense band with increased thickness, which is contrasted by the normal reflectivity and thickness of the corresponding layers of the unaffected macular regions. Prolonged ischemia results in consecutive atrophy of these layers with each layer exhibiting differential sensitivity to the underlying hypoxia. Animal experiments have revealed retinal ganglion cells to be relatively resistant to the ischemia compared to the other retinal neurons.[209] Similar findings in vivo using SD-OCT imaging revealed the relative preservation of the

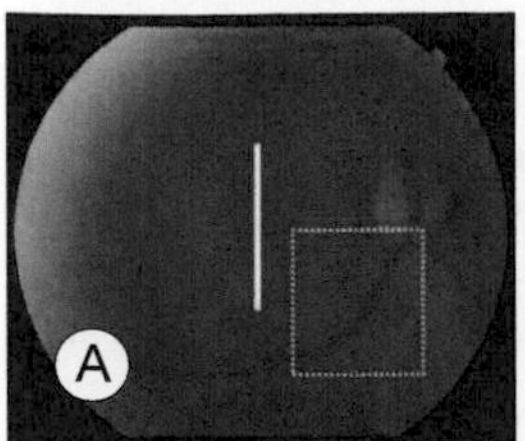

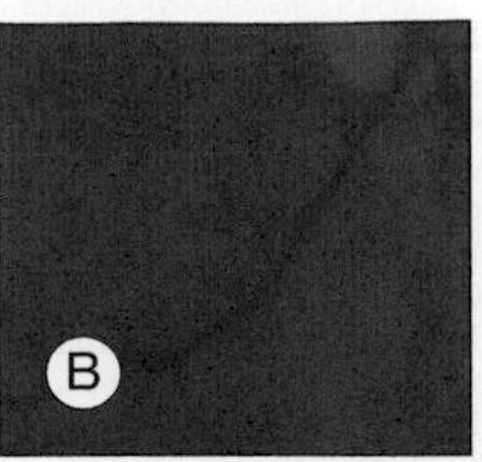

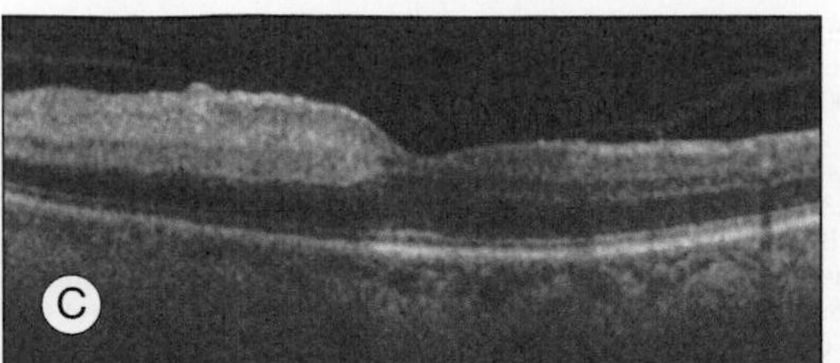

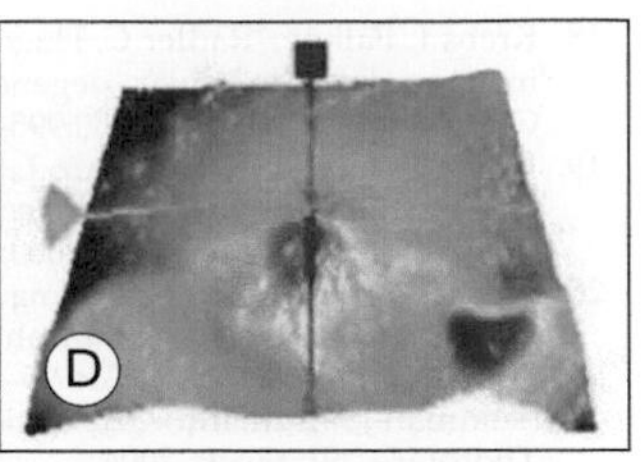

Fig. 3.36 Branch retinal artery occlusion. (A) Color photo of the right eye shows area of whitening in the distribution of an inferotemporal retinal arteriole: white vertical line represents location of B-scan; square dotted line represents area of embolus in arteriole which is magnified. (B) Embolus was appreciated in the inferior retinal arteriole next to the optic nerve. (C) Spectral domain optical coherence tomography (OCT) vertical scan through the fovea illustrates increased thickness and hyperreflectivity of the inner retinal layers in the inferior perifoveolar area, denoting the presence of intracellular edema, with decreased reflectivity of photoreceptor and retinal pigment epithelial layers. The asymmetry of optical reflectivity in perifoveal region is an important finding; OCT findings in the superior perifoveolar area are normal. (D) Retinal thickness map shows increased thickness in the inferior perifoveal area.

ganglion cell layer as opposed to the thinning of the inner plexiform and nuclear layers (Fig. 3.36).[210]

FUTURE DIRECTIONS

The recent advances in OCT technology have clearly revolutionized the assessment of patients with retinal disorders. Although SD-OCT has changed the way we image macular diseases, the future of OCT holds even more promise with the use of longer-wavelength light sources, faster scan times, functional assessments, and higher image resolution.

Current commercial available SD-OCT instruments allow dense scanning of the macula with high axial resolution (approximately 5–8 µm). Ultrahigh-resolution OCT may achieve axial image resolution of 2–3 µm enabling better visualization of retinal structures. However, the price-versus-performance trade-off remains, limiting the use of this technology to research applications.[2] The use of adaptive optics to correct the ocular aberrations may increase not only the axial resolution, but also the transverse resolution of OCT systems and provide cellular level detail.[211]

Swept-source OCT systems allow significant increases in imaging sensitivity and speed (>300 000 A-scans per second), with decreased motion artifacts, through the use of a tunable laser and a photodetector. While swept-source OCT can achieve extremely high imaging speeds, the axial image resolution is less than that achieved using SD-OCT.[2,212]

Clinically available SD-OCT instruments operate with a light source of approximately 840 nm. This wavelength is highly scattered and absorbed by the melanin in the RPE and choroid, reducing the light penetration into deeper tissues. Imaging the retina with a wavelength of 1050 nm enables greater light penetration and thus a better visualization of choroidal structures.[213,214] The use of this wavelength also has the advantage of less interference by media opacities such as cataract.[215]

In the field of functional OCT, Doppler OCT systems are able to detect the retinal blood flow by the assessment of light reflectivity in multiple successive datasets over short time periods.[216] Polarization-sensitive OCT uses tissue birefringence properties to detect the health of different retinal layers. The combination of birefringence and thickness measurements may provide a more sensitive diagnostic tool than either alone.[217,218]

Much has been learned since the development of the first OCT instrument, and OCT holds the promise for continuing advances in fundamental research and improvements in clinical care.

Disclosures

Drs Garcia Filho, Rosenfeld, and Yehoshua received research support from Carl Zeiss Meditec. Dr Gregori and the University of Miami co-own a patent that is licensed to Carl Zeiss Meditec. Dr Rosenfeld has received honoraria for lectures from Carl Zeiss Meditec.

REFERENCES

1. Gabriele ML, Wollstein G, Ishikawa H, et al. Optical coherence tomography: history, current status, and laboratory work. Invest Ophthalmol Vis Sci 2011;52:2425–36.
2. Drexler W, Fujimoto JG. State-of-the-art retinal optical coherence tomography. Prog Retin Eye Res 2008;27:45–88.
3. Li Y, Gregori G, Knighton RW, et al. Registration of OCT fundus images with color fundus photographs based on blood vessel ridges. Opt Express 2011;19:7–16.
4. Jiao S, Knighton R, Huang X, et al. Simultaneous acquisition of sectional and fundus ophthalmic images with spectral-domain optical coherence tomography. Opt Express 2005;13:444–52.
5. Han IC, Jaffe GJ. Evaluation of artifacts associated with macular spectral-domain optical coherence tomography. Ophthalmology 2010;117:1177–89 e4.
6. Ho J, Sull AC, Vuong LN, et al. Assessment of artifacts and reproducibility across spectral- and time-domain optical coherence tomography devices. Ophthalmology 2009;116:1960–70.
7. Mylonas G, Ahlers C, Malamos P, et al. Comparison of retinal thickness measurements and segmentation performance of four different spectral and time domain OCT devices in neovascular age-related macular degeneration. Br J Ophthalmol 2009;93:1453–60.
8. Wolf-Schnurrbusch UE, Ceklic L, Brinkmann CK, et al. Macular thickness measurements in healthy eyes using six different optical coherence tomography instruments. Invest Ophthalmol Vis Sci 2009;50:3432–7.
9. Srinivasan VJ, Monson BK, Wojtkowski M, et al. Characterization of outer retinal morphology with high-speed, ultrahigh-resolution optical coherence tomography. Invest Ophthalmol Vis Sci 2008;49:1571–9.
10. Krebs I, Smretschnig E, Moussa S, et al. Quality and reproducibility of retinal thickness measurements in two spectral-domain optical coherence tomography machines. Invest Ophthalmol Vis Sci 2011;52:6925–33.
11. Mwanza JC, Oakley JD, Budenz DL, et al. Macular ganglion cell-inner plexiform layer: automated detection and thickness reproducibility with spectral domain-optical coherence tomography in glaucoma. Invest Ophthalmol Vis Sci 2011;52:8323–9.
12. Yehoshua Z, Rosenfeld PJ, Gregori G, et al. Progression of geographic atrophy in age-related macular degeneration imaged with spectral domain optical coherence tomography. Ophthalmology 2011;118:679–86.
13. Gregori G, Wang F, Rosenfeld PJ, et al. Spectral domain optical coherence tomography imaging of drusen in nonexudative age-related macular degeneration. Ophthalmology 2011;118:1373–9.
14. Yehoshua Z, Wang F, Rosenfeld PJ, et al. Natural history of drusen morphology in age-related macular degeneration using spectral domain optical coherence tomography. Ophthalmology 2011;118:2434–41.
15. Malamos P, Ahlers C, Mylonas G, et al. Evaluation of segmentation procedures using spectral domain optical coherence tomography in exudative age-related macular degeneration. Retina 2011;31:453–63.
16. Matt G, Sacu S, Buehl W, et al. Comparison of retinal thickness values and segmentation performance of different OCT devices in acute branch retinal vein occlusion. Eye (Lond) 2011;25:511–8.
17. Krebs I, Haas P, Zeiler F, et al. Optical coherence tomography: limits of the retinal-mapping program in age-related macular degeneration. Br J Ophthalmol 2008;92:933–5.

18. Krebs I, Falkner-Radler C, Hagen S, et al. Quality of the threshold algorithm in age-related macular degeneration: Stratus versus Cirrus OCT. Invest Ophthalmol Vis Sci 2009;50:995–1000.
19. Patel PJ, Chen FK, da Cruz L, et al. Segmentation error in Stratus optical coherence tomography for neovascular age-related macular degeneration. Invest Ophthalmol Vis Sci 2009;50:399–404.
20. Drexler W, Sattmann H, Hermann B, et al. Enhanced visualization of macular pathology with the use of ultrahigh-resolution optical coherence tomography. Arch Ophthalmol 2003;121:695–706.
21. Schuman JS, Pulliafito CA. Optical coherence tomography of ocular diseases. Thorofare, NJ: Slack; 2004.
22. Gloesmann M, Hermann B, Schubert C, et al. Histologic correlation of pig retina radial stratification with ultrahigh-resolution optical coherence tomography. Invest Ophthalmol Vis Sci 2003;44:1696–703.
23. Anger EM, Unterhuber A, Hermann B, et al. Ultrahigh resolution optical coherence tomography of the monkey fovea. Identification of retinal sublayers by correlation with semithin histology sections. Exp Eye Res 2004;78: 1117–25.
24. Lujan BJ, Roorda A, Knighton RW, et al. Revealing Henle's fiber layer using spectral domain optical coherence tomography. Invest Ophthalmol Vis Sci 2010;52:1486–92.
25. Spaide RF, Curcio CA. Anatomical correlates to the bands seen in the outer retina by optical coherence tomography: literature review and model. Retina 2011;31:1609–19.
26. Srinivasan VJ, Ko TH, Wojtkowski M, et al. Noninvasive volumetric imaging and morphometry of the rodent retina with high-speed, ultrahigh-resolution optical coherence tomography. Invest Ophthalmol Vis Sci 2006;47:5522–8.
27. Toth CA, Narayan DG, Boppart SA, et al. A comparison of retinal morphology viewed by optical coherence tomography and by light microscopy. Arch Ophthalmol 1997;115:1425–8.
28. Manjunath V, Taha M, Fujimoto JG, et al. Choroidal thickness in normal eyes measured using Cirrus HD optical coherence tomography. Am J Ophthalmol 2010;150:325–9 e1.
29. Spaide RF, Koizumi H, Pozzoni MC. Enhanced depth imaging spectral-domain optical coherence tomography. Am J Ophthalmol 2008;146:496–500.
30. Chen Y, Burnes DL, de Bruin M, et al. Three-dimensional pointwise comparison of human retinal optical property at 845 and 1060 nm using optical frequency domain imaging. J Biomed Opt 2009;14:024016.
31. Margolis R, Spaide RF. A pilot study of enhanced depth imaging optical coherence tomography of the choroid in normal eyes. Am J Ophthalmol 2009;147:811–5.
32. Ouyang Y, Heussen FM, Mokwa N, et al. Spatial distribution of posterior pole choroidal thickness by spectral domain optical coherence tomography. Invest Ophthalmol Vis Sci 2011;52:7019–26.
33. Ikuno Y, Kawaguchi K, Nouchi T, et al. Choroidal thickness in healthy Japanese subjects. Invest Ophthalmol Vis Sci 2009;51:2173–6.
34. Ikuno Y, Maruko I, Yasuno Y, et al. Reproducibility of retinal and choroidal thickness measurements in enhanced depth imaging and high-penetration optical coherence tomography. Invest Ophthalmol Vis Sci 2011;52:5536–40.
35. Giammaria D, Ioni A, Bartoli B, et al. Comparison of macular thickness measurements between time-domain and spectral-domain optical coherence tomographies in eyes with and without macular abnormalities. Retina 2011;31:707–16.
36. Gass J. Stereoscopic atlas of macular diseases: diagnosis and treatment. St Louis: Mosby-Year Book; 1997. p. 903–14.
37. Uchino E, Uemura A, Ohba N. Initial stages of posterior vitreous detachment in healthy eyes of older persons evaluated by optical coherence tomography. Arch Ophthalmol 2001;119:1475–9.
38. Smiddy WE, Michels RG, Green WR. Morphology, pathology, and surgery of idiopathic vitreoretinal macular disorders. A review. Retina 1990;10:288–96.
39. Johnson MW. Perifoveal vitreous detachment and its macular complications. Trans Am Ophthalmol Soc 2005;103:537–67.
40. Witkin AJ, Patron ME, Castro LC, et al. Anatomic and visual outcomes of vitrectomy for vitreomacular traction syndrome. Ophthalm Surg Lasers Imaging 2010;41:425–31.
41. Gallemore RP, Jumper JM, McCuen BW, 2nd, et al. Diagnosis of vitreoretinal adhesions in macular disease with optical coherence tomography. Retina 2000;20:115–20.
42. Johnson MW. Tractional cystoid macular edema: a subtle variant of the vitreomacular traction syndrome. Am J Ophthalmol 2005;140:184–92.
43. Do DV, Cho M, et al. Impact of optical coherence tomography on surgical decision making for epiretinal membranes and vitreomacular traction. Retina 2007;27:552–6.
44. Chang LK, Fine HF, Spaide RF, et al. Ultrastructural correlation of spectral-domain optical coherence tomographic findings in vitreomacular traction syndrome. Am J Ophthalmol 2008;146:121–7.
45. Hikichi T, Yoshida A, Trempe CL. Course of vitreomacular traction syndrome. Am J Ophthalmol 1995;119:55–61.
46. Sulkes DJ, Ip MS, Baumal CR, et al. Spontaneous resolution of vitreomacular traction documented by optical coherence tomography. Arch Ophthalmol 2000;118:286–7.
47. Yamada N, Kishi S. Tomographic features and surgical outcomes of vitreomacular traction syndrome. Am J Ophthalmol 2005;139:112–7.
48. Sonmez K, Capone A, Jr, Trese MT, et al. Vitreomacular traction syndrome: impact of anatomical configuration on anatomical and visual outcomes. Retina 2008;28:1207–14.
49. Pearlstone AD. The incidence of idiopathic preretinal macular gliosis. Ann Ophthalmol 1985;17:378–80.
50. McCarty DJ, Mukesh BN, Chikani V, et al. Prevalence and associations of epiretinal membranes in the visual impairment project. Am J Ophthalmol 2005;140:288–94.
51. Smiddy WE, Maguire AM, Green WR, et al. Idiopathic epiretinal membranes. Ultrastructural characteristics and clinicopathologic correlation. Ophthalmology 1989;96:811–20; discussion 821.
52. Vinores SA, Campochiaro PA, Conway BP. Ultrastructural and electron-immunocytochemical characterization of cells in epiretinal membranes. Invest Ophthalmol Vis Sci 1990;31:14–28.
53. Appiah AP, Hirose T. Secondary causes of premacular fibrosis. Ophthalmology 1989;96:389–92.
54. Wilkins JR, Puliafito CA, Hee MR, et al. Characterization of epiretinal membranes using optical coherence tomography. Ophthalmology 1996;103: 2142–51.
55. Gass JD. Reappraisal of biomicroscopic classification of stages of development of a macular hole. Am J Ophthalmol 1995;119:752–9.
56. Takahashi A, Nagaoka T, Yoshida A. Stage 1-A macular hole: a prospective spectral-domain optical coherence tomography study. Retina 2011;31:127–47.
57. Takahashi A, Yoshida A, Nagaoka T, et al. Macular hole formation in fellow eyes with a perifoveal posterior vitreous detachment of patients with a unilateral macular hole. Am J Ophthalmol 2011;151:981–9 e4.
58. Kelly NE, Wendel RT. Vitreous surgery for idiopathic macular holes. Results of a pilot study. Arch Ophthalmol 1991;109:654–9.
59. Brooks HL, Jr. Macular hole surgery with and without internal limiting membrane peeling. Ophthalmology 2000;107:1939–48; discussion 1948–9.
60. Bottoni F, De Angelis S, Luccarelli S, et al. The dynamic healing process of idiopathic macular holes after surgical repair: a spectral-domain optical coherence tomography study. Invest Ophthalmol Vis Sci 2011;52:4439–46.
61. Hee MR, Puliafito CA, Wong C, et al. Optical coherence tomography of macular holes. Ophthalmology 1995;102:748–56.
62. Ko TH, Witkin AJ, Fujimoto JG, et al. Ultrahigh-resolution optical coherence tomography of surgically closed macular holes. Arch Ophthalmol 2006;124: 827–36.
63. Sano M, Shimoda Y, Hashimoto H, et al. Restored photoreceptor outer segment and visual recovery after macular hole closure. Am J Ophthalmol 2009;147:313–8 e1.
64 Oh J, Smiddy WE, Flynn HW, Jr, et al. Photoreceptor inner/outer segment defect imaging by spectral domain OCT and visual prognosis after macular hole surgery. Invest Ophthalmol Vis Sci 2009;51:1651–8.
65. Ooka E, Mitamura Y, Baba T, et al. Foveal microstructure on spectral-domain optical coherence tomographic images and visual function after macular hole surgery. Am J Ophthalmol 2011;152:283–90 e1.
66. Muqit MM, Akram I, Turner GS, et al. Fourier-domain optical coherence tomography imaging of gas tamponade following macular hole surgery. Ophthalmic Surg Lasers Imaging 2011;41 Online: e1–6.
67. Sano M, Inoue M, Taniuchi S, et al. Ability to determine postoperative status of macular hole in gas-filled eyes by spectral domain-optical coherence tomography. Clin Exp Ophthalmol 2011;39:885–892.
68. Eckardt C, Eckert T, Eckardt U, et al. Macular hole surgery with air tamponade and optical coherence tomography-based duration of face-down positioning. Retina 2008;28:1087–96.
69. Bressler NM, Bressler SB, Congdon NG, et al. Potential public health impact of Age-Related Eye Disease Study results: AREDS report no. 11. Arch Ophthalmol 2003;121:1621–4.
70. Congdon N, O'Colmain B, Klaver CC, et al. Causes and prevalence of visual impairment among adults in the United States. Arch Ophthalmol 2004;122: 477–85.
71. Friedman DS, O'Colmain BJ, Munoz B, et al. Prevalence of age-related macular degeneration in the United States. Arch Ophthalmol 2004;122:564–72.
72. Klein R, Peto T, Bird A, et al. The epidemiology of age-related macular degeneration. Am J Ophthalmol 2004;137:486–95.
73. Bird AC, Bressler NM, Bressler SB, et al. An international classification and grading system for age-related maculopathy and age-related macular degeneration. The International ARM Epidemiological Study Group. Surv Ophthalmol 1995;39:367–74.
74. Hirvela H, Luukinen H, Laara E, et al. Risk factors of age-related maculopathy in a population 70 years of age or older. Ophthalmology 1996;103:871–7.
75. Vingerling JR, Hofman A, Grobbee DE, et al. Age-related macular degeneration and smoking. The Rotterdam Study. Arch Ophthalmol 1996;114:1193–6.
76. Seddon JM, Sharma S, Adelman RA. Evaluation of the clinical age-related maculopathy staging system. Ophthalmology 2006;113:260–6.
77. Bartlett H, Eperjesi F. Use of fundus imaging in quantification of age-related macular change. Surv Ophthalmol 2007;52:655–71.
78. Seddon JM, Sharma S, Adelman RA, et al. Optical coherence tomography of age-related macular degeneration and choroidal neovascularization. Ophthalmology 1996;103:1260–70.
79. Pieroni CG, Witkin AJ, Ko TH, et al. Ultrahigh resolution optical coherence tomography in non-exudative age related macular degeneration. Br J Ophthalmol 2006;90:191–7.
80. Sikorski BL, Bukowska D, Kaluzny JJ, et al. Drusen with accompanying fluid underneath the sensory retina. Ophthalmology 2010;118:82–92.
81. Spaide RF, Curcio CA. Drusen characterization with multimodal imaging. Retina 2010;30:1441–54.
82. Roquet W, Roudot-Thoraval F, Coscas G, et al. Clinical features of drusenoid pigment epithelial detachment in age related macular degeneration. Br J Ophthalmol 2004;88:638–42.
83. Schuman SG, Koreishi AF, Farsiu S, et al. Photoreceptor layer thinning over drusen in eyes with age-related macular degeneration imaged in vivo with

spectral-domain optical coherence tomography. Ophthalmology 2009;116: 488–96 e2.
84. Davis MD, Gangnon RE, Lee LY, et al. The Age-Related Eye Disease Study severity scale for age-related macular degeneration: AREDS report no. 17. Arch Ophthalmol 2005;123:1484–98.
85. Ferris FL, Davis MD, Clemons TE, et al. A simplified severity scale for age-related macular degeneration: AREDS report no. 18. Arch Ophthalmol 2005;123:1570–4.
86. Ho J, Witkin AJ, Liu J, et al. Documentation of intraretinal retinal pigment epithelium migration via high-speed ultrahigh-resolution optical coherence tomography. Ophthalmology 2010;118:687–93.
87. Zweifel SA, Imamura Y, Spaide TC, et al. Prevalence and significance of subretinal drusenoid deposits (reticular pseudodrusen) in age-related macular degeneration. Ophthalmology 2010;117:1775–81.
88. Zweifel SA, Spaide RF, Curcio CA, et al. Reticular pseudodrusen are subretinal drusenoid deposits. Ophthalmology 2009;117:303–12 e1.
89. Sarks JP, Sarks SH, Killingsworth MC. Evolution of geographic atrophy of the retinal pigment epithelium. Eye (Lond) 1988;2:552–77.
90. Sunness JS. The natural history of geographic atrophy, the advanced atrophic form of age-related macular degeneration. Mol Vis 1999;5:25.
91. Sunness JS, Bressler NM, Tian Y, et al. Measuring geographic atrophy in advanced age-related macular degeneration. Invest Ophthalmol Vis Sci 1999;40:1761–9.
92. Sunness JS, Margalit E, Srikumaran D, et al. The long-term natural history of geographic atrophy from age-related macular degeneration: enlargement of atrophy and implications for interventional clinical trials. Ophthalmology 2007;114:271–7.
93. Schmitz-Valckenberg S, Fleckenstein M, Gobel AP, et al. Optical coherence tomography and autofluorescence findings in areas with geographic atrophy due to age-related macular degeneration. Invest Ophthalmol Vis Sci 2010;52:1–6.
94. Fleckenstein M, Charbel Issa P, Helb HM, et al. High-resolution spectral domain-OCT imaging in geographic atrophy associated with age-related macular degeneration. Invest Ophthalmol Vis Sci 2008;49:4137–44.
95. Bearelly S, Chau FY, Koreishi A, et al. Spectral domain optical coherence tomography imaging of geographic atrophy margins. Ophthalmology 2009;116:1762–9.
96. Spaide RF. Age-related choroidal atrophy. Am J Ophthalmol 2009;147: 801–10.
97. Wood A, Binns A, Margrain T, et al. Retinal and choroidal thickness in early age-related macular degeneration. Am J Ophthalmol 2011;152: 1030–8.
98. Lujan BJ, Wang F, Gregori G, et al. Calibration of fundus images using spectral domain optical coherence tomography. Ophthalmic Surg Lasers Imaging 2008;39(Suppl):S15–20.
99. Lujan BJ, Rosenfeld PJ, Gregori G, et al. Spectral domain optical coherence tomographic imaging of geographic atrophy. Ophthalmic Surg Lasers Imaging 2009;40:96–101.
100. Green WR. Clinicopathologic studies of treated choroidal neovascular membranes. A review and report of two cases. Retina 1991;11:328–56.
101. Green WR. Histopathology of age-related macular degeneration. Mol Vis 1999;5:27.
102. Keane PA, Aghaian E, Ouyang Y, et al. Acute severe visual decrease after photodynamic therapy with verteporfin: spectral-domain OCT features. Ophthalmic Surg Lasers Imaging 2010;41(Suppl):S85–8.
103. Keane PA, Liakopoulos S, Chang KT, et al. Relationship between optical coherence tomography retinal parameters and visual acuity in neovascular age-related macular degeneration. Ophthalmology 2008;115:2206–14.
104. Yannuzzi LA, Hope-Ross M, Slakter JS, et al. Analysis of vascularized pigment epithelial detachments using indocyanine green videoangiography. Retina 1994;14:99–113.
105. Jager RD, Mieler WF, Miller JW. Age-related macular degeneration. N Engl J Med 2008;358:2606–17.
106. Zayit-Soudry S, Moroz I, Loewenstein A. Retinal pigment epithelial detachment. Surv Ophthalmol 2007;52:227–43.
107. Bloom SM, Singal IP. The outer Bruch membrane layer: a previously undescribed spectral-domain optical coherence tomography finding. Retina 2010; 31:316–23.
108. Coscas G, Coscas F, Zourdani A, et al. [Optical coherence tomography and ARMD.] J Fr Ophtalmol 2004;27:3S7–30.
109. Pepple K, Mruthyunjaya P. Retinal pigment epithelial detachments in age-related macular degeneration: classification and therapeutic options. Semin Ophthalmol 2011;26:198–208.
110. Spaide RF. Enhanced depth imaging optical coherence tomography of retinal pigment epithelial detachment in age-related macular degeneration. Am J Ophthalmol 2009;147:644–52.
111. Joeres S, Tsong JW, Updike PG, et al. Reproducibility of quantitative optical coherence tomography subanalysis in neovascular age-related macular degeneration. Invest Ophthalmol Vis Sci 2007;48:4300–7.
112. Lee SY, Stetson PF, Ruiz-Garcia H, et al. Automated characterization of pigment epithelial detachment using optical coherence tomography. Invest Ophthalmol Vis Sci 2012;53:164–70.
113. Hoskin A, Bird AC, Sehmi K. Tears of detached retinal pigment epithelium. Br J Ophthalmol 1981;65:417–22.
114. Chang LK, Sarraf D. Tears of the retinal pigment epithelium: an old problem in a new era. Retina 2007;27:523–34.
115. Levin LA, Seddon JM, Topping T. Retinal pigment epithelial tears associated with trauma. Am J Ophthalmol 1991;112:396–400.
116. Ishida Y, Kato T, Minamoto A, et al. Retinal pigment epithelial tear in a patient with central serous chorioretinopathy treated with corticosteroids. Retina 2004;24:633–6.
117. Gelisken F, Inhoffen W, Partsch M, et al. Retinal pigment epithelial tear after photodynamic therapy for choroidal neovascularization. Am J Ophthalmol 2001;131:518–20.
118. Pece A, Introini U, Bottoni F, et al. Acute retinal pigment epithelial tear after photodynamic therapy. Retina 2001;21:661–5.
119. Meyer CH, Mennel S, Schmidt JC, et al. Acute retinal pigment epithelial tear following intravitreal bevacizumab (Avastin) injection for occult choroidal neovascularisation secondary to age related macular degeneration. Br J Ophthalmol 2006;90:1207–8.
120. Carvounis PE, Kopel AC, Benz MS. Retinal pigment epithelium tears following ranibizumab for exudative age-related macular degeneration. Am J Ophthalmol 2007;143:504–5.
121. Gelisken F, Ziemssen F, Voelker M, et al. Retinal pigment epithelial tears after single administration of intravitreal bevacizumab for neovascular age-related macular degeneration. Eye (Lond) 2009;23:694–702.
122. Gass JD. Pathogenesis of tears of the retinal pigment epithelium. Br J Ophthalmol 1984;68:513–9.
123. Chan CK, Abraham P, Meyer CH, et al. Optical coherence tomography-measured pigment epithelial detachment height as a predictor for retinal pigment epithelial tears associated with intravitreal bevacizumab injections. Retina 2009;30:203–11.
124. Chiang A, Chang LK, Yu F, et al. Predictors of anti-VEGF-associated retinal pigment epithelial tear using FA and OCT analysis. Retina 2008;28: 1265–9.
125 Landa G, Su E, Garcia PM, et al. Inner segment–outer segment junctional layer integrity and corresponding retinal sensitivity in dry and wet forms of age-related macular degeneration. Retina 2011;31:364–70.
126. Oishi A, Hata M, Shimozono M, et al. The significance of external limiting membrane status for visual acuity in age-related macular degeneration. Am J Ophthalmol 2010;150:27–32 e1.
127. Yannuzzi LA, Negrao S, Iida T, et al. Retinal angiomatous proliferation in age-related macular degeneration. Retina 2001;21:416–34.
128. Gass JD, Agarwal A, Lavina AM, et al. Focal inner retinal hemorrhages in patients with drusen: an early sign of occult choroidal neovascularization and chorioretinal anastomosis. Retina 2003;23:741–51.
129. Truong SN, Alam S, Zawadzki RJ, et al. High resolution Fourier-domain optical coherence tomography of retinal angiomatous proliferation. Retina 2007;27:915–25.
130. Freund KB, Ho IV, Barbazetto IA, et al. Type 3 neovascularization: the expanded spectrum of retinal angiomatous proliferation. Retina 2008;28: 201–11.
131. Querques G, Atmani K, Berboucha E, et al. Angiographic analysis of retinal-choroidal anastomosis by confocal scanning laser ophthalmoscopy technology and corresponding (eye-tracked) spectral-domain optical coherence tomography. Retina 2009;30:222–34.
132. Krebs I, Glittenberg C, Hagen S, et al. Retinal angiomatous proliferation: morphological changes assessed by Stratus and Cirrus OCT. Ophthalmic Surg Lasers Imaging 2009;40:285–9.
133. Yannuzzi LA, Sorenson J, Spaide RF, et al. Idiopathic polypoidal choroidal vasculopathy (IPCV). Retina 1990;10:1–8.
134. Costa RA, Navajas EV, Farah ME, et al. Polypoidal choroidal vasculopathy: angiographic characterization of the network vascular elements and a new treatment paradigm. Prog Retin Eye Res 2005;24:560–86.
135. Saito M, Iida T, Nagayama D. Cross-sectional and en face optical coherence tomographic features of polypoidal choroidal vasculopathy. Retina 2008;28:459–64.
136. Ojima Y, Hangai M, Sakamoto A, et al. Improved visualization of polypoidal choroidal vasculopathy lesions using spectral-domain optical coherence tomography. Retina 2009;29:52–9.
137. Harding SP. Neovascular age-related macular degeneration: decision making and optimal management. Eye (Lond) 2010;24:497–505.
138. Brown DM, Kaiser PK, Michels M, et al. Ranibizumab versus verteporfin for neovascular age-related macular degeneration. N Engl J Med 2006;355: 1432–44.
139. Rosenfeld PJ, Brown DM, Heier JS, et al. Ranibizumab for neovascular age-related macular degeneration. N Engl J Med 2006;355:1419–31.
140. Engelbert M, Zweifel SA, Freund KB. Long-term follow-up for type 1 (sub-retinal pigment epithelium) neovascularization using a modified "treat and extend" dosing regimen of intravitreal antivascular endothelial growth factor therapy. Retina 2010;30:1368–75.
141. Martin DF, Maguire MG, Ying GS, et al. Ranibizumab and bevacizumab for neovascular age-related macular degeneration. N Engl J Med 2011;364: 1897–908.
142. Fung AE, Lalwani GA, Rosenfeld PJ, et al. An optical coherence tomography-guided, variable dosing regimen with intravitreal ranibizumab (Lucentis) for neovascular age-related macular degeneration. Am J Ophthalmol 2007;143: 566–83.
143. Engelbert M, Zweifel SA, Freund KB. "Treat and extend" dosing of intravitreal antivascular endothelial growth factor therapy for type 3 neovascularization/ retinal angiomatous proliferation. Retina 2009;29:1424–31.
144. Lalwani GA, Rosenfeld PJ, Fung AE, et al. A variable-dosing regimen with intravitreal ranibizumab for neovascular age-related macular degeneration: year 2 of the PrONTO Study. Am J Ophthalmol 2009;148:43–58 e1.
145. Zweifel SA, Engelbert M, Laud K, et al. Outer retinal tubulation: a novel optical coherence tomography finding. Arch Ophthalmol 2009;127:1596–602.

146. Gass JD. Pathogenesis of disciform detachment of the neuroepithelium. Am J Ophthalmol 1967;63:Suppl:1–139.
147. Spaide RF, Campeas L, Haas A, et al. Central serous chorioretinopathy in younger and older adults. Ophthalmology 1996;103:2070–9; discussion 2079–80.
148. Kitaya N, Nagaoka T, Hikichi T, et al. Features of abnormal choroidal circulation in central serous chorioretinopathy. Br J Ophthalmol 2003;87:709–12.
149. Jalkh AE, Jabbour N, Avila MP, et al. Retinal pigment epithelium decompensation. I. Clinical features and natural course. Ophthalmology 1984;91:1544–8.
150. Yannuzzi LA, Shakin JL, Fisher YL, et al. Peripheral retinal detachments and retinal pigment epithelial atrophic tracts secondary to central serous pigment epitheliopathy. Ophthalmology 1984;91:1554–72.
151. Scheider A, Nasemann JE, Lund OE. Fluorescein and indocyanine green angiographies of central serous choroidopathy by scanning laser ophthalmoscopy. Am J Ophthalmol 1993;115:50–6.
152. Guyer DR, Yannuzzi LA, Slakter JS, et al. Digital indocyanine green videoangiography of central serous chorioretinopathy. Arch Ophthalmol 1994;112:1057–62.
153. Piccolino FC, Borgia L. Central serous chorioretinopathy and indocyanine green angiography. Retina 1994;14:231–42.
154. Prunte C, Flammer J. Choroidal capillary and venous congestion in central serous chorioretinopathy. Am J Ophthalmol 1996;121:26–34.
155. Kamppeter B, Jonas JB. Central serous chorioretinopathy imaged by optical coherence tomography. Arch Ophthalmol 2003;121:742–3.
156. Montero JA, Ruiz-Moreno JM. Optical coherence tomography characterisation of idiopathic central serous chorioretinopathy. Br J Ophthalmol 2005;89:562–4.
157. van Velthoven ME, Verbraak FD, Garcia PM, et al. Evaluation of central serous retinopathy with en face optical coherence tomography. Br J Ophthalmol 2005;89:1483–8.
158. Hussain N, Baskar A, Ram LM, et al. Optical coherence tomographic pattern of fluorescein angiographic leakage site in acute central serous chorioretinopathy. Clin Experiment Ophthalmol 2006;34:137–40.
159. Hirami Y, Tsujikawa A, Sasahara M, et al. Alterations of retinal pigment epithelium in central serous chorioretinopathy. Clin Experiment Ophthalmol 2007;35:225–30.
160. Wang MS, Sander B, Larsen M. Retinal atrophy in idiopathic central serous chorioretinopathy. Am J Ophthalmol 2002;133:787–93.
161. Stock G, Ahlers C, Sayegh R, et al. [Three-dimensional imaging in central serous chorioretinopathy]. Ophthalmologe 2008;105:1127–34.
162. Eandi CM, Chung JE, Cardillo-Piccolino F, et al. Optical coherence tomography in unilateral resolved central serous chorioretinopathy. Retina 2005;25:417–21.
163. Furuta M, Iida T, Kishi S. Foveal thickness can predict visual outcome in patients with persistent central serous chorioretinopathy. Ophthalmologica 2009;223:28–31.
164. Maruko I, Iida T, Sekiryu T, et al. Morphologic changes in the outer layer of the detached retina in rhegmatogenous retinal detachment and central serous chorioretinopathy. Am J Ophthalmol 2009;147:489–94 e1.
165. Fujimoto H, Gomi F, Wakabayashi T, et al. Morphologic changes in acute central serous chorioretinopathy evaluated by Fourier-domain optical coherence tomography. Ophthalmology 2008;115:1494–500, 1500 e1–2.
166. Matsumoto H, Kishi S, Otani T, et al. Elongation of photoreceptor outer segment in central serous chorioretinopathy. Am J Ophthalmol 2008;145:162–8.
167. Hee MR, Puliafito CA, Wong C, et al. Optical coherence tomography of central serous chorioretinopathy. Am J Ophthalmol 1995;120:65–74.
168. Kon Y, Iida T, Maruko I, et al. The optical coherence tomography-ophthalmoscope for examination of central serous chorioretinopathy with precipitates. Retina 2008;28:864–9.
169. Mitarai K, Gomi F, Tano Y. Three-dimensional optical coherence tomographic findings in central serous chorioretinopathy. Graefes Arch Clin Exp Ophthalmol 2006;244:1415–20.
170. Gupta P, Gupta V, Dogra MR, et al. Morphological changes in the retinal pigment epithelium on spectral-domain OCT in the unaffected eyes with idiopathic central serous chorioretinopathy. Int Ophthalmol 2009;30:175–81.
171. Ojima Y, Hangai M, Sasahara M, et al. Three-dimensional imaging of the foveal photoreceptor layer in central serous chorioretinopathy using high-speed optical coherence tomography. Ophthalmology 2007;114:2197–207.
172. Matsumoto H, Sato T, Kishi S. Outer nuclear layer thickness at the fovea determines visual outcomes in resolved central serous chorioretinopathy. Am J Ophthalmol 2009;148:105–10 e1.
173. Imamura Y, Fujiwara T, Margolis R, et al. Enhanced depth imaging optical coherence tomography of the choroid in central serous chorioretinopathy. Retina 2009;29:1469–73.
174. Maruko I, Iida T, Sugano Y, et al. Subfoveal choroidal thickness in fellow eyes of patients with central serous chorioretinopathy. Retina 2011;31:1603–8.
175. Maruko I, Iida T, Sugano Y, et al. One-year choroidal thickness results after photodynamic therapy for central serous chorioretinopathy. Retina 2011;31:1921–7.
176. Henderson BA, Kim JY, Ament CS, et al. Clinical pseudophakic cystoid macular edema. Risk factors for development and duration after treatment. J Cataract Refract Surg 2007;33:1550–8.
177. Wolf EJ, Braunstein A, Shih C, et al. Incidence of visually significant pseudophakic macular edema after uneventful phacoemulsification in patients treated with nepafenac. J Cataract Refract Surg 2007;33:1546–9.
178. Irvine SR. A newly defined vitreous syndrome following cataract surgery. Am J Ophthalmol 1953;36:499–619.
179. Schepens CL, Avila MP, Jalkh AE, et al. Role of the vitreous in cystoid macular edema. Surv Ophthalmol 1984;28(Suppl):499–504.
180. Moss SE, Klein R, Klein BE. Ten-year incidence of visual loss in a diabetic population. Ophthalmology 1994;101:1061–70.
181. Moss SE, Klein R, Klein BE. The 14-year incidence of visual loss in a diabetic population. Ophthalmology 1998;105:998–1003.
182. Strom C, Sander B, Larsen N, et al. Diabetic macular edema assessed with optical coherence tomography and stereo fundus photography. Invest Ophthalmol Vis Sci 2002;43:241–5.
183. Brown JC, Solomon SD, Bressler SB, et al. Detection of diabetic foveal edema: contact lens biomicroscopy compared with optical coherence tomography. Arch Ophthalmol 2004;122:330–5.
184. Browning DJ, Apte RS, Bressler SB, et al. Association of the extent of diabetic macular edema as assessed by optical coherence tomography with visual acuity and retinal outcome variables. Retina 2009;29:300–5.
185. Al-latayfeh MM, Sun JK, Aiello LP. Ocular coherence tomography and diabetic eye disease. Semin Ophthalmol 2010;25:192–7.
186. Browning DJ, McOwen MD, Bowen RM, Jr, et al. Comparison of the clinical diagnosis of diabetic macular edema with diagnosis by optical coherence tomography. Ophthalmology 2004;111:712–5.
187. Virgili G, Menchini F, Dimastrogiovanni AF, et al. Optical coherence tomography versus stereoscopic fundus photography or biomicroscopy for diagnosing diabetic macular edema: a systematic review. Invest Ophthalmol Vis Sci 2007;48:4963–73.
188. Davis MD, Bressler SB, Aiello LP, et al. Comparison of time-domain OCT and fundus photographic assessments of retinal thickening in eyes with diabetic macular edema. Invest Ophthalmol Vis Sci 2008;49:1745–52.
189. Otani T, Kishi S, Maruyama Y. Patterns of diabetic macular edema with optical coherence tomography. Am J Ophthalmol 1999;127:688–93.
190. Kim BY, Smith SD, Kaiser PK. Optical coherence tomographic patterns of diabetic macular edema. Am J Ophthalmol 2006;142:405–12.
191. Soliman W, Sander B, Hasler PW, et al. Correlation between intraretinal changes in diabetic macular oedema seen in fluorescein angiography and optical coherence tomography. Acta Ophthalmol 2008;86:34–9.
192. Early Treatment Diabetic Retinopathy Study research group. Photocoagulation for diabetic macular edema. Early Treatment Diabetic Retinopathy Study report number 1. Arch Ophthalmol 1985;103:1796–806.
193. Early Treatment Diabetic Retinopathy Study Research Group. Photocoagulation for diabetic macular edema: Early Treatment Diabetic Retinopathy Study report no. 4. Int Ophthalmol Clin 1987;27:265–72.
194. Early Treatment Diabetic Retinopathy Study Research Group. Treatment techniques and clinical guidelines for photocoagulation of diabetic macular edema. Early Treatment Diabetic Retinopathy Study report no. 2. Ophthalmology 1987;94:761–74.
195. Elman MJ, Bressler NM, Qin H, et al. Expanded 2-year follow-up of ranibizumab plus prompt or deferred laser or triamcinolone plus prompt laser for diabetic macular edema. Ophthalmology 2011;118:609–14.
196. Michaelides M, Kaines A, Hamilton RD, et al. A prospective randomized trial of intravitreal bevacizumab or laser therapy in the management of diabetic macular edema (BOLT study) 12-month data: report 2. Ophthalmology 2010;117:1078–86 e2.
197. Kim NR, Kim YJ, Chin HS, et al. Optical coherence tomographic patterns in diabetic macular oedema: prediction of visual outcome after focal laser photocoagulation. Br J Ophthalmol 2009;93:901–5.
198. Soliman W, Sander B, Soliman KA, et al. The predictive value of optical coherence tomography after grid laser photocoagulation for diffuse diabetic macular oedema. Acta Ophthalmol 2008;86:284–91.
199. Kaiser PK, Riemann CD, Sears JE, et al. Macular traction detachment and diabetic macular edema associated with posterior hyaloidal traction. Am J Ophthalmol 2001;131:44–9.
200. Ghazi NG, Ciralsky JB, Shah SM, et al. Optical coherence tomography findings in persistent diabetic macular edema: the vitreomacular interface. Am J Ophthalmol 2007;144:747–54.
201. Haller JA, Qin H, Apte RS, et al. Vitrectomy outcomes in eyes with diabetic macular edema and vitreomacular traction. Ophthalmology 2010;117:1087–93 e3.
202. Maheshwary AS, Oster SF, Yuson RM, et al. The association between percent disruption of the photoreceptor inner segment–outer segment junction and visual acuity in diabetic macular edema. Am J Ophthalmol 2010;150:63–7 e1.
203. Otani T, Yamaguchi Y, Kishi S. Correlation between visual acuity and foveal microstructural changes in diabetic macular edema. Retina 2010;30:774–80.
204. Sakamoto A, Nishijima K, Kita M, et al. Association between foveal photoreceptor status and visual acuity after resolution of diabetic macular edema by pars plana vitrectomy. Graefes Arch Clin Exp Ophthalmol 2009;247:1325–30.
205. Hayreh SS. Classification of central retinal vein occlusion. Ophthalmology 1983;90:458–74.
206. Ota M, Tsujikawa A, Murakami T, et al. Foveal photoreceptor layer in eyes with persistent cystoid macular edema associated with branch retinal vein occlusion. Am J Ophthalmol 2008;145:273–80.
207. Shroff D, Mehta DK, Arora R, et al. Natural history of macular status in recent-onset branch retinal vein occlusion: an optical coherence tomography study. Int Ophthalmol 2008;28:261–8.

208. Falkenberry SM, Ip MS, Blodi BA, et al. Optical coherence tomography findings in central retinal artery occlusion. Ophthalmic Surg Lasers Imaging 2006;37:502–5.
209. Goldenberg-Cohen N, Dadon S, Avraham BC, et al. Molecular and histological changes following central retinal artery occlusion in a mouse model. Exp Eye Res 2008;87:327–33.
210. Murthy RK, Grover S, Chalam KV. Sequential spectral domain OCT documentation of retinal changes after branch retinal artery occlusion. Clin Ophthalmol 2010;4:327–9.
211. Fernandez EJ, Hermann B, Povazay B, et al. Ultrahigh resolution optical coherence tomography and pancorrection for cellular imaging of the living human retina. Opt Express 2008;16:11083–94.
212. Huber R, Adler DC, Srinivasan VJ, et al. Fourier domain mode locking at 1050 nm for ultra-high-speed optical coherence tomography of the human retina at 236 000 axial scans per second. Opt Lett 2007;32:2049–51.
213. Unterhuber A, Povazay B, Hermann B, et al. In vivo retinal optical coherence tomography at 1040 nm – enhanced penetration into the choroid. Opt Express 2005;13:3252–8.
214. Povazay B, Hermann B, Hofer B, et al. Wide-field optical coherence tomography of the choroid in vivo. Invest Ophthalmol Vis Sci 2009;50:1856–63.
215. Povazay B, Hermann B, Unterhuber A, et al. Three-dimensional optical coherence tomography at 1050 nm versus 800 nm in retinal pathologies: enhanced performance and choroidal penetration in cataract patients. J Biomed Opt 2007;12:041211.
216. Wang Y, Lu A, Gil-Flamer J, et al. Measurement of total blood flow in the normal human retina using Doppler Fourier-domain optical coherence tomography. Br J Ophthalmol 2009;93:634–7.
217. Ahlers C, Gotzinger E, Pircher M, et al. Imaging of the retinal pigment epithelium in age-related macular degeneration using polarization-sensitive optical coherence tomography. Invest Ophthalmol Vis Sci 2010;51:2149–57.
218. Cense B, Chen TC, Park BH, et al. Thickness and birefringence of healthy retinal nerve fiber layer tissue measured with polarization-sensitive optical coherence tomography. Invest Ophthalmol Vis Sci 2004;45:2606–12.

Chapter 4

Autofluorescence Imaging

Monika Fleckenstein, Steffen Schmitz-Valckenberg, Frank G. Holz

BASIC PRINCIPLES

Fundus autofluorescence

Fundus autofluorescence (FAF) imaging is a noninvasive imaging method for in vivo mapping of naturally or pathologically occurring fluorophores of the ocular fundus. The dominant sources are fluorophores accumulating in lipofuscin (LF) granules in the retinal pigment epithelium (RPE).[1] In the absence of RPE cells, minor fluorophores including collagen and elastin, e.g., in choroidal blood vessel walls, may also become visible. Bleaching phenomena and loss of photopigment may result in increased FAF by reduced absorbance anterior to the RPE level.

Retinal pigment epithelium and lipofuscin

The RPE constitutes a polygonal monolayer between the neurosensory retina and the choroid and is essential for vision. Given multiple essential physiological functions of the RPE, it is not surprising that RPE dysfunction has been implicated in a variety of retinal diseases (reviewed by Schmitz-Valckenberg et al.[2]).

A hallmark of aging is the gradual accumulation of LF granules in the cytoplasm of RPE cells. It is thought that progressive LF accumulation is mainly a byproduct of the constant phagocytosis of shed photoreceptor outer-segment discs.[3–5] Several lines of evidence indicate that adverse effects of excessive LF accumulation represent a common downstream pathogenetic mechanism in various monogenic macular and retinal dystrophies as well as in multifactorial complex retinal disease entities, including age-related macular degeneration (AMD).[3,4,6–8]

Apparently, once formed, the RPE cell has no means of either degrading or transporting LF material and granules into the extracellular space via exocytosis. Subsequently, these granules are trapped in the cytoplasmic space of the postmitotic RPE cells. Previous studies have shown that various LF components such as A2-E (*N*-retinylidene-*N*-retinylethanol-amine), a dominant fluorophore, possess toxic properties which may interfere with normal cell function via various molecular mechanisms, including impairment of lysosomal degradation due to inhibition of the lysosomal adenosine triphosphate-dependent proton pump.[9–12] Other components of LF include precursors of A2-E, molecules formed by the mixture of oxygen-containing moieties within photo-oxidized A2-E, reactions between retinoids and other constituents other than ethanolamine, and peroxidation products of proteins and lipids.[13,14] The molecular composition of LF may possibly be dependent on specific underlying molecular mechanisms. Zhou and associates demonstrated with an in vitro assay a link between inflammation, activation of the complement system, oxidative damage, drusen, and RPE LF.[15] They suggested that products of the photo-oxidation of RPE LF components could serve as a trigger for the complement system which could predispose the macular area to a chronic, low-grade inflammatory process over time.

Detection of LF and its constituents is facilitated by its autofluorescent properties. When stimulated with light in the blue range, LF granules typically emit a green–yellow fluorescence.[16,17] The distribution of LF in postmitotic human RPE cells and its accumulation with age have been extensively studied in vitro, applying fluorescence microscopic techniques.[5,6,8]

Near-infrared autofluorescence

Near-infrared autofluorescence (NIA) images can also be obtained in vivo, most commonly and easily by using the indocyanine green angiography mode of the scanning laser ophthalmoscope, i.e., without dye injection.[18,19] Due to the excitation and emission in the red end of the spectrum, the topographic distribution of fluorophores other than LF may be studied by this technique. It has been suggested that the NIA signal is largely melanin-derived.[18–20] As such, Keilhauer and Delori[18] further speculated that, to varying degrees, choroidal sources contributed to this signal. Gibbs et al.[21] investigated NIA in humans and mice and suggested that melanosomes in the RPE and choroid were likely the dominant origin of the signal. Except for measurements in cell cultures at low magnification, their analyses were limited to excitation at 633 nm, in contrast to in vivo NIA, which is generated at 795 nm. Using a customized magnification lens attached to the front of the confocal scanning laser ophthalmoscope (cSLO), Schmitz-Valckenberg and coworkers studied the distribution of the NIA signal in retinal cross-sections of a human donor eye and correlated ex vivo autofluorescence measurements to in vivo findings in a rat animal model.[22] They observed that the NIA signal was spatially confined to the RPE monolayer and melanin in the choroid.

Macular pigment imaging

Macular pigment, consisting of lutein and zeaxanthin, extensively accumulates along the axons of the cone photoreceptors in the central retina.[23–25] As has been reported, a number of functions have been proposed for macular pigment,[24,25] including filtration of blue light which may reduce photo damage and glare, minimization of the effects of chromatic aberration on visual acuity, improvement in fine-detail discrimination, and enhancement of contrast sensitivity. Neutralization of reactive oxygen species by macular pigment may have a protective effect on the neurosensory retina. Although there may be a large variation with regard to the concentration of macular pigment, the pattern of distribution is relatively uniform in the normal population. It generally shows a peak concentration at the foveal center and rapidly decreases with eccentricity, with very little present at about 8° of eccentricity.

Peak absorption of luteal pigment is at 460 nm. These absorption properties can be readily recorded in vivo by blue-light autofluorescence imaging.[26] Therefore, blue FAF imaging can also be used to determine the topographic distribution of macular pigment. Compared to other methods, including heterochromatic flicker photometry, the advantage of FAF imaging is its objective acquisition technique which is not dependent on psychophysical cooperation by the examined individual.

TECHNIQUES OF FUNDUS AUTOFLUORESCENCE IMAGING

Recording of autofluorescence images is noninvasive and requires relatively little time.

The intensity of naturally occurring fluorescence of the ocular fundus is about 2 orders of magnitude lower than the background of a fluorescein angiogram at the most intense part of the dye transit.[1] Absorption of light with reduction of the fluorescence signal, or excitation and emission of light with an increase in the fluorescence signal by anatomical structures anterior to the retina, may further complicate or interfere with the detection of the FAF signal. In the eye, the principal barrier is the crystalline lens which has highly fluorescent properties in the short-wavelength range (excitation between 400 and 600 nm results in peak emission at c. 520 nm). With increasing age and particularly the development of nuclear lens opacities, the fluorescence of the lens becomes even more prominent.

Pioneering work on the spectral analysis of the origin of the autofluorescence signal was performed by Delori and coworkers[1] using a fundus spectrometer. In parallel, von Rückmann et al., in their landmark paper, described the use of cSLO for FAF imaging.[27]

Fundus spectrophotometer

The fundus spectrophotometer by Delori and coworkers[1] was designed to analyse systematically the excitation and emission spectra of the autofluorescence signals originating from small retinal areas (2° diameter) of the fundus. By incorporating an image intensifier diode array as a detector, a beam separation in the pupil, and confocal detection to minimize contribution of autofluorescence from the crystalline lens, this device allowed the absolute measurements of autofluorescence. These authors showed that fundus fluorescence is emitted across a broad band from 500 to 800 nm. Both at the center of the fovea and at 7° temporally, optimal excitation occurred at 510 nm with peak emission at approximately 630 nm, indicating the predominance of a fluorophore at these excitation and emission spectra. There was a significant increase with age and the recording along a horizontal line through the fovea showed a minimum fluorescence at the fovea, a maximum intensity at 7–15° from the fovea, and a decrease toward the periphery, most likely reflecting the concomitant distribution of macular pigment and melanin interfering with the emission of the dominant fluorophore. The optic disc was characterized by a less intense signal. The relationship with age and the topographic distribution of the dominant fundus fluorophore were consistent with those of RPE LF as measured in the RPE of human donor eyes.[3,5]

Along with autofluorescence recordings in patients with several pathological conditions, the initial work by Delori et al.[1] demonstrated that LF is the dominant source of intrinsic fluorescence of the ocular fundus. However, the small area sampled by the fundus spectrometer as well as the customized relatively complex instrumentation and techniques were not practical for recording fundus autofluorescence from patients in a clinical setting.

Scanning laser ophthalmoscopy

Confocal scanning laser ophthalmoscopy (cSLO) optimally addresses the limitations of the low intensity of the autofluorescence signal and the interference of the crystalline lens. It was used initially by von Rückmann and coworkers in a clinical imaging system.[27] The confocal scanning laser ophthalmoscope projects a low-power laser beam on the retina which is swept across the fundus in a raster pattern.[28] The intensity of the reflected light at each point, after passing through the confocal pinhole, is registered by means of a detector, and a two-dimensional image is subsequently generated. Confocal optics insure that out-of-focus light (i.e., light originating outside the adjusted focal plane, but within the light beam) is suppressed and, thus, the image contrast is enhanced. This suppression increases with the distance from the focal plane and signals from sources anterior to the retina, i.e., the lens or the cornea, are effectively reduced.

In contrast to the 2° retinal field of the fundus spectrophotometer, the cSLO allows imaging over larger retinal areas. To reduce background noise and to enhance image contrast, a series of several single images is usually recorded (reviewed by Schmitz-Valckenberg et al.[2]). For the final fundus autofluorescence image, a number of these frames (usually out of 4–32) are averaged and pixel values are normalized. Given the high sensitivity of the cSLO and the high frame rate of up to 16 frames per second, FAF imaging can be performed within seconds and at low excitation energies which are well below the maximum retinal irradiance limits of lasers established by the American National Standards Institute and other international standards.[29]

With the cSLO, excitation is usually induced in the blue range ($\lambda = 488$ nm), and an emission filter between 500 and 700 nm is used to detect emission of the autofluorescence signal. The most widely used cSLO system for FAF imaging is the Heidelberg retina angiograph/Heidelberg Spectralis. One key advantage of the Spectralis system is the simultaneous acquisition of optical coherence tomography (OCT) recordings that allow for both averaging of several OCT B-scans in order to enhance the signal-to-noise ratio and the synchronous topographic alignment of FAF intensities with OCT findings.[30] Other previous systems, such as the Rodenstock cSLO and the Zeiss prototype SM 30 4024 for FAF imaging, are no longer commercially available. Nidek has recently introduced the F-10 cSLO platform that also allows for FAF imaging (Fig. 4.1).

Fundus camera

The relatively weak fundus autofluorescence signal, absorption effects of the crystalline lens, nonconfocality, and light-scattering effects are important limitations of fundus camera-based systems for FAF recordings. Delori and coworkers described a modified fundus camera for FAF imaging.[31] Their design included the insertion of an aperture in the illumination optics of the camera in order to minimize the loss of contrast caused by light scattering and fluorescence from the crystalline lens. However, the modification also resulted in the restriction of the field of view to a 13° diameter circle; this, together with the complex design, is the likely reason why this configuration has not been further pursued. In 2003, Spaide[32] reported the modification of a commercially available fundus camera system by shifting the excitation and emission wavelengths for fundus autofluorescence imaging towards the red end of the spectrum in order to suppress the fluorescence originating from the lens (Fig. 4.2). The relatively inexpensive purchase of an additional filter set, together with the broad availability of the flash fundus camera, may make this an attractive alternative. These operate with excitation in the green spectrum and emission is recorded in the yellow–orange spectrum.[33]

In addition to the different excitation light (green versus blue) for FAF recording, other major technical differences between fundus camera systems and the cSLO setup must be considered (Table 4.1). In particular, the absence of confocal optics makes the fundus camera prone to light scattering and generation of secondary reflectance light that interferes with the FAF detection. The visualization of subtle FAF alterations is challenging with the modified fundus camera, as shown in one study of patients with geographic atrophy (GA) secondary to AMD.[34]

Wide-field imaging

The standard image field of the typical cSLO encompasses a retinal field of 30° × 30°. Additional lenses allow for imaging of a 55° field or, using the composite mode, imaging over even larger retinal areas. Using the fundus camera, so-called montage images can be manually generated using image analysis software on the basis of a seven-field panorama survey.

Peripheral FAF images can also be recorded with a recently introduced wide-field scanning laser ophthalmoscope (P200Tx, Optos). This system allows for FAF acquisition in less than 2 seconds by using green light excitation (532 nm). FAF recordings beyond the vascular arcades may be particularly helpful for assessment of the peripheral extension of retinal diseases (Fig. 4.3).

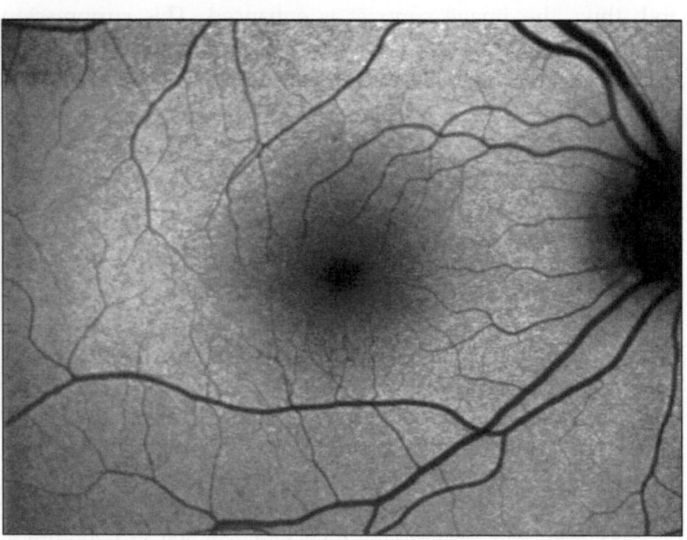

Fig. 4.1 Normal fundus autofluorescence image obtained with a Nidek F-10 scanning laser ophthalmoscope.

Table 4.1 Summary of technical differences between the confocal scanning laser ophthalmoscope (cSLO) and the modified fundus camera for fundus autofluorescence imaging

cSLO	Modified fundus camera
One excitation wavelength (laser source) Large emission spectrum (cutoff filter)	Bandwidth filters for excitation and emission
Continuous scanning at low light intensities in a raster pattern	One single flash at maximum intensities
Confocal system	Entire cone of light
Laser power fixed by manufacturer, detector sensitivity adjustable	Flash light intensity, gain and gamma of detector adjustable
Imaging processing with averaging of single frames and pixel normalization	Manual contrast and brightness

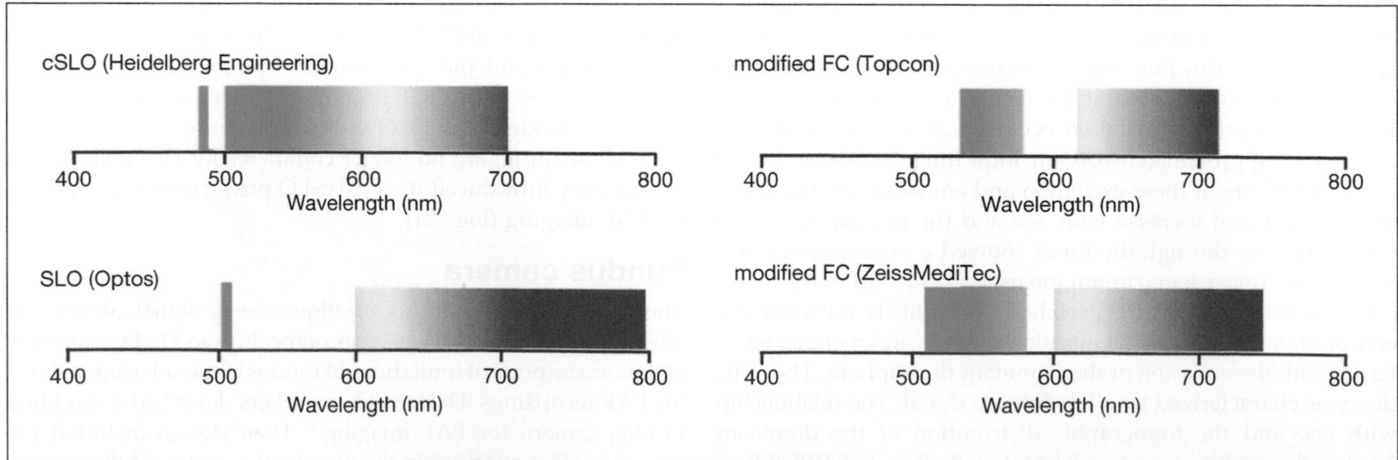

Fig. 4.2 Range of excitation and emission for different camera systems. cSLO, confocal scanning laser ophthalmoscopy; FC, fundus camera.

INTERPRETATION OF FUNDUS AUTOFLUORESCENCE IMAGES

The FAF image shows the spatial distribution of the intensity of the FAF signal for each pixel in gray values (arbitrary values from 0 to 255). Per definition, low pixel values (dark) illustrate low intensities and high pixel values (bright) illustrate high intensities. The topographical distribution of FAF in normal eyes demonstrates a consistent pattern, as illustrated in Fig. 4.4.[27] A diffuse FAF signal over the posterior pole can be seen, while retinal vessels (due to an absorption phenomenon by blood contents, i.e., hemoglobin) and the optic nerve head (absence of autofluorescent material) are characterized by a very low signal and appear dark. Showing a high degree of inter-individual variability, decreased FAF intensities at the macular area with a minimum in the fovea are observed; these are caused by absorption of short-wavelength light due to luteal pigment (lutein and zeaxanthin).

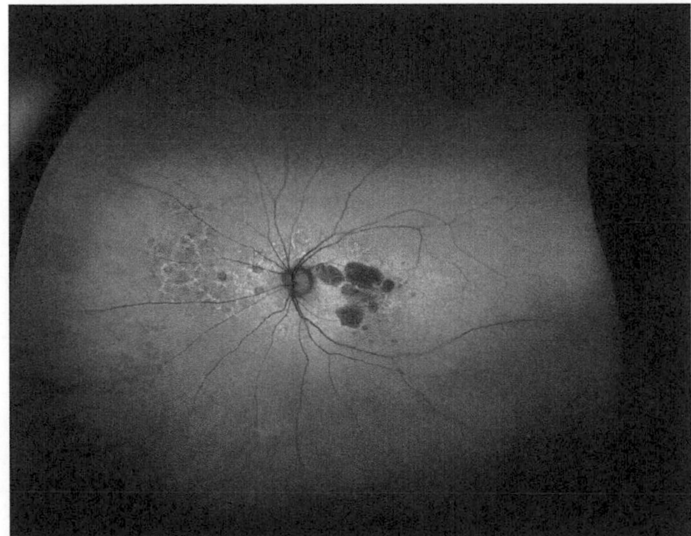

Fig. 4.3 Patient with geographic atrophy due to age-related macular degeneration. The image was recorded by a wide-field scanning laser ophthalmoscope (P200Tx, Optos). This system allows for fundus autofluorescence acquisition in less than 2 seconds by using green light excitation (532 nm). Note the peripheral extension of abnormal fundus autofluorescence signal nasal to the optic disc.

Using pixel gray values, typical ratios between the intensity of the fovea and perifoveal macula have been established in normal subjects (reviewed by Schmitz-Valckenberg et al.[2]). Based on these findings, qualitative descriptions of localized FAF changes are widely used. Usually, the FAF signal over a certain retinal location is categorized in decreased, normal, or increased intensities in comparison to the background signal of the same image.

In contrast, the quantification of absolute intensities and their comparison between subjects or within longitudinal observation in the same subject are more complicated and remain a challenge in FAF imaging. Of note, as the pixel histogram in the usual available cSLO images is normalized in order to visualize better the topographic distribution of the FAF intensity (see above), the pixel values are not absolute and these images must not be used for absolute intensity analyses from the outset. Furthermore, when interpreting FAF images, one should take into account that the digital resolution of the detector in current imaging devices exceeds the maximum spatial resolution of ocular media and the optics of the system, mainly due to high-order aberrations. Therefore, single pixel values of a standard FAF image do not reflect the actual anatomical resolution of the image and should not be used to compare intensities between different locations. This also explains why increasing the digital resolution of the detector does not improve the resolution of the actual image, but rather results in an artificially high-resolution, posterized image.

When analyzing absolute intensities on averaged but non-normalized FAF images (after ensuring that the normalization of the pixel histogram is turned off), a great variability of the mean gray value for a certain retinal location is usually noted when FAF images are subsequently acquired from the same subject directly one after the other using the same imaging device. A systematic analysis by Lois and coworkers[35] reported good intraobserver and moderate interobserver reproducibility when comparing the absolute mean pixel value of a 16 × 16 pixel square on the retina. In this report, the image resolution is not provided. When assuming an image resolution of 256 × 256 pixels and a 40° × 30° field (as these settings were published in previous studies using the same cSLO by the same group), the 16 × 16 pixel box would encompass a retinal area of c. 2° × 1.9°. Hence, moderate interobserver reproducibility would just have been achieved over a rather large retinal area, but was not shown for the anatomical resolution of the imaging system.

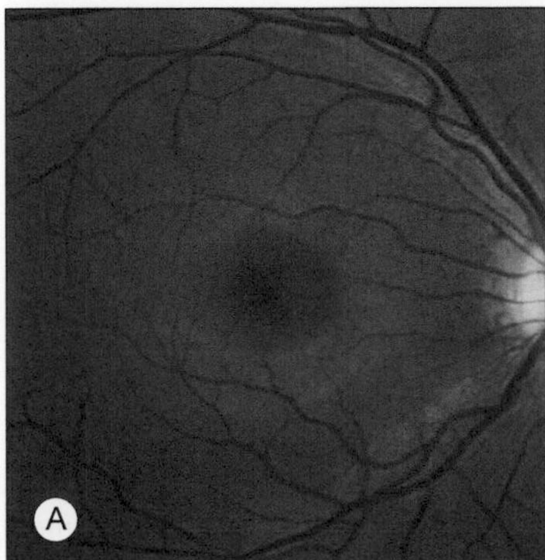

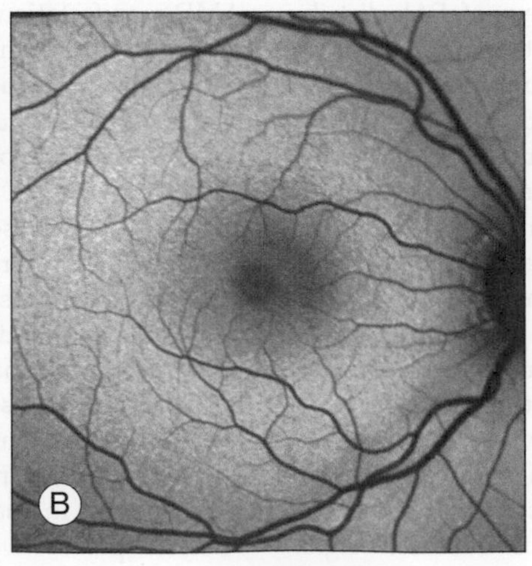

Fig. 4.4 Color fundus photograph (A) and fundus autofluorescence image (B) of the right eye of a normal subject imaged with the confocal scanning laser ophthalmoscope (Heidelberg retina angiograph, HRA 2, Heidelberg Engineering, Heidelberg, Germany). Topographical distribution of fundus autofluorescence intensity shows typical background signal with a dark optic disc (absence of autofluorescent material) and retinal vessels (absorption). Further, intensity is markedly decreased over the fovea due to the absorption of the blue light by yellow macular pigment. (Reproduced with permission from Schmitz-Valckenberg S, Fleckenstein M, Scholl HP, et al. Fundus autofluorescence and progression of age-related macular degeneration. Surv Ophthalmol 2009;54:96–117.)

Several confounding factors have to be taken into account when comparing absolute FAF intensities between different examinations and different individuals. This not only includes standardization of settings (laser power, detector sensitivity, correction of refractive errors, and image-processing steps, including the number of averaged images), but also eye movements, position of the patient in the chin rest, orientation of the camera, distance between the camera and the cornea, fluctuations of laser power, and short-term dynamic changes in FAF intensities caused by prolonged exposure to the excitation light or previous dark adaption (reviewed by Schmitz-Valckenberg et al.[2]).

Recently, Delori and coworkers introduced a method for quantitative autofluorescence measurements by insertion of an internal FAF reference to account for variable laser power and detector sensitivity.[36] Quantified autofluorescence is calculated accounting for the calibrated reference, the zero gray level, and the magnification (refractive error). For retinal degenerations and related diseases, this approach may enhance the understanding of disease processes, and may serve as a diagnostic aid, as a more sensitive marker of natural disease progression, and as a tool to monitor the effects of therapeutic interventions targeting LF accumulations.

CLINICAL APPLICATIONS

Age-related macular degeneration

Early AMD

Early manifestation of AMD include focal hypo- and hyperpigmentation at the level of the RPE as well as drusen with extracellular material accumulating in the inner aspects of Bruch's membrane.[37] Drusen may be distinguished based on size (small versus large) and morphology (hard versus soft). Postmortem analyses demonstrated that some molecular species in drusen material possess autofluorescent properties.

In vivo FAF changes in early AMD have been described by several authors using the cSLO and the fundus camera, respectively (reviewed by Schmitz-Valckenberg et al.[2]). Interestingly, drusen visible on fundus photography are not necessarily correlated with notable FAF changes and areas of increased FAF may or may not correspond with areas of hyperpigmentation or soft or hard drusen (Fig. 4.5). Overall, larger drusen are more frequently associated with notable FAF abnormalities than smaller ones, with the exception of basal laminar drusen. Crystalline drusen typically demonstrate a corresponding decreased FAF signal.

Delori and coworkers described a pattern of FAF distribution associated with drusen which consists of decreased FAF in the center of the druse with a surrounding annulus of increased FAF.[31] It has been speculated that this appearance is caused by attenuated RPE at the center and tangential orientation of RPE cells at the edges of the druse. A reduced turnover and a net increase in the amount of LF of the RPE cells at the edges would lead to the increased signal. Interestingly, this ring-like appearance of drusen with FAF imaging is much more pronounced when imaged with a flash fundus camera. Several authors have consistently reported that confluent drusen and large foveal soft drusen (drusenoid RPE detachments) topographically correspond well with mildly increased FAF using cSLO.[38–40] With a fundus camera-based system, large soft drusen have a slightly decreased FAF signal at their centers and are surrounded by a faint ring of increased signal. Multiple foci and/or irregular areas of FAF are observed when several small, hard or soft drusen coalesce. Focal areas of increased FAF are typically found in the vicinity of drusen with overlying areas of pigment-clumping or adjacent to long-standing and crystalline drusen.

Increased FAF signal adjacent to drusen fundoscopically corresponding to focal hyperpigmentation and pigment figures has been attributed to the presence of melanolipofuscin or changes in the metabolic activity of the RPE. Areas of hypopigmentation on fundus photographs tend to be associated with a corresponding decreased FAF signal, suggesting the absence of RPE cells or degenerating RPE cells with reduced content of LF granules.

So-called reticular pseudodrusen have been identified as a risk factor for the development of late-stage AMD. In patients with GA this specific phenotypic pattern, which is best recognized by infrared reflectance and FAF imaging, can be detected in over 60% of eyes with GA.[41] The precise morphological correlate of this distinct pattern is controversial. Speculations range from abnormalities in the inner choroid[42] to subretinal deposits[43]; the latter speculation is based on the spectral domain (SD)-OCT changes recorded in the presence of reticular pseudodrusen.[30,43,44]

The variability of the FAF phenotye in AMD contrasts with young patients with monogenic disorders in whom the drusen typically autofluoresce brightly, presumably reflecting a composition of the accumulating material distinctly different from age-related drusen.

The spectrum of FAF findings in patients with early AMD was classified by an international expert group.[40] Pooling data from several retinal centers, a system with eight different FAF patterns was developed, including normal, minimal change, focal increased, patchy, linear, lace-like, reticular, and speckled pattern (Fig. 4.5). This classification demonstrates the relatively poor correlation between visible alterations on fundus photography and notable FAF changes. Based on these results, it was speculated that FAF findings in early AMD may indicate more widespread abnormalities and a greater extent of disease than is ophthalmoscopically visible. The changes seen in FAF imaging at the RPE cell level may precede the occurrence of visible lesions as the disease progresses. This classification system may help to identify specific high-risk characteristics for disease progression and may be of value in future interventional trials. Furthermore, it may be of use in molecular genetic analysis to identify one or several genes conferring risk for the development of certain AMD manifestations.

Recent approaches to investigate FAF findings in AMD patients have included the use of image analysis software to compare pixel values and topographically map and register alterations visible on FAF images with fundus photographs or reflectance images.[32,38] Differences in the percentage of areas with focally increased FAF intensity between eyes with various AMD manifestations have been reported. One study reported that the fellow eyes of patients with unilateral exudative AMD in the other eye tended not to exhibit FAF abnormalities. Another analysis showed that patients with exudative AMD in one eye had larger amounts of areas with abnormal autofluorescence in the fellow eye than did the eyes of patients with early disease and without a history of exudative AMD. Unfortunately, because of differences in imaging devices and the use of different image analysis protocols, comparisons between these studies are

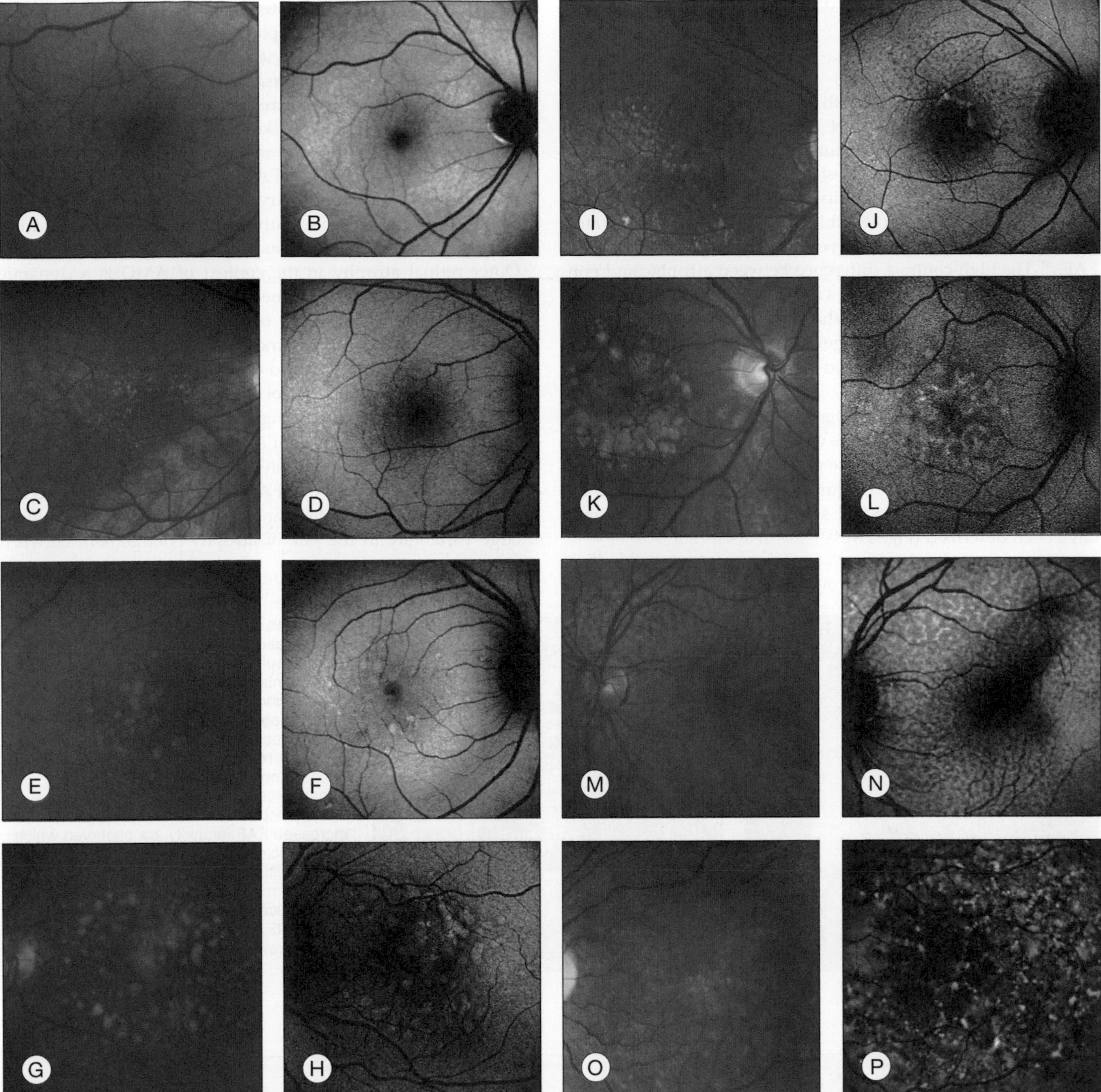

Fig. 4.5 Classification of abnormal autofluorescence patterns in early age-related macular disease. Corresponding color fundus photographs and fundus autofluorescence (FAF) images are shown. Eight phenotypic patterns are differentiated: (1) Normal (A, B): homogeneous-background FAF and a gradual decrease in the inner macula toward the fovea due to the masking effect of macular pigment. Only small hard drusen are visible in the corresponding fundus photograph. (2) Minimal change (C, D): only minimal variations from normal background FAF. There is limited irregular increase or decrease in FAF intensity due to multiple small hard drusen. (3) Focal (E, F): several well-defined spots with markedly increased FAF. Fundus photograph of the same eye with multiple hard and soft drusen. (4) Patchy (G, H): multiple large areas (over 200 µm in diameter) of increased FAF corresponding to large, soft drusen and/or hyperpigmentation on the fundus photograph. (5) Linear (I, J): characterized by the presence of at least one linear area of markedly increased FAF. A corresponding hyperpigmented line is visible on the fundus photograph. (6) Lace-like (K, L): multiple branching linear structures of increased FAF. This pattern may correspond to hyperpigmentation on the fundus photograph or to no visible abnormalities. (7) Reticular (M, N): multiple, specific small areas of decreased FAF with brighter lines in between. The reticular pattern not only occurs in the macular area but is found more typically in a superotemporal location. There may be visible reticular drusen in the corresponding fundus photograph. (8) Speckled (O, P): a variety of FAF abnormalities are noted to occupy a larger area of the FAF image. There seem to be fewer pathologic areas in the corresponding fundus. (Reproduced with permission from Bindewald A, Bird AC, Dandekar SS, et al. Classification of fundus autofluorescence patterns in early age-related macular disease. Invest Ophthalmol Vis Sci 2005;46:3309–14.)

difficult and further investigation is required (reviewed by Schmitz-Valckenberg et al.[2]).

Geographic atrophy

Areas of GA are associated with RPE cell death as well as with loss or attenuation of adjacent layers, in particular the outer neurosensory retina and the choriocapillaris. [45] With disappearance of the RPE, LF is also lost, resulting in a corresponding marked decrease in FAF intensity (Figs 4.6 and 4.7).[27] Compared to drusen which may also exhibit a decreased FAF signal, atrophic areas typically show an even more profound reduction of FAF. [31] The high-contrast difference between atrophic and nonatrophic regions of retina allows more easy and reliable delineation of the area of atrophy than from conventional fundus photographs. [46] These advantages of documenting and studying GA by FAF imaging have been used in many natural history studies[47,48] (Figs 4.6 and 4.7).

An even more striking finding of FAF imaging in GA patients is the frequent presence of areas of hyperautoflourescence in the junctional zone surrounding the patch of atrophy.[49] Distinct patterns of abnormal FAF in the junctional zone of atrophy and a high degree of intraindividual symmetry between fellow eyes have been described (Fig. 4.8).[50,51]

Recently, a classification system of FAF patterns in the junctional zone of atrophy in GA patients has been proposed (Fig. 4.9).[52] Studies of retinal sensitivity have underscored the importance of increased FAF surrounding areas of GA and, thus, the pathophysiological role of increased RPE LF accumulation in such patients. Scholl and coworkers have demonstrated that rod photoreceptor function is more severely affected than cone function over areas with increased FAF using fine matrix mapping.[53] Combining SLO microperimetry and FAF imaging in another study, impaired photopic sensitivity has been observed in areas of abnormal FAF in the junctional zone[54].

Outer retinal atrophy in the context of AMD is a dynamic process with gradual enlargement of atrophic areas over time. Initial natural history studies on atrophy progression in GA patients using FAF imaging demonstrated the occurrence of new atrophic patches and the spread of pre-existing atrophy in areas with abnormally high levels of FAF at baseline.[49] Looking at larger patient groups with longer review periods, the significance of increased junctional FAF for foreshadowing atrophy enlargement has been highlighted.[47,48] In accordance with other natural history studies, the FAM (Fundus Autofluorescence Imaging in Age-related Macular Degeneration) study identified a large variability in the rate of atrophy enlargement between

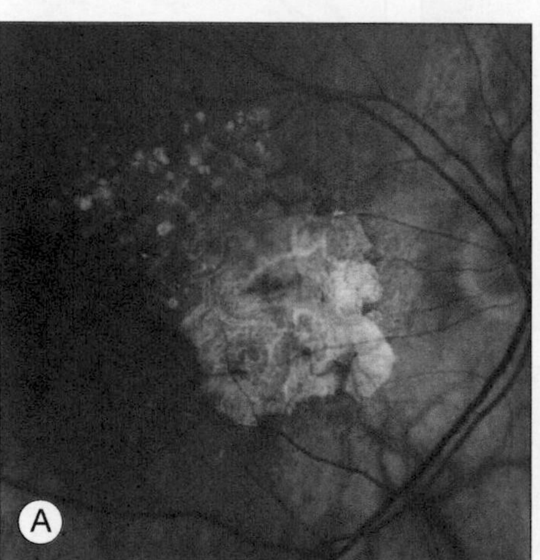

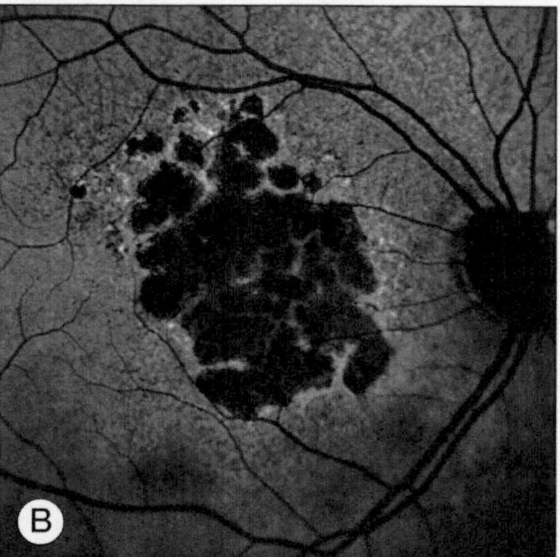

Fig. 4.6 In atrophic age-related macular degeneration, geographic atrophy appears as a sharply demarcated area with depigmentation and enhanced visualization of deep choroidal vessels on the color fundus photograph (A). On the corresponding fundus autofluorescence (FAF) image (B), atrophic patches are clearly delineated by decreased intensity and high-contrast to adjacent nonatrophic retina. Surrounding the atrophy, in the junctional zone, foci and areas of increased FAF intensity are observed which are invisible on fundus photography. These abnormalities tend to precede atrophy over time and may serve as disease markers. (Reproduced with permission from Holz FG, Spaide RF. Essentials in ophthalmology: Medical retina. Berlin: Springer; 2007, Fig. 5.3.)

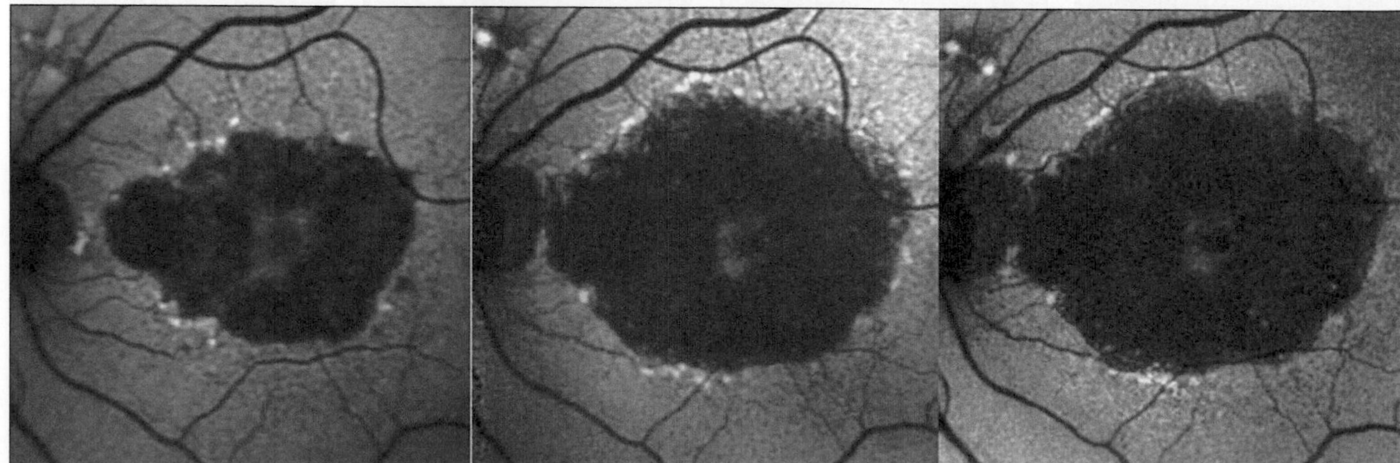

Fig. 4.7 Monitoring of atrophic progression over time with fundus autofluorescence imaging, showing the natural course of the disease over 5 years. (Reproduced with permission from Holz FG, Spaide RF. Essentials in ophthalmology: Medical retina. Berlin: Springer; 2007, Fig. 5.4.)

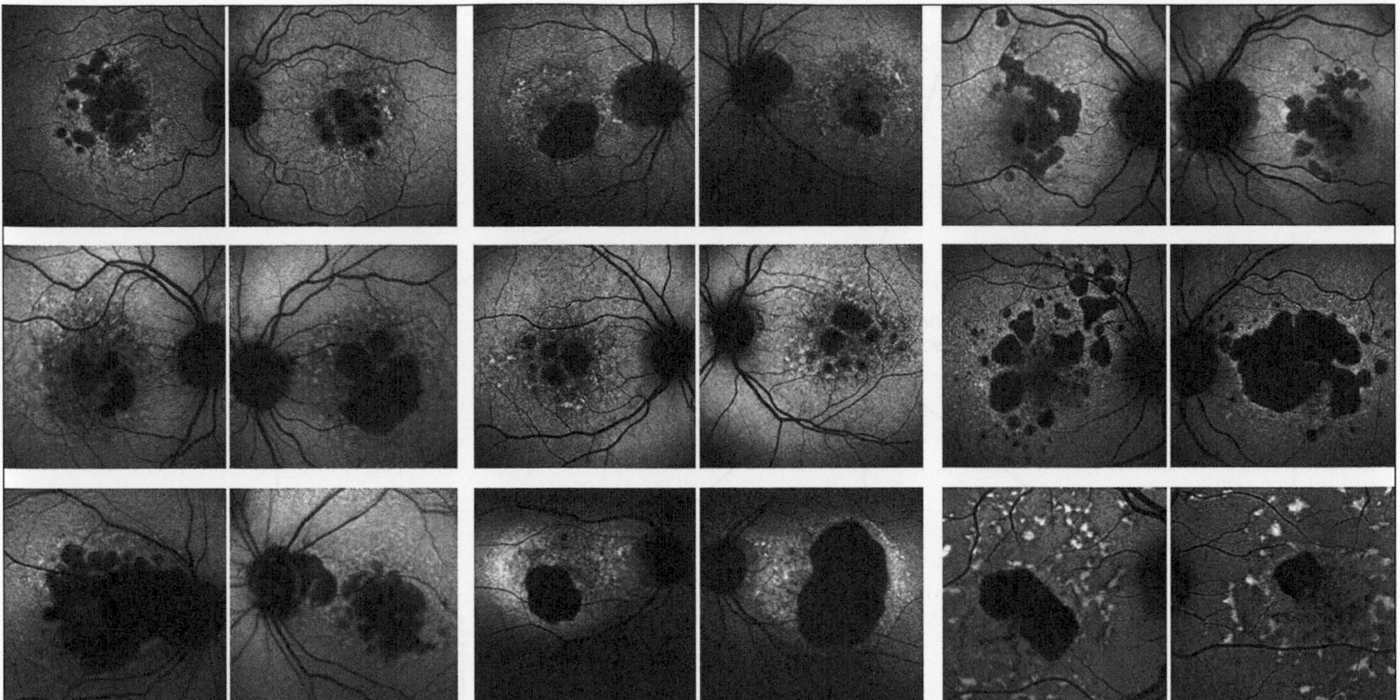

Fig. 4.8 Fundus autofluorescence images of patients with bilateral geographic atrophy (images of the right and left eye are taken at the same time point). There is a high degree of symmetry with respect of the configuration of atrophy while there is a high degree of interindividual variability. (Reproduced with permission from Fleckenstein M, Adrion C, Schmitz-Valckenberg S, et al. Concordance of disease progression in bilateral geographic atrophy due to AMD. Invest Ophthalmol Vis Sci 2010;51:637–42. Copyright ARVO.org.)

patients, which was neither explained by the extent of baseline atrophy nor by any other comorbid factor such as smoking, lens status, or family history. Interestingly, the initial studies using FAF imaging on patients with GA have already reported various patterns of changes in FAF in the junctional zone of GA (reviewed by Schmitz-Valckenberg et al.[2]). These investigators speculated that their observations might reflect heterogeneity of the underlying disease process. In addition, Bellmann and coworkers reported a high degree of symmetry of abnormal FAF patterns in patients with bilateral GA in the presence of a high degree of interindividual variability, suggesting that genetic determinants rather than nonspecific aging changes may be involved.[50]

A more recent analysis of the FAM study of 195 eyes of 129 patients shows that variable rates of progression of GA are dependent on the specific phenotype of abnormal FAF pattern at baseline.[48] Atrophy enlargement was the slowest in eyes with no abnormal FAF pattern (median 0.38 mm^2/year), followed by eyes with the focal FAF pattern (median 0.81 mm^2/year), then by eyes with the diffuse FAF pattern (median 1.77 mm^2/year), and finally, by eyes with the banded FAF pattern (1.81 mm^2/year). The difference in atrophy progression between the groups of no abnormal and focal FAF patterns and the groups of the diffuse and banded FAF patterns was statistically significant ($P < 0.0001$). These results have subsequently been confirmed in another large-scale study (the Natural History of Geographic Atrophy Progression (GAP)).[55,56] These findings underscore the importance of abnormal FAF intensities around atrophy and the pathophysiological role of increased RPE LF accumulation in patients with GA due to AMD.

Pigment epithelium detachment

FAF imaging in eyes with pigment epithelium detachment (PED) secondary to AMD show variable FAF phenotypes which are not always detectable using conventional imaging techniques such as fundus photography, fluorescein, or indocyanine green angiography (Fig. 4.10). The majority of PEDs show a corresponding marked, evenly distributed increase of the FAF signal over the lesion surrounded by a well-defined, less autofluorescent halo delineating the entire border of the lesion. There are also PEDs with an intermediate or a decreased FAF signal over the lesion which may or may not correspond to areas of RPE atrophy or fibrovascular scarring. Additional investigation, however, is necessary to categorize fully the FAF features of PEDs and to correlate these findings with other imaging studies. Rarely, a PED shows a cartwheel pattern of increased autofluorescence corresponding with hyperpigmented radial lines. The hyperpigmented lines correlate with subretinal hyperreflective structures, as demonstrated by OCT.

However, a systematic analysis of these FAF alterations with correlation to the underlying causes of PED such as choroidal neovascularization (CNV), retinal angiomatous proliferation, polypoidal vasculopathy, or serous, nonexudative PED is lacking to date. These changes are probably not only caused by increased or decreased amounts of LF, but may derive from other dominant fluorophores with similar excitation and emission spectra, such as extracellular fluid or degraded photoreceptors (Fig. 4.10).

Choroidal neovascularization

Theoretical considerations would suggest that FAF imaging may provide important clues to our understanding of CNV secondary to AMD. For example, it may be helpful to assess the integrity of the RPE which may influence the development and behavior of new vascular complexes as well as photoreceptor viability and potential therapeutic success.

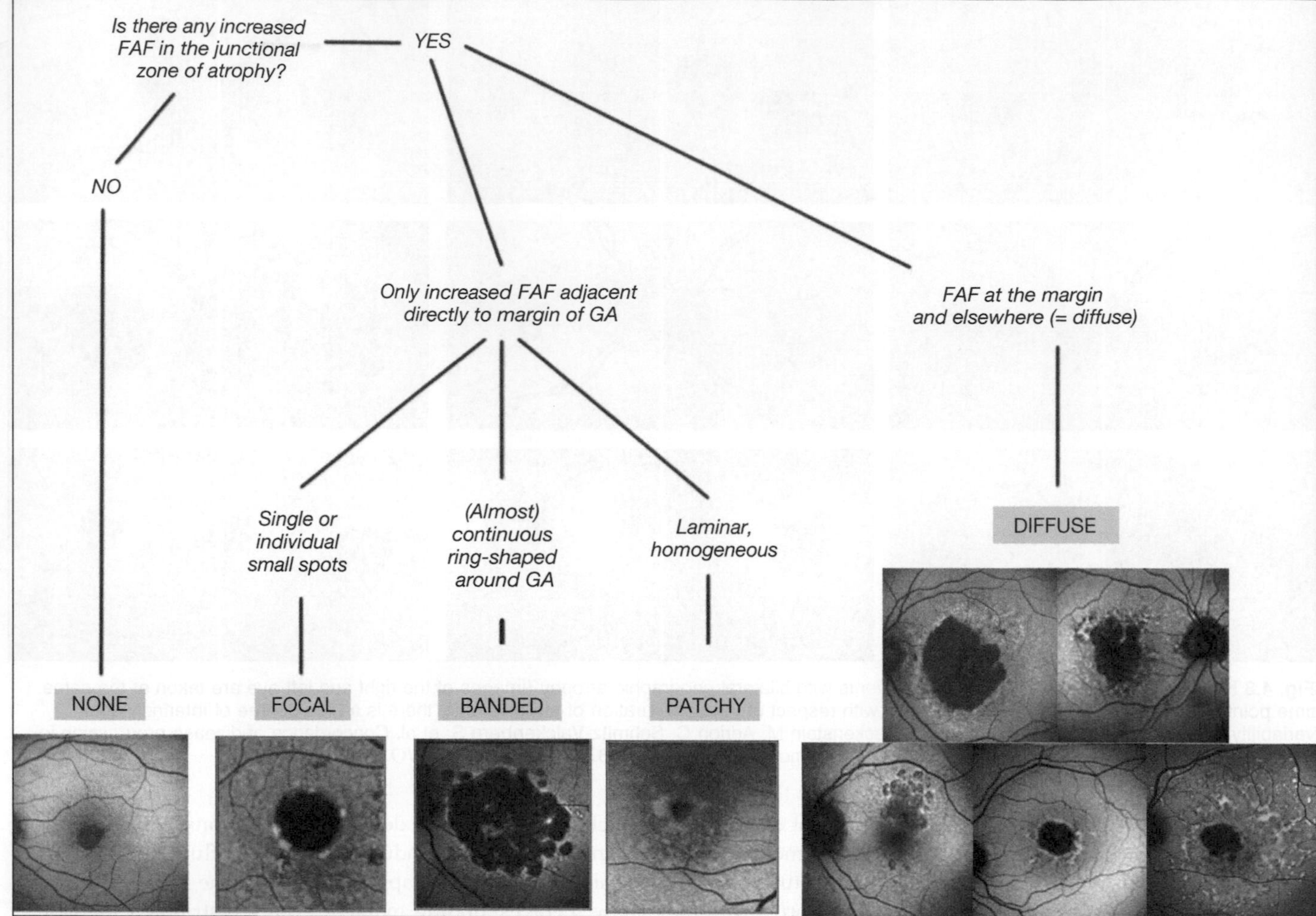

Fig. 4.9 Classification of fundus autofluorescence (FAF) patterns in the junctional zone in patients with geographic atrophy (GA) due to age-related macular degeneration. Eyes with no apparent increased FAF intensity are graded as "none" (slow progressor). The eyes with increased FAF are divided into two groups depending on the configuration of increased FAF surrounding atrophy. Eyes showing areas with increased FAF directly adjacent to the margin of the atrophic patch(es) and elsewhere are called "diffuse" (rapid progressors) and are subdivided into five groups. From left to right: (top row) fine granular, branching, (bottom row) trickling, reticular, and fine granular with punctuated spots. Eyes with increased FAF only at the margin of GA are divided into three subtypes (focal (slow progressor), banded (rapid progressor), and patchy (no data, occurs rarely)) according to their typical FAF pattern around atrophy. (Reproduced with permission from Schmitz-Valckenberg S, Fleckenstein M, Scholl HP, et al. Fundus autofluorescence and progression of age-related macular degeneration. Surv Ophthalmol 2009;54:96–117.)

Patients with early CNV secondary to AMD tend to have patches of "continuous" or "normal" autofluorescence corresponding with areas of hyperfluorescence on the corresponding fluorescein angiograms, implying that RPE viability is preserved at least initially in CNV development (Fig. 4.11).[57] By contrast, eyes with long-standing CNV typically exhibit more areas of decreased FAF signal, which could be explained by photoreceptor loss and scar formation with increased melanin deposition (Fig. 4.11).

One other important finding in eyes with CNV is that abnormal FAF intensities typically extend beyond the edge of the angiographically defined lesion, indicating a more widespread involvement than is apparent from conventional imaging studies. Increased FAF signal has also been described around the edge of lesions. It has been speculated that this observation may reflect the proliferation of RPE cells around the CNV.[58] As in other exudative retinal diseases, such as central serous chorioretinopathy, areas with increased FAF adjacent to CNV are commonly found inferior to the leakage on fluorescein angiography, most likely representing gravitational effects of fluid tracking. In contrast to fluid, hemorrhages and intraretinal exudates typically show a decreased FAF signal because of light absorption obscuring the underlying retinal details. When retinal hemorrhages undergo organization and evolve into an ocher color on fundoscopy, they may become intensely autofluorescent. Later, with disappearance of the yellowish material seen on biomicroscopy, a large RPE scar and atrophy with decreased autofluorescence may be visible.[59] Other imaging studies, such as fundus photography, are often required to differentiate between hemorrhages, exudates, and RPE atrophy.

Comparing FAF findings with the classification of occult and classic CNV based on fluorescein angiography, Spital et al.[59a] reported that focal areas of decreased FAF are more prevalent in classic CNV in comparison to larger occult CNVs. McBain and associates confirmed this finding and speculated that typical decreased FAF signals at the site of the CNV are related to absorption phenomena caused by the CNV growing in the subretinal space, rather than being related to severe damage to the

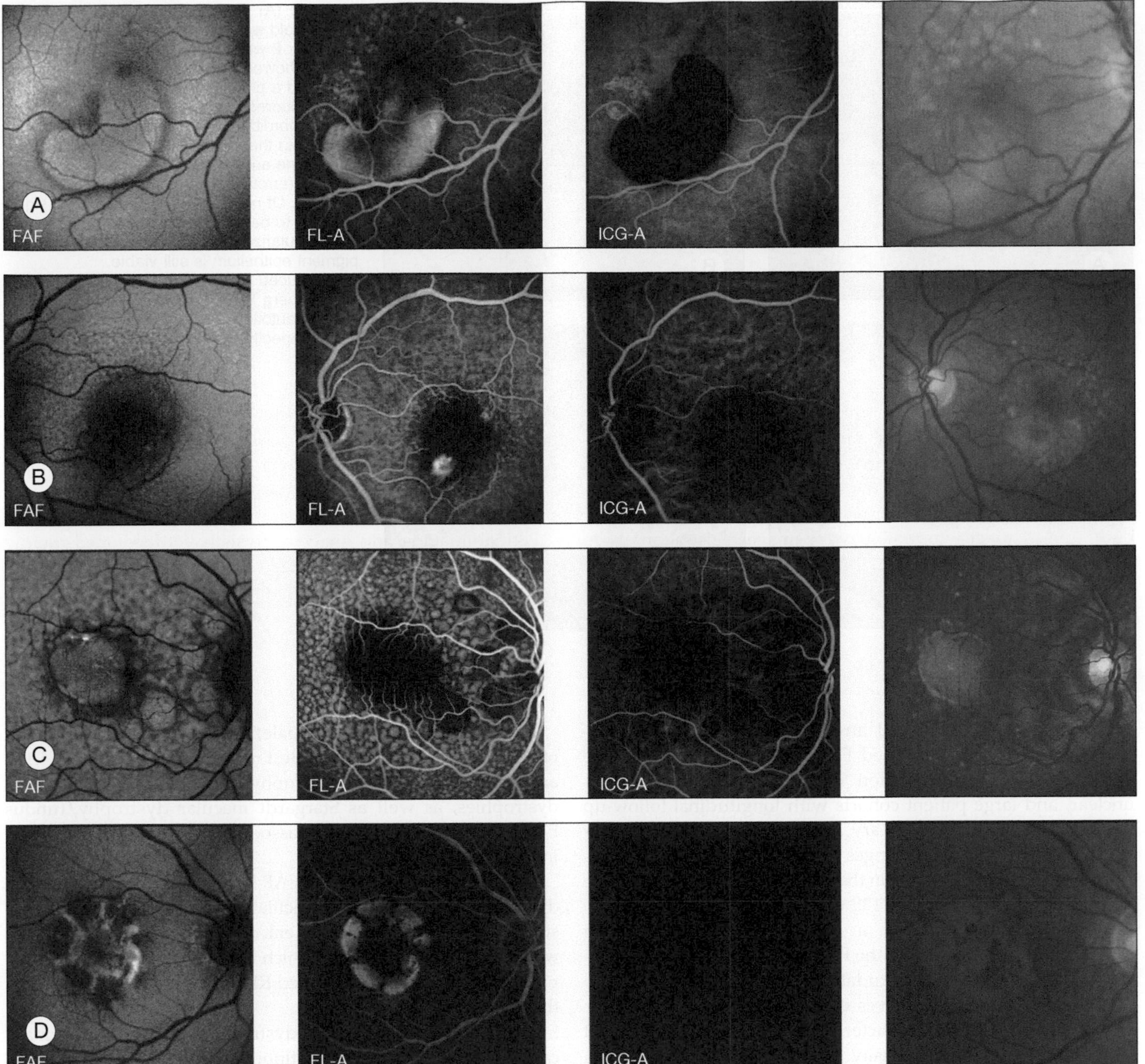

Fig. 4.10 Pigment epithelium detachment classification based on fundus autofluorescence (FAF) characteristics. (A) Increased FAF; (B) decreased FAF; (C) FAF; and (D) cartwheel FAF. FL-A, fluorescein angiography; ICG-A, indocyanine green angiography. (Reproduced with permission from Roth F, et al. Fundus autofluorescence imaging of pigment epithelial detachments. ARVO Meet Abstracts 2004;45:2962.)

RPE. [58] These observations would be in accordance with histopathological studies which have shown that classic CNV membranes are composed of predominantly subretinal fibrovascular changes as opposed to most occult lesions, which remain external to the RPE. However, a more recent study could not demonstrate any significant difference in FAF alterations between occult and classic CNVs secondary to AMD.[57] A continuous pattern of preserved autofluorescence in the central macula was observed in most patients and this was correlated with better visual acuity, shorter symptom length, and smaller lesion size. These observations would suggest that the new vessel complex, regardless of whether classic or occult, was either external (sclerad) to the RPE or had little impact on the attenuation of the FAF signal.

Recently, Heimes and coworkers analyzed the prognostic value of RPE autofluorescence with respect to the therapeutic outcome of anti-vascular endothelial growth factor therapy in exudative AMD.[60] The analysis of 95 eyes showed a significant difference in visual acuity outcomes in eyes with changes in FAF within the central 500 and 1000 μm.

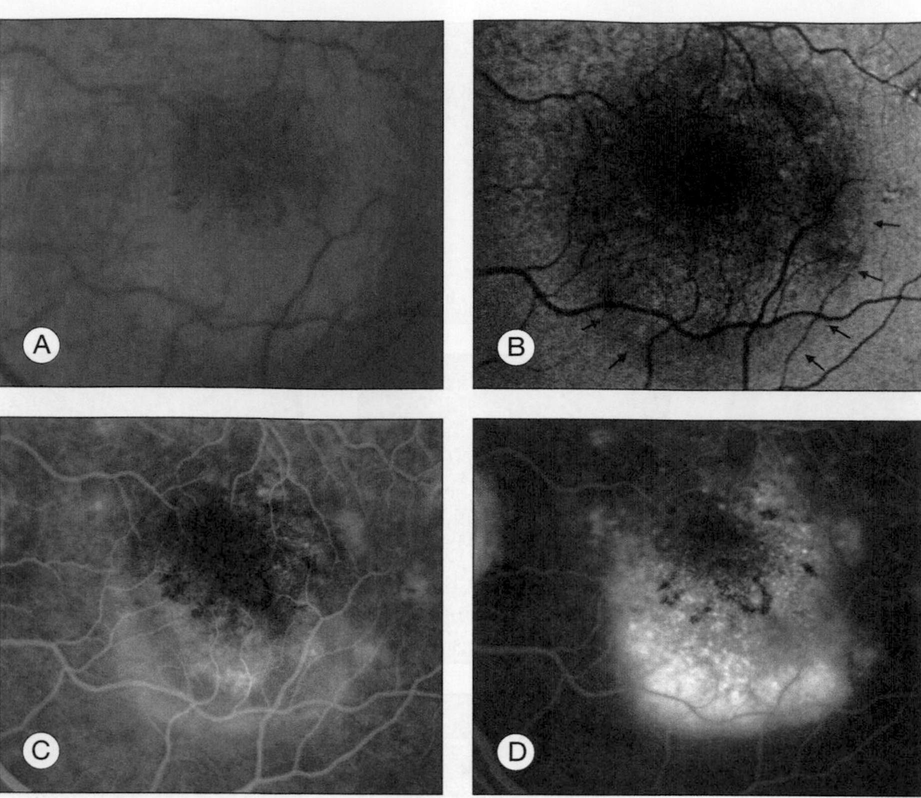

Fig. 4.11 (A) The right central macula of this 73-year-old woman with a history of blurred vision for 2 weeks (central visual acuity 20/30) showed fresh hemorrhages, subretinal fluid, and a pigment epithelium detachment. (C, D) Fluorescein angiography reveals an active choroidal neovascular membrane with leakage in the inferior part of the lesion. (B) On the autofluorescence image, the borders (arrows) of the subretinal fluid can be seen. Of note, the autofluorescence signal appears to be normal at the site of the active neovascularization, suggesting that the retinal pigment epithelium is still viable. (Reproduced with permission from Schmitz-Valckenberg S, Holz FG, Bird AC, et al. Fundus autofluorescence imaging: review and perspectives. Retina 2008;28:385–409.)

In patients with advanced atrophic AMD, the role of surrounding areas with increased FAF signal with regard to the development and progression of exudative AMD remains unclear, and large patient cohorts with longitudinal follow-up are still lacking. In a secondary analysis of one study of four eyes,[58] no abnormal FAF changes were observed prior to development of CNV at the site or in the vicinity where the membrane later developed. Looking at 125 eyes with soft drusen and no history of laser treatment, a longitudinal analysis (mean follow-up 18 months) within the FAM study disclosed nine eyes which developed advanced exudative AMD during the follow-up period.[61] Six of these nine eyes exhibited the so-called patchy FAF pattern at baseline, characterized by a homogeneous broad zone of increased FAF intensity. This finding, if confirmed in other studies, would suggest that the "patchy" FAF pattern in early AMD may represent a high-risk marker for progression to advanced AMD.

Macular and diffuse retinal dystrophies

In macular and diffuse retinal dystrophies, various associated abnormalities in FAF have been described (reviewed by von Rückmann et al.[62]). In areas of atrophy, the FAF signal is typically markedly decreased due to loss of the RPE and consequently a lack of autofluorescent LF. It is well established that autofluorescent material excessively accumulates in the RPE in association with various genetically determined retinal diseases. Increased FAF due to excessive LF accumulation in RPE cells may result from abnormally high turnover of photoreceptor outer segments or impaired RPE lysosomal degradation of normal or altered phagocytosed molecular substrates.

The extent and pattern of increased FAF may show characteristic abnormal distributions in retinal dystrophy disease entities.

The fundoscopically visible pale/yellowish lesions at the level of RPE/Bruch's membrane in Best macular dystrophy (Fig. 4.12), adult vitelliform macular dystrophy (Fig. 4.13), and other pattern dystrophies, as well as Stargardt macular dystrophy/fundus flavimaculatus (Fig. 4.14), are associated with an intense focally increased FAF signal.

The flecks with increased FAF signal in Stargardt macular dystrophy and fundus flavimaculatus may fade over time, with subsequent atrophy development. This finding is in accordance with histopathological data which have shown that these flecks represent aggregates of enlarged RPE cells engorged to 10 times their normal size with LF.

As in all forms of macular dystrophies examined systematically to date, background autofluorescence in Stargardt macular dystrophy appears to be elevated, implying a generalized abnormality of the RPE. This observation confirms the impression derived from histological studies that inherited macular dystrophies affect the entire RPE.

Lorenz and coworkers[63] described absent or minimal FAF intensities in patients with early-onset severe retinal dystrophy associated with mutations on both alleles of RPE65. The lack or severe decrease of FAF signal would be consistent with the biochemical defect and could be used as a clinical marker of this genotype. Another study demonstrated that patients with Leber congenital amaurosis having vision reduced to light perception and undetectable electroretinograms (ERGs) may still exhibit normal or minimally decreased FAF intensities.[64] This suggests that the RPE–photoreceptor complex is, at least in part, functionally and anatomically intact. This finding would have implications for future treatment, suggesting that photoreceptor function may still be rescuable in such patients.

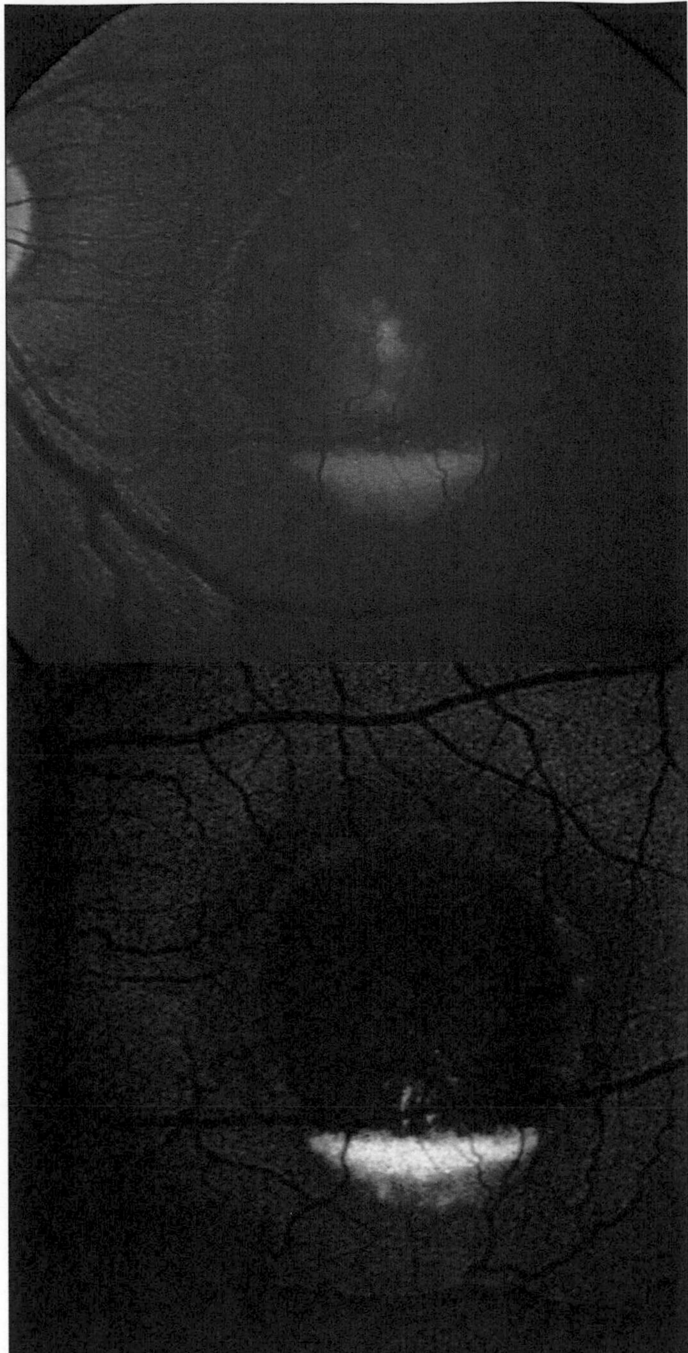

Fig. 4.12 Best macular dystrophy. Vitelliruptive stage. There is prominent increased fundus autofluorescence (FAF) in the lower part of the original vitelliform lesion that is still demarcated by a faint ring of increased FAF. (Reproduced with permission from Ho AC, Brown GC, McNamara JA, et al. Color atlas and synopsis of clinical ophthalmology: Retina. New York: McGraw Hill; 2003.)

Discrete, well-defined lines of increased FAF may occur in various forms of retinal dystrophies.[65–67] These lines have no prominent correlate on fundus biomicroscopy, although there is evidence that these lines precisely reflect the border of the regions of retinal dysfunction.[65,67,68] Despite the variable orientation of this line in different entities, e.g., orientation along the retinal veins in pigmented paravenous chorioretinal atrophy (PPCRA) or as a ring-like structure in retinitis pigmentosa (RP) or macular dystrophies (Fig. 4.15), the similar appearance on FAF images and the concordance of functional findings indicate that these lines in heterogeneous diseases share a common underlying pathophysiological mechanism.[67]

In RP it could be demonstrated that patients with a larger-diameter FAF ring also had larger preserved central visual fields.[65] Furthermore, Robson et al. firstly showed a high correlation between the pattern ERG P50 amplitude – a valuable indicator of macula function – and the size of the abnormal ring. Later, they could demonstrate by fine matrix mapping that photopic sensitivity was preserved over the central macular areas, but there was a gradient of sensitivity loss over high-density segments of the ring and severe threshold elevation outside the arc of the ring. Scotopic sensitivity losses were more severe, and they encroached on areas within the ring.[65]

Popovic et al.[68] confirmed by fundus perimetry, among other methods, that retinal sensitivity was preserved within the ring and was lost outside the ring, regardless of whether the FAF pattern was normal or whether atrophic lesions of the RPE were already present or not. Figure 4.16A shows fundus perimetry in a patient with autosomal dominant RP.

It has been concluded that the ring of increased FAF in RP demarcates areas of preserved central photopic function and that constriction of the ring may mirror progressive visual field loss by advancing dysfunction that encroaches over areas of central macular.[65]

Functional assessment in CRD, CD (cone dystrophy), and macular dystrophies exhibiting a parafoveal ring of increased FAF revealed inverted results compared to RP: Robson et al. could demonstrate that the pattern ERG P50 amplitude was inversely related to the size of the FAF ring; by fine matrix mapping they revealed a gradient of sensitivity loss across the arc of increased FAF.[65]

By fundus perimetry, in patients with macular dystrophy (Fig. 4.16), it could be demonstrated, that within the ring – independent of a normal or abnormal FAF signal – there was severe retinal dysfunction.[67] Outside the ring, the FAF signal and retinal sensitivity were almost normal.

Despite a different orientation of the line in PPCRA, fundus perimetry revealed that photoreceptor dysfunction exceeded the area of RPE cell loss and was precisely delineated (Fig. 4.17). In the central retina and in the periphery that was not circumscribed by the FAF signal line, the FAF signal was normal and photoreceptor sensitivity was preserved. Within the area outlined by increased FAF, independently of whether a normal or abnormal FAF signal was present, there was severe photoreceptor impairment. Despite the variable orientation and morphology of the line, these observations reflect the findings in RP and CD whereby the ring or line of increased FAF represented the border between functional and dysfunctional retinal sensitivity.

Fleckenstein and coworkers[69] first described the SD-OCT correlate of these lines of increased FAF. Specifically, these corresponded with a discrete junctional zone between an area with preserved OCT layers and an area where the outer aspects of the retina are lost and the external limiting membrane band appeared to rest directly on the RPE (Figs 4.18 and 4.19).

More recently, the same SD-OCT correlate has been demonstrated in patients with RP.[70] This junction might be characterized by progressively altered photoreceptor outer and inner segments. While the pathophysiological mechanism is unknown, it may be hypothesized that the increased FAF signal, observed in various retinal dystrophies, might result from an increased metabolic burden of corresponding RPE cells and subsequent

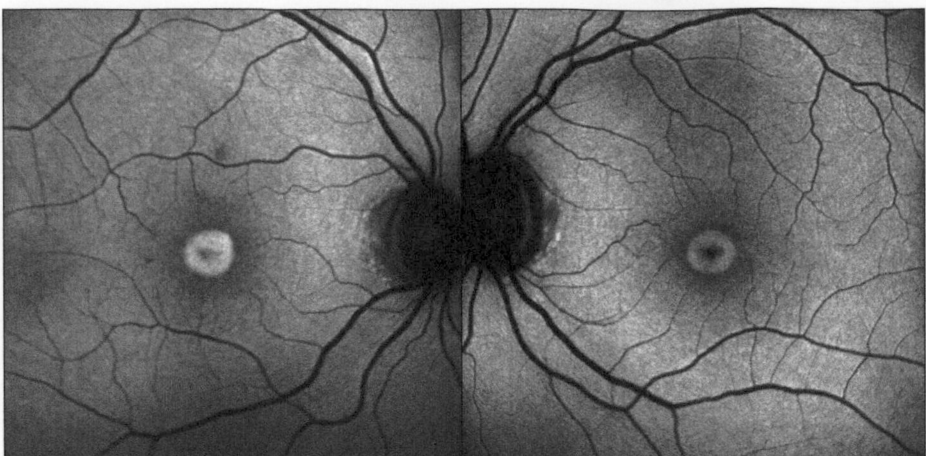

Fig. 4.13 Adult vitelliform macular dystrophy. A sharply demarcated area of increased fundus autofluorescence (FAF) is visible in the macular area. In the center of the lesion there is reduced FAF. (Reproduced with permission from Ho AC, Brown GC, McNamara JA, et al. Color atlas and synopsis of clinical ophthalmology: Retina. New York: McGraw Hill; 2003.)

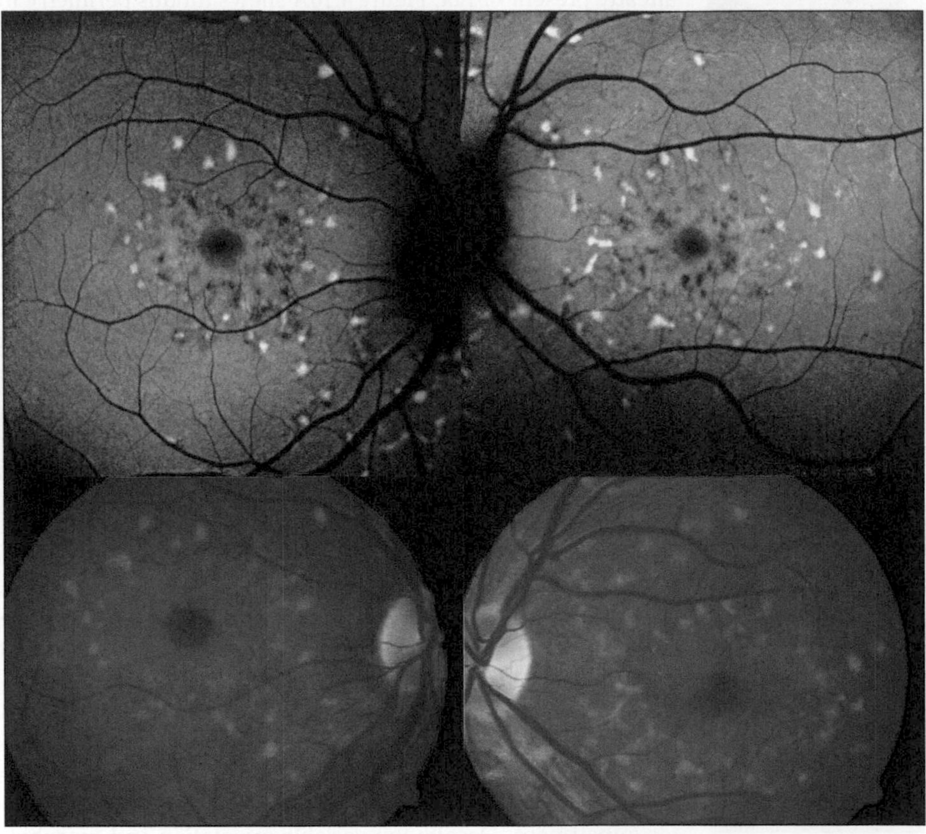

Fig. 4.14 Stargardt macular dystrophy/fundus flavimaculatus. Fundoscopically visible focal flecks show a bright, increased fundus autofluorescence (FAF) signal. Focal areas of decreased FAF seem to correspond with retinal pigment epithelial atrophy. (Reproduced with permission from Ho AC, Brown GC, McNamara JA, et al. Color atlas and synopsis of clinical ophthalmology: Retina. New York: McGraw Hill; 2003.)

excessive accumulation of fluorophores in the lysosomal compartment due to phagocytosis of components of severely altered photoreceptors in such junctional zones. Changes in absorbtion of the FAF signal due to loss of photoreceptor outer segments may also contribute to this phenomenon. In the zone with a normal FAF signal but impaired retinal sensitivity, the structure of the photoreceptors seems to be severely distorted. A normal FAF signal, therefore, does not necessarily reflect an intact photoreceptor–RPE complex, but may rather correspond to a structurally intact-appearing RPE cell monolayer with or without the presence of intact photoreceptors.

Macular telangiectasia

Macular telangiectasia (MacTel) type 2 is a bilateral disease of unknown cause with characteristic alterations of the macular capillary network and progressive retinal cell death.[71–73] The disease typically manifests temporal to the fovea, and may later encompass an oval-shaped area centered on the foveola.

As outlined above, normal eyes show masking of the foveal 488-nm blue-light FAF due to the accumulation of luteal pigment. Reduced macular pigment density in MacTel type 2 affects this masking. Eyes with MacTel type 2 show an abnormally increased signal in the macular area to a variable degree with blue-light FAF imaging (Figs 4.20 and 4.21).[74] A loss of luteal pigment may initially occur in the area temporal to the foveal center (Fig. 4.22).[74,75] Quantitative analysis confirmed that the loss of luteal pigment was more pronounced in the temporal compared with the nasal parafoveolar area and suggested that zeaxanthin would be more reduced than lutein.[75]

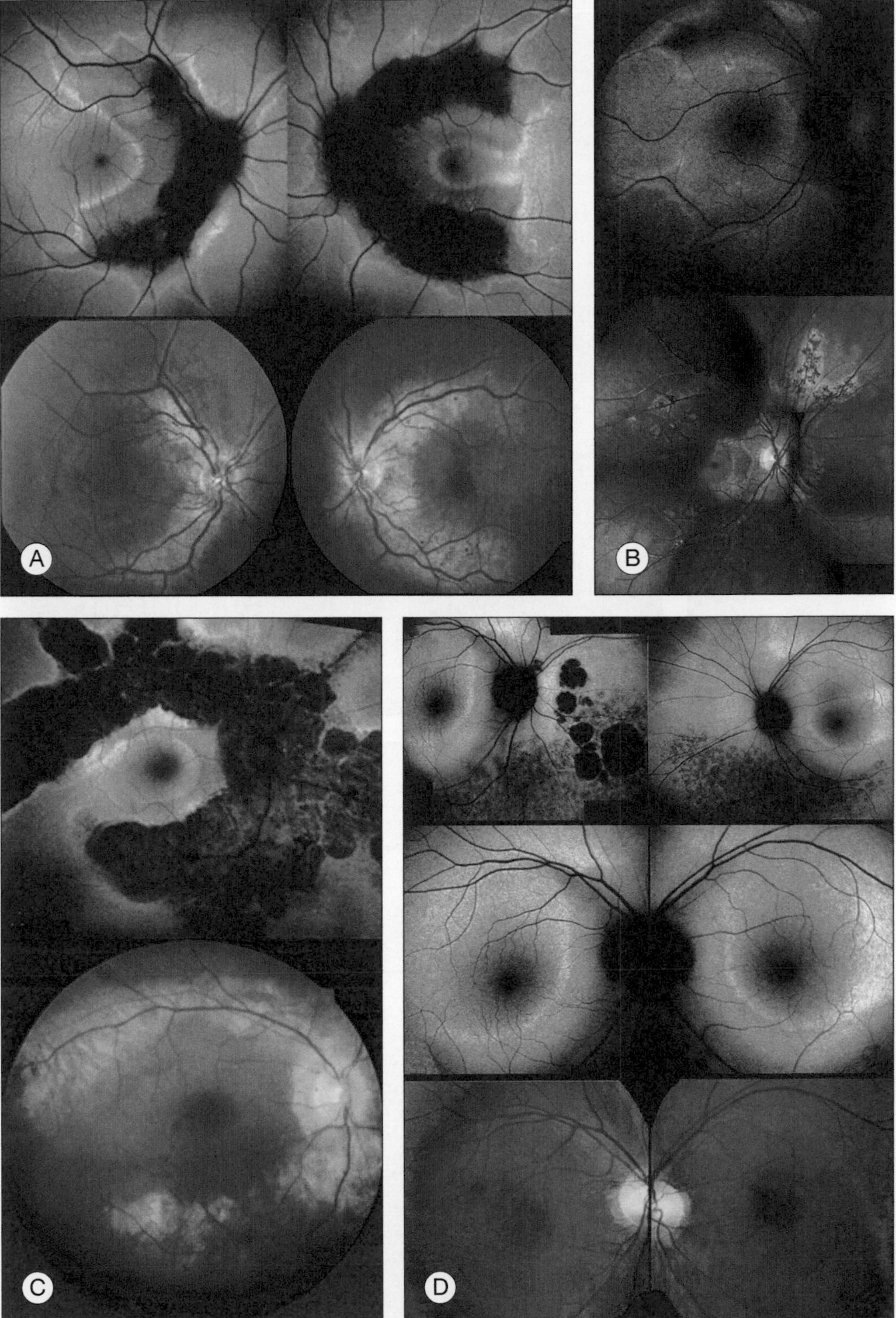

Fig. 4.15 Arcs and rings of increased fundus autofluorescence (FAF) in patients with various forms of retinal dystrophies. Patients 1–3 (A–C), diagnosed with pigmented paravenous chorioretinal atrophy, demonstrates an arc of increased FAF orienting along the retinal veins. There is a normal FAF signal between this arc and the atrophic areas (i.e., decreased FAF) and in the area that is not circumscribed by the line. In the left eye of patient 1 (A) and the right eye of patient 3 (C), the arc of increased FAF almost merges to a parafoveal ring with a temporal opening. In patient 4 (D) with sector retinitis pigmentosa, there is an arc with a semicircular configuration in the parafoveal region.

Continued

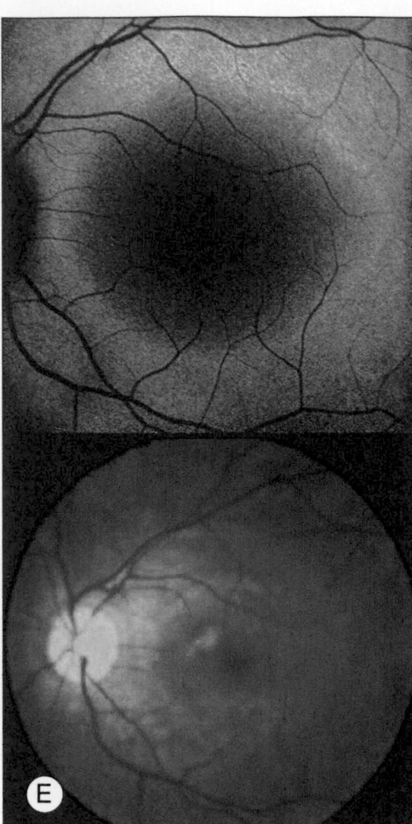

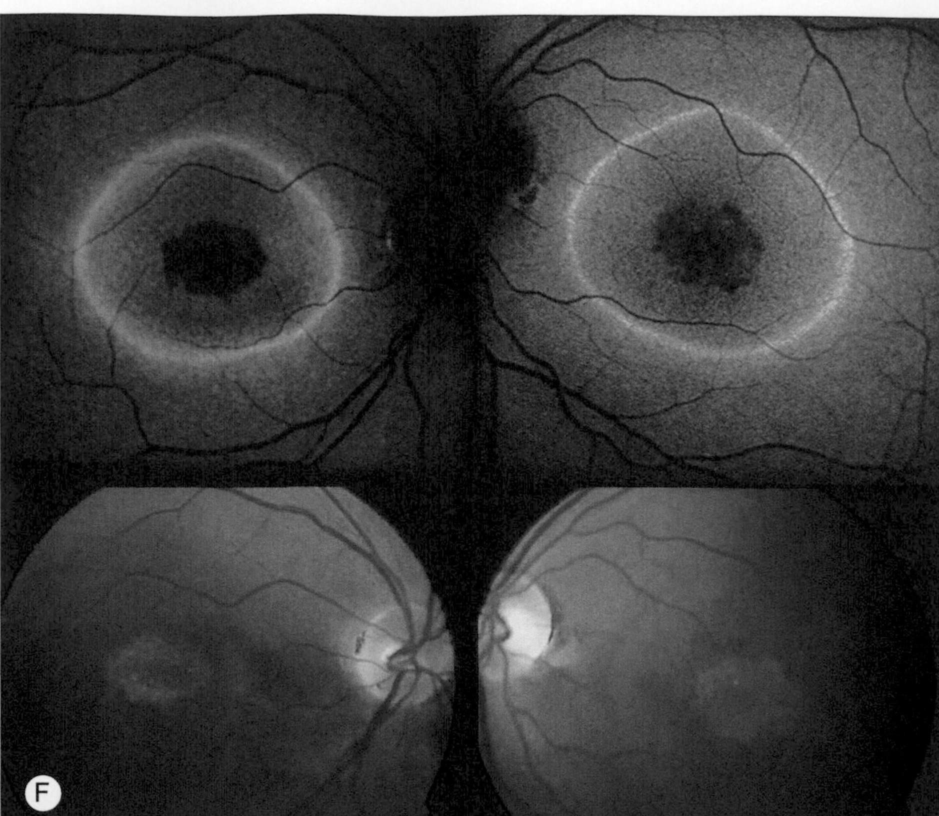

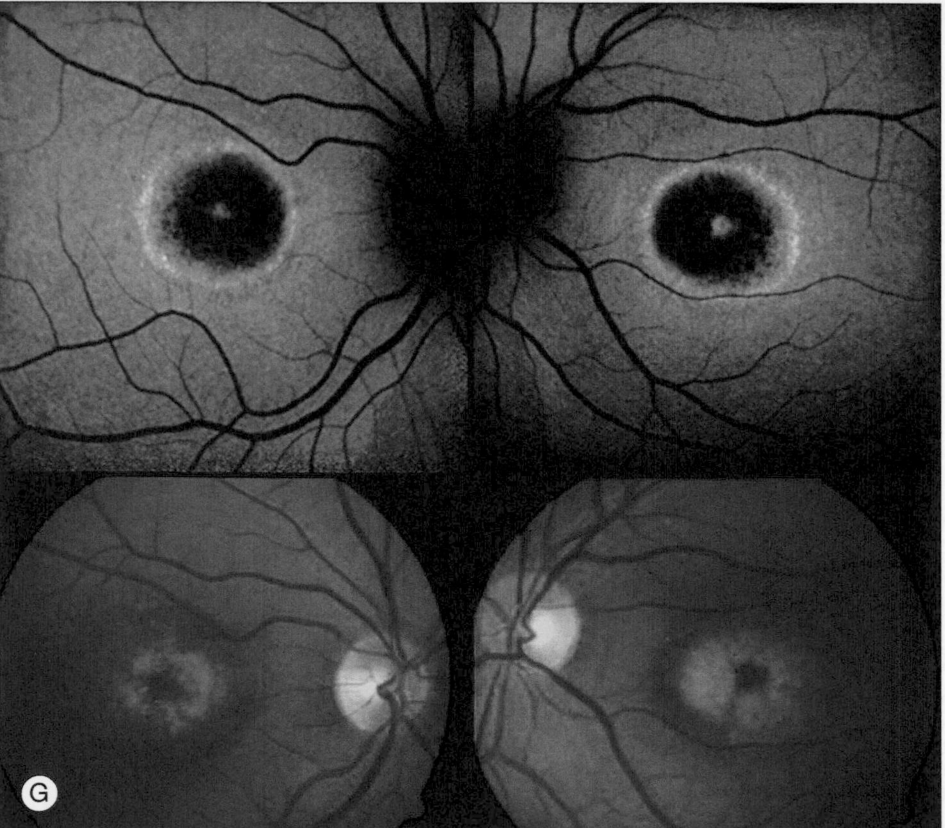

Fig. 4.15 Cont'd In typical retinitis pigmentosa (patient 5, E), there is a ring of increased FAF. Within and outside the ring, there is a normal FAF signal. In patient 6 (F), who is diagnosed with macular dystrophy, there is a parafoveal ring of increased FAF. Centrally, there is reduced FAF corresponding to the fundoscopically visible lesion. On both sides of the ring, there is a normal FAF signal. In patient 7 (G) with another bull's-eye macular dystrophy, a ring of increased FAF directly borders the central lesion. In the very center, there is a spot of preserved FAF. Note that there is no significant correlate of the arc of increased FAF in the conventional color fundus photograph. (Reproduced with permission from Fleckenstein M, Charbel Issa P, Fuchs HA, et al. Discrete arcs of increased fundus autofluorescence in retinal dystrophies and functional correlate on microperimetry. Eye (Lond) 2009;23:567–75.)

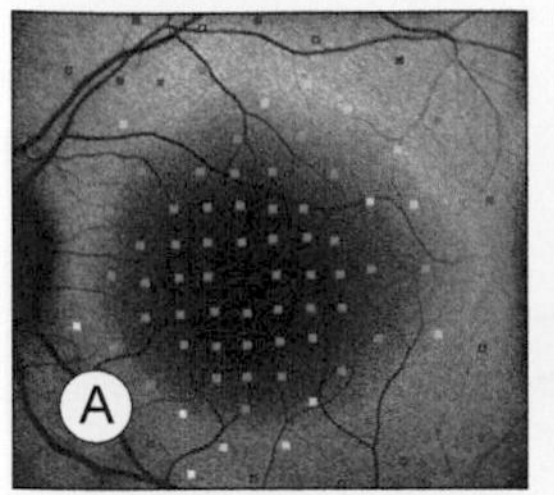

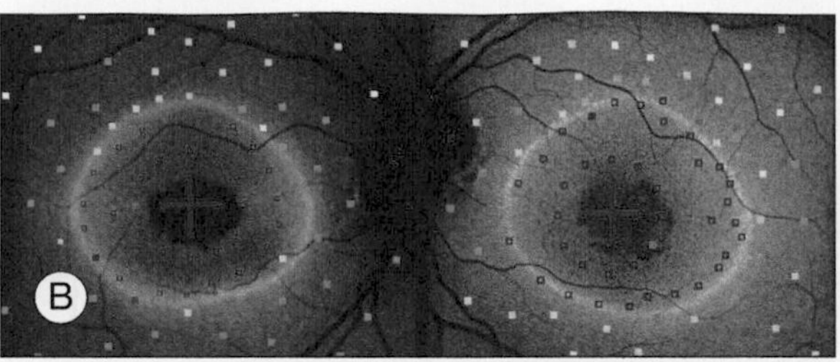

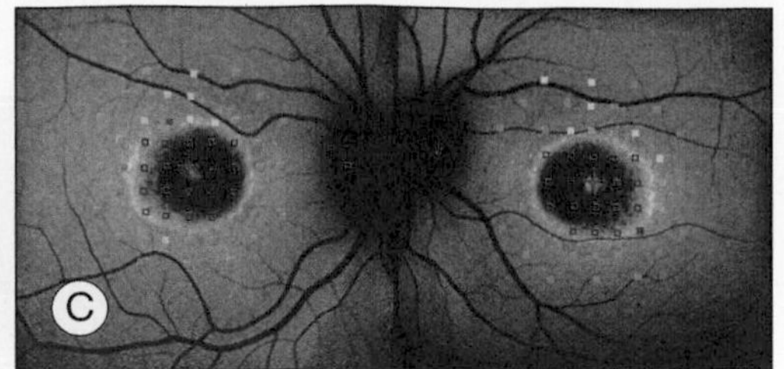

Fig. 4.16 Fundus-controlled microperimetric assessment of rings of increased fundus autofluorescence (FAF). The sensitivity map is superimposed on the FAF image. Light increment sensitivity (LIS) varies from 0 to 20 dB (attenuation scale). Hollow red squares indicate testing points where the brightest stimulus was not seen. (A) In the patient with autosomal dominant retinitis pigmentosa, LIS is preserved within the ring; outside, there is severely impaired LIS despite a normal FAF signal. In patients with macular dystrophy exhibiting a ring of increased FAF (B, C), LIS is significantly impaired within the ring independently of a normal or decreased FAF signal; outside, LIS is preserved. These findings are the inverse of the findings in patients diagnosed with retinitis pigmentosa (A). (Reproduced with permission from Fleckenstein M, Charbel Issa P, Fuchs HA, et al. Discrete arcs of increased fundus autofluorescence in retinal dystrophies and functional correlate on microperimetry. Eye (Lond) 2009;23:567–75.)

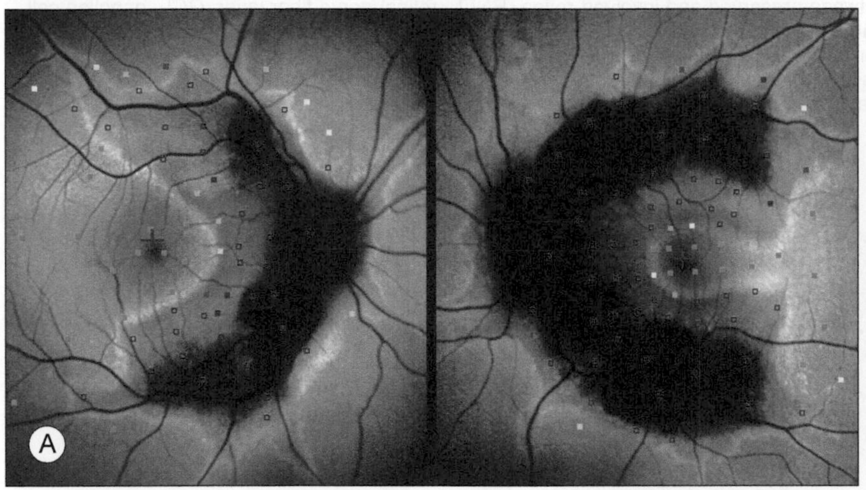

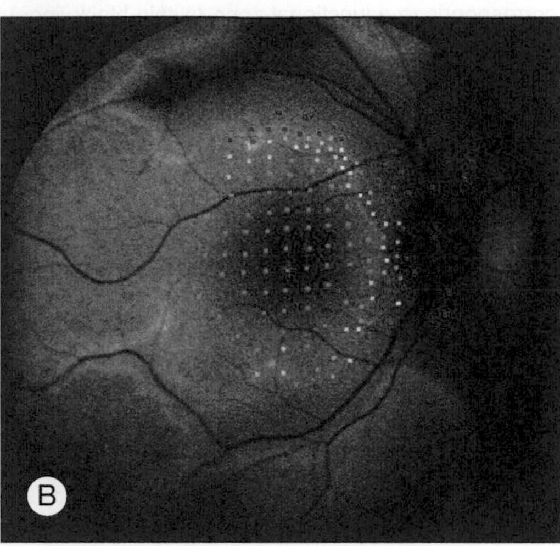

Fig. 4.17 Fundus-controlled microperimetric assessment in pigmented paravenous chorioretinal atrophy. The sensitivity map is superimposed on the fundus autofluorescence (FAF) image. Light increment sensitivity (LIS) varies from 0 to 20 dB (attenuation scale). Hollow red squares indicate testing points where the brightest stimulus was not seen. In the area that is framed by the arc of increased FAF, LIS is severely impaired independently of a normal or abnormal FAF signal. The arc of increased FAF demarcates the area of preserved LIS. (Reproduced with permission from Fleckenstein M, Charbel Issa P, Fuchs HA, et al. Discrete arcs of increased fundus autofluorescence in retinal dystrophies and functional correlate on microperimetry. Eye (Lond) 2009;23:567–75.)

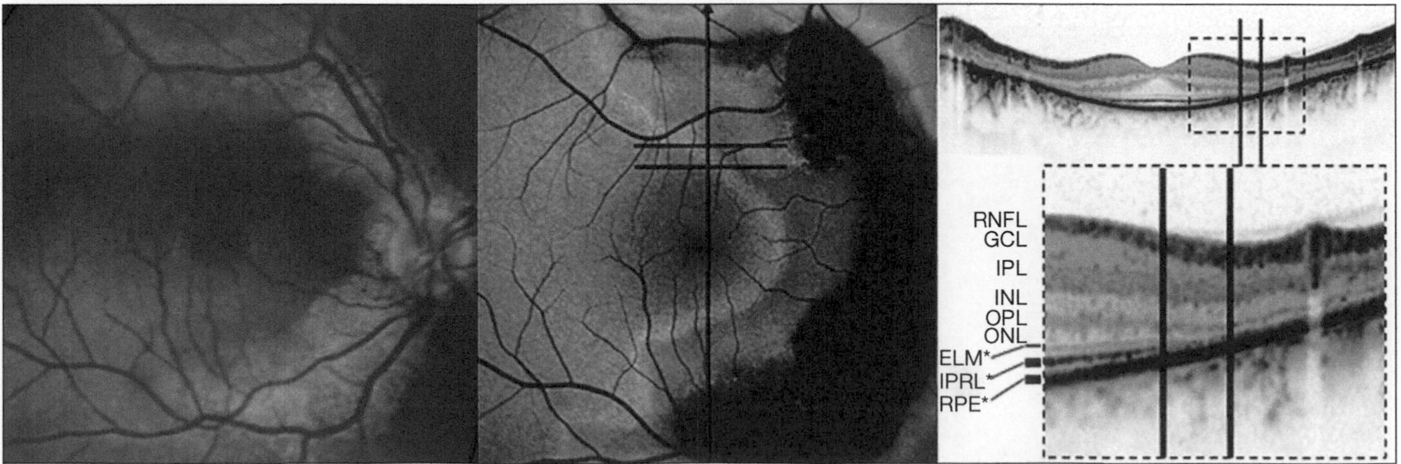

Fig. 4.18 Simultaneous fundus autofluorescence (FAF) and spectral domain-optical coherence tomography imaging. The line of increased FAF corresponds to a junctional zone (within black lines) between involved and preserved retina. RNFL, retinal nerve fiber layer; GCL, ganglion cell layer; IPL, inner plexiform layer; INL, inner nuclear layer; OPL, outer plexiform layer; ONL, outer nuclear layer; ELM*, presumed correspondence of the external limiting membrane; IPRL*, presumed correspondence of the interface of the inner/outer segments of photoreceptors; RPE*, presumed correspondence of the retinal pigment epithelium. (Reproduced with permission from Fleckenstein M, Charbel Issa P, Helb HM, et al. Correlation of lines of increased autofluorescence in macular dystrophy and pigmented paravenous retinochoroidal atrophy by optical coherence tomography. Arch Ophthalmol 2008;126:1461–3.)

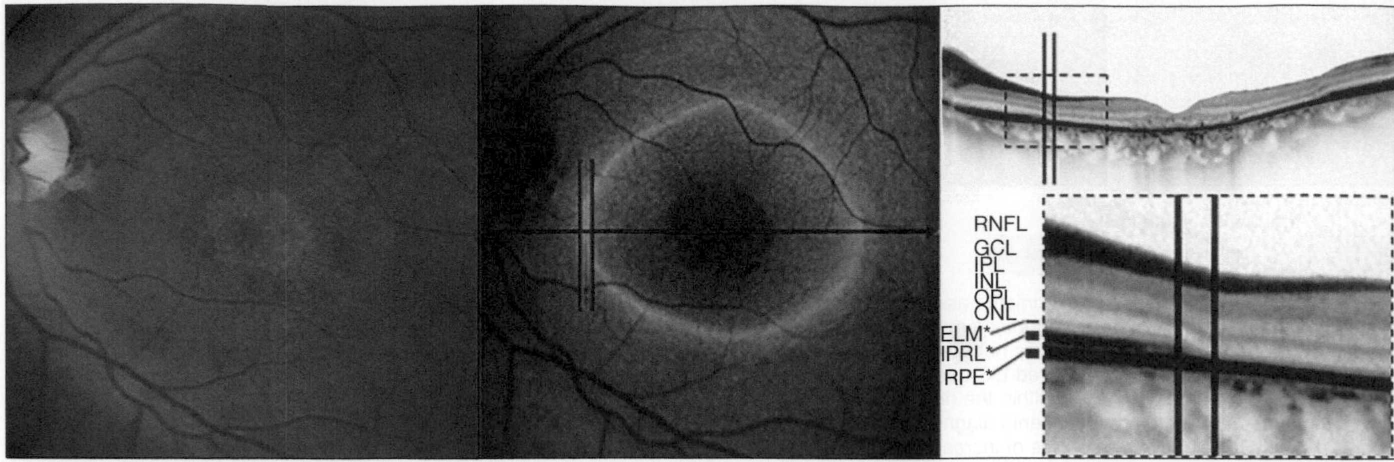

Fig. 4.19 Simultaneous fundus autofluorescence (FAF) and spectral domain optical coherence tomography imaging. The line of increased FAF corresponds to a junctional zone (within black lines) between preserved and involved retina. RNFL, retinal nerve fiber layer; GCL, ganglion cell layer; IPL, inner plexiform layer; INL, inner nuclear layer; OPL, outer plexiform layer; ONL, outer nuclear layer; ELM*, presumed correspondence of the external limiting membrane; IPRL*, presumed correspondence of the interface of the inner/outer segments of photoreceptors; RPE*, presumed correspondence of the retinal pigment epithelium. (Reproduced with permission from Fleckenstein M, Charbel Issa P, Helb HM, et al. Correlation of lines of increased autofluorescence in macular dystrophy and pigmented paravenous retinochoroidal atrophy by optical coherence tomography. Arch Ophthalmol 2008;126:1461–3.)

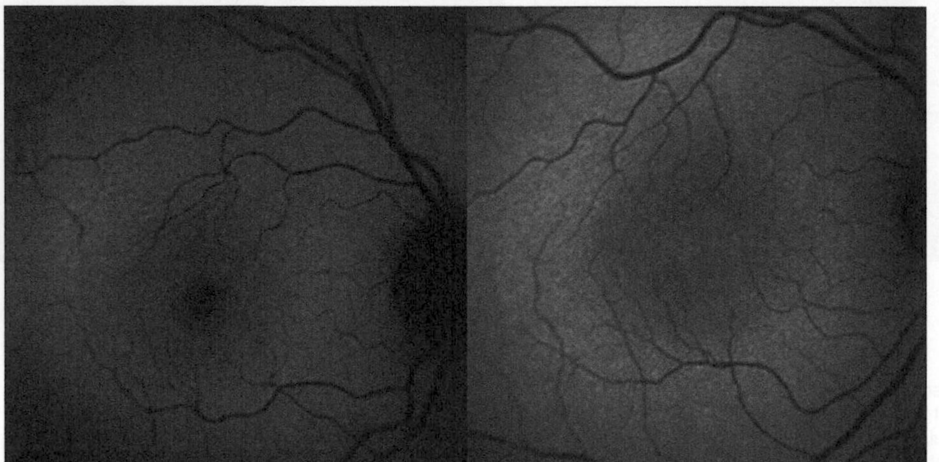

Fig. 4.20 Fundus autofluorescence image obtained at 488 nm (excitation) of a normal eye (left) and of a 59-year-old woman with type 2 idiopathic macular telangiectasis (right). (Reproduced with permission from Helb HM, Charbel Issa P, van der Veen RLP, et al. Macular pigment density and distribution in patients with type II macular telangiectasia. Retina 2008;28:808–16.)

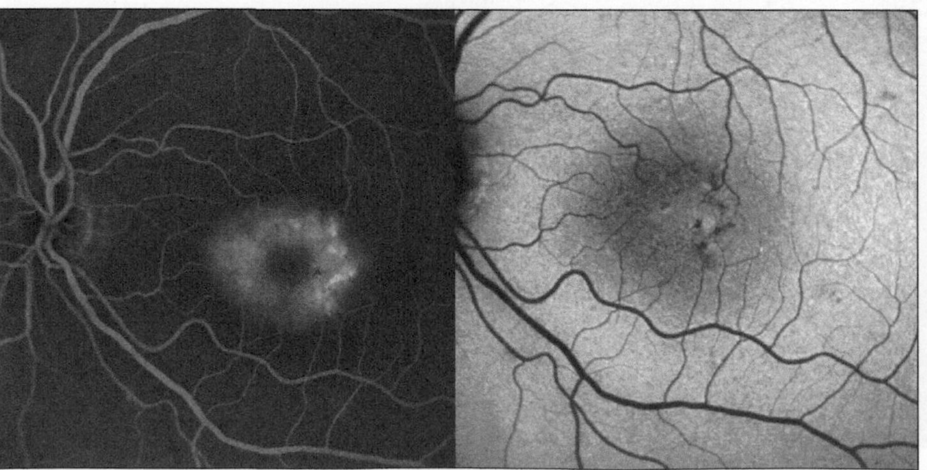

Fig. 4.21 Fluorescein angiogram frame (left) and fundus autofluorescence (FAF) image obtained at 488 nm (right) of a patient with type 2 idiopathic macular telangiectasia showing an abnormal FAF distribution in the macular area due to depletion of luteal pigment. (Reproduced with permission from Helb HM, Charbel Issa P, van der Veen RLP, et al. Macular pigment density and distribution in patients with type II macular telangiectasia. Retina 2008;28:808–16.)

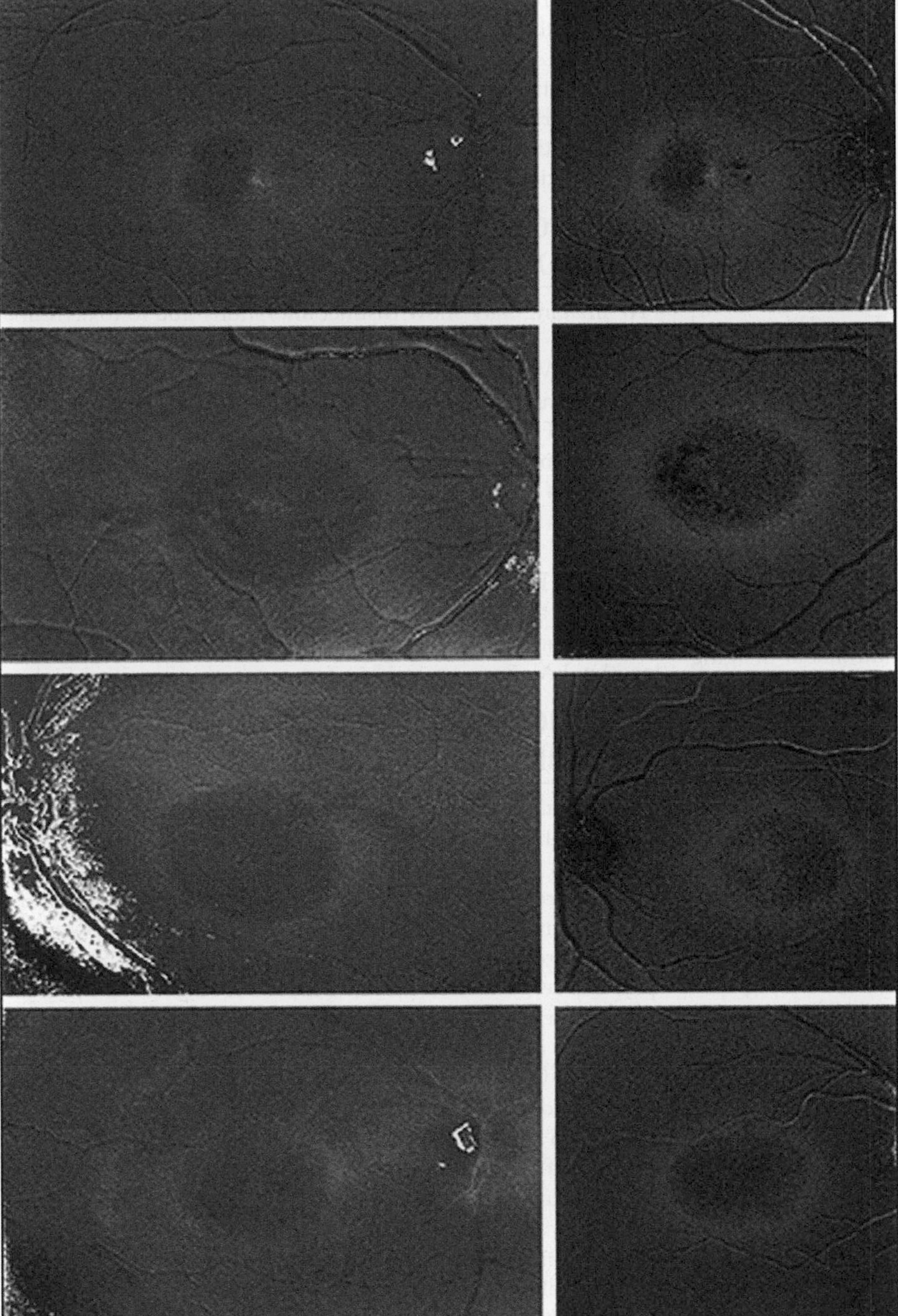

Fig. 4.22 Macular pigment optical density (MPOD) maps obtained by digital subtraction of log fundus reflectance maps (left column) compared with corresponding fundus autofluorescence maps (right column). The independent measurement techniques demonstrated the same rings of MPOD at 5–7° eccentricity. (Reproduced with permission from Helb HM, Charbel Issa P, van der Veen RLP, et al. Macular pigment density and distribution in patients with type II macular telangiectasia. Retina 2008;28:808–16.)

Further proof for the depletion in macular pigment derived from a postmortem analysis of an eye with MacTel type 2. Macroscopic examination disclosed the absence of the central yellowish spot.[76] A yellow ring of residual macular pigment was present eccentrically in accordance with the in vivo imaging observations. The loss of macular pigment was subsequently divided into three classes based on a cross-sectional analysis of two-wavelength (blue-light and green-light) FAF images[77]: Class 1 shows a wedge-shaped loss of macular pigment restricted to an area temporal to the foveal center. In class 2, the area is larger and also involves the foveal center. Class 3 is characterized by loss of luteal pigment within an oval-shaped area centered on the foveola. There was a significant association of these three classes of macular pigment loss with the consecutive disease stages of MacTel type 2 described by Gass and Blodi.[71] Correlation studies with microperimetric data revealed a trend towards worse retinal function with increasing class of macular pigment changes.

Pseudoxanthoma elasticum

Pseudoxanthoma elasticum (PXE) is caused by a mutation in the *ABCC6* gene. More than 300 distinct loss-of-function mutations representative of over 1000 mutant alleles in *ABCC6* have been found. Many of the missense mutations occur at locations in the protein involving domain–domain interactions in the *ABCC6* transporter. Even heterozygotes can show manifestations of disease. FAF abnormalities are common in eyes affected by PXE. Typical phenotypic alterations, including angioid streak, and drusen of the optic nerve, have autofluorescence correlates. Peau d'orange is hardly detectable on FAF, whereas comet-tail lesions are typically apparent. RPE atrophy can be widespread and heterogeneous, located mostly adjacent to angioid streaks or CNV.[78,79]

Furthermore, irregular patterns of increased FAF at the posterior pole with an appearance similar to that of pattern dystrophies can be found in eyes with PXE. In these eyes, areas of yellowish deposits and hyperpigmentation on color photography corresponded to areas of increased FAF (Fig. 4.23). Agarwal et al.[80] suggested the following classification: a fundus appearance similar to a pattern dystrophy of the fundus flavimaculatus, the reticular, the vitelliform and the fundus pulverulentus types, respectively. The pattern dystrophy-like changes in PXE may occur unilaterally or bilaterally.

Abnormalities of the RPE–photoreceptor complex detected by FAF imaging are more diverse and widespread than expected from conventional fundus imaging. Such extensive alteration of the RPE suggests an important role of pathological RPE changes in the evolution of visual loss in PXE.

Recently, the abnormalities detected by multimodal imaging suggest a centrifugal spread of the retinal pathologic features of the Bruch's membrane–RPE complex in PXE. These results suggest that three different areas centered on the posterior pole can be defined in the fundus of patients with PXE. These areas are separated by two consecutive transition zones. The central two areas may indicate different stages of pathologic fundus alterations.[81]

Central serous chorioretinopathy

Central serous chorioretinopathy is a condition characterized by idiopathic leaks at the level of the RPE leading to serous pigment epithelial and neurosensory retinal detachments. In the early phases of the disease, the visual acuity may be good despite the presence of the macular detachment, and after resolution the acuity often shows improvement. More chronic forms of central serous chorioretinopathy are associated with atrophic and degenerative changes of the retina and RPE and consequently with visual acuity decline.[82]

Accordingly, FAF findings in central serous chorioretinopathy are dependent on the extent of involvement of the RPE and the stage of the disease.[83] Patients with acute leaks imaged within the first month have minimal abnormalities other than a slight increase in autofluorescence in the area of the serous retinal detachment. Over time, the area of the detachment increasingly exhibits more irregular increased autofluorescence. In some patients, discrete granules with increased intensity within the detachment are observed which correspond with the pinpoint subretinal precipitates seen on fundoscopy. It has been suggested that these dots may represent macrophages engorged with phagocytosed outer segments. Patients with chronic disease have irregular levels of autofluorescence with markedly decreased intensity over areas of atrophy. A typical finding also includes the visualization of fluid tracks in the inferior retina (Fig. 4.24). The area of the leak also undergoes change in autofluorescence over time. Soon after the development of central serous chorioretinopathy, little or no change in the autofluorescence pattern in the area around the leak is seen, although the leak site may be somewhat hypoautofluorescent. Patients with more chronic leaks can have decreased autofluorescence surrounding the known leaks. This area of hypoautofluorescence appears to expand in size with increasing chronicity of the leak. Patients who were known to have a history of chronic central serous chorioretinopathy that had been inactive for several years are left with hypoautofluorescent areas and no hyperautofluorescent regions.

CHLOROQUINE AND HYDROXYCHLOROQUINE RETINOPATHY

FAF imaging may show distinct alterations due to toxic retinal effects of long-term chloroquine and hydroxychloroquine therapy.[84] Various methods have been proposed to detect early stages of chloroquine retinopathy. Early on, a pericentral ring of increased FAF intensity may occur associated with pericentral reduction in multifocal ERG amplitudes and pericentral interruption of the photoreceptor inner-segment–outer-segment junction on SD-OCT imaging.[85] More advanced stages are associated with a more mottled appearance with increased and decreased FAF intensity in the pericentral macula (Fig. 4.25). While electrophysiological examination has been thought to represent an adequate tool to diagnose early chloroquine maculopathy, FAF imaging can be used as a highly sensitive tool.

FUNCTIONAL CORRELATES OF FAF ABNORMALITIES

The relevance of alterations in FAF images can further be addressed by assessing corresponding retinal sensitivity. Severe damage to the RPE such as atrophy, melanin pigment migration, or fibrosis leading to compromised photoreceptor function are confirmed by microperimetry to correspond topographically to areas of decreased autofluorescence.[53,54] In patients with GA secondary to AMD, it has been shown that, in addition to absence of retinal sensitivity over atrophic areas, retinal function is relatively and significantly reduced over areas with increased FAF intensities compared to areas with normal background signal.[54] Localized functional impairment over areas with increased FAF has also been recently confirmed in patients with early AMD. Using fine matrix mapping, it has been demonstrated that, interestingly, rod function is more severely affected than cone function over areas with increased FAF in patients with AMD.[53] These studies are in accordance with the observation of increased accumulation of autofluorescent material at the level of the RPE prior to the occurrence of cell death. As normal photoreceptor function is dependent on normal RPE function, in particular with regard to the constant phagocytosis of shed distal outer-segment stacks for photoreceptor cell renewal, a negative-feedback mechanism has been proposed, whereby cells with LF-loaded secondary lysosomes would less efficiently phagocytose newly shed photoreceptor outer segments, subsequently leading to impaired retinal sensitivity. This would also be in line with experimental data showing that compounds of LF, such as A2-E, possess toxic properties and may interfere with normal RPE cell function.[10]

In patients with different retinal dystrophies, lines and rings of increased FAF have been noted (see above).[65] Interestingly, functional testing by microperimetry and electrophysiology indicates that these rings circumscribe areas of preserved photoreceptor function (Fig. 4.16A).[65,67,68]

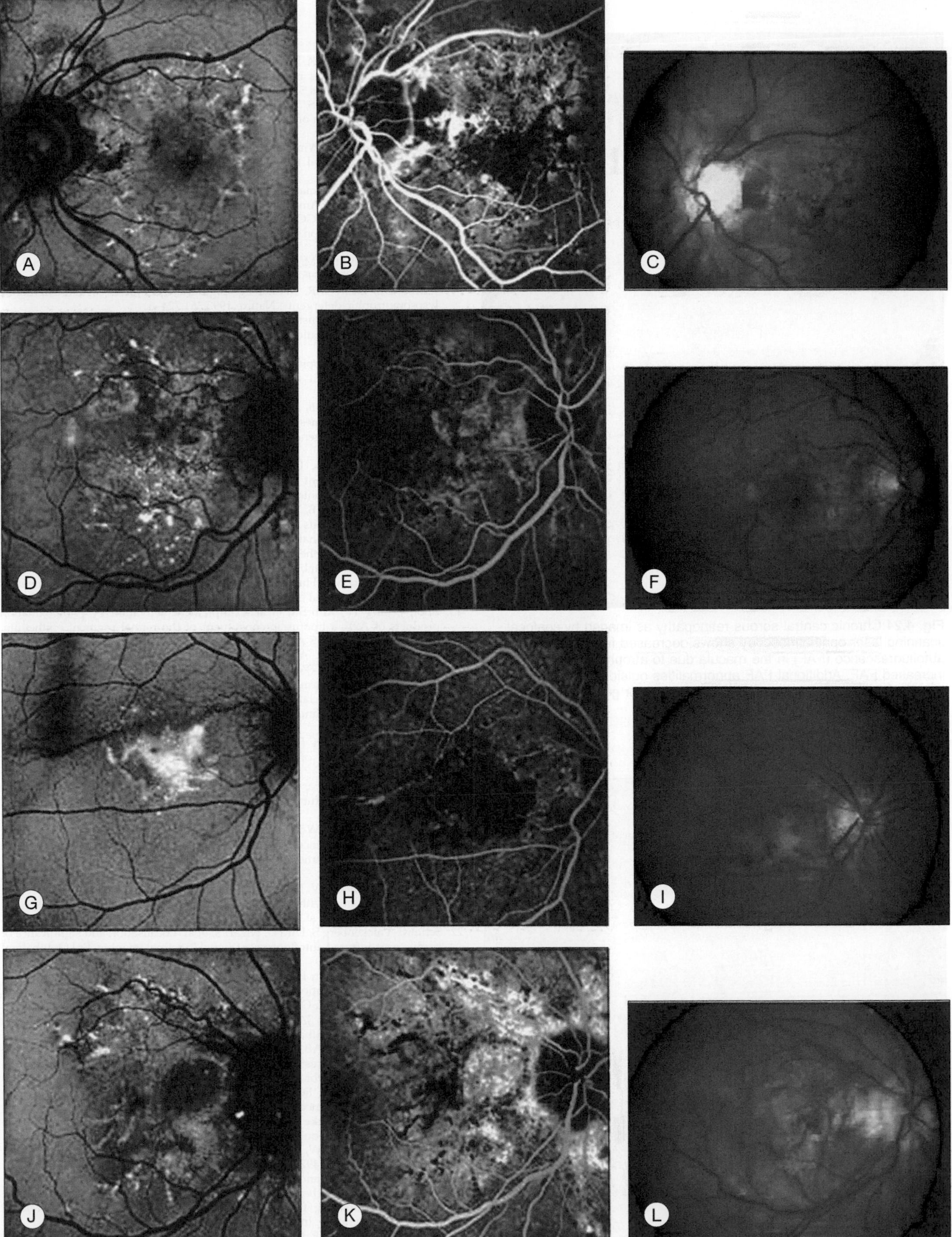

Fig. 4.23 Various types of retinal pigment epithelium degenerative patterns of the macula observed in pseudoxanthoma elasticum (first column: fundus autofluorescence; second column: fluorescein angiography; third column: color fundus photograph). (A–C) Fundus changes resembling reticular dystrophy; (D–F) fundus changes resembling fundus flavimaculatus; (G–I) fundus changes resembling vitelliform dystrophy; (J–L) fundus changes resembling fundus pulverulentus. (Reproduced with permission from Finger RP, Charbel Issa P, Ladewig M, et al. Fundus autofluorescence in pseudoxanthoma elasticum. Retina 2009;29:1496–505.)

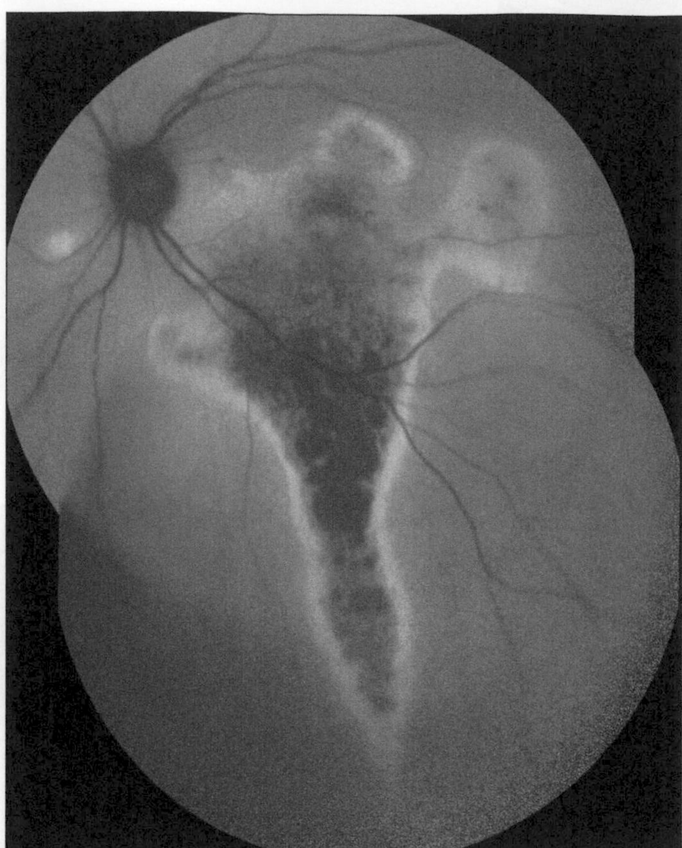

Fig. 4.24 Chronic central serous retinopathy as imaged by confocal scanning laser ophthalmoscopy shows decreased fundus autofluorescence (FAF) in the macula due to atrophy with surrounding increased FAF. Additional FAF abnormalities outside the central macula, including prominent descending tracts or gutters, are also observed.

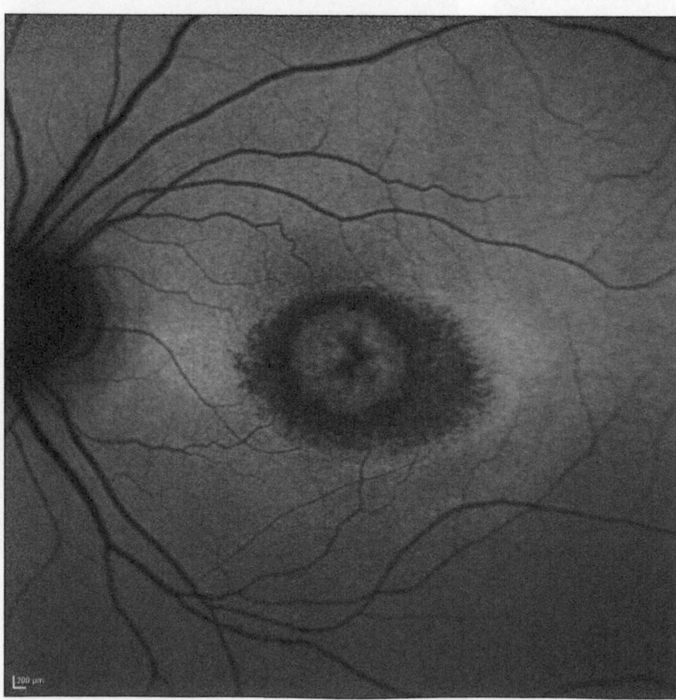

Fig. 4.25 Advanced stage of chloroquine retinopathy. There is a mottled appearance with increased and decreased fundus autofluorescence intensity in the pericentral macula.

REFERENCES

1. Delori FC, Dorey CK, Staurenghi G, et al. In vivo fluorescence of the ocular fundus exhibits retinal pigment epithelium lipofuscin characteristics. Invest Ophthalmol Vis Sci 1995;36:718–29.
2. Schmitz-Valckenberg S, Fleckenstein M, Scholl HP, et al. Fundus autofluorescence and progression of age-related macular degeneration. Surv Ophthalmol 2009;54:96–117.
3. Weiter JJ, Delori FC, Wing GL, et al. Retinal pigment epithelial lipofuscin and melanin and choroidal melanin in human eyes. Invest Ophthalmol Vis Sci 1986;27:145–52.
4. Feeney-Burns L, Berman ER, Rothmann H. Lipofuscin of human retinal pigment epithelium. Am J Ophthalmol 1980;90:783–91.
5. Wing GL, Blanchard GC, Weiter JJ. The topography and age relationship of lipofuscin concentration in the retinal pigment epithelium. Invest Ophthalmol Vis Sci 1978;17:601–7.
6. Sparrow JR, Boulton M. RPE lipofuscin and its role in retinal pathobiology. Exp Eye Res 2005;80:595–606.
7. Eldred GE, Lasky MR. Retinal age-pigments generated by self-assembling lysosomotrophic detergents. Nature 1993;361:724–6.
8. Dorey CK, Wu G, Ebenstein D, et al. Cell loss in the aging retina. Relationship to lipofuscin accumulation and macular degeneration. Invest Ophthalmol Vis Sci 1989;30:1691–9.
9. Schütt F, Davies S, Kopitz J, et al. Photodamage to human RPE cells by A2-E, a retinoid component of lipofuscin. Invest Ophthalmol Vis Sci 2000;41: 2303–8.
10. Bergmann M, Schutt F, Holz FG, et al. Inhibition of the ATP-driven proton pump in RPE lysosomes by the major lipofuscin fluorophore A2-E may contribute to the pathogenesis of age-related macular degeneration. FASEB J 2004;18:562–4.
11. Brunk UT, Wihlmark U, Wrigstad A, et al. Accumulation of lipofuscin within retinal pigment epithelial cells results in enhanced sensitivity to photo-oxidation. Gerontology 1995;41(Suppl 2):201–12.
12. Hammer M, Richter S, Guehrs KH, et al. Retinal pigment epithelium cell damage by A2-E and its photo-derivatives. Mol Vis 2006;12:1348–54.
13. Liu J, Itagaki Y, Ben-Shabat S, et al. The biosynthesis of A2E, a fluorophore of aging retina, involves the formation of the precursor, A2-PE, in the photoreceptor outer segment membrane. J Biol Chem 2000;275:29354–60.
14. Eldred GE, Katz ML. Fluorophores of the human retinal pigment epithelium: separation and spectral characterization. Exp Eye Res 1988;47:71–86.
15. Zhou J, Jang YP, Kim SR, et al. Complement activation by photooxidation products of A2E, a lipofuscin constituent of the retinal pigment epithelium. Proc Natl Acad Sci U S A 2006;103:16182–7.
16. Lamb LE, Simon JD. A2E: a component of ocular lipofuscin. Photochem Photobiol 2004;79:127–36.
17. Marmorstein AD, Marmorstein LY, Sakaguchi H, et al. Spectral profiling of autofluorescence associated with lipofuscin, Bruch's membrane, and sub-RPE deposits in normal and AMD eyes. Invest Ophthalmol Vis Sci 2002;43: 2435–41.
18. Keilhauer CN, Delori FC. Near-infrared autofluorescence imaging of the fundus: visualization of ocular melanin. Invest Ophthalmol Vis Sci 2006; 47:3556–64.
19. Weinberger AW, Lappas A, Kirschkamp T, et al. Fundus near infrared fluorescence correlates with fundus near infrared reflectance. Invest Ophthalmol Vis Sci 2006;47:3098–108.
20. Kellner U, Kellner S, Weinitz S. Fundus autofluorescence (488 nm) and near-infrared autofluorescence (787 nm) visualize different retinal pigment epithelium alterations in patients with age-related macular degeneration. Retina 2010;30:6–15.
21. Gibbs D, Cideciyan AV, Jacobson SG, et al. Retinal pigment epithelium defects in humans and mice with mutations in MYO7A: imaging melanosome-specific autofluorescence. Invest Ophthalmol Vis Sci 2009;50:4386–93.
22. Schmitz-Valckenberg S, Lara D, Nizari S, et al. Localisation and significance of in vivo near-infrared autofluorescent signal in retinal imaging. Br J Ophthalmol 2011;95:1134–9.
23. Snodderly DM, Brown PK, Delori FC, et al. The macular pigment. I. Absorbance spectra, localization, and discrimination from other yellow pigments in primate retinas. Invest Ophthalmol Vis Sci 1984;25:660–73.
24. Whitehead AJ, Mares JA, Danis RP. Macular pigment: a review of current knowledge. Arch Ophthalmol 2006;124:1038–45.
25. Davies NP, Morland AB. Macular pigments: their characteristics and putative role. Prog Retin Eye Res 2004;23:533–59.
26. Wolf S, Wolf-Schnurrbusch U. Macular pigment measurement – theoretical background. In: Holz FG, Schmitz-Valckenberg S, Spaide RF, et al. editors. Atlas of autofluorescence imaging. Berlin: Springer; 2007.
27. von Rückmann A, Fitzke FW, Bird AC. Distribution of fundus autofluorescence with a scanning laser ophthalmoscope. Br J Ophthalmol 1995;79:407–12.
28. Webb RH, Hughes GW, Delori FC. Confocal scanning laser ophthalmoscope. Appl Optics 1987;26:1492–9.
29. American National Standard for the Safe Use of Lasers Z136.1; 1993.
30. Fleckenstein M, Charbel Issa P, Helb HM, et al. High-resolution spectral domain-OCT imaging in geographic atrophy associated with age-related macular degeneration. Invest Ophthalmol Vis Sci 2008;49:4137–44.
31. Delori FC, Fleckner MR, Goger DG, et al. Autofluorescence distribution associated with drusen in age-related macular degeneration. Invest Ophthalmol Vis Sci 2000;41:496–504.
32. Spaide RF. Fundus autofluorescence and age-related macular degeneration. Ophthalmology 2003;110:392–9.

33. Spaide RF. Autofluorescence Imaging with the fundus camera. In: Holz FG, Schmitz-Valckenberg S, Spaide RF, et al, editors. Atlas of autofluorescence imaging. Berlin: Springer; 2007. p. 49–53.
34. Schmitz-Valckenberg S, Fleckenstein M, Gobel AP, et al. Evaluation of autofluorescence imaging with the scanning laser ophthalmoscope and the fundus camera in age-related geographic atrophy. Am J Ophthalmol 2008;146: 183–92.
35. Lois N, Halfyard AS, Bunce C, et al. Reproducibility of fundus autofluorescence measurements obtained using a confocal scanning laser ophthalmoscope. Br J Ophthalmol 1999;83:276–9.
36. Delori F, Greenberg JP, Woods RL, et al. Quantitative measurements of autofluorescence with the scanning laser ophthalmoscope. Invest Ophthalmol Vis Sci 2011;52:9379–90.
37. Bird A. Age-related macular disease. Br J Ophthalmol 1996;80:2–3.
38. Smith RT, Chan JK, Busuoic M, et al. Autofluorescence characteristics of early, atrophic, and high-risk fellow eyes in age-related macular degeneration. Invest Ophthalmol Vis Sci 2006;47:5495–504.
39. Lois N, Owens SL, Coco R, et al. Fundus autofluorescence in patients with age-related macular degeneration and high risk of visual loss. Am J Ophthalmol 2002;133:341–9.
40. Bindewald A, Bird AC, Dandekar SS, et al. Classification of fundus autofluorescence patterns in early age-related macular disease. Invest Ophthalmol Vis Sci 2005;46:3309–14.
41. Schmitz-Valckenberg S, Alten F, Steinberg JS, et al. Reticular drusen associated with geographic atrophy in age-related macular degeneration. Invest Ophthalmol Vis Sci 2011;52:5009–15.
42. Arnold JJ, Sarks SH, Killingsworth MC, et al. Reticular pseudodrusen. A risk factor in age-related maculopathy. Retina 1995;15:183–91.
43. Zweifel SA, Spaide RF, Curcio CA, et al. Reticular pseudodrusen are subretinal drusenoid deposits. Ophthalmology 2010;117:303–12 e1.
44. Schmitz-Valckenberg S, Steinberg JS, Fleckenstein M, et al. Combined confocal scanning laser ophthalmoscopy and spectral-domain optical coherence tomography imaging of reticular drusen associated with age-related macular degeneration. Ophthalmology 2010;117:1169–76.
45. Sarks SH. Ageing and degeneration in the macular region: a clinico-pathological study. Br J Ophthalmol 1976;60:324–41.
46. Schmitz-Valckenberg S, Jorzik J, Unnebrink K, et al. Analysis of digital scanning laser ophthalmoscopy fundus autofluorescence images of geographic atrophy in advanced age-related macular degeneration. Graefes Arch Clin Exp Ophthalmol 2002;240:73–8.
47. Schmitz-Valckenberg S, Bindewald-Wittich A, Dolar-Szczasny J, et al. Correlation between the area of increased autofluorescence surrounding geographic atrophy and disease progression in patients with AMD. Invest Ophthalmol Vis Sci 2006;47:2648–54.
48. Holz FG, Bindewald-Wittich A, Fleckenstein M, et al. Progression of geographic atrophy and impact of fundus autofluorescence patterns in age-related macular degeneration. Am J Ophthalmol 2007;143:463–72.
49. Holz FG, Bellman C, Staudt S, et al. Fundus autofluorescence and development of geographic atrophy in age-related macular degeneration. Invest Ophthalmol Vis Sci 2001;42:1051–6.
50. Bellmann C, Jorzik J, Spital G, et al. Symmetry of bilateral lesions in geographic atrophy in patients with age-related macular degeneration. Arch Ophthalmol 2002;120:579–84.
51. Holz FG, Bellmann C, Margaritidis M, et al. Patterns of increased in vivo fundus autofluorescence in the junctional zone of geographic atrophy of the retinal pigment epithelium associated with age-related macular degeneration. Graefes Arch Clin Exp Ophthalmol 1999;237:145–52.
52. Bindewald A, Schmitz-Valckenberg S, Jorzik JJ, et al. Classification of abnormal fundus autofluorescence patterns in the junctional zone of geographic atrophy in patients with age related macular degeneration. Br J Ophthalmol 2005;89: 874–8.
53. Scholl HP, Bellmann C, Dandekar SS, et al. Photopic and scotopic fine matrix mapping of retinal areas of increased fundus autofluorescence in patients with age-related maculopathy. Invest Ophthalmol Vis Sci 2004;45:574–83.
54. Schmitz-Valckenberg S, Bultmann S, Dreyhaupt J, et al. Fundus autofluorescence and fundus perimetry in the junctional zone of geographic atrophy in patients with age-related macular degeneration. Invest Ophthalmol Vis Sci 2004;45:4470–6.
55. Schmitz-Valckenberg S, Jaffe GJ, Fleckenstein M, et al. and GAP Study Group. Lesion characteristics and progression in the Natural History of Geographic Atrophy (GAP) Study. ARVO Meeting Abstracts 2009;50:3914.
56. Holz FG, Schmitz-Valckenberg S, Fleckenstein M, et al. Lesion characteristics and progression in the Natural History of Geographic Atrophy (GAP) Study. ARVO Meeting Abstracts 2010;51:94.
57. Vaclavik V, Vujosevic S, Dandekar SS, et al. Autofluorescence imaging in age-related macular degeneration complicated by choroidal neovascularization: a prospective study. Ophthalmology 2008;115:342–6.
58. McBain VA, Townend J, Lois N. Fundus autofluorescence in exudative age-related macular degeneration. Br J Ophthalmol 2007;91:491–6.
59. Sawa M, Ober MD, Spaide RF. Autofluorescence and retinal pigment epithelial atrophy after subretinal hemorrhage. Retina 2006;26:119–20.
59a. Spital G, Redermacher M, Müller C, et al. [Autofluorescence characteristics of lipofuscin components in different forms of late senile macular degeneration.] Klin Monabl Augenheilkd 1998;213:23–31.
60. Heimes B, Lommatzsch A, Zeimer M, et al. Foveal RPE autofluorescence as a prognostic factor for anti-VEGF therapy in exudative AMD. Graefes Arch Clin Exp Ophthalmol 2008;246:1229–34.
61. Einbock W, Moessner A, Schnurrbusch UE, et al. Changes in fundus autofluorescence in patients with age-related maculopathy. Correlation to visual function: a prospective study. Graefes Arch Clin Exp Ophthalmol 2005;243:300–5.
62. von Rückmann A, Fitzke F, Schmitz-Valckenberg S, et al. Macular and retinal dystrophies. In: Holz FG, Schmitz-Valckenberg S, Spaide R, et al, editors. Atlas of fundus and fluorescence imaging. Berlin: Springer; 2007.
63. Lorenz B, Wabbels B, Wegscheider E, et al. Lack of fundus autofluorescence to 488 nanometers from childhood on in patients with early-onset severe retinal dystrophy associated with mutations in RPE65. Ophthalmology 2004;111: 1585–94.
64. Scholl HP, Chong NH, Robson AG, et al. Fundus autofluorescence in patients with leber congenital amaurosis. Invest Ophthalmol Vis Sci 2004;45:2747–52.
65. Robson AG, Michaelides M, Saihan Z, et al. Functional characteristics of patients with retinal dystrophy that manifest abnormal parafoveal annuli of high density fundus autofluorescence; a review and update. Doc Ophthalmol 2008;116:79–89.
66. von Ruckmann A, Fitzke FW, Bird AC. In vivo fundus autofluorescence in macular dystrophies. Arch Ophthalmol 1997;115:609–15.
67. Fleckenstein M, Charbel Issa P, Fuchs HA, et al. Discrete arcs of increased fundus autofluorescence in retinal dystrophies and functional correlate on microperimetry. Eye (Lond) 2009;23:567–75.
68. Popovic P, Jarc-Vidmar M, Hawlina M. Abnormal fundus autofluorescence in relation to retinal function in patients with retinitis pigmentosa. Graefes Arch Clin Exp Ophthalmol 2005;243:1018–27.
69. Fleckenstein M, Charbel Issa P, Helb HM, et al. Correlation of lines of increased autofluorescence in macular dystrophy and pigmented paravenous retinochoroidal atrophy by optical coherence tomography. Arch Ophthalmol 2008; 126:1461–3.
70. Lima LH, Cella W, Greenstein VC, et al. Structural assessment of hyperautofluorescent ring in patients with retinitis pigmentosa. Retina 2009;29:1025–31.
71. Gass JD, Blodi BA. Idiopathic juxtafoveolar retinal telangiectasis. Update of classification and follow-up study. Ophthalmology 1993;100:1536–46.
72. Hutton WL, Snyder WB, Fuller D, et al. Focal parafoveal retinal telangiectasis. Arch Ophthalmol 1978;96:1362–7.
73. Gass JDM. Stereoscopic atlas of macular diseases: diagnosis and treatment. 2nd ed. St Louis: Mosby; 1977.
74. Helb HM, Charbel Issa P, van der Veen RL, et al. Abnormal macular pigment distribution in type 2 idiopathic macular telangiectasia. Retina 2008;28:808–16.
75. Charbel Issa P, van der Veen RL, Stijfs A, et al. Quantification of reduced macular pigment optical density in the central retina in macular telangiectasia type 2. Exp Eye Res 2009;89:25–31.
76. Powner MB, Gillies MC, Tretiach M, et al. Perifoveal muller cell depletion in a case of macular telangiectasia type 2. Ophthalmology 2010;117:2407–16.
77. Zeimer MB, Padge B, Heimes B, et al. Idiopathic macular telangiectasia type 2: distribution of macular pigment and functional investigations. Retina 2010;30:586–95.
78. Charbel Issa P, Finger RP, Holz FG, et al. Multimodal imaging including spectral domain OCT and confocal near infrared reflectance for characterisation of outer retinal pathology in pseudoxanthoma elasticum. Invest Ophthalmol Vis Sci 2009;50:5913–8.
79. Finger RP, Charbel Issa P, Ladewig M, et al. Fundus autofluorescence in pseudoxanthoma elasticum. Retina 2009;29:1496–505.
80. Agarwal A, Patel P, Adkins T, et al. Spectrum of pattern dystrophy in pseudoxanthoma elasticum. Arch Ophthalmol 2005;123:923–8.
81. Charbel Issa P, Finger RP, Gotting C, et al. Centrifugal fundus abnormalities in pseudoxanthoma elasticum. Ophthalmology 2010;117:1406–14.
82. Spaide RF, Campeas L, Haas A, et al. Central serous chorioretinopathy in younger and older adults. Ophthalmology 1996;103:2070–9; discussion 9-80.
83. Spaide RF, Klancnik JM, Jr. Fundus autofluorescence and central serous chorioretinopathy. Ophthalmology 2005;112:825–33.
84. Kellner U, Renner AB, Tillack H. Fundus autofluorescence and mfERG for early detection of retinal alterations in patients using chloroquine/ hydroxychloroquine. Invest Ophthalmol Vis Sci 2006;47:3531–8.
85. Kellner S, Weinitz S, Kellner U. Spectral domain optical coherence tomography detects early stages of chloroquine retinopathy similar to multifocal electroretinography, fundus autofluorescence and near-infrared autofluorescence. Br J Ophthalmol 2009;93:1444–7.

Chapter 5

Advanced Imaging Technologies

Pearse A. Keane, Humberto Ruiz-Garcia, SriniVas R. Sadda

INTRODUCTION – RETINAL IMAGING TO DATE

Assessment of chorioretinal disease is dependent on the ability to visualize pathologic changes occurring in the posterior segment of the eye using optical instruments, termed ophthalmoscopy (Fig. 5.1A).[1] Ophthalmoscopy, in turn, has been greatly enhanced by the development of techniques that allow recording of these changes.[2] By the end of the 19th century the first images of the living human retina had been obtained (Fig. 5.1B) and, by the 1950s, with the advent of electronic flashes and 35-mm cameras, the field of modern retinal/fundal imaging had been born.[3]

As well as documenting pathology, fundal imaging facilitates the identification of morphologic features not visible to the clinician on biomicroscopy. For example, from an early stage in its development, fundus photography has incorporated angiographic methodologies for the visualization of blood vessels.[1,4] In the 1960s, the assessment of retinal disease was revolutionized by the introduction of fluorescein angiography (Fig. 5.2A). In the 1970s, evaluation of the choroidal circulation was also improved through the use of indocyanine green dye. The development of these angiographic techniques has also led, at least in part, to the discovery that certain fundal structures fluoresce in the absence of contrast. The subsequent evolution of fundus autofluorescence imaging has greatly extended our ability to evaluate retinal degenerative and other disorders.[2]

Since the 1990s, fundus photographic systems have also made the transition from "analogue" image capture using film to digital image capture using charge-coupled devices (CCDs), allowing for improved image processing and analysis.[2] In parallel with this, new image capture technologies have emerged such

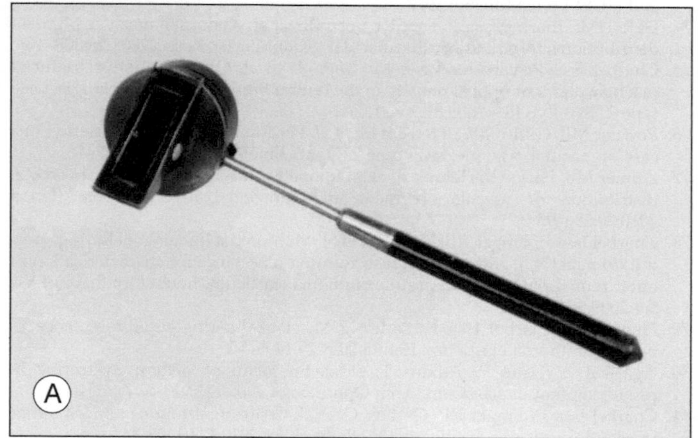

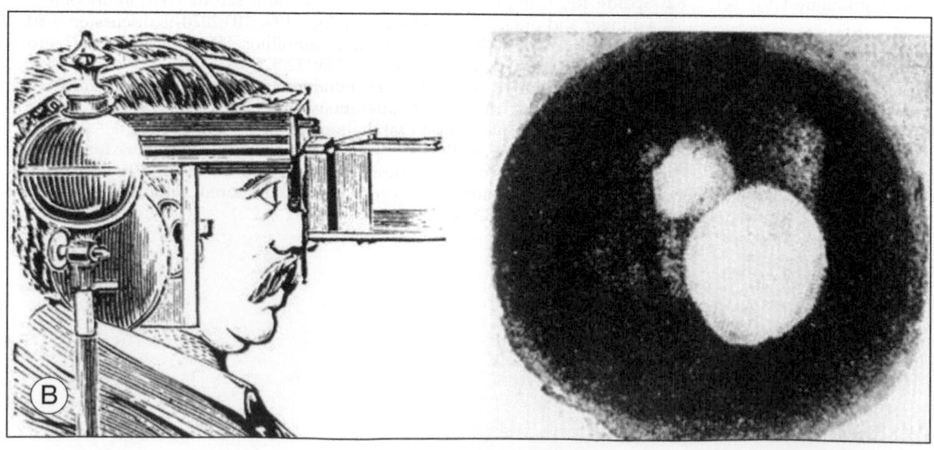

Fig. 5.1 Early attempts at retinal visualization and image capture. (A) Early model of the Helmholtz ophthalmoscope, 1851. (Alcon Laboratories Museum of Ophthalmology, The Sherman Collection, Fort Worth, TX, USA. Historical image: Helmholtz ophthalmoscope, 1851. Ophthalmology 2002;109:729. Reproduced with permission.) (B) The first published human fundus photograph involved this apparatus, an albocarbon burner, and a 2½-minute exposure. Blood vessels cannot be defined, but the optic disc can be seen as a white area superiorly, while inferiorly, the larger light area is an artifact. (Reproduced with permission from Same PJ. Landmarks in the historical development of fluorescein angiography. J Ophthalm Photography 1993;15:18.)

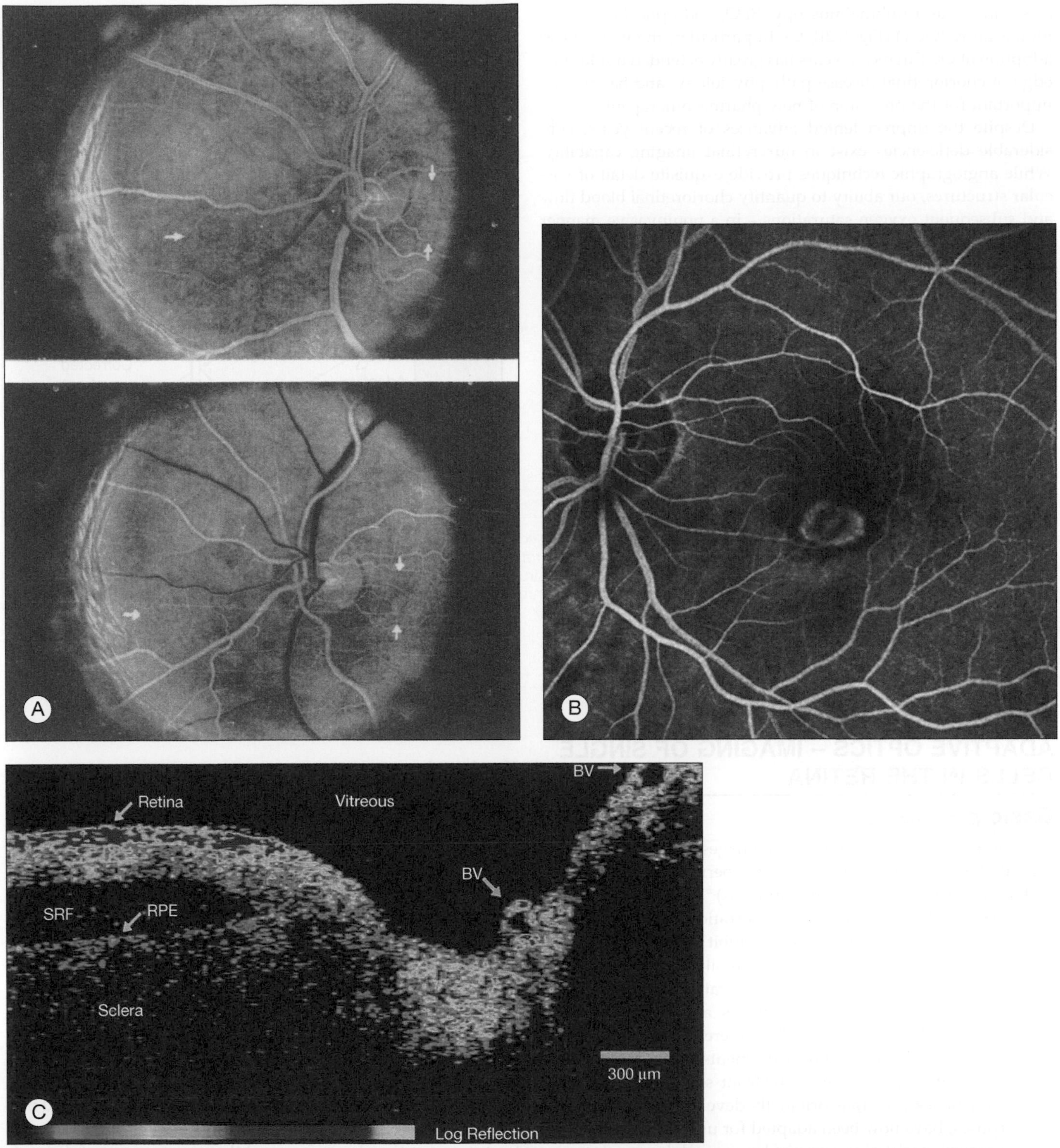

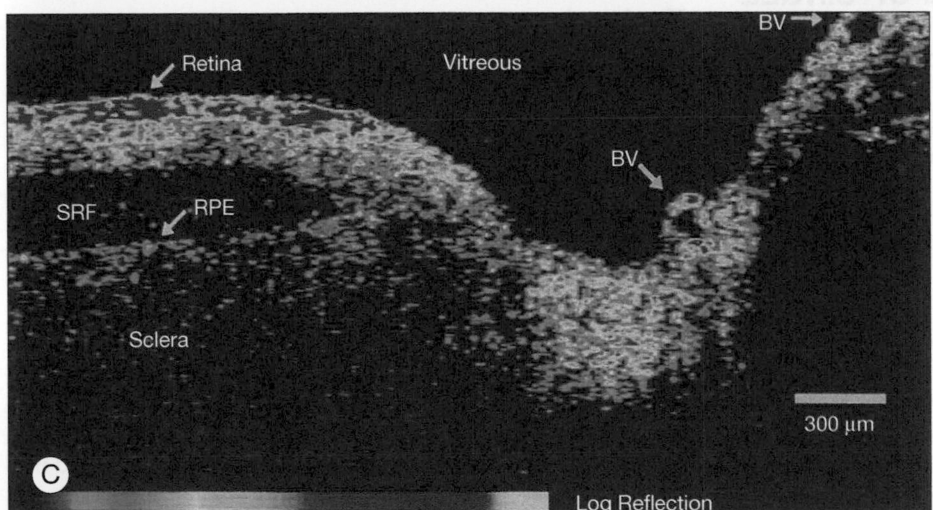

Fig. 5.2 Fluorescein angiography, scanning laser ophthalmoscopy, and optical coherence tomography (OCT). (A) Early attempt at fundus fluorescein angiography in a normal subject. (Reproduced with permission from Novotny HR, Alvis DL. A method of photographing fluorescence in circulating blood in the human retina. Circulation 1961;24:82–6.) (B) A single frame from a fluorescein angiogram taken with a confocal scanning laser ophthalmoscope (cSLO) showing a choroidal neovascular membrane. (Reproduced with permission from Bennett PJ, Barry CJ. Ophthalmic imaging today: an ophthalmic photographer's viewpoint – a review. Clin Exp Ophthalmol 2009;37:2–13.) (C) Early attempt at OCT imaging of the human retina and optic nerve, obtained in vitro. SRF, subretinal fluid; RPE, retinal pigment epithelium; BV, blood vessel. (Reproduced with permission from Huang D, Swanson EA, Lin CP, et al. Optical coherence tomography. Science 1991;254:1178–81.)

as scanning laser ophthalmoscopy (SLO) and optical coherence tomography (OCT) (Fig. 5.2B, C). In particular, the widespread adoption of OCT in recent years has greatly extended our knowledge of chorioretinal disease pathophysiology, and has proven important for the provision of new pharmacotherapeutics.[1]

Despite the unprecedented advances of recent years, considerable deficiencies exist in our retinal imaging capability. While angiographic techniques provide exquisite detail of vascular structures, our ability to quantify chorioretinal blood flow and subsequent oxygen saturations – in a noninvasive manner – remains inadequate. While OCT provides cross-sectional images of the neurosensory retina (and more recently the choroid) with high axial resolution, its transverse resolution is limited, and our ability to assess many retinal cell types remains poor (e.g., Müller cells, microglia, astrocytes, and individual neuronal elements). Furthermore, many advances in microscopic techniques that permit "molecular" imaging in basic science research have yet to make the transition to human clinical studies.

In this chapter, we discuss the attempts that are underway to address the shortcomings of current retinal imaging technologies. We begin by describing the use of adaptive optics to provide cellular-level image resolution, before moving on to describe Doppler and spectral imaging techniques for the assessment of retinal blood flow and oxygenation. We then describe a number of technologies with the potential for assessment of novel functional parameters, such as photoacoustic and magnetic resonance imaging (MRI). We conclude by introducing the emerging field of nanotechnology and describing how the use of targeted nanoparticles may ultimately allow molecular-level imaging in clinical practice.

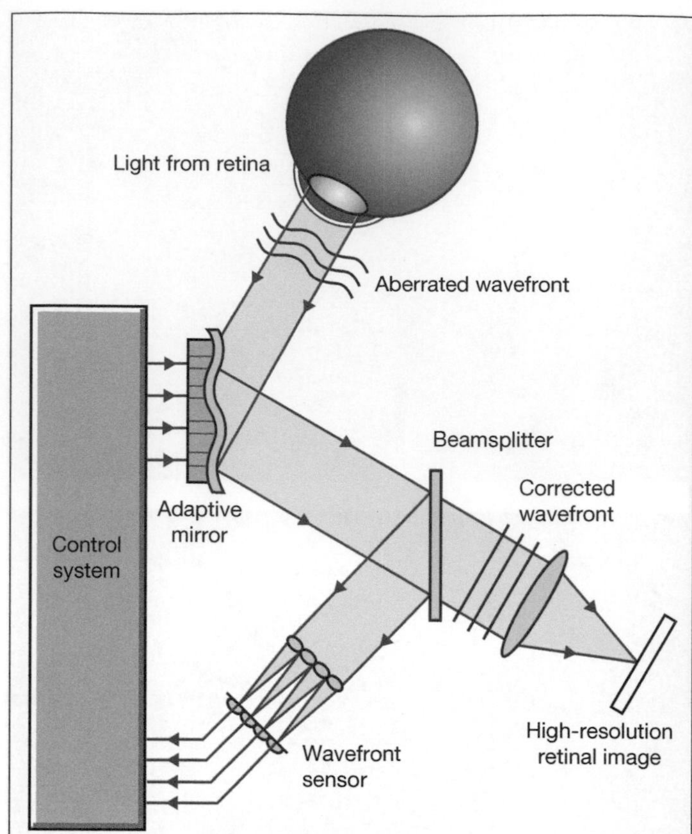

Fig. 5.3 Schematic representation of a typical adaptive optics system. (Courtesy of Joseph Carroll, Williams Laboratory, University of Rochester.)

ADAPTIVE OPTICS – IMAGING OF SINGLE CELLS IN THE RETINA

Basic principles

Our ability to obtain high-resolution images of the human retina is limited by the presence of defects, or aberrations, in the optical system of the eye (i.e., the cornea and lens).[5] In addition to exhibiting lower-order monochromatic aberrations such as defocus and astigmatism, normal eyes also exhibit higher-order monochromatic aberrations such as coma, trefoil, and spherical aberration. The combined effects of these aberrations limit the quality of images obtainable for the diagnosis and management of retinal disease. Until the early 1990s, there existed no effective way to obtain rapid, precise measurements of the human eye's optical aberrations. However, wavefront sensors based on the Hartmann–Shack principle, originally developed for astronomical purposes, have now been adapted for use in the human eye. These sensors consist of an array of lenses, each having the same focal length, which can be used to approximate the whole wavelength of incident light. Once measured, the detected aberrations can then be corrected (i.e., rendered flat) using one or more deformable mirrors: the mirrors have large numbers of small electronically controlled actuators on their rear surface that can push and pull the mirror within a range of ±2 μm, allowing it to adopt any desired configuration (Fig. 5.3). By incorporating wavefront sensing and correction into existing optical imaging platforms – "adaptive optics" – it is now possible to acquire images of the retina with cellular-level resolution, and in a noninvasive fashion.[5,6]

Technology

The adaptive optics devices first developed for ophthalmic use were conventional fundus cameras modified to incorporate wavefront sensing and correction.[7,8] These systems typically focus a laser beam on the retina at a location of interest. The light reflected from the retina is then distorted by the optical system of the eye before returning to the wavefront sensor. Information obtained from the wavefront sensor is then used to alter the shape of the deformable mirrors and compensate for the aberration. This process continues in a closed loop until the ocular aberrations have been reduced to near diffraction-limited levels; at this point, a flash from a separate incoherent light source is triggered by the wavefront sensor, illuminating the retina as an image is captured by the digital fundus camera.

Adaptive optics components have also been incorporated into confocal SLO systems, offering the advantage of increased contrast, cross-sectional imaging, and the measurement of dynamic changes such as blood flow.[5,9] In an adaptive optics SLO, light returning from the retina is split into a light detection path and a wavefront-sensing path. Again, deformable mirrors are used to provide closed-loop dynamic compensation for ocular aberrations. In contrast to flood-illuminated adaptive optics devices, the adaptive optics SLO uses the same source of light for the wavefront sensor as for the retinal illumination; as a result, the wavefront sensor is able to measure aberrations from the entire scanned area of the retina. When imaging the retina, SLO devices provide a transverse resolution of approximately 15 μm but are limited to an axial resolution of approximately 300 μm. With the addition of adaptive optics correction to an SLO, the transverse resolution may be increased to less than 3 μm while the axial resolution may be improved to 40 μm.

Adaptive optics devices have also been incorporated into prototype OCT systems.[10,11] The axial resolution achievable using OCT is many orders of magnitude greater than that achievable using an SLO device, with commercially available devices commonly achieving axial resolutions of approximately 5 μm. However, the transverse resolution of OCT systems is determined by the size of the laser spot that can be focused on the retina – a factor limited by ocular aberrations. A successful combination of OCT and adaptive optics could potentially demonstrate, therefore, the narrowest point-spread function of all in vivo retinal-imaging techniques (Fig. 5.4). However, a number of technical challenges remain, in particular, the reductions in image quality that occur as a result of chromatic aberrations when large-bandwidth light sources are used.[12,13]

Finally, adaptive optics may be useful for the performance of fundus perimetry ("microperimetry") in the study of macular

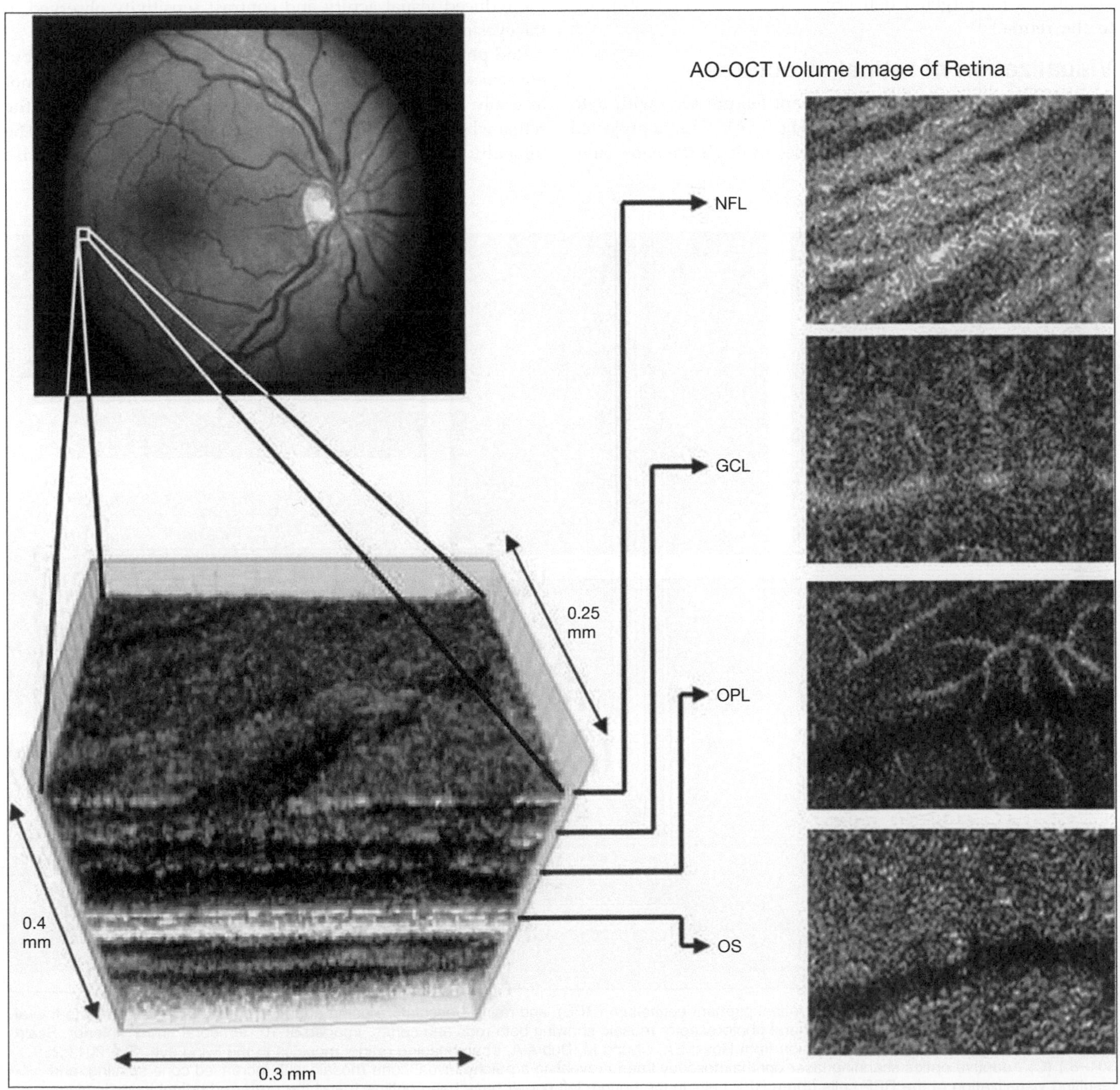

Fig. 5.4 Adaptive optics optical coherence tomography (AO-OCT) volume acquired over a 1° retinal region located temporal of the fovea, as illustrated by the rectangle in the fundus photograph. The images on the right are en face views of particular retinal layers extracted from the AO-OCT volume. Retinal layers from top to bottom are: nerve fiber layer (NFL), ganglion cell layer (GCL), outer plexiform layer (OPL), and outer-segment (OS) layer of photoreceptors. (Reproduced with permission from Miller DT, Kocaoglu OP, Wang Q, et al. Adaptive optics and the eye (super resolution OCT). Eye 2011;25:321–30.)

disease.[1] In current microperimetry systems, macular light sensitivity is measured using a stimulus size that covers an area containing in excess of 150 cones at the foveal center. As with the imaging modalities described above, further reductions in stimulus size are hindered by aberrations of the optical systems in the human eye, a shortcoming that may be overcome through the incorporation of adaptive optics.[14] In addition, by analyzing the warping that occurs both within individual SLO frames and between frames, adaptive optics can be used to resolve the effects of eye movements at a fine spatial scale. As a consequence, in adaptive optics microperimetry, real-time stabilization of the retinal image is possible, and allows for targeted delivery of the small visual stimulus to the retina.[15,16]

Visualization of retinal structures

Cone photoreceptors are the dominant feature seen with both flood-illuminated and SLO devices (Fig. 5.5A).[6,17] Light projected into the eye from these devices passes through the cone outer segment and is reflected by the retinal pigment epithelium (RPE), the most highly reflective surface in the retina. As light is reflected out of the eye, it is guided toward a small area of the pupil by the cone inner segments (in this respect cones act as "optical fibers," rejecting stray light in the retina and maximizing efficiency in light collection). The human eye has three classes of cone photoreceptors: blue (S), green (M), and red (L). Adaptive optics has supplied the first data regarding the proportion, and arrangement, of each cone class in the human eye.[18] By quantifying cone receptor density, it has also been demonstrated that the density of cone packing appears to be lower in highly myopic eyes versus emmetropic eyes – a finding consistent with the reduced visual acuity and contrast sensitivity observed in the eyes of axial myopes.[19]

Rod photoreceptors are abundant in the peripheral retina but are also seen in the macular region of human eyes. Rods are not as easily visualized in the normal retina, even in areas of the retina where they outnumber cones approximately 10-fold.[6] The difficulty in imaging rods is consistent with their smaller size

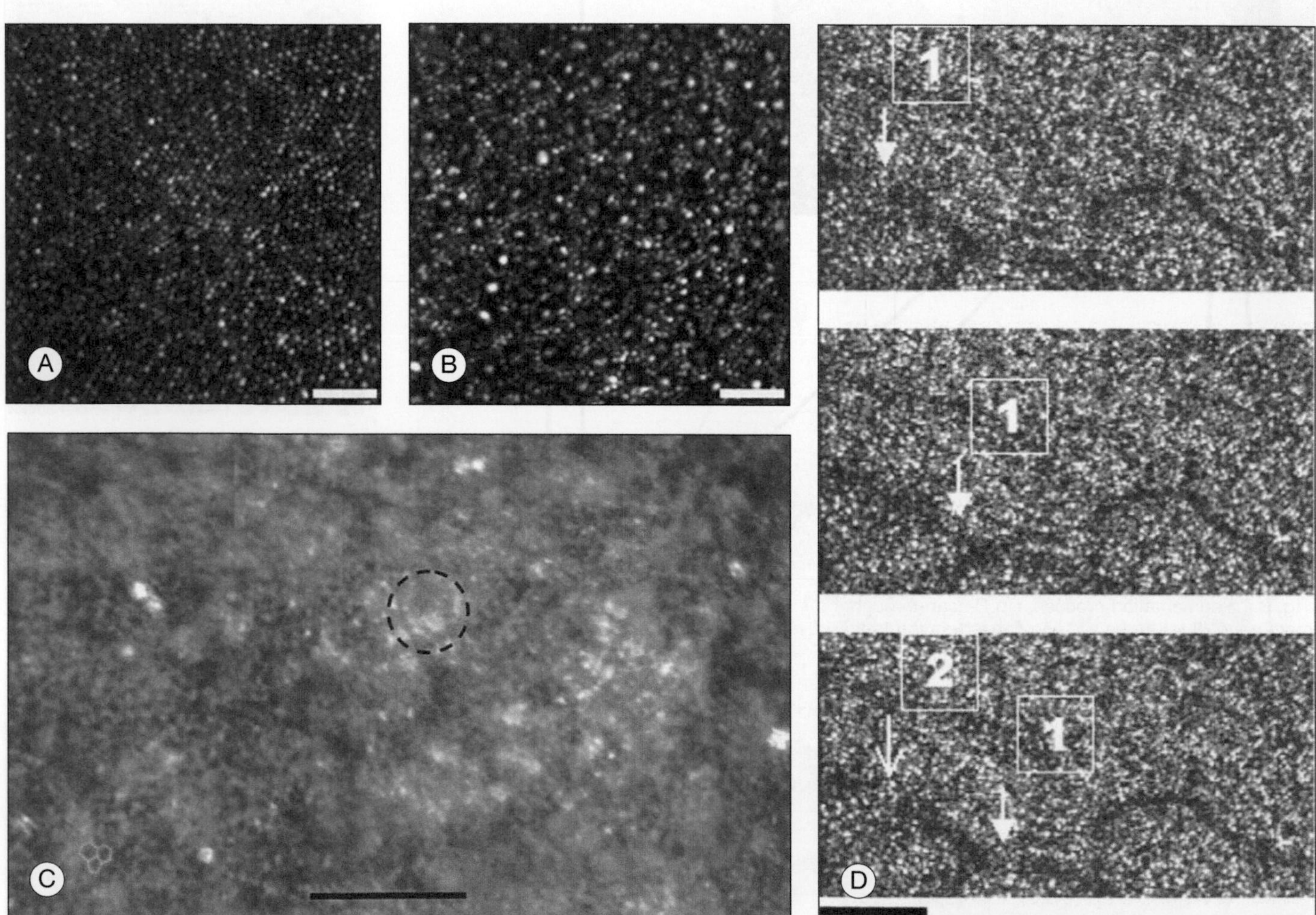

Fig. 5.5 Visualization of photoreceptors, retinal pigment epithelium (RPE), and retinal vasculature using adaptive optics. (A) The complete foveal cone mosaic and (B) the complete peripheral photoreceptor mosaic showing both rods and cones, imaged at 10° temporal and 1° inferior. Scale bars = 20 µm. (Reproduced with permission from Rossi EA, Chung M, Dubra A, et al. Imaging retinal mosaics in the living eye. Eye 2011;25: 301–8.) (C) Adaptive optics scanning laser ophthalmoscopy image revealing a patchy foveal cone mosaic with increased cone spacing, and resulting visualization of the RPE cells (three RPE cells in the bottom left corner have been outlined, and the preferred retinal locus is also indicated by the dashed circle in the image). (Reproduced with permission from Roorda A, Zhang Y, Duncan JL. High-resolution in vivo imaging of the RPE mosaic in eyes with retinal disease. Invest Ophthalmol Vis Sci 2007;48:2297–303.) (D) Three successive frames demonstrate a single leukocyte's (1) change in position from left to right in each frame. A second leukocyte (2) has just come into view in the last frame. Scale bar = 100 µm. (Reproduced with permission from Martin JA, Roorda A. Direct and noninvasive assessment of parafoveal capillary leukocyte velocity. Ophthalmology 2005;112:2219–24.)

(approximately 2 μm in diameter), and their broad angular tuning, which reflects less light back through the pupil where it can be collected for imaging. However, recent advances, including the use of smaller confocal pinholes and improvements in registration algorithms, have now allowed clear images of single rods to be obtained in the living human eye (as well as aiding visualization of the smallest cones at the foveal center) (Fig. 5.5A).[20]

Rod and cone photoreceptors rest on a monolayer of RPE cells. Each RPE cell in the monolayer has an approximate diameter of 10 μm, dimensions well within the resolution limits of adaptive optics systems; however, direct in vivo visualization of single RPE cells remains challenging. Unlike cone photoreceptors, the intrinsic contrast of RPE cells is poor. In addition, much of the light scattered by the RPE is masked by the overlying photoreceptors, which are also highly scattering. To date, direct imaging of the RPE has only been possible in human subjects with retinal disease where absence of cone photoreceptors has allowed visualization of the underlying RPE (Fig. 5.5B).[21] However, by the incorporation of adaptive optics with fundus autofluorescence, images of the RPE cell mosaic have been achieved in primate eyes.[22]

The high scanning speed of SLO systems allows retinal images to be captured at video rates, thus allowing measurement of dynamic retinal changes, such as blood flow. The use of an adaptive optics SLO thus allows direct visualization of white blood cells as they transit through retinal capillaries (the smaller size and different absorption characteristic of red blood cells make them more difficult to visualize) (Fig. 5.5C).[23,24] As a consequence, direct noninvasive measurement of the velocity of retinal blood flow becomes possible. Retinal imaging with adaptive optics may also be useful for detection of structural changes in the retinal vasculature not visible with other imaging modalities, such as microaneurysms and hard exudates in diabetic retinopathy.[25]

Although cone photoreceptors offer high contrast and can now routinely be imaged using adaptive optics, other cell types in the retina are not as easily visualized. Unlike cones, other neurons are not highly reflective of light and do not exhibit high contrast (the reflected signal from ganglion cells is 60 times lower than that from cones). These difficulties are especially difficult to surmount given the safe limits for laser usage in humans, and the effects of involuntary eye movements. Despite these obstacles, recent animal studies have made progress toward in vivo visualization of retinal ganglion cells using fluorescent markers, and the development of similar capabilities in humans may lead to improved understanding of optic neuropathies such as glaucoma.[26]

Early clinical applications

The cellular-level resolution provided by adaptive optics retinal imaging allows direct measurement of photoreceptor density and diameter and is, therefore, an ideal tool for the examination of patients with inherited retinal degenerations (Fig. 5.6). On examination with adaptive optics, diseased cones do not show the same reflectance pattern as healthy photoreceptors, resulting in dark gaps or areas of "drop-out" within the cone photoreceptor mosaic.[27] Significant correlations have been found between parafoveal cone density and a number of functional parameters, including best-corrected visual acuity, contrast sensitivity, and detection sensitivities for visual stimuli recorded using multifocal electroretinography.[28–30] In a recent phase II clinical trial where patients with inherited retinal degenerations were treated with sustained-release ciliary neurotrophic factor, no changes in visual acuity, visual field, or electroretinography responses were observed. However, using an adaptive optics SLO, significant differences in both cone density and spacing were detected between treatment and control groups.[31]

High-resolution adaptive optics imaging has also been used to aid the examination of patients with "macular microholes,"[32]

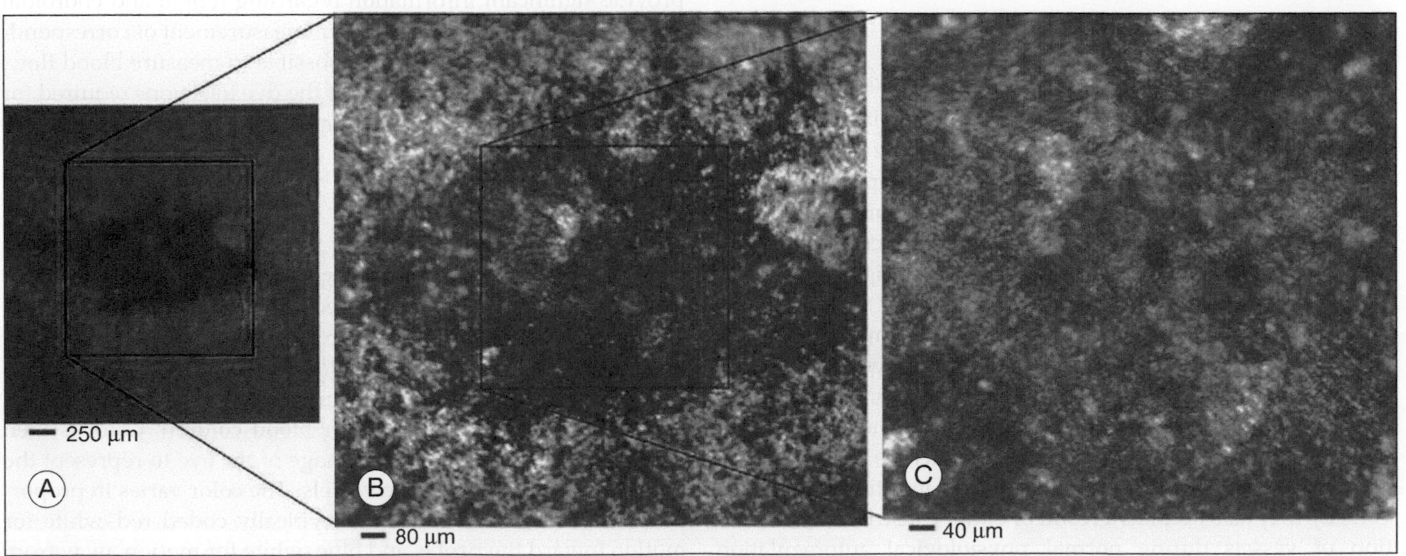

Fig. 5.6 Adaptive optics scanning laser ophthalmoscope (AOSLO) images at different magnifications with corresponding features on the fundus photograph (A). (B) Six-degree montage from 3° adaptive optics images of the central macula of the cone–rod dystrophy patient's right eye. In addition to the features detected in the fundus photograph, detailed structures in the granular pattern of the retinal pigment epithelium in the atrophic bull's-eye lesion are observed. Within the central relatively spared region (box), photoreceptors are seen as gray dots. (C) Three-degree montage from 1.5° images. The photoreceptors are visible in the central relatively spared area of the retina. (Reproduced with permission from Wolfing JI, Chung M, Carroll J, et al. High-resolution retinal imaging of cone–rod dystrophy. Ophthalmology 2006;113:1019.)

color blindness,[33] foveal hypoplasia,[34] and otherwise unexplained visual disturbances.[35] In patients with glaucoma and other optic neuropathies, adaptive optics has also revealed evidence of structural changes in cone photoreceptors when there is permanent damage to the overlying inner retinal layers.[36]

Conclusions

It is clear that the addition of adaptive optics to existing retinal imaging platforms is an important step for clinical ophthalmology, particularly when such devices can be made inexpensive, user-friendly, and reliable. In fact, the first commercially available adaptive optics system, for ophthalmic research purposes only, has recently been launched (the rtx1 Adaptive Optics Retinal Camera, Imagine Eyes, France). Rapid progress is also being made on the use of adaptive optics with other imaging systems, and, although significant technical challenges must still be overcome, the inclusion of adaptive optics in OCT systems seems particularly promising.

DOPPLER IMAGING – ASSESSMENT OF BLOOD FLOW

Basic principles

The Doppler effect, first described in the 19th century by the Austrian physicist Christian Doppler, is the change in frequency of a wave as it is reflected off a moving object: if the reflecting object is moving away from the observer/transducer, the frequency of the reflected waves is lower than that of the waves emitted, and vice versa. As the frequency shift is dependent on the velocity of the moving object, this effect can be used to measure the velocity of blood flowing in the eye.[37] Importantly, the Doppler effect is also dependent on the angle between the axis of the wave and the axis of movement of the object. Therefore, if the observer/transducer is not parallel to the axis of the moving object calculations must be performed using a Doppler angle correction formula:

$$V = \Delta FC / 2F_0 \cos\alpha$$

where V is the velocity of the moving object, ΔF is the Doppler (frequency) shift, C is the velocity of the wave in the medium, F_0 is the frequency of the wave source, and $\cos\alpha$ is the Doppler angle. Of note, accurate measurement of the Doppler angle is a significant obstacle to the noninvasive assessment of ocular blood flow. Furthermore, as the Doppler angle increases between 60° and 90°, velocity calculations are subject to significant errors (cosine 90° is equal to zero).

Utilization of the Doppler effect in ocular imaging systems allows calculation of ocular blood flow velocities.[37] Reductions in blood flow velocity may occur as a result of vascular degenerative changes in diseases such as diabetic retinopathy, or as a result of vascular occlusion in diseases such as central retinal vein occlusion (CRVO). However, changes in retinal blood flow velocity may also occur as a result of either constriction or dilatation of vessels during normal physiological autoregulation (according to Bernoulli's principle, constriction of a blood vessel causes a conversion of pressure into kinetic energy, thereby increasing the velocity of the blood, but decreasing its pressure). Therefore, measurements of the absolute quantities of "blood flow" may represent a more clinically relevant parameter.

Blood flow (Q) is the volume of blood passing through a vessel in a given time, and is determined by the velocity of the blood (V) multiplied by the cross-sectional area of the blood vessel through which it passes (πr^2).[38] Consequently, if blood flow velocity can be measured using the Doppler effect, and the diameter of the blood vessel can also be measured, then absolute values for blood flow may be determined. Measurements of retinal vascular diameter can be acquired from fundus images obtained with standard optical imaging techniques (e.g., fundus photography).[39,40] However, in order to measure retinal vascular diameters in real units of length, the magnification of the image induced by the eye, as well as the magnification of the camera, must be known (failure to account for such magnification will result in significant errors).

Non-Doppler assessment of retinal blood flow

Measurement of retinal blood flow is possible using quantitative angiography, based on use of dye dilution techniques.[37,39,40] In this method, the concentration of fluorescent dye within the blood at a specific observation point is graphed over time, producing a dye dilution curve. The enhanced contrast provided by SLO systems is particularly suited to this approach, and it can be used to evaluate vascular parameters such as retinal arteriovenous passage time and mean dye velocity. The increased contrast provided by SLO images also allows measurement of blood velocities in the small vessels surrounding the fovea and the optic nerve head (in the future, this technique is likely to be enhanced through the incorporation of adaptive optics).[40] Indocyanine green angiography may also be used to evaluate the choroidal circulatory flow, as the infrared light sources employed penetrate the RPE more efficiently than the shorter wavelengths used in fluorescein angiography. In one analysis method, the choroid is divided into six regions, and dye dilution curves are created for each region (Fig. 5.7A). Parameters such as 10% filling time, and maximum brightness, can then be calculated.[40] SLO-based fluorescein and indocyanine green angiography provide significant information regarding retinal and choroidal blood velocities. However, without measurement of corresponding vascular diameters, it is not possible to measure blood flow. In addition, the invasive nature of the dye injections required for these approaches precludes their routine use in many clinical scenarios.

Doppler ultrasound

Color Doppler imaging (CDI) is an ultrasound technique that combines B-scan gray-scale imaging of tissue structure, color representation of blood flow based on Doppler shifted frequencies, and pulsed-Doppler measurement of blood flow velocities (Fig. 5.7B).[37,40] As in other Doppler-based methods, blood flow velocity is determined by the shift in the frequency of sound waves reflected from the moving blood column. Color is then added to the B-scan gray-scale image of the eye to represent the motion of blood through the vessels. The color varies in proportion to the flow velocity and is typically coded red–white for motion toward the probe, and blue–white for motion away from the probe. Using the color Doppler image, the operator can then identify the vessel of interest and place the sampling window for pulsed Doppler measurements (this window is generally situated in the center of the vessel). At this point, the general flow axis of the blood flow is detected simply by observation to

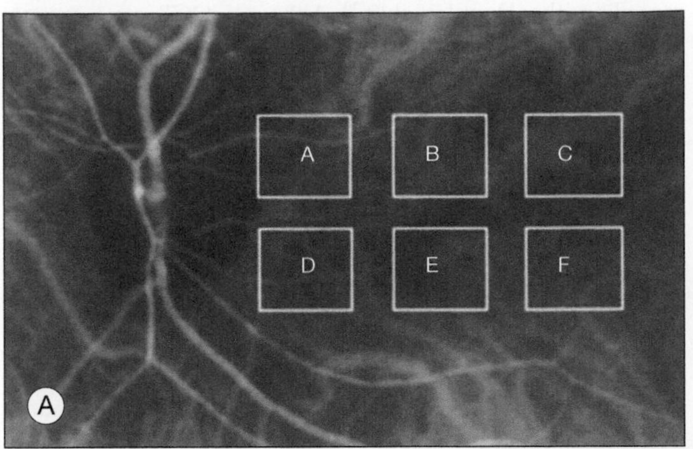

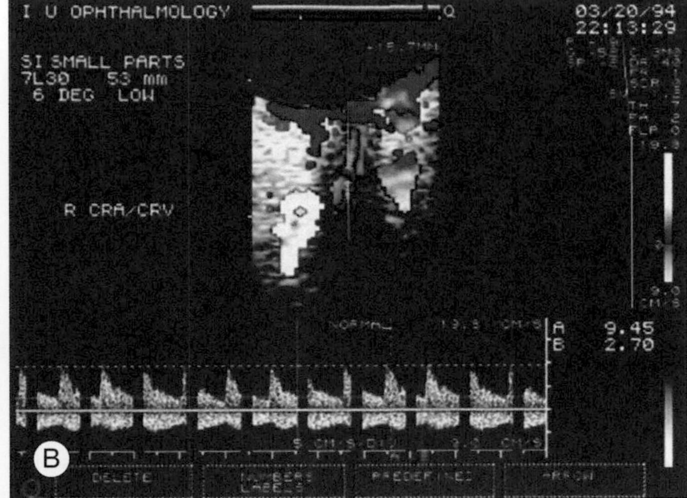

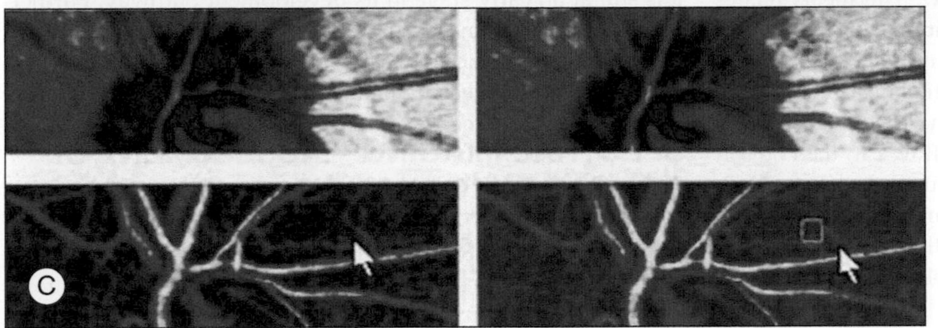

Fig. 5.7 Evaluation of chorioretinal blood flow. (A) Quantification of choroidal blood flow using indocyanine green angiography. Six locations, each a 6° square, are identified on the image for dye dilution analysis. (B) Color Doppler image (CDI) of the central retinal artery and vein. The Doppler shifted spectrum (time–velocity curve) is displayed at the bottom of the image. Red and blue pixels represent blood movement towards and away from the transducer, respectively. (C) Confocal scanning laser Doppler flowmetry (Heidelberg retinal flowmeter) of optic nerve head and peripapillary retina. The left arrow indicates a 1 × 1-pixel measurement window, which collects flow values from the entire retina except for large vessels, for new pixel-by-pixel analysis. The right arrow indicates a 10 × 10-pixel measurement window used for conventional analysis. (Reproduced with permission from Harris A, Chung HS, Ciulla TA, et al. Progress in measurement of ocular blood flow and relevance to our understanding of glaucoma and age-related macular degeneration. Prog Retin Eye Res 1999;18:673–7.)

determine the Doppler flow angle for the appropriate calculation of velocity. Flow–velocity data are then plotted against time, and the computer identifies the peak and trough of the waves.

Current CDI analysis focuses primarily on the arteries located behind the globe: ophthalmic artery, central retinal artery, and posterior ciliary arteries. CDI can be used to describe blood flow to the eye in terms of a set of well-defined parameters including: (1) peak systolic velocity (PSV); (2) end-diastolic velocity; and (3) resistance index.[37,40] It does not provide absolute measurements of blood flow (no quantitative information on vessel diameter is obtained). With a 7.5-MHz probe, CDI is able to resolve structures of 0.2 mm (200 µm) or larger, but can also be used to measure Doppler shifts in smaller vessels such as the posterior ciliary arteries (diameter of approximately 40 µm). CDI may be of particular use for the primary evaluation and follow-up of orbital vascular lesions, such as varices, arteriovenous malformations, and carotid-cavernous sinus fistulas. It has also been used for the semiquantitative assessment of perfusion in retinal and choroidal vascular disease. Specifically, in patients with CRVO, the central retinal artery PSV and end-diastolic velocity have been found to be much lower than in unaffected fellow eyes and in healthy control subjects.[41] Patients with ocular ischemic syndromes also present reduced PSVs in the central retinal and posterior ciliary arteries, as well as increased resistance.[42]

Laser Doppler velocimetry

Bidirectional laser Doppler velocimetry (LDV) is a technique used to quantify maximum blood velocity in large retinal vessels.[37,43] Instruments based on this principle typically consist of a modified fundus camera where the body of the camera has been replaced by a fiberoptic unit. A low-powered laser light source casts a beam on to the ocular fundus which is positioned by the operator on the retinal vessel of interest. The Doppler shifted frequency spectra of the returning light can then be measured. These spectra exhibit large fluctuations up to a clearly measurable maximum shift – this maximum shift arises from scattered light from red blood cells flowing at the maximum speed at the center of the vessel. If the Doppler angles are then known, the maximum frequency shift can be used to calculate the maximum vessel velocity; however, these angles are difficult to measure reproducibly. Therefore, a bidirectional technique was developed to expand the capability of LDV to provide absolute measurements of maximum velocity.[43] In the bidirectional technique, one incident beam is used to illuminate a sight along a retinal vessel. The light scattered by the blood cells at the illuminated site is then detected simultaneously in two distinct directions separated by a known, fixed angle. Two Doppler shifted frequency spectra are measured and the difference between their maximum shifts is then used to calculate the maximum velocity in units of speed.

By combining an eye-tracking system with a retinal laser instrument based on bidirectional LDV, Canon has developed a commercially available instrument (Canon Laser Blood Flowmeter (CLBF)-100, Tokyo, Japan).[44] This device allows concomitant measurement of blood vessel diameter; as a result, total retinal blood flow in a single vessel can be calculated in absolute units. Thus far, the smallest vessels in which the blood flow rate has been measured were approximately 40 μm in diameter.[44]

Laser Doppler flowmetry

Laser Doppler flowmetry (LDF) is a technique where laser light is not directed at a retinal vessel, but on an area of vascularized retinal tissue with no large vessels visible.[37,39] LDF instruments are based on the theories of Bonner and Nossal, which describe the characteristics of laser light injected at one point into capillary tissue and collected at an adjacent point.[43] This theory relates the Doppler shift of the light to the total number of blood cells moving in the illuminated tissue volume, and to the flow rate of the moving cells. By using this theory, relative measurements of the mean velocity of the red blood cells, and the blood volume, can be obtained. Relative values of blood flow can then be calculated as the product of velocity and volume. However, such measurements are not absolute, and variations in vascular density and vessel orientation, even within relatively small volumes of tissue, can lead to considerable differences in the scattering properties between subjects.

Scanning LDF combines the principles of scanning laser tomography and LDF, with the commercially available Heidelberg retina flowmeter (HRF) providing two-dimensional flow maps of the retina and optic nerve head (Fig. 5.7C).[45] In this system, the HRF images a 2880 × 720 μm area of the retina or optic nerve, at a resolution of approximately 10 μm/pixel. After the scan is performed, the HRF computer performs a fast Fourier transform to extract the Doppler shift spectrum from each measured pixel of reflected light. The HRF device is simple to use and sensitive to small changes over time in the same eye. However, the flow measurements are displayed in arbitrary units and there is a lack of accuracy when dealing with very high and very low blood speeds. Furthermore, contributions to blood flow measurements from the underlying choriocapillaris cannot be excluded and previous experimental tests of the instrumentation have demonstrated that large-flow readings can be obtained from sample volumes even when they contain no moving cells.[43]

Doppler optical coherence tomography

OCT, first described by Huang et al. in 1991, uses interferometry to generate high-resolution cross-sectional images of the neurosensory retina.[46] Since the mid-1990s, Doppler measurements have been incorporated into prototype OCT imaging systems (Fig. 5.8).[10] In the original time-domain OCT systems, the blood velocity can be determined by measurement of the Doppler shift of the interference fringe frequency after Fourier transformation of the data, whereas, in newer spectral domain OCT systems, direct recording of the interference fringe frequency is possible. However, in this approach, blood velocity sensitivity and image spatial resolution are coupled and inversely related (increasing the velocity sensitivity decreases the spatial resolution). In order to overcome this limitation, a number of Doppler OCT prototypes utilize the phase change between sequential A-scans in order to generate information regarding the Doppler shift.[10] Although OCT can generate cross-sectional images of retinal blood flow, accurate quantification of this flow remains challenging: to achieve this it is necessary to measure the geometry of the vessel and, in particular, the Doppler angle. Furthermore, current Doppler OCT systems are limited in terms of the maximal velocities measurable, and in terms of the smallest vessel diameters measurable (capillary flow involves single erythrocyte movement rather than continuous fluid flow).

Conclusions

A number of commercial devices, allowing assessment of retinal blood flow, have been introduced. However, these devices have significant issues which have prevented their widespread adoption as of yet. The prospects for Doppler OCT appear good, yet it is still at an early stage in its development pathway. Furthermore, due to the complexity of retinal hemodynamics, extensive validation and reproducibility studies are required before acceptance of any new measurement approach.

SPECTRAL IMAGING – ASSESSMENT OF RETINAL OXYGENATION

Basic principles

Spectroscopy is the study of the interaction between any form of matter and radiated energy (e.g., visible light). By measuring radiation intensity as a function of wavelength, and through the identification of characteristic signatures, it is possible to determine the constituents of a material. For example, in astronomy, spectral analysis can be used to derive many properties of distant stars and galaxies. As well as its uses in remote sensing, spectroscopy has also been adapted for a number of laboratory-based applications. In biological systems, the combination of spectroscopy with conventional imaging techniques – "spectral imaging" – allows determination of the spatial distribution of spectroscopic data.[47] In clinical settings, the application of spectroscopic principles has been of particular use for oximetry – the measurement of oxygen saturation in a patient's blood. From as early as 1935, transillumination of the ear has been used as a method of continuously measuring oxygen saturation in human blood. The subsequent incorporation of plethysmography (the analysis of pulsatile components of the arterial cycle) has facilitated the development of pulse oximeters capable of measuring arterial oxygen saturation in isolation.

The use of spectral imaging to perform blood oximetry is dependent on assumptions about the relationship between light transmittance through the blood and its oxygen saturation.[47] According to the Lambert–Beer law, for any given wavelength of light, its transmittance through blood is dependent on the extinction coefficient of the blood (ε), the concentration of blood (c), and the path length (d) through which the light travels:

$$I_T = I_O 10^{-\varepsilon c d},$$

where I_T is the intensity of the light transmitted through the blood, and I_o is the intensity of incident light. By rearranging the equation, the extinction coefficient of blood (ε) can be seen to be proportional to the logarithm of (I_o/I_T), i.e., the optical density (OD):

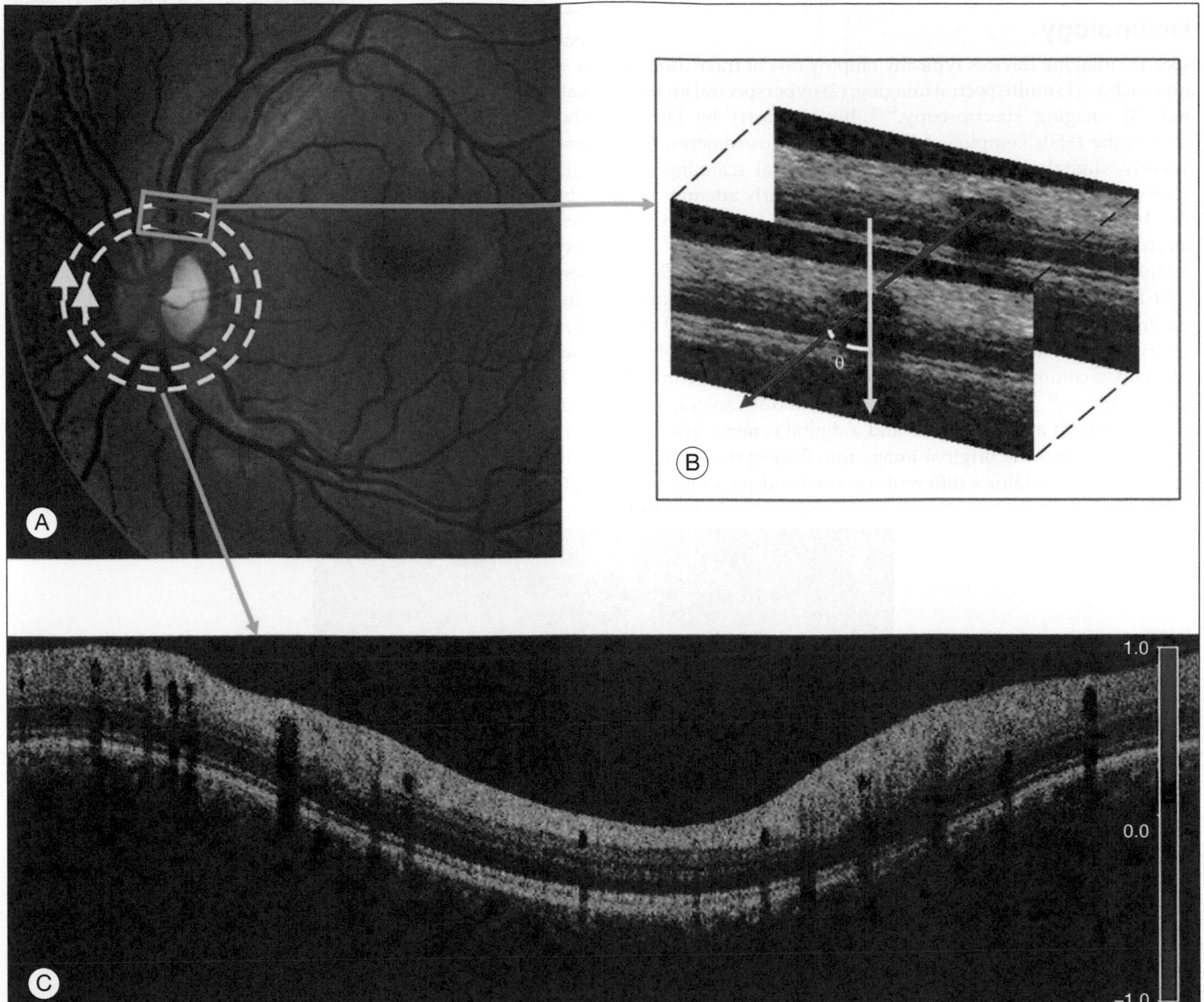

Fig. 5.8 Doppler optical coherence tomography (OCT). (A) Fundus photograph showing the double circular pattern of the OCT beam scanning retinal blood vessels emerging from the optic disc. (B) The relative position of a blood vessel in the two OCT cross-sections is used to calculate the Doppler angle θ between the beam and the blood vessel. (C) Color Doppler OCT image showing the unfolded cross-section from a circular scan. Arteries and veins can be distinguished by the direction of flow as determined by the signs (blue or red) of the Doppler shift and the angle θ. (Reproduced with permission from Wang Y, Fawzi AA, Varma R, et al. Pilot study of optical coherence tomography measurement of retinal blood flow in retinal and optic nerve diseases. Invest Ophthalmol Vis Sci 2011;52:841.)

$$\varepsilon cd = \log(I_O / I_T)$$
$$\varepsilon cd = OD$$

The extinction coefficient of blood (ε) is dependent on its main absorbing component, hemoglobin, which, in turn, is dependent on its oxygen concentration. As the extinction coefficient of blood varies with wavelength, analyzing the optical density of blood at multiple wavelengths compensates for variables such as the concentration and path length and ultimately allows estimation of oxygen levels in the blood (the exact details of these calculations are beyond the scope of this chapter, but have been reviewed in detail by Harris et al.).[48] However, in retinal oximetry, it is impractical to determine optical densities (and thus oxygen concentrations) through the measurement of light transmittance. Instead, measurements of light reflected from the retina are typically used:

$$OD_{vessel} = \log(I_V / I_R)$$

where I_V and I_R are the intensity of light reflected from the retinal vessel and adjacent retina respectively (retinal oximetry assumes that a large fraction of incident light is reflected back from the tissues surrounding the vessels). Although the principles described above require a number of assumptions that may not hold true in the real world, measurement of light reflected from the retina at multiple wavelengths, in this manner, forms the basis for a number of noninvasive retinal oximetry technologies.

Technology

Spectral imaging devices typically employ one of three different approaches: (1) multispectral imaging; (2) hyperspectral imaging; and (3) imaging spectroscopy.[47,48] Initial efforts by Hickam et al. in the 1950s[49] employed film-based fundus cameras; more recently, digital fundus cameras and confocal scanning laser ophthalmoscopes have also been employed. Early attempts have also been made at the utilization of OCT in association with spectral analysis techniques.

Multispectral imaging involves the measurement of reflected light from images obtained at discrete and somewhat narrow spectral bands. Adopting a similar approach to that first described by Beach et al.,[50] Hardarson et al. have developed Oxymap, a commercially available device approved for investigational usage.[51] This device consists of a fundus camera, which is coupled with a beam splitter and a digital camera. The beam splitter separates the original image into four optical channels, each of which contains a different narrow band-pass filter (each band-pass filter only allows light of specific wavelengths to pass). This simultaneously yields four fundus images, each with a specific wavelength of light. Specialized software automatically selects measurement points on these images and calculates the optical density of retinal vessels at two wavelengths, 605 nm and 586 nm (optical density is sensitive to oxygen saturation at 605 nm but not at 586 nm). The ratio of these optical densities is approximately linearly related to the hemoglobin oxygen concentration. The oximeter is then calibrated to yield relative oxygen saturation values. This approach has been shown to be sensitive to changes in oxygen concentration and to yield reproducible results. Other commercially available multispectral devices have also recently been described (Imedos UG, Jena, Germany).

Hyperspectral imaging involves the measurement of light from images obtained at narrow spectral bands over a contiguous spectral range. Mordant et al. have recently described the validation of a hyperspectral fundus camera for noninvasive retinal oximetry (Fig. 5.9).[52] In their system, a commercial fundus

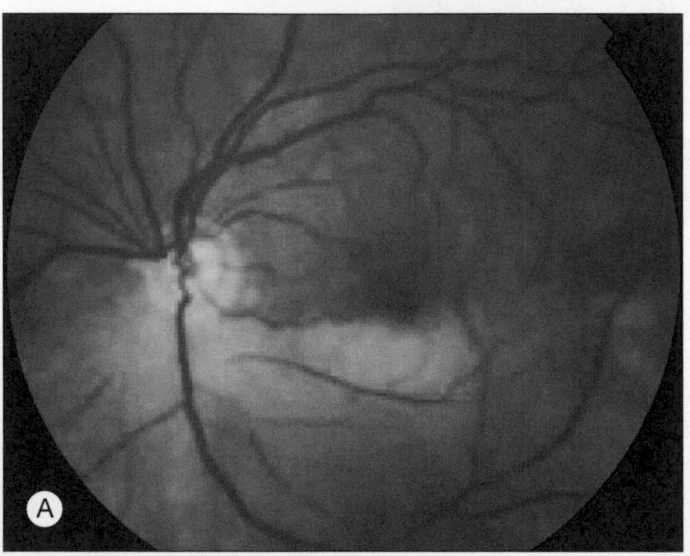

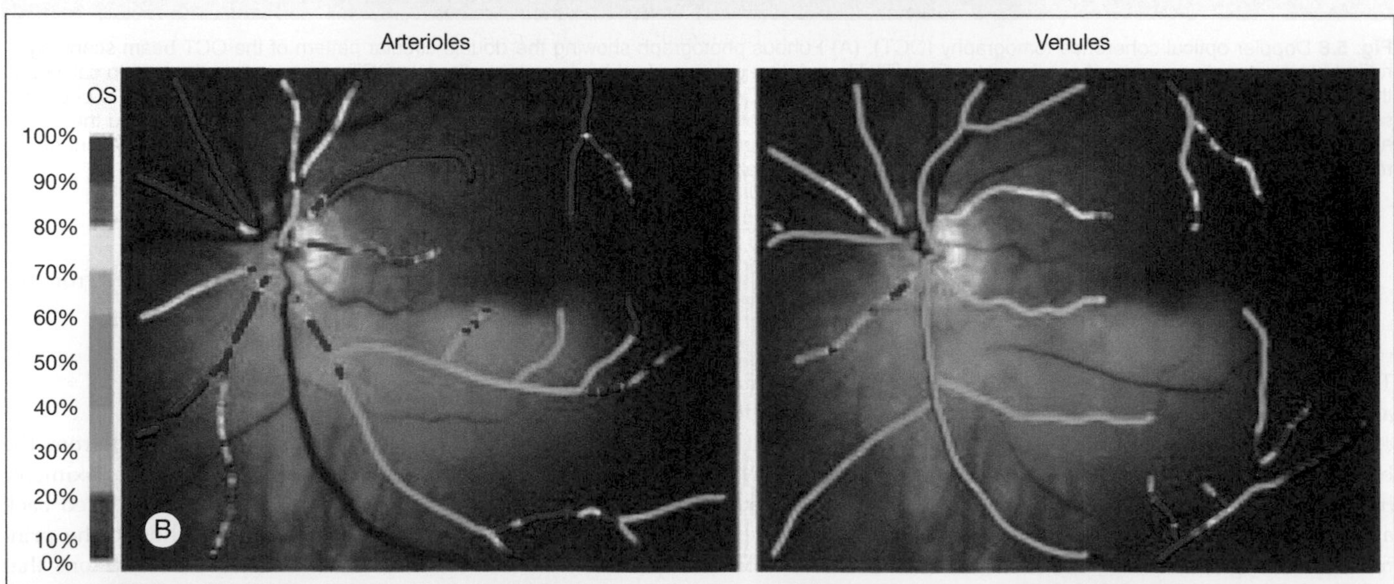

Fig. 5.9 Spectral imaging of the retina. (A) Color fundus photograph demonstrating a left inferotemporal branch retinal arteriole occlusion. (B) Pseudocolor oxim map showing abnormally low oxygen saturation within the affected inferotemporal retinal arteriole in contrast to the normal oxygen saturation levels in the unaffected superotemporal arteriole. The corresponding inferotemporal retinal venule has a normal level of oxygen saturation. (Reproduced with permission from Mordant DJ, Al-Abboud I, Muyo G, et al. Spectral imaging of the retina. Eye 2011;25:317.)

camera is linked to a liquid crystal tunable filter in the optical path of the camera's light source; this enables the electronic selection of a combination of desired wavelengths between 400 and 700 nm. A CCD camera is then used to record a sequence of spectral images between 500 and 650 nm in 2-nm increments (this process takes approximately 10–15 minutes in healthy volunteers). Further image processing and analysis then take place: the images are registered, the retinal vessel profiles extracted, and their optical densities estimated. Oxygen saturations can then be calculated. Use of hyperspectral imaging in this manner may provide more accurate measurements of oxygen saturation than two-wavelength multispectral approaches (such approaches have been reported to overestimate oxygen saturation). However, such an approach requires the use of sensitive detectors and powerful computers to enable fast and accurate processing of images.

A third method utilized for the noninvasive measurement of retinal oxygen saturation involves imaging spectroscopy. Schweitzer et al. have described an imaging ophthalmospectrometer, which consists of a modified fundus camera and an attached spectrograph.[53] The instrument illuminates the retina with a small slit of light and then simultaneous measurements are made at 76 different wavelengths in this discrete area using a spectrometer. This approach may be the most accurate; however, a major limitation is that measurements are made at one single cross-section of one or two retinal vessels. By contrast, a complete two-dimensional mapping of oxygen saturation in the retinal vascular tree is needed for clinical diagnostics.

Clinical applications

Using the Oxymap system, Hardarson and Stéfansson have evaluated retinal vasculature oxygen saturations in patients following CRVO and branch retinal vein occlusion (BRVO).[54,55] In patients with CRVO, they demonstrated that retinal venular oxygen saturation is lower than in fellow eyes. However, they also demonstrated considerable variability within and between CRVO eyes. Similarly, in patients with BRVO, they found considerable variability in oxygen saturation between patients. They found evidence of hypoxia in some patients but not others and speculated that this reflected variable disease severity in terms of degree of occlusion, recanalization, collateral circulation, and coexistent tissue atrophy. Hardarson et al. have also used this system to examine the effects of glaucoma filtration surgery, and topical antiglaucoma medications, on retinal vascular oxygen concentrations.[56]

Using the Imedos system, Hammer et al. found that, in patients with diabetes, increasing severity of retinopathy was associated with increased retinal venous oxygen saturations (from 63 ± 5% for mild nonproliferative retinopathy to 75 ± 8% for proliferative retinopathy). They suggest that these changes may occur secondary to the degeneration of capillary vascular beds with formation of arteriovenous shunt vessels.[57] Conversely, earlier work by Tiedeman et al. demonstrated evidence of increased oxygen consumption (i.e., decreased retinal venous oxygen saturation) in diabetic patients with acute hyperglycemia.[58]

Conclusions

Although major progress has been made in recent years, there is currently no consensus on the optimal method for measurement of oxygen saturation in the retinal vasculature. A number of spectral imaging devices provide relative, rather than absolute, measurements of oxygen saturation. Furthermore, all devices rely, to a certain extent, on biophotonic assumptions that may not hold true for in vivo imaging. Therefore, it is vital that detailed validation and reproducibility assessments be performed on all new retinal oximeters before such devices can be widely adopted for clinical or research purposes.

PHOTOACOUSTIC IMAGING – ASSESSMENT OF RETINAL ABSORPTION

Basic principles

In large part, contemporary retinal imaging modalities are based on the measurement of light reflected from the retina, e.g., fundus photography, SLO, OCT systems.[2] In contrast, no ophthalmic imaging modality exists that can directly measure the absorption of light by retinal tissues – information of potentially great significance. Assessment of optical absorption profiles at multiple wavelengths may improve the accuracy of retinal vascular oxygen saturation measurements (current "spectral imaging" determines optical density ratios indirectly, through the measurement of reflected light). Retinal absorption characteristics may also provide contrast for generation of enhanced retinal angiographic maps. Assessment of optical absorption could also be useful for providing contrast when imaging the highly pigmented RPE cell mosaic. Fortunately, through recent advances in microscopy, utilizing the photoacoustic effect, it has become possible to acquire optical absorption profiles in the context of noninvasive ophthalmic imaging – photoacoustic ophthalmoscopy (PAOM).[59,60]

The photoacoustic effect was first recognized by Alexander Graham Bell in the 1880s when he discovered that thin discs of selenium emit sound when exposed to a rapidly interrupted beam of sunlight. This phenomenon occurs as energy absorbed from the incident light is converted into kinetic energy, which results in local heating and, thus, generation of a pressure wave or sound. In the recently described photoacoustic microscopy (PAM),[61] a laser is used to irradiate a target tissue and thus induce ultrasonic pressure waves as a result of specific optical absorption. These pressure waves can then be recorded using a high-resolution ultrasonic transducer, and images generated. Through the integration of OCT technology with a laser-scanning, optical-resolution PAM, Jiao et al. have recently reported the use of PAOM in small animals.[59,60]

Technology

In the system developed by Jiao et al. the illumination source is a frequency-doubled, Q-switched, Nd:YAG laser, combined with the output laser beam of a fiber-based spectral domain OCT system, and then scanned across the retina using a galvanometer.[59] The photoacoustic waves induced from the retina are then detected by an ultrasonic transducer placed in contact with the eyelid (coupled by ultrasound gel). The resulting photoacoustic images can then be registered with the images generated from the integrated OCT system (Fig. 5.10). As with conventional OCT image sets, maximum-amplitude "projection" images can be generated from photoacoustic datasets allowing two-dimensional visualization of the retinal vasculature. Volumetric images can also be generated following automated segmentation of the RPE and retinal vessels. More recently, the same group has tested the acquisition of photoacoustic images in association with fundus autofluorescence signals (apart from generating heat, the

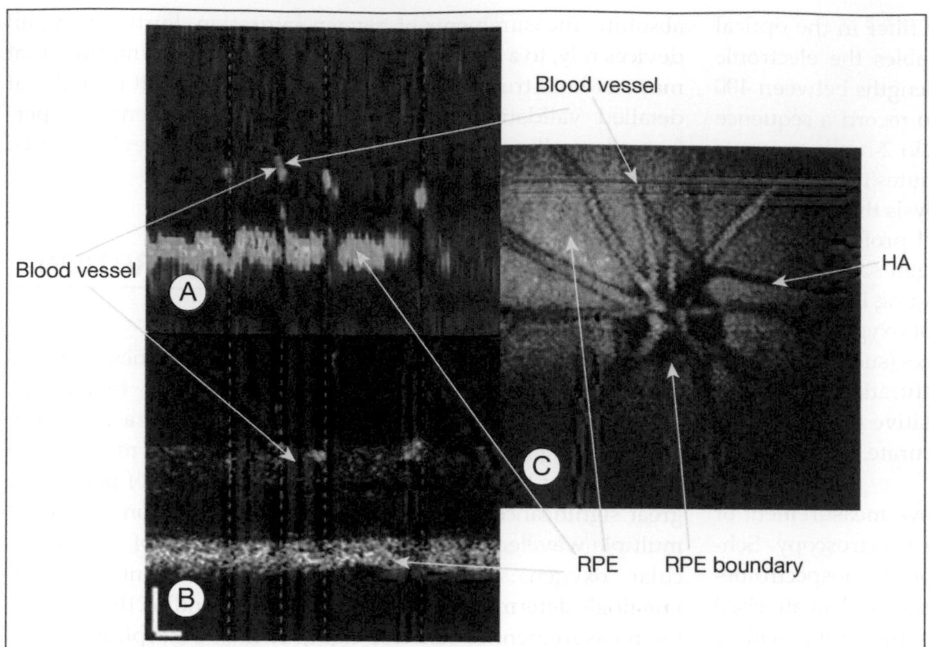

Fig. 5.10 Comparison of optical coherence tomography (OCT) and photoacoustic ophthalmoscopy (PAOM) images acquired simultaneously in vivo. (A) PAOM B-scan image in pseudocolor; (B) OCT B-scan image; (C) projection image of the PAOM data set. Scale: 100 μm. HA, hyaloid artery; RPE, retinal pigment epithelium. (Reproduced with permission from Jiao S, Jiang M, Hu J, et al. Photoacoustic ophthalmoscopy for in vivo retinal imaging. Optics Express 2010;18:3971.)

absorbed photons may undergo other physical processes, such as stimulating autofluorescence when fluorophores are present). Multimodal imaging in this manner may thus provide spatial information on the distribution of both melanin and lipofuscin via photoacoustic and autofluorescent signals respectively.[62]

Conclusions

The development of photoacoustic imaging techniques may greatly extend the scope of future retinal imaging; however, at present, the technology remains at an early stage in the development process. Much of the work to date, on photoacoustic imaging in the eye, has been performed in tissue samples or in animals. A number of technical hurdles remain before images will be obtained from living human subjects, or commercial, clinical devices introduced.

MAGNETIC RESONANCE IMAGING

As previously described, the acquisition of retinal images is largely dependent on optical techniques such as fundus photography. However, many such techniques are constrained by a relatively small field of view, and are often limited when there is disease-induced opacification of the ocular media, such as lens opacity or vitreous hemorrhage. In the clinical setting, these limitations are addressed, at least in part, by acoustic imaging techniques such as ultrasonography. More recently, however, advances in MRI offer the prospect of retinal application in humans.[63,64] In addition to a wide field of view, and the ability to acquire images despite media opacification, retinal MRI may also enable evaluation of novel functional parameters.

Basic principles

In MRI systems, a powerful magnetic field is applied to the body leading to alignment of the magnetization of its hydrogen nuclei or protons (the human body is largely made up of water molecules which contain two hydrogen atoms). Radiofrequency fields are then used to alter this alignment systematically, causing the protons to spin and producing a rotating magnetic field detectable by the scanner. Detectors in the MRI system then evaluate a number of parameters (e.g., spin density, spin–lattice relaxation time (T_1), spin–spin relaxation times (T_2)), which vary depending on the local tissue environment. As a result, soft tissue images can be generated. Image contrast may be further enhanced through the use of exogenous paramagnetic contrast agents such as gadolinium. In this manner, clinical MRI scanners can produce high-resolution images of the entire body, both noninvasively and in a single setting.[63]

As well as its anatomical imaging capability, MRI scanning can be used to measure blood flow.[63] MRI-derived quantification of blood flow may be performed by the use of exogenous intravenous contrast agents. However, it may also be performed noninvasively by magnetically labeling blood as a means of providing endogenous contrast. These techniques have been widely used to quantify blood flow to the brain and have been cross-validated using positron emission tomography. Relative blood oxygen saturations can also be measured using the blood oxygenation level-dependent (BOLD) technique. This technique detects differences in magnetic resonance signal intensity that arise from changes in the oxygen saturation of hemoglobin during brain activation – a local decrease in concentration of deoxygenated hemoglobin will increase the BOLD signal, while an increase will decrease the BOLD signal. In the brain, when a specific region is activated in response to stimulation, local blood flow increases in response to the increased metabolic demand; such increases in blood flow will provide a boost in oxygen delivery and thus decrease the concentration of deoxygenated hemoglobin. Techniques that measure blood flow and oxygenation can thus be used to image brain function noninvasively – functional MRI (fMRI).[63]

Retinal imaging

To date, most work on retinal imaging using magnetic resonance has been reported in animal studies (Fig. 5.11).[63] As the spatial resolution of MRI is limited compared to that of OCT and other

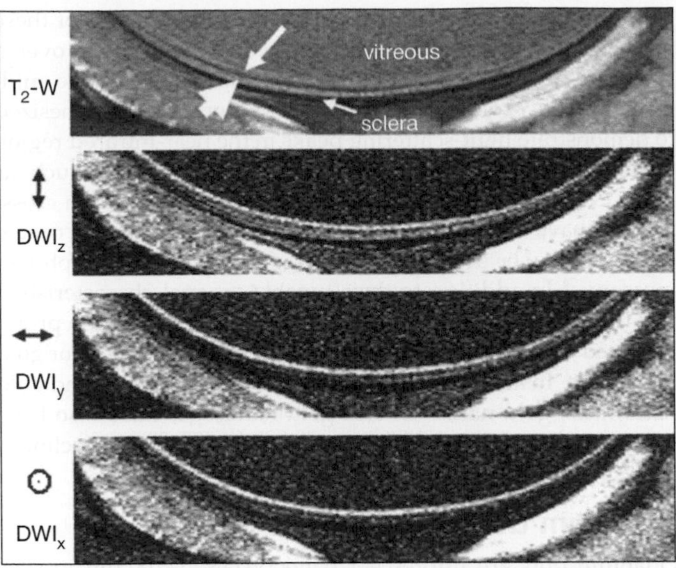

Fig. 5.11 Magnetic resonance imaging (MRI) of the retina in vivo. Higher-resolution T_2-weighted (TE = 40 ms) and diffusion-weighted (b = 504 s/mm^2) images at 50 × 100 μm resolution. Diffusion-sensitizing gradients were placed along the *x*, *y*, or *z* axis separately. The small and large white arrows indicate the "inner" and "outer" strips, respectively. (Reproduced with permission from Shen Q, Cheng H, Pardue MT, et al. Magnetic resonance imaging of tissue and vascular layers in the cat retina. J Magn Reson Imaging 2006;23:470.)

optical imaging modalities, current magnetic resonance-derived retinal imaging only allows delineation of three to four distinct retinal layers. Using gadolinium for contrast provides increased signal from the retinal and choroidal vasculature and thus aids in correlation of MRI retinal scans with histological sections (the avascular photoreceptor layers do not show any enhancements using this method). Manganese has also been used as a contrast agent to improve the anatomic contrast between layers; using this approach, it has been possible to reveal seven distinct retinal bands of alternating hypo- and hyperintensity.[63]

In 2008, the first report of retinal blood flow assessment in rats, using MRI, was published.[65] In this study, arterial spin labeling was used to quantify basal blood flow levels and their responses to physiological stimulation. With the improvements in spatial resolution afforded by new MRI devices, visualization of both retinal and choroidal blood flow has become possible. In animals, using BOLD fMRI techniques, differential responses of the retinal and choroidal circulations to physiological stimuli (e.g., hyperoxia versus hypercapnia) have been demonstrated.[63] In animal studies, BOLD fMRI responses have also been assessed in response to visual stimuli. The results of these studies suggest evidence that retinal vessels were very responsive to visual stimulation but choroidal vessels only showed small percentage changes.

Conclusions

Translation of retinal MRI from animal studies to human research and clinical practice faces a number of obstacles. The MRI scanners available in clinical environments currently have limited spatial resolutions and low signal-to-noise ratios. In addition, the issue of eye movements in awake humans is a major limiting factor. As a first step in addressing these issues, the feasibility of multimodal MRI has recently been tested on anesthetized large, nonhuman primates (baboons) using a standard clinical scanner.[66] Studies of this nature allow optimization of MRI scanning parameters and represent a first step towards magnetic resonance-derived retinal imaging in humans. Zhang et al. have recently demonstrated, for the first time, the use of BOLD fMRI to examine the changes associated with oxygen and carbogen challenges in the unanesthetized human retina.[67] Although much work has still to be done, such imaging may prove a useful adjunct to more established optical imaging methods, particularly when assessing the differential regulation of the retinal and choroidal circulations.

NANOTECHNOLOGY

Basic principles

Nanotechnology involves the creation and use of materials and devices on a nanometer scale, i.e., at the size scale of intracellular structures and molecules.[68] To comprehend the implications of nanotechnology adequately, it is necessary to appreciate the relative sizes of important biological structures. For example: macrophages are approximately 21 000 nm in diameter; red blood cells are approximately 7000 nm in diameter; cone photoreceptors measure between 500 and 4000 nm in diameter; the smallest single cellular organisms (bacteria of the genus *Mycoplasma*) are 200 nm in diameter; a strand of DNA is approximately 2 nm in diameter; and the smallest molecule, H_2, is less than 1/10 of 1 nm in size. According to the National Nanotechnology Initiative, nanoparticles are those with a diameter ranging from 1 to 100 nm (within the biomedical community, slightly larger particles are often defined as nanoparticles owing to a similarity in size to important naturally occurring agents, such as viruses).[69] At these dimensions, nanoparticles show unique properties that seem surprising but are, in fact, attributable to the principles of quantum mechanics. As a result of these effects, slight deviations in the size, shape, and organization of nanoparticles can have profound effects on their properties.

The engineering of nanomaterials and/or devices, and their application in "nanomedicine," are likely to alter profoundly our approach to disease, with significant advances in biopharmaceuticals (e.g., drug design and delivery), implantable materials and devices (e.g., tissue regeneration scaffolds), and diagnostic tools (e.g., genetic testing and imaging).[68,69] In ophthalmology, the use of nanoparticles shows particular promise for use as contrast agents in retinal imaging. Nanoparticles can be "functionalized" (i.e., conjugated with targeting ligands) to facilitate their precise and specific targeting. During their synthesis, the properties of nanoparticles can also be finely tuned for use with multiple imaging modalities. Finally, the biocompatibility of many nanoparticles has been established and, thus, the potential exists for their translation to clinical settings. In this section, we provide an overview of the properties and translation imaging potential for a number of nanoparticle groups.

Iron oxide nanoparticles

Magnetic nanoparticles are particularly attractive for magnetic resonance-derived imaging.[68,69] MRI is based on the behavior, alignment, and interaction of protons in the presence of a magnetic field (see above). Within a strong magnetic field, protons are perturbed; magnetic nanoparticles can then be used to alter their longitudinal (T_1) or transverse (T_2) relaxation times and, thus, image contrast is generated. Superparamagnetic iron oxide

(SPIO) nanoparticles have large magnetic moments and are well suited as T_2 contrast agents in this context. A significant benefit associated with SPIO nanoparticles is their biocompatibility and ready detection at moderate concentrations; as a result, SPIO nanoparticles have been approved by the Food and Drug Administration for use in clinical practice and are now commercially available (e.g., ferucarbotran: Resovist, Bayer, Germany).

Gold nanoparticles

Due to the phenomenon of localized surface plasmon resonance – the collective oscillation of their conduction electrons in the presence of an incident light – gold nanoparticles can show strong extinction peaks in the visible and near-infrared regions of the electromagnetic spectrum (in simple terms, they are capable of scattering or absorbing large amounts of light when illuminated). As a result, gold nanoparticles are particularly well suited for use as contrast agents in optical imaging.[70]

Colloidal gold (suspensions of gold nanoparticles in fluid) has been used for hundreds of years to impart vibrant colors to the stained-glass windows of Gothic churches, and for many decades in the treatment of patients with rheumatoid arthritis.[68] Since 1971, when Faulk and Taylor[71] invented the immunogold staining procedure, colloidal gold has also been widely used in laboratory settings, with the optical (and electron beam) contrast qualities of gold providing excellent detection qualities for techniques such as immunoblotting, flow cytometry, and hybridization assays.[72] More recently, the creation of a new form of nanoparticle – gold nanoshells – has reignited interest in gold nanoparticles as contrast agents for clinical imaging (Fig. 5.12).[73] Gold nanoshells consist of a dielectric core (typically silica), surrounded by a thin gold shell. Unlike colloidal gold, the optical resonance of these nanoshells can be precisely and systematically varied over a broad range, extending from the near-ultraviolet to the mid-infrared. Thus, gold nanoshells can be designed and synthesized to demonstrate light-scattering peaks in the near-infrared region commonly utilized by ophthalmic imaging systems such as OCT. Conversely, gold nanoshells with large absorption cross-sections have been used for photothermal destruction of cancer cells, and may be useful in the future for photoacoustic ophthalmoscopy.[74] In addition to their tunable spectral characteristics, and their putative biocompatibility, the same conjugation protocols used to functionalize colloidal gold can also be used for gold nanoshells. In addition to spherical gold nanoparticles and gold nanoshells, gold nanorods and gold nanocages have also been investigated as contrast agents for optical imaging in preclinical settings.[75]

Quantum dots

Quantum dots are fluorescent nanocrystals, 1–100 nm in size, with unique optical and electrical properties, and with a synthetic history of approximately 20 years.[68,69] Quantum dots commonly consist of a metalloid crystalline core (e.g., cadmium selenide) surrounded by a shell (e.g., zinc sulfide). The fluorescent properties of quantum dots offer a number of advantages for their use in optical imaging. The brightness of quantum dots is 10–100 times greater than most organic dyes or proteins. Quantum dots also show broad absorption characteristics with narrow-emission spectra that are continuous and tunable due to quantum size effects. Quantum dots also possess a long fluorescence lifetime and undergo negligible photobleaching. Most importantly perhaps, quantum dots can be labeled to allow

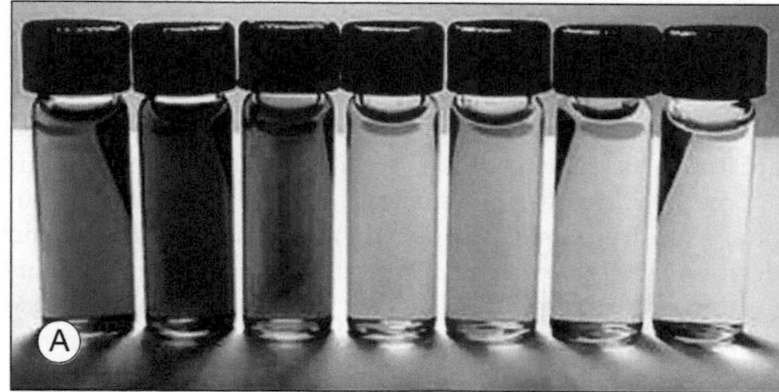

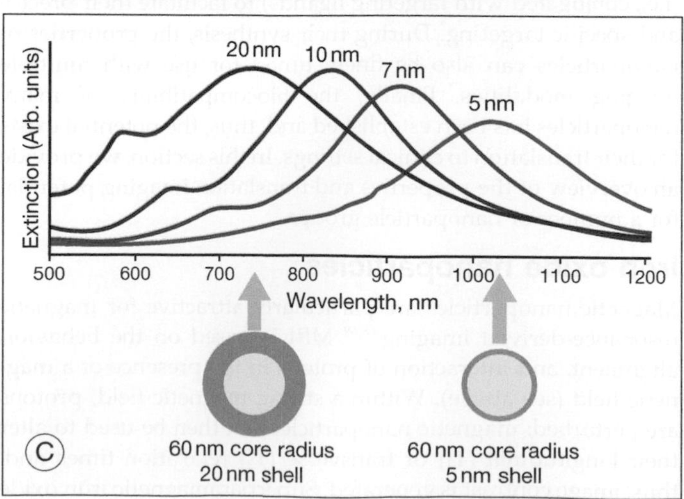

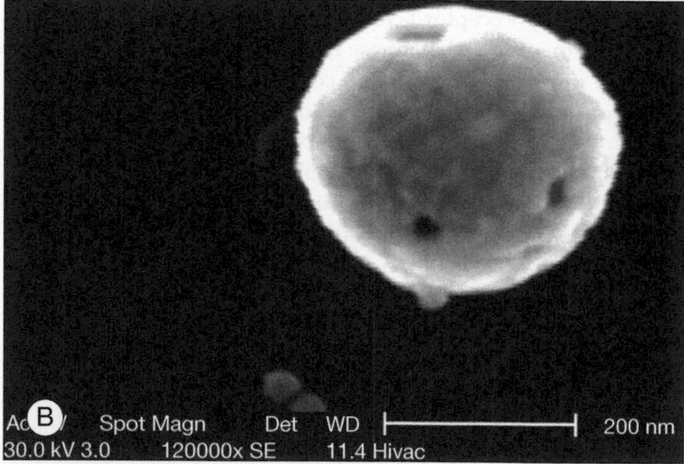

Fig. 5.12 Gold nanoparticles, such as nanoshells, may be of use as contrast agents for clinical imaging. (A) Visual demonstration of the tunability of metal nanoshells. (Reproduced with permission from Loo C, Lin A, Hirsch L, et al. Nanoshell-enabled photonics-based imaging and therapy of cancer. Technol Cancer Res Treat 2004;3:34.) (B) Scanning electron microscopy image of nanoshell with 291-nm core diameter and 15-nm shell thickness. (Reproduced with permission from Agrawal A, Huang S, Wei Haw Lin A, et al. Quantitative evaluation of optical coherence tomography signal enhancement with gold nanoshells. J Biomed Opt 2006;11:041121–2.) (C) Optical resonances of gold shell-silica core nanoshells as a function of their core/shell ratio. Respective spectra correspond to the nanoparticles depicted beneath. (Reproduced with permission from Loo C, Lin A, Hirsch L, et al. Nanoshell-enabled photonics-based imaging and therapy of cancer. Technol Cancer Res Treat 2004;3:34.)

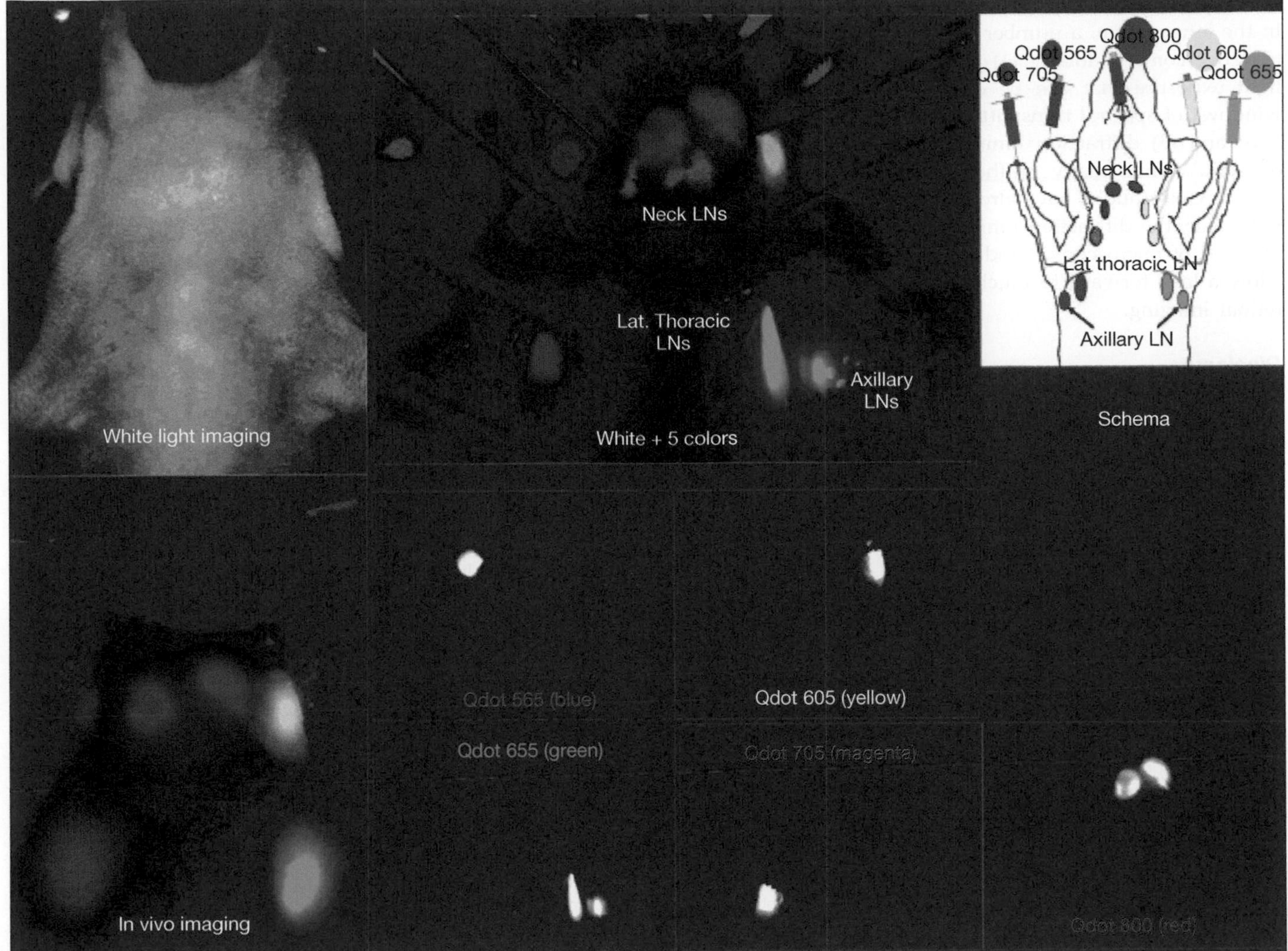

Fig. 5.13 In vivo and intrasurgical spectral fluorescence imaging of a mouse injected with five-carboxyl quantum dots (565, blue; 605, yellow; 655, green; 705, magenta; 800, red), intracutaneously into the middle digits of the bilateral upper extremities, the bilateral ears, and at the median chin, as shown in the schema. Five primary draining lymph nodes were simultaneously visualized with different colors through the skin in the in vivo image and are more clearly seen in the image taken at the surgery. (Reproduced with permission from Kobayashi H, Hama Y, Koyama Y, et al. Simultaneous multicolor imaging of five different lymphatic basins using quantum dots. Nano Lett 2007;7:1714.)

precise targeting of cellular structures. As a result of these features, quantum dots are increasingly being used for in vivo imaging in animal studies (Fig. 5.13), although concerns about cytotoxicity must be addressed before they will be suitable for use in humans.

Conclusions

A large number of other nanoparticle groups are currently being investigated for their biomedical potential, with examples including carbon nanotubes, dendrimers, perfluorocarbons, and lipid-based nanoparticles.[69] The unique and tunable optical properties of many nanoparticles, along with their small size and capacity for cellular targeting, make them strong candidates for use as contrast agents in retinal imaging. Using these agents in combination with techniques such as OCT may ultimately allow visualization of many retinal structures (e.g., Müller cells) and cellular processes (e.g., apoptosis) in clinical practice. While such usage has yet to be demonstrated in humans, the previous commercialization of magnetic nanoparticles for MRI and the early clinical trials of gold nanoparticle therapy in humans provide grounds for optimism in this regard.

CONCLUSIONS AND FUTURE DIRECTIONS

In the past 25 years, advances in retinal imaging have revolutionized the diagnosis and management of retinal disease. As recently as 1990, the conventional wisdom held that axial image resolution was fundamentally constrained by geometric optics and the depth of focus.[6] However, with the advent of OCT, axial resolution has now been improved 1000-fold over that previously thought possible. In the short to medium term, continued advances in OCT will be coupled with advances in adaptive optics technology to provide unprecedented noninvasive cellular imaging. In parallel with this, functional extensions of these and other imaging modalities will provide greatly enhanced information regarding parameters such as retinal blood flow and oxygenation. Increasing use of nanotechnology may provide "molecular" imaging capabilities, and allow evaluation of biochemical processes such as apoptosis. In the longer term, a number of fundamental limits will need to be overcome, including: (1) constraints imposed by maximum light exposure that can be delivered safely to the eye; (2) windows of spectral transmittance imposed by the cornea and lens; and (3) diffraction limits imposed by the wave nature of light.[6] While many of these barriers seem impenetrable, early breakthroughs have already taken place in each area. In particular, the diffraction limit has already been surpassed in the field of microscopy,[75] and the use of such techniques may allow a leap forward to much smaller spatial scales in future retinal imaging.

Disclosure

Dr Keane has received a proportion of his funding from the UK Department of Health's National Institute for Health Research Biomedical Research Centre for Ophthalmology at Moorfields Eye Hospital and University College London Institute of Ophthalmology. The views expressed in the publication are those of the authors and not necessarily those of the Department of Health.

Dr Sadda is a co-inventor of Doheny intellectual property related to optical coherence tomography that has been licensed by Topcon Medical Systems, and is a member of the scientific advisory board for Heidelberg Engineering. Dr Sadda also receives research support from Carl Zeiss Meditec, Optos, and Optovue, Inc.

REFERENCES

1. Keane PA, Sadda SR. Imaging chorioretinal vascular disease. Eye (Lond) 2010;24:422–7.
2. Yannuzzi LA, Ober MD, Slakter JS, et al. Ophthalmic fundus imaging: today and beyond. Am J Ophthalmol 2004;137:511–24.
3. Bennett TJ, Barry C. Ophthalmic imaging today: an ophthalmic photographer's viewpoint - a review. Clin Exp Ophthalmol 2009;37:2–13.
4. Yannuzzi LA. Indocyanine green angiography: a perspective on use in the clinical setting. Am J Ophthalmol 2011;151:745–51.
5. Roorda A. Adaptive optics ophthalmoscopy. J Refract Surg 2000;16:S602–607.
6. Williams DR. Imaging single cells in the living retina. Vision Res 2011;51: 1371–96.
7. Liang J, Williams DR, Miller DT. Supernormal vision and high-resolution retinal imaging through adaptive optics. J Opt Soc Am A 1997;14: 2884–92.
8. Kitaguchi Y, Fujikado T, Bessho K, et al. Adaptive optics fundus camera to examine localized changes in the photoreceptor layer of the fovea. Ophthalmology 2008;115:1771–7.
9. Roorda A, Romero-Borja F, Donnelly W III. Adaptive optics scanning laser ophthalmoscopy. Optics Express 2002;10:405–12.
10. Drexler W, Fujimoto JG. State-of-the-art retinal optical coherence tomography. Progr Retinal eye res 2008;27:45–88.
11. Miller DT, Kocaoglu OP, Wang Q, et al. Adaptive optics and the eye (super resolution OCT). Eye (Lond) 2011;25:321–30.
12. Fernández EJ, Hermann B, Povazay B, et al. Ultrahigh resolution optical coherence tomography and pancorrection for cellular imaging of the living human retina. Optics Express 2008;16:11083–94.
13. Zawadzki RJ, Cense B, Zhang Y, et al. Ultrahigh-resolution optical coherence tomography with monochromatic and chromatic aberration correction. Optics Express 2008;16:8126–43.
14. Poonja S, Patel S, Henry L, et al. Dynamic visual stimulus presentation in an adaptive optics scanning laser ophthalmoscope. J Refract Surg 2005;21: S575–580.
15. Vogel CR, Arathorn DW, Roorda A, et al. Retinal motion estimation in adaptive optics scanning laser ophthalmoscopy. Optics Express 2006;14: 487–97.
16. Arathorn DW, Yang Q, Vogel CR, et al. Retinally stabilized cone-targeted stimulus delivery. Optics Express 2007;15:13731–44.
17. Miller DT, Williams DR, Morris GM, et al. Images of cone photoreceptors in the living human eye. Vision Res 1996;36:1067–79.
18. Roorda A, Williams DR. The arrangement of the three cone classes in the living human eye. Nature 1999;397:520–2.
19. Chui TY, Song H, Burns SA. Individual variations in human cone photoreceptor packing density: variations with refractive error. Invest Ophthalmol Vis Sci 2008;49:4679–87.
20. Doble N, Choi SS, Codona JL, et al. In vivo imaging of the human rod photoreceptor mosaic. Optics lett 2011;36:31–3.
21. Roorda A, Zhang Y, Duncan JL. High-resolution in vivo imaging of the RPE mosaic in eyes with retinal disease. Invest Ophthalmol Vis Sci 2007;48: 2297–303.
22. Gray DC, Merigan W, Wolfing JI, et al. In vivo fluorescence imaging of primate retinal ganglion cells and retinal pigment epithelial cells. Optics Express 2006;14:7144–58.
23. Martin J, Roorda A. Direct and noninvasive assessment of parafoveal capillary leukocyte velocity. Ophthalmology 2005;112:2219–24.
24. Zhong Z, Petrig BL, Qi X, et al. In vivo measurement of erythrocyte velocity and retinal blood flow using adaptive optics scanning laser ophthalmoscopy. Optics Express 2008;16:12746–56.
25. Doble N. High-resolution, in vivo retinal imaging using adaptive optics and its future role in ophthalmology. Expert Rev Med Devices 2005;2: 205–16.
26. Gray DC, Wolfe R, Gee BP, et al. In vivo imaging of the fine structure of rhodamine-labeled macaque retinal ganglion cells. Invest Ophthalmol Vis Sci 2008;49:467–73.
27. Wolfing JI, Chung M, Carroll J, et al. High-resolution retinal imaging of cone-rod dystrophy. Ophthalmology 2006;113:1019 e1011.
28. Duncan JL, Talcott KE, Ratnam K, et al. Cone structure in retinal degeneration associated with mutations in the peripherin/RDS gene. Invest Ophthalmol Vis Sci 2011;52:1557–66.
29. Duncan JL, Zhang Y, Gandhi J, et al. High-resolution imaging with adaptive optics in patients with inherited retinal degeneration. Invest Ophthalmol Vis Sci 2007;48:3283–91.
30. Carroll J. Adaptive optics retinal imaging: applications for studying retinal degeneration. Arch Ophthalmol 2008;126:857–8.
31. Talcott KE, Ratnam K, Sundquist SM, et al. Longitudinal study of cone photoreceptors during retinal degeneration and in response to ciliary neurotrophic factor treatment. Invest Ophthalmol Vis Sci 2011;52:2219–26.
32. Kitaguchi Y, Bessho K, Yamaguchi T, et al. In vivo measurements of cone photoreceptor spacing in myopic eyes from images obtained by an adaptive optics fundus camera. Jpn J Ophthalmol 2007;51:456–61.
33. Carroll J, Neitz M, Hofer H, et al. Functional photoreceptor loss revealed with adaptive optics: an alternate cause of color blindness. Proc Natl Acad Sci U S A 2004;101:8461–6.
34. Marmor MF, Choi SS, Zawadzki RJ, et al. Visual insignificance of the foveal pit: reassessment of foveal hypoplasia as fovea plana. Arch Ophthalmol 2008;126:907–13.
35. Joeres S, Jones SM, Chen DC, et al. Retinal imaging with adaptive optics scanning laser ophthalmoscopy in unexplained central ring scotoma. Arch Ophthalmol 2008;126:543–7.
36. Choi SS, Zawadzki RJ, Keltner JL, et al. Changes in cellular structures revealed by ultra-high resolution retinal imaging in optic neuropathies. Invest Ophthalmol Vis Sci 2008;49:2103–19.
37. Ciulla TA, Regillo CD, Harris A. Retina and optic nerve imaging. Philadelphia: Lippincott Williams & Wilkins; 2003.
38. Williamson TH, Harris A. Ocular blood flow measurement. Br J Ophthalmol 1994;78:939–45.
39. Schmetterer L, Garhofer G. How can blood flow be measured? Surv Ophthalmol 2007;52(Suppl 2):S134–138.
40. Harris A, Chung H, Ciulla T, et al. Progress in measurement of ocular blood flow and relevance to our understanding of glaucoma and age-related macular degeneration. Prog Retin Eye Res 1999;18:669–87.
41. Keyser BJ, Flaharty PM, Sergott RC, et al. Color Doppler imaging of arterial blood flow in central retinal vein occlusion. Ophthalmology 1994;101: 1357–61.
42. Ho AC, Lieb WE, Flaharty PM, et al. Color Doppler imaging of the ocular ischemic syndrome. Ophthalmology 1992;99:1453–62.
43. Feke G, Yoshida A. Laser based instruments for ocular blood flow assessment. J Biomed Optics 1998;3:415–22.
44. Yoshida A, Feke GT, Mori F, et al. Reproducibility and clinical application of a newly developed stabilized retinal laser Doppler instrument. Am J Ophthalmol 2003;135:356–61.
45. Sehi M. Basic technique and anatomically imposed limitations of confocal scanning laser Doppler flowmetry at the optic nerve head level. Acta Ophthalmol 2011;89:e1–11.
46. Huang D, Swanson E, Lin C, et al. Optical coherence tomography. Science 1991;254:1178–81.
47. Mordant DJ, Al-Abboud I, Muyo G, et al. Spectral imaging of the retina. Eye (Lond) 2011;25:309–20.
48. Harris A, Dinn RB, Kagemann L, et al. A review of methods for human retinal oximetry. Ophthalm Surg Lasers Imaging 2003;34:152–64.
49. Hickam JB, Sieker HO, Frayser R. . Studies of retinal circulation and A-V oxygen difference in man. Trans Am Clin Climatol Assoc 1959;71:34–44.
50. Beach JM, Schwenzer KJ, Srinivas S, et al. Oximetry of retinal vessels by dual-wavelength imaging: calibration and influence of pigmentation. J Appl Physiol 1999;86:748–58.
51. Hardarson SH, Harris A, Karlsson RA, et al. Automatic retinal oximetry. Invest Ophthalmol Vis Sci 2006;47:5011–6.
52. Mordant DJ, Al-Abboud I, Muyo G, et al. Validation of human whole blood oximetry, using a hyperspectral fundus camera with a model eye. Invest Ophthalmol Vis Sci 2011;52:2851–9.
53. Schweitzer D, Hammer M, Kraft J, et al. In vivo measurement of the oxygen saturation of retinal vessels in healthy volunteers. IEEE Trans Biomed Eng 1999;46:1454–65.
54. Hardarson SH, Stefánsson E. Oxygen saturation in central retinal vein occlusion. Am J Ophthalmol 2010;150:871–5.

55. Hardarson SH, Stefánsson E. Oxygen saturation in branch retinal vein occlusion. Acta Ophthalmol 2011. Epub ahead of print April 21, 2011; doi: 10.1111/j.1755-3768.2011.02109.x.
56. Hardarson SH, Gottfredsdottir MS, Halldorsson GH, et al. Glaucoma filtration surgery and retinal oxygen saturation. Invest Ophthalmol Vis Sci 2009;50: 5247–50.
57. Hammer M, Vilser W, Riemer T, et al. Diabetic patients with retinopathy show increased retinal venous oxygen saturation. Graefe's Arch Clin Exp Ophthalmol 2009;247:1025–30.
58. Tiedeman JS, Kirk SE, Srinivas S, et al. Retinal oxygen consumption during hyperglycemia in patients with diabetes without retinopathy. Ophthalmology 1998;105:31–6.
59. Jiao S, Jiang M, Hu J, et al. Photoacoustic ophthalmoscopy for in vivo retinal imaging. Optics Express 2010;18:3967–72.
60. Jiao S, Xie Z, Zhang HF, et al. Simultaneous multimodal imaging with integrated photoacoustic microscopy and optical coherence tomography. Optics Lett 2009;34:2961–3.
61. Zhang HF, Maslov K, Stoica G, et al. Functional photoacoustic microscopy for high-resolution and noninvasive in vivo imaging. Nature Biotechnol 2006;24: 848–51.
62. Zhang X, Jiang M, Fawzi AA, et al. Simultaneous dual molecular contrasts provided by the absorbed photons in photoacoustic microscopy. Optics lett 2010;35:4018–20.
63. Duong TQ. Magnetic resonance imaging of the retina: a brief historical and future perspective. Saudi J Ophthalmol 2011;25:137–43.
64. Duong TQ, Muir ER. Magnetic resonance imaging of the retina. Jpn J Ophthalmol 2009;53:352–67.
65. Li Y, Cheng H, Duong TQ. Blood-flow magnetic resonance imaging of the retina. Neuroimage 2008;39:1744–51.
66. Zhang Y, Wey HY, Nateras OS, et al. Anatomical, blood oxygenation level-dependent, and blood flow MRI of nonhuman primate (baboon) retina. Magn Resonance Med 2011;66:546–54.
67. Zhang Y, Peng Q, Kiel JW, et al. Magnetic resonance imaging of vascular oxygenation changes during hyperoxia and carbogen challenges in the human retina. Invest Ophthalmol Vis Sci 2011;52:286–91.
68. Zarbin MA, Montemagno C, Leary JF, et al. Nanomedicine in ophthalmology: the new frontier. Am J Ophthalmol 2010;150:144–62.
69. Nune SK, Gunda P, Thallapally PK, et al. Nanoparticles for biomedical imaging. Expert Opin Drug Deliv 2009;6:1175–94.
70. Arvizo R, Bhattacharya R, Mukherjee P. Gold nanoparticles: opportunities and challenges in nanomedicine. Expert Opin Drug Deliv 2010;7:753–63.
71. Faulk WP, Taylor GM. An immunocolloid method for the electron microscope. Immunochemistry 1971;8:1081–3.
72. Roth J. The silver anniversary of gold: 25 years of the colloidal gold marker system for immunocytochemistry and histochemistry. Histochem Cell Biol 1996;106:1–8.
73. Loo C, Lin A, Hirsch L, et al. Nanoshell-enabled photonics-based imaging and therapy of cancer. Technol Cancer Res Treat 2004;3:33–40.
74. Gobin AM, Lee MH, Halas NJ, et al. Near-infrared resonant nanoshells for combined optical imaging and photothermal cancer therapy. Nano Lett 2007;7:1929–34.
75. Murphy CJ, Gole AM, Stone JW, et al. Gold nanoparticles in biology: beyond toxicity to cellular imaging. Acc Chem Res 2008;41:1721–30.
76. Betzig E, Patterson GH, Sougrat R, et al. Imaging intracellular fluorescent proteins at nanometer resolution. Science 2006;313:1642–5.

Chapter 6

Image Processing

Michael Abràmoff, Christine N. Kay

INTRODUCTION

In this review, we discuss quantitative approaches to retinal image analysis. Special emphasis is placed on familiarizing the reader with basic concepts in imaging and image analysis. Fundus and optical coherence tomography (OCT) image analysis are reviewed as well as the use of these modalities in providing comprehensive descriptions of retinal morphology and function. We discuss screening-motivated computer-aided detection of retinal lesions as well as translational clinical applications in diagnosis and therapy.

After reading this chapter the reader should be able to understand concepts in retinal image analysis, and critically review the clinical impact of the research in this field.

HISTORY OF RETINAL IMAGING

The optical properties of the eye that allow image formation prevent direct inspection of the retina. Though existence of the red reflex has been known for centuries, special techniques are needed to obtain a focused image of the retina. The first attempt to image the retina, in a cat, was completed by the French physician Jean Mery, who showed that if a live cat is immersed in water, its retinal vessels are visible from the outside.[1] The impracticality of such an approach for humans led to the invention of the principles of the ophthalmoscope in 1823 by Czech scientist Jan Evangelista Purkyně (frequently spelled Purkinje) and its reinvention in 1845 by Charles Babbage.[2,3] Finally, the ophthalmoscope was reinvented yet again and reported by von Helmholtz in 1851.[4] Thus, inspection and evaluation of the retina became routine for ophthalmologists, and the first images of the retina (Fig. 6.1) were published by the Dutch ophthalmologist van Trigt in 1853.[5] The first useful photographic images of the retina, showing blood vessels, were obtained in 1891 by the German ophthalmologist Gerloff.[6] In 1910, Gullstrand developed the fundus camera, a concept still used to image the retina today[7]; he later received the Nobel Prize for this invention. Because of its safety and cost-effectiveness at documenting retinal abnormalities, fundus imaging has remained the primary method of retinal imaging.

In 1961, Novotny and Alvis published their findings on fluorescein angiographic imaging.[8] In this imaging modality, a fundus camera with additional narrow-band filters is used to image a fluorescent dye injected into the bloodstream that binds to leukocytes. It remains widely used, because it allows an understanding of the functional state of the retinal circulation.

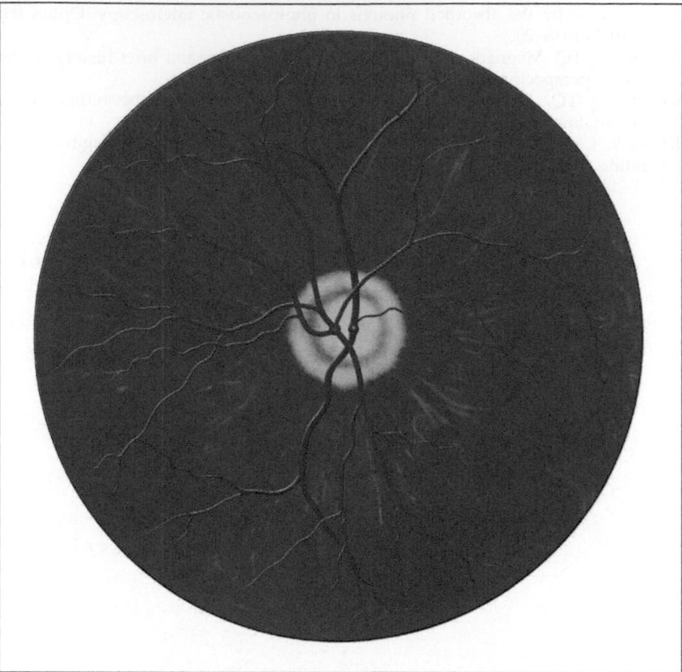

Fig. 6.1 First known image of human retina, as drawn by van Trigt in 1853. (Reproduced from Trigt AC. Dissertatio ophthalmologica inauguralis de speculo oculi. Utrecht: Universiteit van Utrecht, 1853.)

The initial approach to depict the three-dimensional (3D) shape of the retina was stereo fundus photography, as first described by Allen in 1964, where multiangle images of the retina are combined by the human observer into a 3D shape.[9] Subsequently, confocal scanning laser ophthalmoscopy (SLO) was developed, using the confocal aperture to obtain multiple images of the retina at different confocal depths, yielding estimates of 3D shape. However, the optics of the eye limit the depth resolution of confocal imaging to approximately 100 µm, which is poor when compared with the typical 300–500 µm thickness of the whole retina.[10]

OCT, first described in 1987 as a method for time-of-flight measurement of the depth of mechanical structures,[11,12] was later extended to a tissue-imaging technique. This method of determining the position of structures in tissue, described by Huang et al. in 1991,[13] was termed OCT. In 1993 in vivo retinal OCT was accomplished for the first time.[14] Today, OCT has become a prominent biomedical tissue-imaging technique, especially in the eye, because it is particularly suited to ophthalmic applications and other tissue imaging requiring micrometer resolution.

HISTORY OF RETINAL IMAGE PROCESSING

Matsui et al. were the first to publish a method for retinal image analysis, primarily focused on vessel segmentation.[15] Their approach was based on mathematical morphology and they used digitized slides of fluorescein angiograms of the retina. In the following years, there were several attempts to segment other anatomical structures in the normal eye, all based on digitized slides. The first method to detect and segment abnormal structures was reported in 1984, when Baudoin et al. described an image analysis method for detecting microaneurysms, a characteristic lesion of diabetic retinopathy (DR).[16] Their approach was also based on digitized angiographic images. They detected microaneurysms using a "top-hat" transform, a step-type digital image filter.[17] This method employs a mathematical morphology technique that eliminates the vasculature from a fundus image yet leaves possible microaneurysm candidates untouched. The field dramatically changed in the 1990s with the development of digital retinal imaging and the expansion of digital filter-based image analysis techniques. These developments resulted in an exponential rise in the number of publications, which continues today.

CURRENT STATUS OF RETINAL IMAGING

Retinal imaging has developed rapidly during the last 160 years and is a now a mainstay of the clinical care and management of patients with retinal as well as systemic diseases. Fundus photography is widely used for population-based, large-scale detection of DR, glaucoma, and age-related macular degeneration. OCT and fluorescein angiography are widely used in the daily management of patients in a retina clinic setting. OCT has also become an increasingly helpful adjunct in preoperative planning and postoperative evaluation of vitreoretinal surgical patients.[18] The overview below is partially based on an earlier review paper.[19]

FUNDUS IMAGING

We define fundus imaging as the process whereby reflected light is used to obtain a two-dimensional (2D) representation of the 3D, semitransparent, retinal tissues projected on to the imaging plane. Thus, any process that results in a 2D image where the image intensities represent the amount of a reflected quantity of light is fundus imaging. Consequently, OCT imaging is not fundus imaging, while the following modalities/techniques all belong to the broad category of fundus imaging:

1. fundus photography (including so-called red-free photography): image intensities represent the amount of reflected light of a specific waveband
2. color fundus photography: image intensities represent the amount of reflected red (R), green (G), and blue (B) wavebands, as determined by the spectral sensitivity of the sensor
3. stereo fundus photography: image intensities represent the amount of reflected light from two or more different view angles for depth resolution
4. SLO: image intensities represent the amount of reflected single-wavelength laser light obtained in a time sequence
5. adaptive optics SLO: image intensities represent the amount of reflected laser light optically corrected by modeling the aberrations in its wavefront
6. fluorescein angiography and indocyanine angiography: image intensities represent the amounts of emitted photons from the fluorescein or indocyanine green fluorophore that was injected into the subject's circulation.

There are several technical challenges in fundus imaging. Since the retina is normally not illuminated internally, both external illumination projected into the eye as well as the retinal image projected out of the eye must traverse the pupillary plane. Thus the size of the pupil, usually between 2 and 8 mm in diameter, has been the primary technical challenge in fundus imaging.[7] Fundus imaging is complicated by the fact that the illumination and imaging beams cannot overlap because such overlap results in corneal and lenticular reflections diminishing or eliminating image contrast. Consequently, separate paths are used in the pupillary plane, resulting in optical apertures on the order of only a few millimeters. Because the resulting imaging setup is technically challenging, fundus imaging historically involved relatively expensive equipment and highly trained ophthalmic photographers. Over the last 10 years or so, there have been several important developments that have made fundus imaging more accessible, resulting in less dependence on such experience and expertise. There has been a shift from film-based to digital image acquisition, and as a consequence the importance of picture archiving and communication systems (PACS) has substantially increased in clinical ophthalmology, also allowing integration with electronic medical records. Requirements for population-based early detection of retinal diseases using fundus imaging have provided the incentive for effective and user-friendly imaging equipment. Operation of fundus cameras by nonophthalmic photographers has become possible due to nonmydriatic imaging, digital imaging with near-infrared focusing, and standardized imaging protocols to increase reproducibility.

Though standard fundus imaging is widely used, it is not suitable for retinal tomography, because of the mixed backscatter caused by the semitransparent retinal layers.

OPTICAL COHERENCE TOMOGRAPHY IMAGING

OCT is a noninvasive optical medical diagnostic imaging modality which enables in vivo cross-sectional tomographic visualization of the internal microstructure in biological systems. OCT is analogous to ultrasound B-mode imaging, except that it measures the echo time delay and magnitude of light rather than sound, therefore achieving unprecedented image resolutions (1–10 μm).[20] OCT is an interferometric technique, typically employing near-infrared light. The use of relatively long-wavelength light with a very wide-spectrum range allows OCT to penetrate into the scattering medium and achieve micrometer resolution.

The principle of OCT is based upon low-coherence interferometry, where the backscatter from more outer retinal tissues can be differentiated from that of more inner tissues, because it takes longer for the light to reach the sensor. Because the differences between the most superficial and the deepest layers in the retina are around 300–400 μm, the difference in time of arrival is very small and requires interferometry to measure.[21]

The principle of low coherence, or low correlation, means that the light coming from the light source is only correlating for a short amount of time. In other words, the autocorrelation function of the light wave is only large for a short duration, and at all other times it is essentially zero. If the light is fully coherent, the autocorrelation is high forever, and it becomes impossible to create an interference pattern and determine when the light was emitted; if the light was entirely incoherent, there would be no interference at all. A smaller coherence duration thus results in a better depth resolution, but at lower intensity.

Thus, the low coherence of the light essentially "labels," with its autocorrelogram, each short duration of the light wave, with the next duration having a different "label." Though we use the term "label," it is important to understand that the light wave is actually continuous and not pulsed.

This label uniquely indicates when reflected light was emitted. The low coherent light is optically split into two bundles, called arms, before being sent into the eye. One arm, the reference arm, is aimed at a mirror with a known distance, and thereby reflected; the other, the sample arm, is sent into the eye and reflects back from the different tissues, at yet unknown depth.

If the distance to the mirror is exactly the same as the distance to the tissue, and we optically combine the two reflected (reference and sample) arm light waves, their interference will be nonzero. This is because the more the two light waves resemble each other at a moment in time, the higher the interference; remember that, after splitting, each carried the same low coherence "label." Because the optical properties of the eye add noise and thus slightly change the reflected reference arm light wave, the interference will never be perfect. Though the coherence pattern or label changes continuously over time, once they are split they have the same "label" (but change rapidly over time), so that the interference will be high as long as the reference and sample distances stay the same. The energy or envelope of the interferogram is measured as intensity at the sensor and is then displayed as the OCT signal intensity. Of course, by changing the position of the mirror, we can "interrogate" the amount of interference at different sample tissue depths.

We see the importance of the choice of a good low-coherence source – with either an incoherent or fully coherent source, interferometry is impossible. Such light can be generated by using superluminescent diodes (superbright light-emitting diodes) or lasers with extremely short pulses, femtosecond lasers. The optical setup typically consists of a Michelson interferometer with a low-coherence, broad-bandwidth light source (Fig. 6.2). By scanning the mirror in the reference arm, as in time domain OCT, modulating the light source, as in swept source OCT, or decomposing the signal from a broadband source into spectral

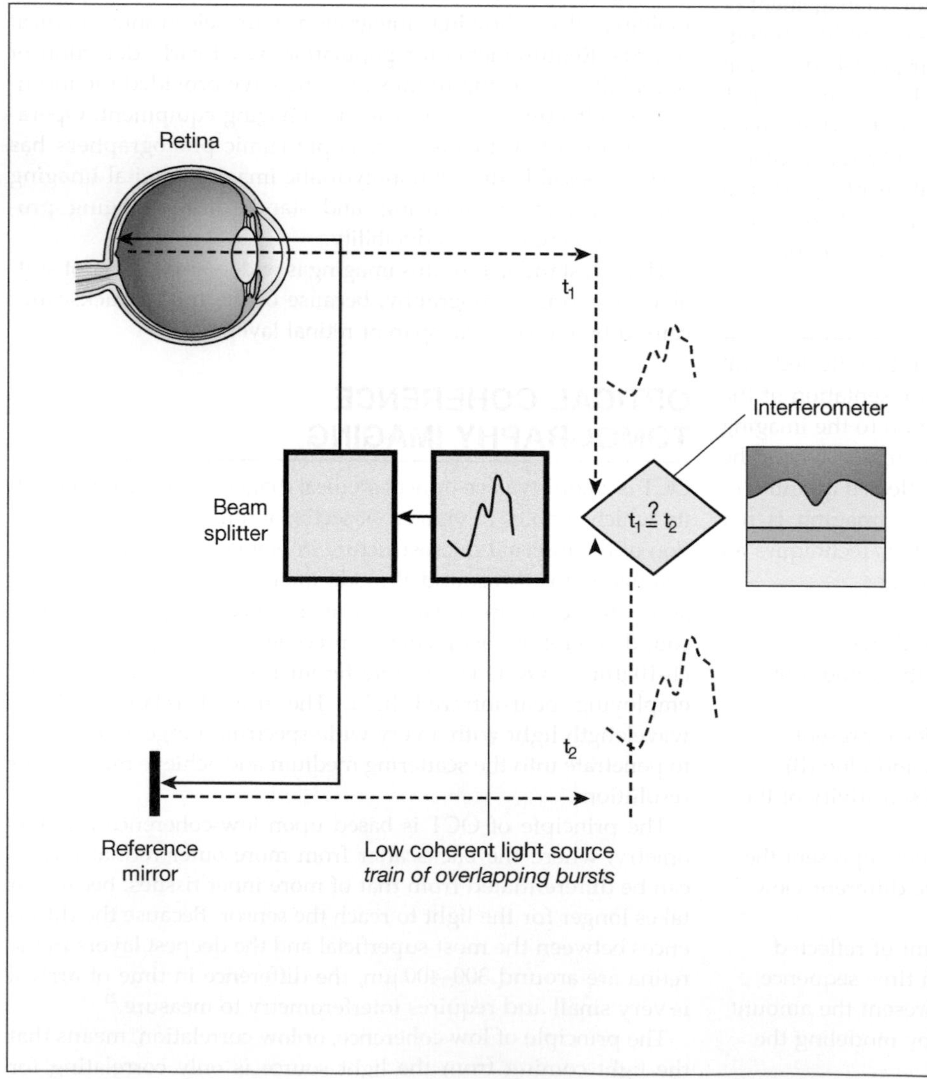

Fig. 6.2 Schematic diagram of the operation of an optical coherence tomography instrument, emphasizing splitting of the light in two arms, overlapping train of bursts "labeled" based on their autocorrelogram, and their interference after being reflected from retinal tissue as well as from the reference mirror (assuming the time delays of both paths are equal).

components, as in spectral domain OCT (SD-OCT), a reflectivity profile of the sample can be obtained, as measured by the interferogram. The reflectivity profile, called an A-scan, contains information about the spatial dimensions and location of structures within the retina. A cross-sectional tomograph (B-scan) may be achieved by laterally combining a series of these axial depth scans (A-scan). En face imaging (C-scan) at an acquired depth is possible depending on the imaging engine used.

The transverse resolution of OCT scans (x, y) depends on the speed and quality of the galvanic scanning mirrors and the optics of the eye, and is typically 20–40 μm. The resolution of the A-scans along the z direction depends on the coherence of the light source and is currently 4–8 μm in commercially available scanners. Isotropic (or isometric) means that the size of each imaged element, or voxel, is the same in all three dimensions. Current commercially available OCT devices routinely offer voxel sizes of 30 × 30 × 2 μm, achieving isometricity in the x–y plane only. Available SD-OCT scanners are never truly isotropic, because the retinal tissue in each A-scan is sampled at much smaller intervals in depth than are the distances between A- and/or B-scans. The resolution in depth, or what we call the z-dimension, is currently always higher than the resolution in the x–y plane. The primary advantage of x–y isotropic imaging when quantifying properties of the retina is that fewer assumptions have to be made about the tissue between the measured samples, thus potentially leading to more accurate indices of retinal morphology.

Time domain OCT

With time domain OCT, the reference mirror is moved mechanically to different positions, resulting in different flight time delays for the reference arm light. Because the speed at which the mirror can be moved is mechanically limited, only thousands of A-scans can be obtained per second. The envelope of the interferogram determines the intensity at each depth.[13] The ability to image the retina two-dimensionally and three-dimensionally depends on the number of A-scans that can be acquired over time. Because of motion artifacts such as saccades, safety requirements limiting the amount of light that can be projected on to the retina, and patient comfort, 1–3 seconds per image or volume is essentially the limit of acceptance. Thus, the commercially available time domain OCT, which allowed collecting of up to 400 A-scans per second, has not yet been suitable for 3D imaging.

Frequency domain OCT

In frequency domain OCT, broadband interference is acquired with spectrally separated detectors, either by encoding the optical frequency in time with a spectrally scanning source or with a dispersive detector, like a grating and a linear detector array. The depth scan can be immediately calculated by Fourier transform from the acquired spectra, without movement of the reference arm. This feature improves imaging speed dramatically, while the reduced losses during a single scan improve the signal to noise proportional to the number of detection elements. The parallel detection at multiple-wavelength ranges limits the scanning range, while the full spectral bandwidth sets the axial resolution.

Spectral domain OCT

A broadband light source is used, broader than in time domain OCT, and the interferogram is decomposed spectrally using a diffraction grating and a complementary metal oxide semiconductor or charged couple device linear sensor. The Fourier transform is again applied to the spectral correlogram intensities to determine the depth of each scatter signal.[22] With SD-OCT, tens of thousands of A-scans can be acquired each second, and thus true 3D imaging is routinely possible. Consequently, 3D OCT is now in wide clinical use, and has become the standard of care.

Swept source OCT

Instead of moving the reference arm, as with time domain OCT imaging, in swept source OCT the light source is rapidly modulated over its center wavelength, essentially attaching a second label to the light, its wavelength. A photo sensor is used to measure the correlogram for each center wavelength over time. A Fourier transform on the multiwavelength or spectral interferogram is performed to determine the depth of all tissue scatters at the imaged location.[22] With swept source OCT, hundreds of thousands of A-scans can be obtained every second, with additional increase in scanning density when acquiring 3D image volumes.

AREAS OF ACTIVE RESEARCH IN RETINAL IMAGING

Retinal imaging is rapidly evolving and newly completed research findings are quickly translated into clinical use.

Portable, cost-effective fundus imaging

For early detection and screening, the optimal place for positioning fundus cameras is at the point of care: primary care clinics, public venues (e.g., drug stores, shopping malls). Though the transition from film-based to digital fundus imaging has revolutionized the art of fundus imaging and made telemedicine applications feasible, the current cameras are still too bulky, expensive, and may be difficult to use for untrained staff in places lacking ophthalmic imaging expertise. Several groups are attempting to create more cost-effective and easier-to-use handheld fundus cameras, employing a variety of technical approaches.[23,24]

Functional imaging

For the patient as well as for the clinician, the outcome of disease management is mainly concerned with the resulting organ function, not its structure. In ophthalmology, current functional testing is mostly subjective and patient-dependent, such as assessing visual acuity and utilizing perimetry, which are all psychophysical metrics. Among more recently developed "objective" techniques, oxymetry is a hyperspectral imaging technique in which multispectral reflectance is used to estimate the concentration of oxygenated and deoxygenated hemoglobin in the retinal tissue.[25] The principle allowing the detection of such differences is simple: deoxygenated hemoglobin reflects longer wavelengths better than does oxygenated hemoglobin. Nevertheless, measuring absolute oxygenation levels with reflected light is difficult because of the large variety in retinal reflection across individuals and the variability caused by the imaging process. The retinal reflectance can be modeled by a system of equations, and this system is typically underconstrained if this variability is not accounted for adequately. Increasingly sophisticated reflectance models have been developed to correct for the underlying variability, with some reported success.[26] Near-infrared fundus reflectance in response to visual stimuli is another way to determine the retinal function in vivo and has been successful in cats. Initial progress has also been demonstrated in humans.[27]

Adaptive optics

The optical properties of the normal eye result in a point spread function width approximately the size of a photoreceptor. It is therefore impossible to image individual cells or cell structure using standard fundus cameras because of aberrations in the human optical system. Adaptive optics uses mechanically activated mirrors to correct the wavefront aberrations of the light reflected from the retina, and thus has allowed individual photoreceptors to be imaged in vivo.[28] Imaging other cells, especially the clinically highly important ganglion cells, has thus far been unsuccessful in humans.

Longer-wavelength OCT imaging

3D OCT imaging is now the clinical standard of care for several eye diseases. The wavelengths around 840 μm used in currently available devices are optimized for imaging of the retina. Deeper structures, such as the choroidal vessels, which are important for AMD and other choroidal diseases, and the lamina cribrosa, relevant for glaucomatous damage, are not as well depicted. Because longer wavelengths penetrate deeper into the tissue, a major research effort has been undertaken to develop low-coherence swept source lasers with center wavelengths of 1000–1300 μm. Prototypes of these devices are already able to resolve detail in the choroid and lamina cribrosa.[29]

CLINICAL APPLICATIONS OF RETINAL IMAGING

The most obvious example of a retinal screening application is retinal disease detection, in which the patient's retinas are imaged in a remote telemedicine approach. This scenario typically utilizes easy-to-use, relatively low-cost fundus cameras, automated analyses of the images, and focused reporting of the results. This screening application has spread rapidly over the last few years, and, with the exception of the automated analysis functionality, is one of the most successful examples of telemedicine.[30] While screening programs exist for detection of glaucoma, age-related macular degeneration, and retinopathy of prematurity, the most important screening application focuses on early detection of DR.

Early detection of diabetic retinopathy

Early detection of DR via population screening associated with timely treatment has been shown to prevent visual loss and blindness in patients with retinal complications of diabetes.[31,32] Almost 50% of people with diabetes in the USA currently do not undergo any form of regular documented dilated eye exam, in spite of guidelines published by the American Diabetes Association, the American Academy of Ophthalmology, and the American Optometric Association.[33] In the UK, a smaller proportion or approximately 20% of diabetics are not regularly evaluated, as a result of an aggressive effort to increase screening for people with diabetes. Blindness and visual loss can be prevented through early detection and timely management. There is widespread consensus that regular early detection of DR via screening is necessary and cost-effective in patients with diabetes.[34–37] Remote digital imaging and ophthalmologist expert reading have been shown to be comparable or superior to an office visit for assessing DR and have been suggested as an approach to make the dilated eye exam available to unserved and underserved populations that do not receive regular exams by eye care providers.[38,39] If all of these underserved populations were to be provided with digital imaging, the annual number of retinal images requiring evaluation would exceed 32 million in the USA alone (approximately 40% of people with diabetes with at least two photographs per eye).[39,40] In the next decade, projections for the USA are that the average age will increase, the number of people with diabetes in each age category will increase, and there will be an undersupply of qualified eye care providers, at least in the near term. Several European countries have successfully instigated in their health-care systems early detection programs for DR using digital photography with reading of the images by human experts. In the UK, 1.7 million people with diabetes were screened for DR in 2007–2008. In the Netherlands, over 30 000 people with diabetes were screened since 2001 in the same period, through an early-detection project called EyeCheck.[41] The US Department of Veterans Affairs has deployed a successful photo screening program through which more than 120 000 veterans were screened in 2008. While the remote imaging followed by human expert diagnosis approach was shown to be successful for a limited number of participants, the current challenge is to make the early detection more accessible by reducing the cost and staffing levels required, while maintaining or improving DR detection performance. This challenge can be met by utilizing computer-assisted or fully automated methods for detection of DR in retinal images.[42–44]

Early detection of systemic disease from fundus photography

In addition to detecting DR and age-related macular degeneration, it also deserves mention that fundus photography allows certain cardiovascular risk factors to be determined. Such metrics are primarily based on measurement of retinal vessel properties, such as the arterial to venous diameter ratio, and indicate the risk for stroke, hypertension, or myocardial infarct.[45,46]

Image-guided therapy for retinal diseases with 3D OCT

With the introduction of 3D OCT imaging, the wealth of new information about retinal morphology has enabled its usage for close monitoring of retinal disease status and guidance of retinal therapies. The most obvious example of successful image-guided management in ophthalmology is its use in diabetic macular edema. Currently, OCT imaging is widely used to determine the extent and amount of retinal thickening. More detailed analyses of retinal layer morphology and texture from OCT will allow direct image-based treatment to be guided by computer-supported or automated quantitative analysis. This can be subsequently optimized, allowing a personalized approach to retinal disease treatment to become a reality.

Another highly relevant example of a disease that will benefit from image-guided therapy is exudative age-related macular degeneration. With the advent of the anti-vascular endothelial growth factor (VEGF) agents ranibizumab and bevacizumab, it has become clear that outer retinal and subretinal fluid is the main indicator of a need for anti-VEGF retreatment.[47–51] Several studies are under way to determine whether OCT-based quantification of fluid parameters and affected retinal tissue can help improve the management of patients with anti-VEGF agents.

IMAGE ANALYSIS CONCEPTS FOR CLINICIANS

Image analysis is a field that relies heavily on mathematics and physics. The goal of this section is to explain the major clinically relevant concepts and challenges in image analysis, with no use of mathematics or equations. For a detailed explanation of the underlying mathematics, the reader is referred to the appropriate textbooks.[52]

The retinal image

Definition of a retinal image

As interpreted by a computer, an image is a set of elements with values that are organized. The elements, called pixels, each have a single value, the intensity, when the image is a monochrome or an OCT image, and multiple values, when the image is a color image. For example, in an angiogram or OCT image, the intensity value of each pixel is the amount of reflected respectively interfered light that was measured at that pixel position. In a color image, there are usually three intensity values (for red, blue, and green) assigned to a pixel, which combined make up the color of that pixel.

Retinal image quantities

Computers use a binary system (1s and 0s) to store and process information. Because they do not use the decimal system, image intensities typically have values ranging between 0 and 255, 0–65 536, or −32 767 to +32 767, instead of the 0–1000 or 100 000 that one might expect if computers used the decimal system. This can be explained by the fact that, typically, 1, 2, or 3 bytes are used to store the intensity values for a pixel, as combinations of 1s and 0s. Though more bytes take up more space, the precision of the intensity values becomes greater. Psychophysical research has shown that the human visual system can differentiate at most 500 different levels of gray, and at most 10 million different colors, so that increasing the precision of the intensity values beyond these levels will not increase the visual perception of quality of an image. However, there may be some value in increasing the precision despite this fact, since image analysis algorithms can discern a higher number of levels than humans can.

Retinal image compression

Image compression is useful because it decreases the amount of memory required to store images digitally or communicate these images over a network such as the internet. Image compression can be "loss-less" or "lossy," and makes use of the fact that images are always somewhat repetitive. If the intensity value of a pixel has a certain value, the values of the pixels in its surround usually have similar values.

In order to explain the concept of an image compression algorithm, let us proceed with an example. We start with an image in which 50 pixels in an area all have the same intensity value. We will pick the value 128. Instead of storing 50 memory elements, all having the value 50 (typically requiring 50 bytes total), the simple image compression algorithm counts the number of repetitions of an intensity value, reducing this number to two memory elements: the first one, the repeat value 50, and the second one, the repeated intensity, 128 (requiring only two bytes of storage). To restore the original image area, an uncompression algorithm takes the two elements and reconstitutes the 50 pixels each having 128 as intensity.

Because no image information is lost, and the uncompression algorithm can reconstitute the image perfectly, this is loss-less compression.

Lossy image compression

To improve image compression rates even more, lossy compression algorithms make use of the fact that the human visual system does not notice small intensity changes in the image. A lossy compression algorithm would compress the image in the example above in exactly the same manner. However, if we take an image where the 50 pixels in the area did not have exactly the same value, but varied slightly around the value 128, the image compression algorithm would compress the image differently. For the human visual system, this area would be hard to differentiate from the same area where all 50 pixels had intensity values of 128. The simple loss-less algorithm above would not be able to compress this area, because the pixels in the area have different intensities, and would store the 50 pixels as 50 elements. The lossy algorithm is "smarter" and "knows" the limits of human visual perception, and will assign all pixels varying only "a little" from 128 the intensity value of 128, and store the repeat value, and the repeated intensity. The uncompression algorithm would assign all 50 pixels the same 128 as intensity. Thus the original information in the image is lost, though typically this is not noticeable to the human visual system.

Legal issues with lossy image compression

Lossy compression is widely used in ophthalmic imaging, especially for storing acquired images in image databases (see PACS section, below). In theory, but so far not in practice, a medicolegal situation could arise as a result of lossy compression artifact. In a hypothetical case where the diagnosis of a clinician is disputed, that clinician may have seen an abnormality on an image immediately after acquisition, which subsequently underwent lossy compression, was stored, and thus became part of the medical record. Because lossy compression causes irreversible loss of information, that abnormality may no longer be visible on the archived image after uncompression, making it impossible to view the same image that the clinician originally saw and upon which his/her diagnosis was based. One can certainly envision the legal implications and liability of this scenario.

Examples of loss-less compression image formats are compressed TIFF, GIF, and PNG file formats, as well as the "raw" formats that are generated directly by the imaging device. Common lossy compression-based image formats are JPEG and MPEG.

Storing and accessing retinal images: ophthalmology picture-archiving systems

After an image is acquired on a fundus camera or OCT device, it becomes part of the medical record. It therefore should be stored in some form, so that it can be communicated to other clinicians and providers, or consulted at a later date.

Images can be stored directly on the imaging device, but PACS are available that make image storage more practical, allowing images from a variety of imaging devices to be stored and reviewed. PACS may be standalone, or may be integrated into an electronic health record. PACS do not need to be separate, and some are an integral part of an electronic medical record system. Most PACS offer manufacturer independence: the images are stored in such a manner that they can still be viewed even if the device on which they were recorded is no longer available, and are not lost when the "old" device is retired.

With the advent of SD-OCT technology and dense OCT scanning, which can result in image sizes of a gigabyte per exam, deciding how clinical images are stored, and whether all data acquired is stored or just the clinically relevant images, is becoming more and more important for the practitioner, as is choosing the level and type of image compression.

For small practices, keeping images stored on the device can still be a cost-effective solution. For larger practices, storage in a PACS computer network accessible over the clinic allows a patient's images to be accessible in the patient area during clinic. Typically, PACS takes care of compression and uncompression calculations "behind the scenes."

Different strategies for storing ophthalmic images

- Slides and computer printouts stored in the paper chart or photo archive
- Slides and paper printouts scanned and stored in a PACS
- Clinically relevant views stored in a PACS
- All raw data and clinically relevant views stored in a PACS
- Standard for storage and communication of ophthalmology images.

Digital exchange of retinal images and DICOM

DICOM stands for Digital Imaging and Communications in Medicine and is an organization founded in 1983 to create a standard method for the transmission of medical images and their associated information across all fields of medicine. For ophthalmology, Working Group 9 (WG-9) of DICOM is a formal part of the American Academy of Ophthalmology. Until recently, the work of WG-9 has focused on creating standards for fundus, anterior-segment, and external ophthalmic photography, resulting in DICOM Supplement 91 Ophthalmic Photography Image SOP Classes, and on OCT imaging in DICOM Supplement 110: Ophthalmic Tomography Image Storage SOP[53,54] (http://medical.nema.org).

DICOM standards build as much as possible upon other standards. For example, DICOM does not prescribe an image compression standard. Images stored as DICOM images can contain the actual image data. A typical example of this is a JPEG image. DICOM 91 and 110 standardize how metadata for an image, such as patient and visit data, acquisition modes and camera settings, compression settings and data formats, and clinical interpretation, is stored as an integral part of the image.

Retinal image analysis

Image analysis is a process by which meaningful information or measurements can be extracted from digital images, typically by computer algorithms. In ophthalmology, image analysis is primarily used to extract clinically relevant measurements from images of the eye, but also to estimate retinal biomarkers, most commonly from fundus color images and from OCT images. The purpose of this section is to familiarize the reader with the main concepts used in the ophthalmic image analysis literature. Image analysis is best understood as a process consisting of a combination of steps. Not all steps are performed in all image analysis algorithms, and some steps may be explicit as multiple steps in one algorithm and form a combined step in another, different algorithm, but the steps described below are typical.

Common image-processing steps

- Preprocessing: remove variability without losing essential information
- Detection: locate specific structures of interest, or features
- Segmentation: determine precise boundaries of objects
- Registration: find similar regions in two or more images
- Interpretation: output clinically relevant information.

Preprocessing

The purpose of preprocessing is to remove as much variation as possible from the image without losing essential information. There are many sources of variation during image acquisition. Image device manufacturer and type, different sizes of field of view, variations in flash illumination, exposure duration, patient movement, variability in retinal pigmentation or in cornea/lens/vitreous opacities are all examples of variation between images taken for the same purpose. These variations do not contribute to the understanding of the image, but they may alter further image analysis steps.

Preprocessing attempts to eliminate some or all of these sources of variation, as much as possible. A simple example is field of view: by scaling the image, and subtracting unexposed areas of the image, images from different cameras are normalized to a "standard fundus image." Another example is illumination correction, where the pixel intensity values of underexposed areas are increased, and those of overexposed intensities reduced, so that the pixel intensities fall into a narrower and more predictable range.

There are many parallels between image preprocessing using computers and human retinal image processing in ganglion cells.[19]

Detection

The purpose of detection is to locate, typically in a preprocessed image, the specific structures of interest, or features, without yet determining their exact boundaries. Examples of such features can be edges, dark or bright spots, oriented lines, and dark-bright transitions in OCT images. Other terms in use for the concept "structure of interest" are wavelets, textures, or filters. Typically, each individual pixel in the image is examined for the presence of one feature or more, and usually the surrounding area, or context, of each pixel is included in this examination. The examination itself usually involves a mathematical computation of the similarity between prototypes of the feature and each pixel and its surround. Conceptually similar terms used in the image analysis literature resembling similarity computation are "correlation," "convolution," "lifting," "matching," and "comparison." Usually a nonlinearity is utilized to convert the similarity estimate into a discrete value, for example, "present" versus "nonpresent."

The output of the matching process indicates if and where the features were detected in the image. In some image analysis systems, this output is interpreted directly, while in others, a segmentation step (see below) is used to determine the exact boundaries of the object represented by the features.

There are many parallels between the features and the convolution process in digital image analysis, and the filters in the human visual cortex.[55]

Segmentation

The purpose of segmentation is to determine the precise boundaries of objects in the image, when the presence of specific object features has been determined in the detection step. For example, if the ganglion cell layer in an OCT image is detected but still has disjoint boundaries, the segmentation step connects these into a connected boundary. Commonly used segmentation techniques are graph search and dynamic programing, both of which try to find the mathematically best-fitting boundary, given the specific detection output(s). The output of the segmentation step can be used directly for assessment, for example when showing the different layers on a macular OCT scan, or can be the input for an interpretation step.

Registration

The purpose of registration is to find similar regions in two or more images so they can be colocalized. Registration is often used to overlay an angiogram on an OCT image, compare images from the same patient from two different visits, to detect improvement or worsening of the patient's condition between visits, or mosaicing, where several fundus images are stitched together into one image covering a larger area of the retina. The registration step often utilizes similar functions as the detection step.

Interpretation

Usually, when the preceding steps have been completed an interpretation step is used to output clinically relevant information. If the boundaries of the macular retinal layers have been segmented, interpretation involves calculating the distance between the boundaries, so the user can see the thickness of the different layers at specific locations. These thicknesses can even be compared to a database of normal thicknesses at that same location, so that the output represents how likely it is that the retina is thickened at a specific location. Or, after microaneurysms and exudates have been detected and segmented in multiple images from the same patient, these outputs are combined into the clinically relevant information determining whether the patient has more than minimal DR or not.

Unsupervised and supervised image analysis

The design and development of a retinal image analysis system usually involves the combination of some of the steps as explained above, with specific sizes of features and specific operations used to map the input image into the desired interpretation output. The term "unsupervised" is used to indicate such systems. The term "supervised" is used when the algorithm is improved in stepwise fashion by testing whether additional steps or a choice of different parameters can improve performance. This procedure is also called training. The theoretical disadvantage of using a supervised system with a training set is that the provenance of the different settings may not be clear. However, because all retinal image analysis algorithms undergo some optimization of parameters, by the designer or programer, before clinical use, this is only a relative, not absolute, difference. Two distinct stages are required for a supervised learning/classification algorithm to function: a training stage, in which the algorithm "statistically learns" to classify correctly from known classifications, and a testing or classification stage in which the algorithm classifies previously unseen images. For proper assessment of supervised classification method functionality, training data and performance testing data sets must be completely separate.[52]

Pixel feature classification

Pixel feature classification is a machine learning technique that assigns one or more classes to the pixels in an image.[55,57] Pixel classification uses multiple pixel features including numeric properties of a pixel and the surroundings of a pixel. Originally, pixel intensity was used as a single feature. More recently, n-dimensional multifeature vectors are utilized, including pixel contrast with the surrounding region and information regarding the pixel's proximity to an edge. The image is transformed into an n-dimensional feature space and pixels are classified according to their position in space. The resulting hard (categorical) or soft (probabilistic) classification is then used either to assign labels to each pixel (for example "vessel" or "nonvessel" in the case of hard classification), or to construct class-specific likelihood maps (e.g., a vesselness map for soft classification). The number of potential features in the multifeature vector that can be associated with each pixel is essentially infinite. One or more subsets of this infinite set can be considered optimal for classifying the image according to some reference standard. Hundreds of features for a pixel can be calculated in the training stage to cast as wide a net as possible, with algorithmic feature selection steps used to determine the most distinguishing set of features. Extensions of this approach include different approaches to classifying groups of neighboring pixels subsequently by utilizing group properties in some manner, for example cluster feature classification, where the size, shape, and average intensity of the cluster may be used.

Measuring performance of image analysis algorithms

Crucial for the acceptance of image analysis algorithms are evaluations of its performance. Most often performance is compared to human experts, though this raises its own set of issues, as explained below. The agreement between an automatic system and an expert reader may be affected by many influences – system performance may become impaired due to the algorithmic limitations, the imaging protocol, properties of the camera used to acquire the fundus images, and a number of other causes. For example, an imaging protocol that does not allow small lesions to be depicted and thus detected will lead to an artificially overestimated system performance if such small lesions might have been detected with an improved camera or better imaging protocol. Such a system then appears to be performing better than it truly is if human experts and the algorithm both overlook true lesions.

Sensitivity and specificity

The performance of a lesion detection system can be measured by its sensitivity, which is the number of true positives divided by the sum of the total number of (incorrectly missed) false negatives plus the number of (correctly identified) true positives.[52] System specificity is determined as the number of true negatives divided by the sum of the total number of false positives (incorrectly identified as disease) and true negatives. Sensitivity and specificity assessment both require ground truth, which is represented by location-specific discrete values (0 or 1) of disease presence or absence for each subject in the evaluation set. The location-specific output of an algorithm can also be represented by a discrete number (0 or 1). However, the output of the assessment algorithm is often a continuous value determining the likelihood p of local disease presence, with an associated probability value between 0 and 1. Consequently, the algorithm can be made more specific or more sensitive by setting an operating threshold on this probability value, p.

Receiver operator characteristics

If an algorithm outputs a continuous value, as explained above, multiple sensitivity/specificity pairs for different operating thresholds can be calculated. These can be plotted in a graph, which yields a curve, the so-called receiver operator characteristics or ROC curve.[52,56] The area under this ROC curve (AUC, represented by its value Az) is determined by setting a number of different thresholds for the likelihood p. Sensitivity and specificity pairs of the algorithm are then obtained at each of these thresholds. The ground truth is kept constant. The maximum AUC is 1, denoting a perfect diagnostic procedure, with some threshold at which both sensitivity and specificity are 1 (100%).

Repeatability and variability

In addition to the above measures, the performance of an algorithm is also measured by its test–retest variability. With all other variables such as disease state, patient factors, imaging device, and operator held constant while obtaining multiple images, this measure determines how much the algorithm's output remains constant on the "same" input. For an algorithm, test–retest variability is not comparable to intraobserver variability. Almost all image analysis algorithms are deterministic, and if the input image is exactly the same, the output will always be exactly the same.

The reference standard or gold standard

Typically these performance measurements are made by comparing the output of the image analysis system to some standard, usually called the reference standard or gold standard. Because the performance of some image analysis systems, for example for detection of DR, is starting to exceed that of individual clinicians or groups of clinicians, creating the reference standard is an area of active research.[42]

The problem is that the true disease state of the patient is very difficult and in fact, impossible, to measure. For example, at the limit of retinal specialists' detection performance, one specialist may see a microaneurysm in the macula on clinical exam of a patient suspected of having DR, while another only sees some pigmentary variation. In most cases it is impossible to state that one of these clinicians is right and the other is wrong.

Given that determining the true state of disease necessary to create the reference standard is so challenging, the following options have been developed and are in wide use[42]:

1. Using the modality under study. The images are read and adjudicated by multiple trained readers according to a standardized protocol. This is less biased and a better estimate than a single clinician, but has higher cost. This method is often used, but the true disease is not known this way.
2. Using a different modality. In the case of a microaneurysm, an angiogram would be a suitable modality. It requires expert interpretation, and preferably multiple experts. It is less biased towards the imaging modality and may therefore be a better estimate. Because of the added procedure it is less patient-friendly, and has higher cost associated with it.
3. Doing a biopsy. Often this may be ethically unacceptable. It also displaces the problem, because the biopsy would necessarily be interpreted by human expert(s), for example a pathologist, with intra- and interobserver variability. It is more unequivocal, but also more invasive and has higher cost.
4. Outcome-based. If the clinically relevant question is not so much whether a microaneurysm is present or absent, but instead whether the patient is at risk of going blind from proliferative disease, we can wait for that outcome to occur. However, the true state of disease at this moment would still not be known, only the true state at some time in the past. Clinical outcome is maximally unequivocal and minimally subjective.
5. True state of disease, which is an unknowable quantity, as explained above.

As we have seen, in practice the reference standard therefore almost never represents the true state of the disease of a patient.

Clinical safety relevant performance measurement

Performance of a system that has been developed for screening should not be evaluated based solely on its sensitivity and specificity for detection of that disease. Such metrics do not accurately reflect the complete performance in a screening setup. Rare, irregular, or atypical lesions often do not occur frequently enough in standard data sets to affect sensitivity and specificity but can have dramatic health and safety implications. To maximize screening relevance, the system must therefore include a mechanism to detect rare, atypical, or irregular abnormalities, for example in DR detection algorithms.[43] For proper performance assessment, the types of potential false negatives – lesions that can be expected or shown to be incorrectly missed by the automated system – must be determined. While detection of red lesions and bright lesions is widely covered in the literature, detection of rare or irregular lesions, such as hemorrhages, neovascularization, geographic atrophy, scars, and ocular neoplasms has received much less attention, despite the fact that they all can occur in combination with DR and other retinal diseases, as well as in isolation. For example, presence of such lesions in isolated forms and without any co-occurrence of small red lesions is rare in DR; thus missing these does not affect standard metrics of performance to a measurable degree.[41] One suitable approach for detecting such lesions is to use a retinal atlas, where the image is routinely compared to a generic normal retina. After building a retinal atlas by registering the fundus images according to a disc, fovea, and a vessel-based coordinate system, image properties at each atlas location from a previously unseen image can be compared to the atlas-based image properties. Consequently, locations can be identified as abnormal if groups of pixels have values outside the normal atlas range.

FUNDUS IMAGE ANALYSIS

Planar fundus imaging is the most established method of retinal imaging. Until recently, fundus image analysis was the only source of quantitative indices reflecting retinal morphology. Retinal structures that lend themselves for fundus image analysis include: retinal vessels, hemorrhages, microaneurysms, pigment epithelial abnormalities (scars, laser spots), drusen, hyperpigmentation or hypopigmentation, choroid-related abnormalities or lesions, and segmentation of retinal layers. In this section we will discuss retinal vessel detection, retinal lesion detection, construction of fundus imaging-based retinal atlases, and assessment of image analysis algorithms. The previous section on image analysis concepts for clinicians will be helpful in understanding the concepts in this overview. The next section will explain image analysis of OCT images.

Detection of retinal vessels

Automated segmentation of retinal vessels has been highly successful in the detection of large and medium vessels[57–59] (Fig. 6.3). Because retinal vessel diameter and especially the relative diameters of arteries and veins are known to signal the risk of systemic disease, including stroke, accurate determination of retinal vessel diameters, as well as the ability to differentiate veins from arteries, has become more important. Several semiautomated and automated approaches to determining vessel diameter have now been published.[60–62] Other active areas of research include separation of arteries and veins, detection of small vessels with diameters of less than a pixel, and analysis of complete vessel trees using graphs.

Vessel detection approaches can be divided into region-based and edge-based approaches. Region-based segmentation methods label each pixel as either inside or outside a blood vessel. Niemeijer et al. proposed a pixel-based retinal vessel detection method using a gaussian derivative filter bank and k-nearest-neighbor classification.[57,59] Staal et al.[59] proposed a pixel feature-based method that additionally analyzed the vessels as elongated structures. Edge-based methods can be further classified into two categories: window-based methods and tracking-based methods. Window-based methods estimate a match at each pixel against the pixel's surrounding window. The tracking approach exploits local image properties to trace the vessels from an initial point. A tracking approach can better maintain the connectivity of vessel structure. Lalonde et al.[63] proposed a vessel-tracking method by following an edge line while monitoring the connectivity of its twin border on a vessel map computed using a Canny edge operator. Breaks in the connectivity will trigger the creation of seeds that serve as extra starting points for further tracking. Gang et al. proposed a retinal vessel detection using a second-order gaussian filter with adaptive filter width and adaptive threshold.[64]

Detection of fovea and optic disc

Location of the optic disc and fovea benefits retinal image analysis (Fig. 6.4). It is often necessary to mask out the normal anatomy before finding abnormal structures. For instance, the optic disc might be mistaken for a bright lesion if not detected. Secondly, the distribution of the abnormalities is not uniform on fundus photographs. Specific abnormalities occur more often in specific areas on the retina. Most optic disc detection methods are based on the fact that the optic disc is the convergence point of blood vessels and it is normally the brightest structure on a fundus image. Most fovea detection methods depend partially on the result of optic disc detection.

Hoover et al. proposed a method for optic disc detection based on the combination of vessel structure and pixel brightness.[65] If a strong vessel convergence point is found in the image, it is regarded as the optic disc. Otherwise the brightest region is detected. Foracchia et al. proposed an optic disc detection method based on vessel directions.[66] A parabolic model of the main vascular arches is established and the model parameters are the directions associated with different locations on the parabolic model. The point with a minimum sum of square error is reported as the optic disc location. Lowell et al., by matching an optic disc model using the Pearson correlation, determined an initial optic disc location, and then traced the optic disc boundary using a deformable contour model.[67]

Most fovea detection methods use the fact that the fovea is a dark region in the image and that it normally lies in a fixed orientation and location relative to the optic disc and the main vascular arch. In a study by Fleming et al., approximate locations of the optic disc and fovea are obtained using the elliptical form of the main vascular arch.[68] Then, the locations are refined based on the circular edge of the optic disc and the local darkness at the fovea. Li and Chutatape also proposed a method to select the brightest 1% pixels in a gray-level image.[69] The pixels are clustered and principal component analysis based on a trained system is applied to extract a single point as the estimated location of the optic disc. A fovea candidate region is then selected based on the optic disc location and the main vascular arch shape. Within the candidate region, the centroid of the cluster with the lowest mean intensity and pixel number greater than one-sixth disc area is regarded as the foveal location. In a paper by Sinthanayothin et al., the optic disc was located as the area with the highest variation in intensity of adjacent pixels, while the fovea was extracted using intensity information and a

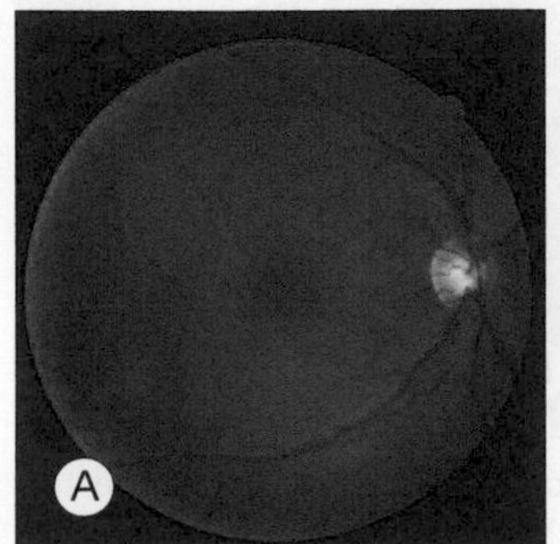

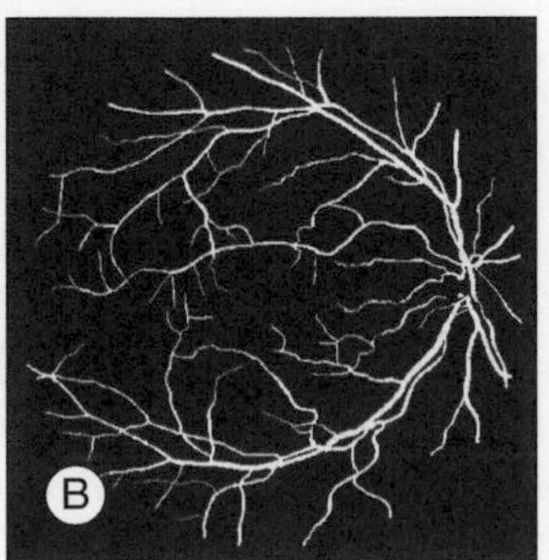

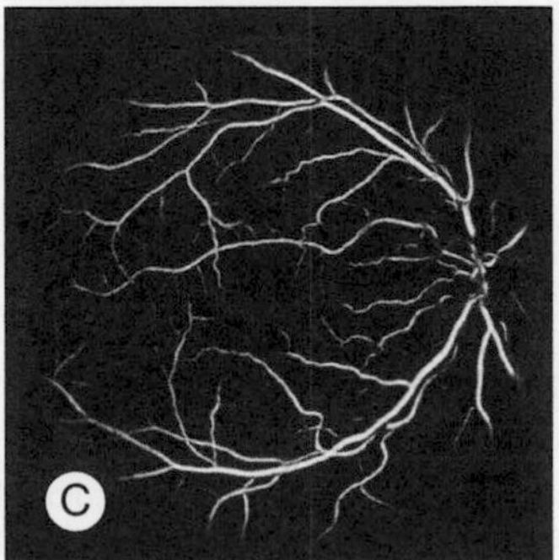

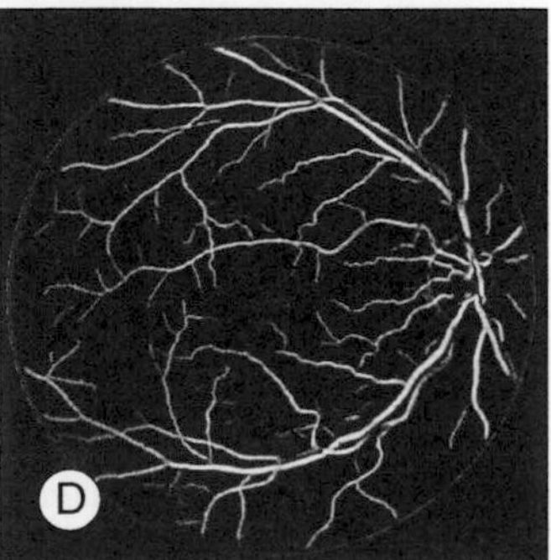

Fig. 6.3 Automated vessel analysis. (A) Fundus image; (B) retinal specialist annotation; (C) vesselness map from Staal algorithm (staal); (D) vesselness map from direct pixel classification. (Reproduced with permission from Niemeijer N, Staal JJ, van Ginneken B, et al. Comparative study of retinal vessel segmentation methods on a new publicly available database. In: Fitzpatrick JM, Sonka, editors. SPIE medical imaging, vol. 5370. SPIE, 2004, p. 648–56.)

relative distance to the optic disc.[70] Tobin et al. proposed a method to detect the optic disc based on blood vessel features, such as density, average thickness, and orientation.[71] Then the fovea location was determined based on the location of the optic disc and a geometry model of the main blood vessel. Niemeijer et al. proposed a method to localize automatically both the optic disc and fovea in 2006.[72,73] For the optic disc detection, a set of features are extracted from the color fundus image. A k-nearest-neighbor classification is used to give a soft label to each pixel on the test image. The probability image is blurred and the pixel with the highest probability is detected as optic disc. Relative position information between the optic disc and the fovea is used to limit the search of fovea into a certain region. For each possible location of the optic disc, a possible location of the fovea is given. The possible locations for the fovea are stored in a separate image and the highest-probability location is detected as the fovea location.

Detection of retinal lesions

In this section we will primarily focus on detection of lesions in DR. DR has the longest history as a research subject in retinal image analysis. Figure 6.4 shows examples of a fundus photograph with the typical lesions automatically detected. After preprocessing, most approaches detect candidate lesions, after which a mathematical morphology template is utilized to segment and characterize the candidates (Fig. 6.5). This approach or a modification thereof is in use in many algorithms for detecting DR and age-related macular degeneration.[74]

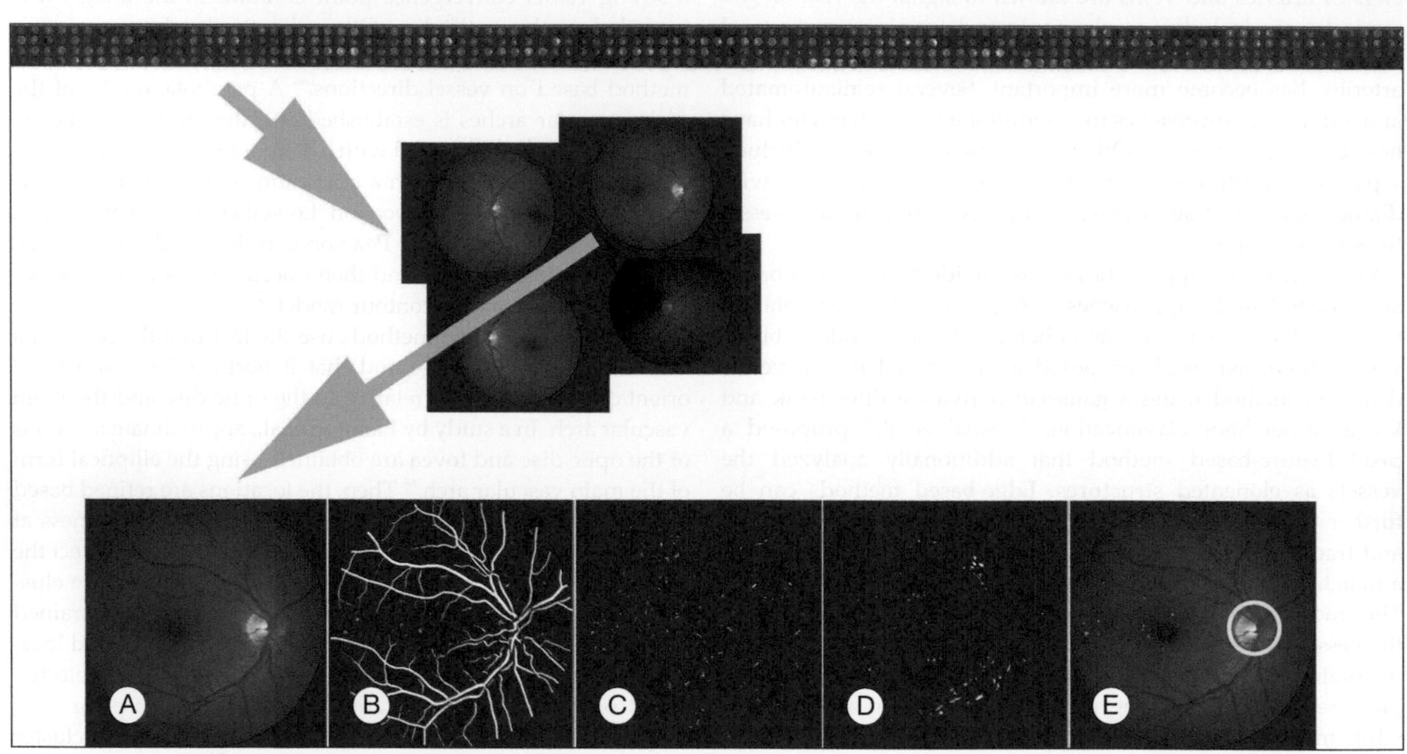

Fig. 6.4 Typical steps necessary for analysis of fundus images, in this case for early diabetic retinopathy. Top row: large sequence of image sets from multiple patients; second row: image set of four retinal images for a single patient; third row: (A) original image; (B) vesselness map; (C) automatically detected red lesions in white; (D) automatically detected bright lesions in white; and (E) detection of fovea (black) and optic disc (yellow) as well as automatically detected red lesions indicated in shades of green; bright lesions in shades of blue superimposed on original image.

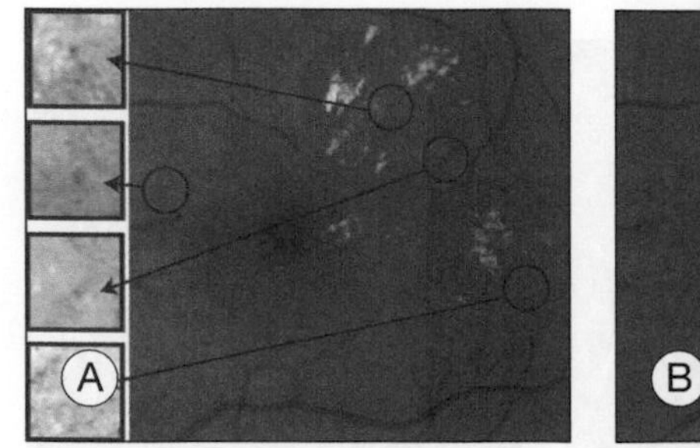

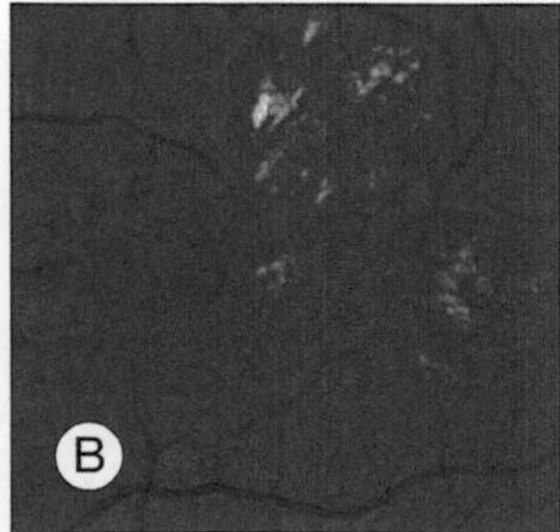

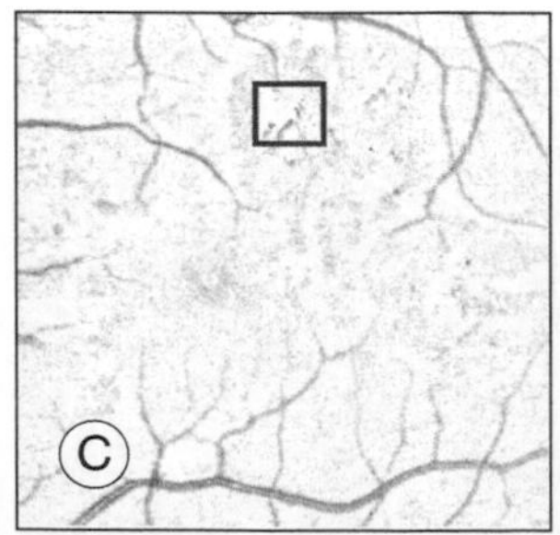

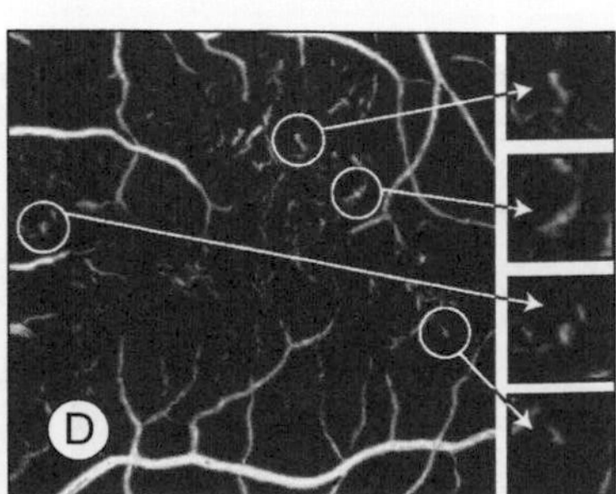

Fig. 6.5 Red lesion pixel feature classification. (A) Part of green color plane of a fundus image. Shown are pieces of vasculature and several red lesions. Circles mark the location of some of the red lesions in the image. (B) After subtracting median filtered version of the green plane, large background gradients are removed. (C) All pixels with a positive value are set to zero to eliminate bright lesions in the image. Note that exudates often partially occlude red lesions. Nonoccluded parts of red lesions show up clearly in this image. An example of this is marked with a rectangle. (D) Pixel classification result produced by contrast enhancement step. Nonoccluded parts of hemorrhages are visible together with the vasculature and a number of red lesions. (Reproduced with permission from Niemeijer M, van Ginneken B, Staal J, et al. Automatic detection of red lesions in digital color fundus photographs. IEEE Trans Med Imaging 2005;24:584–92.)

Additional enhancements include the contributions of Spencer et al.[75] and Frame et al.[76] They added additional preprocessing steps, such as shade correction and matched filter postprocessing, to this basic framework to improve algorithm performance. Algorithms of this kind function by detecting candidate microaneurysms of various shapes, based on their response to specific image filters. A supervised classifier is typically developed to separate valid microaneurysms from spurious or false responses. However, these algorithms were originally developed to detect the high-contrast signatures of microaneurysms in fluorescein angiogram images. An important development was the addition of a more sophisticated filter, a modified version of the top-hat filter, so called because of its cross-section, to red-free fundus photographs rather than angiogram images, as was first described by Hipwell et al.[77] They tested their algorithm on a large set of >3500 images and found a sensitivity/specificity operating point of 0.85/0.76. Once this filter-based approach had been established, development accelerated. The next step was broadening the candidate detection step, originally developed by Baudoin[16] to detect candidate pixels, to a multifilter filter-bank approach.[57,78] The responses of the filters are used to identify pixel candidates using a classification scheme. Mathematical morphology and additional classification steps are applied to these candidates to decide whether they indeed represent microaneurysms and hemorrhages (Fig. 6.6). A similar approach was also successful in detecting other types of DR lesions, including exudates and cotton-wool spots, as well as drusen in AMD.[79]

Small red retinal lesions, namely microaneurysms and small retinal hemorrhages, are typical for multiple retinal disorders, including DR, hypertensive retinopathy, venous occlusive disease, and other less common retinal disorders such as idiopathic juxtafoveal telangiectasia. The primary importance of small red lesions is that they are the leading indicators of DR. Because they are difficult to differentiate for clinicians on standard fundus images from nonmydriatic cameras, hemorrhages and microaneurysms are usually detected together and associated with a single combined label. Historically, red lesion detection algorithms focused on detection of normal anatomical objects, especially the vessels, because they can locally mimic red lesions. Subsequently, a combination of one or more filtering operations combined with mathematical morphology is employed to detect red lesion suspects. In some cases, suspect red lesions are further classified into individual lesion types and refined algorithms are capable of detecting specific retinal structures and abnormalities.

Initially, red lesions were detected in fluorescein angiograms because their contrast against the background is much higher than that of microaneurysms in color fundus photography images.[75,76,80] Hemorrhages mask out fluorescence and present as dark spots in the angiograms. These methods employed a mathematical morphology technique that eliminated the vasculature from a fundus image but left possible microaneurysm candidates untouched, as first described in 1984.[16] Later, this method was extended to high-resolution red-free fundus photographs by Hipwell et al.[77] Instead of using morphology operations, a neural network was used, as demonstrated by Gardner et al.[81] In their work, images are divided into 20 × 20 pixel grids and the grids are individually classified. Sinthanayothin et al. used a detection step to find blood-like regions and to segment both vessels and red lesions in a fundus image.[82] A neural network was used to detect the vessels exclusively, and the remaining objects were labeled as microaneurysms. Niemeijer et al. presented a hybrid scheme that used a supervised pixel classification-based method to detect and segment the microaneurysm candidates in color fundus photographs.[78] This method allowed for the detection of larger red lesions (i.e., hemorrhages) in addition to the microaneurysms using the same system. A large set of additional features, including color, was added to those that had been previously described.[76,80] Using the features in a supervised classifier distinguished between real and spurious candidate lesions. These algorithms can usually distinguish between overlapping microaneurysms because they give multiple candidate responses.

Other recent algorithms only detect microaneurysms and forgo a phase of detecting normal retinal structures like the optic disc, fovea, and retinal vessels, which can act as confounders for abnormal lesions. Instead, the recent approaches find the microaneurysms directly using template matching in wavelet subbands.[83] In this approach, the optimal adapted wavelet transform

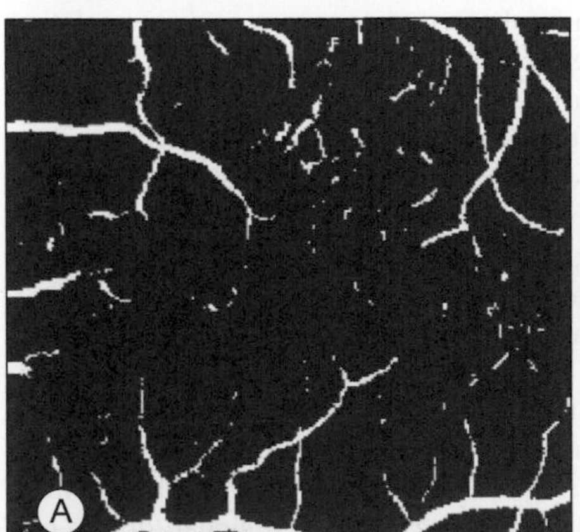

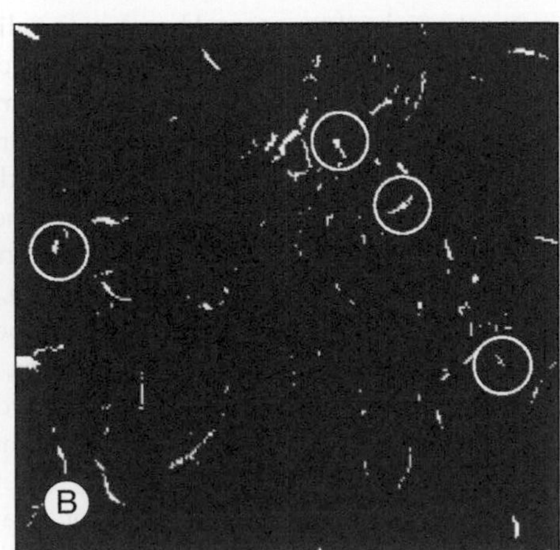

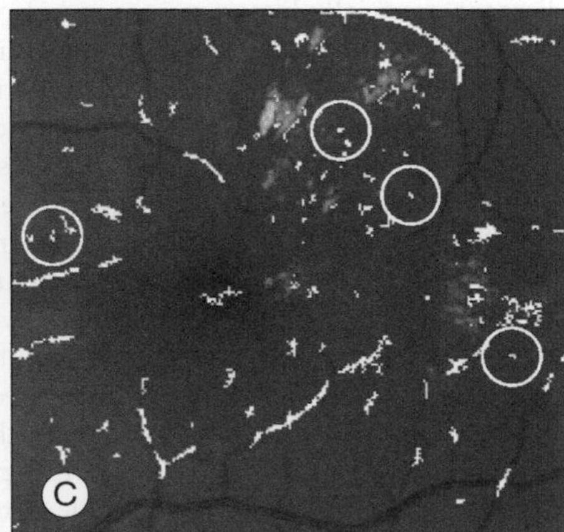

Fig. 6.6 Red lesion detection. (A) Thresholded probability map. (B) Remaining objects after connected component analysis and removal of large vasculature. (C) Shape and size of extracted objects in panel (B) do not correspond well with actual shape and size of objects in original image. Final region growing procedure is used to grow back actual objects in original image, which are shown here. In (B) and (C), the same red lesions as in Figure 6.6A are indicated with a circle. (Reproduced with permission from Niemeijer M, van Ginneken B, Staal J, et al. Automatic detection of red lesions in digital color fundus photographs. IEEE Trans MedImaging 2005;24:584–92.)

is found using a lifting scheme framework. By applying a threshold on the matching result of the wavelet template, the microaneurysms are labeled. This approach has meanwhile been extended explicitly to account for false negatives and false positives.[42] Because it avoids detection of the normal structures, such algorithms can be very fast, on the order of less than a second per image.

Bright lesions, defined as lesions brighter than the retinal background, can be found in the presence of retinal and systemic disease. Some examples of such bright lesions of clinical interest include drusen, cotton-wool spots, and lipoprotein exudates. To complicate the analysis, flash artifacts can be present as false positives for bright lesions. If the lipoprotein exudates only appear in combination with red lesions, they would only be useful for grading DR. The exudates can, however, in some cases appear as isolated signs of DR in the absence of any other lesion. Several computer-based systems to detect exudates have been proposed (Fig. 6.7).[74,79,81,82,84]

Because the different types of bright lesion have different diagnostic importance, algorithms should be capable not only of detecting bright lesions, but also of differentiating among the bright lesion types. One example algorithm capable of detection and differentiation of bright lesions was reported by Niemeijer et al. in 2007.[79] This algorithm is based on an earlier red lesion algorithm presented by Hipwell et al. in 2000[77] and includes the following traditional steps, which are illustrated in Fig. 6.6:

1. lesion candidate cluster detection, where pixels are clustered into highly probable lesion regions
2. true bright lesion detection, where each candidate cluster is classified as a true lesion based on cluster features, including surface area, elongatedness, pixel intensity gradient, standard deviation of pixel values, pixel contrast, and local "vesselness" (as derived from a vessel segmentation map)
3. differentiation of lesions into drusen, exudates, and cotton-wool spots where a third classifier determines the likelihood for the true bright lesion to represent specific lesion types.

Vessel analysis

Vessel measures, such as the average width of arterioles and venules, the ratio of arteriolar to venular widths, and the branching ratio, have been established to be predictive of systemic diseases, especially hypertension, and also have potential value in degenerative retinal diseases such as retinitis pigmentosa. The methods in the section on detection of retinal vessels locate the vessels, but cannot determine vessel width. Additional techniques are needed to measure the vessel width accurately. Al-Diri et al. proposed an algorithm for segmentation and measurement of retinal blood vessels by growing a "ribbon of twins" active contour model. Their approach uses an extraction of segment profiles algorithm, which uses two pairs of contours to capture each vessel edge.[85] The half-height full-width algorithm defines the width as the distance between the points on the intensity curve at which the function reaches half its maximum value to either side of the estimated center point.[86–88] The Gregson algorithm fits a rectangle to the profile, setting the width so that the area under the rectangle is equal to the area under the profile.[33] Xu et al. recently published a method based on graph search showing less variability than human experts (Fig. 6.8).[89]

A fully automated method from the Abramoff group to measure the arteriovenous ratio in disc center retinal images was recently published.[90] This method detects the location of the optic disc, determines an appropriate region of interest, classifies vessels as arteries or veins, estimates vessel widths, and calculates the arteriovenous ratio. The system eliminates all vessels outside the arteriovenous ratio measurement region of interest. A skeletonization operation is then applied to the remaining vessels after which vessel crossings and bifurcation points are removed, leaving a set of vessel segments consisting of only vessel centerline pixels. Features are extracted from each centerline pixel in order to assign these a soft label indicating the likelihood that the pixel is part of a vein. As all centerline pixels in a connected vessel segment should be the same type, the median soft label is assigned to each centerline pixel in the segment. Next, artery vein pairs are matched using an iterative algorithm, and finally, the widths of the vessels are used to calculate the average arteriovenous ratio.

Retinal atlas

The retina has a relatively small number of key anatomic structures (landmarks) visible using planar fundus camera imaging. Additionally, the expected shape, size, and color variations across a population are expected to be high. While there have been a few reports on estimating retinal anatomic structure using a single retinal image,[71] we are not aware of any published work demonstrating the construction of a statistical retinal atlas using data from a large number of subjects. The choice of atlas landmarks in retinal images may vary depending on the view of interest. Regardless, the atlas should represent most retinal image properties in a concise and intuitive way. Three landmarks can be used as the retinal atlas key features: the optic disc center, the fovea, and the main vessel arch defined as the location of the largest vein/artery pairs. The disc and fovea provide landmark points, while the arch is a more complicated two-part curved structure that can be represented by its central axis. The atlas coordinate system then defines an intrinsic, anatomically meaningful framework within which anatomic size, shape, color, and other characteristics can be objectively measured and compared. Choosing either the disc center or fovea alone to define the atlas coordinate system would allow each image from the population to be translated so pinpoint alignment can be achieved. Choosing both disc and fovea allows corrections for translation, scale, and rotational differences across the population. However, nonlinear shape variations across the population would not be considered – this can be accomplished when the vascular arch information is utilized. The end of the arches can be defined as the first major bifurcations of the arch branches. The arch shape and orientation vary from individual to individual and influence the structure of the remaining vessel network. Establishing an atlas coordinate system that incorporates the disc, fovea, and arches allows for translation, rotation, scaling, and nonlinear shape variations to be accommodated across a population.

An isotropic coordinate system is a system in which the size of each imaged element is the same in all three dimensions. This is desirable for a retinal atlas so images can refer to the atlas independent of spatial pixel location by a linear one-to-one mapping. The radial distortion correction (RADIC) model attempts to register images in a distortion-free coordinate system using a planar-to-spherical transformation, so the registered image is isotropic under a perfect registration, and places the registered image in an isotropic coordinate system (Fig. 6.9).[91]

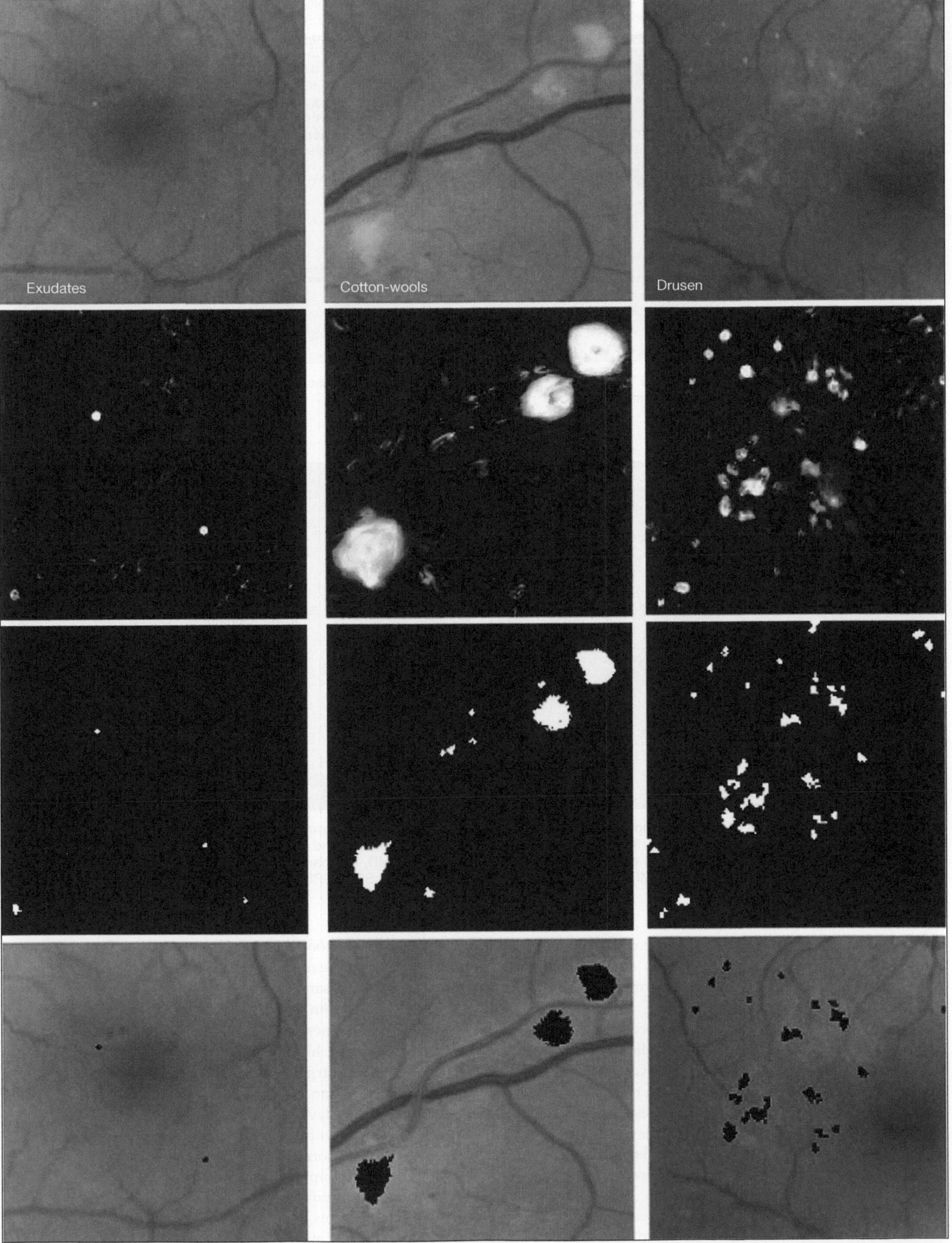

Fig. 6.7 Bright lesion detection algorithm steps performed to detect and differentiate "bright lesions." From left to right: exudates, cotton-wool spots, and drusen. From top to bottom: relevant regions in the retinal color image (all at same scale); a posteriori probability maps after first classification step; pixel clusters labeled as probable bright lesions (potential lesions); bottom row shows final labeling of objects as true bright lesions, overlaid on original image. (Reproduced with permission from Niemeijer M, van Ginneken B, Russell SR, et al. Automated detection and differentiation of drusen, exudates, and cotton-wool spots in digital color fundus photographs for diabetic retinopathy diagnosis. Invest Ophthalmol Vis Sci 2007;48:2260–7.)

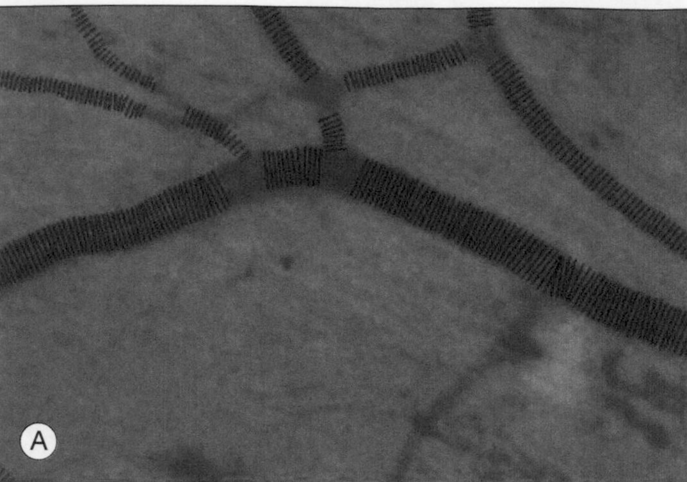

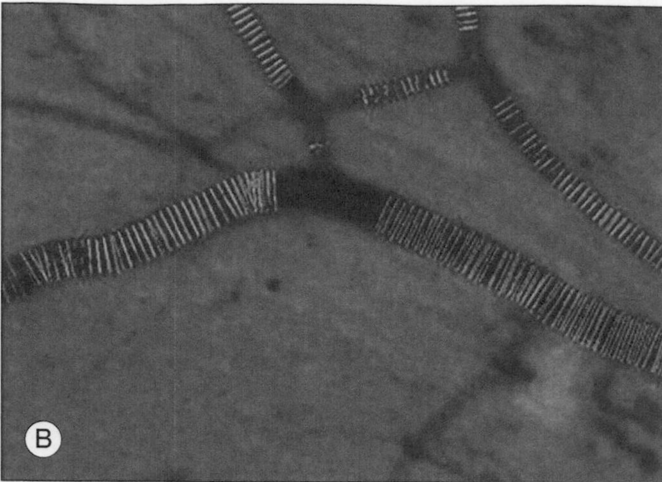

Fig. 6.8 Automated vessel width measurement. (A) Automated measurement of vessel width (black lines); (B) three human experts marking the widths of the vessel manually (in green, blue, and yellow).

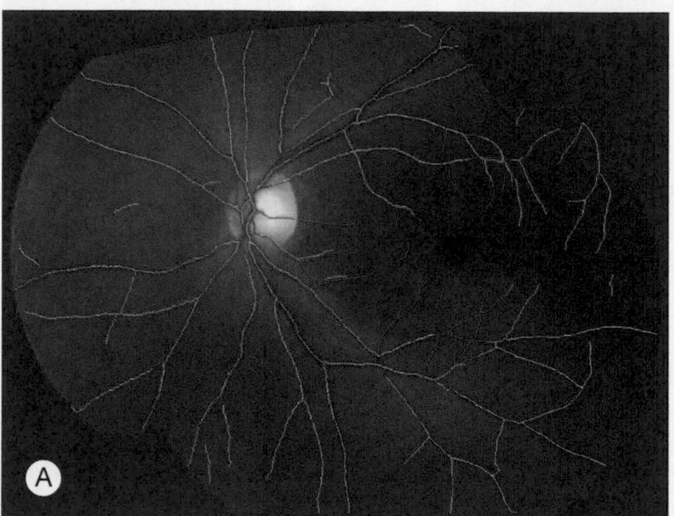

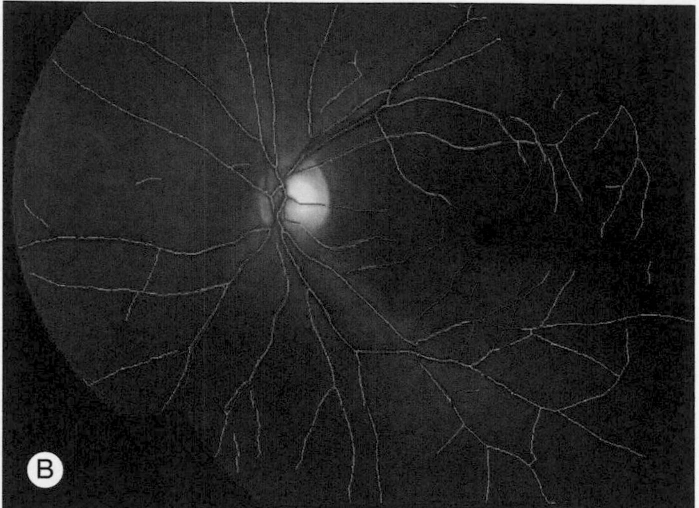

Fig. 6.9 Registration of fundus image pair using (A) quadratic model and (B) radial distortion correction model. Vessel center lines are overlaid for visual assessment of registration accuracy. This registration is performed to disc-centered and macula-centered images to provide an increased anatomic field of view. (Reproduced with permission from Lee S, Abramoff MD, Reinhardt JM. Retinal image mosaicing using the radial distortion correction model. In: Joseph MR, Josien PWP, eds. Proceedings of the SPIE. SPIE, 2008. p 691435.)

An isotropic atlas makes it independent of spatial location to map correspondences between the atlas and test image. The intensities in overlapping area are determined by a distance-weighted blending scheme.[92]

Retinal images in clinical practice are acquired under diverse fundus camera settings subjected to saccadic eye movement, and with variable properties, including focal center, zoom, and tilt. Thus, atlas landmarks from training data need to be aligned to derive any meaningful statistical properties from the atlas. Since the projective distortion within an image is corrected in registration, the interimage variations in the registered images appear as the difference in the rigid coordinate transformation parameters of translation, scale, and rotation.

The atlas landmarks serve as the reference set so each color fundus image can be mapped to the coordinate system defined by the landmarks. As the last step of atlas generation, color fundus images are warped to the atlas coordinate system so that the arch of each image is aligned to the atlas vascular arch (Fig. 6.10).[93] Rigid coordinate alignment is done for each fundus image to register the disc center and the fovea. The control points are determined by sampling points from equidistant locations in radial directions from the disc center. Usually, the sampling uses smoothed trace lines utilizing third-order polynomial curve fitting to eliminate locally high tortuosity of vascular tracings which may cause large geometric distortions (Fig. 6.11).

A retinal atlas can be used as a reference to quantitatively assess the level of deviation from normality. An analyzed image can be compared with the retinal atlas directly in the atlas coordinate space. The normality can thus be defined in several ways depending on the application purpose – using local or global chromatic distribution, degree of vessel tortuosity, presence of pathological features, or presence of artifacts (Fig. 6.12). Other uses for a retinal atlas include image quality detection and disease severity assessment. Retinal atlases can also be employed in content-based image retrieval leading to abnormality detection in retinal images.[94]

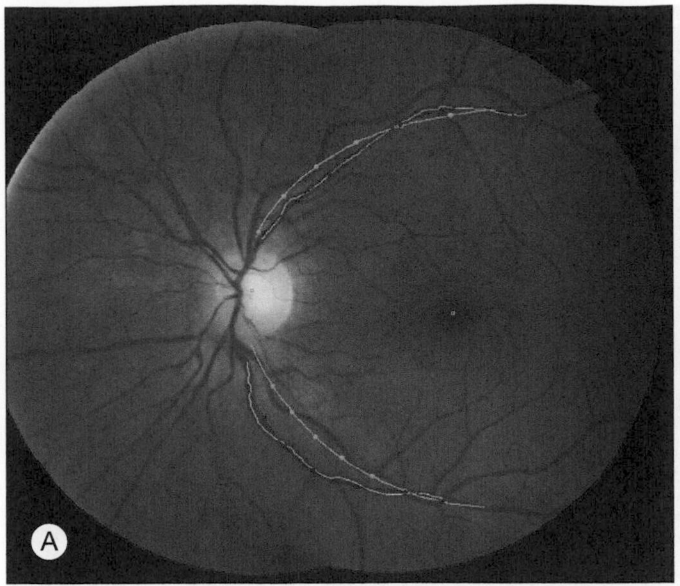

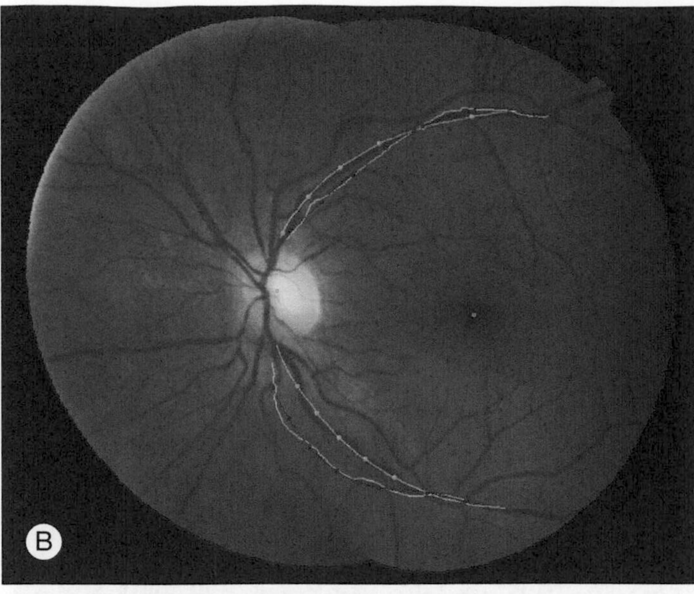

Fig. 6.10 Atlas coordinate mapping by thin plate spline (A) before and (B) after mapping. Naive main arch traces obtained by Dijkstra's line detection algorithm are drawn as yellow lines that undergo polynomial curve fitting to result in blue lines. Atlas landmarks (disc center, fovea, and vascular arch) are drawn in green, and equidistant radial sampling points marked with dots. (Reproduced with permission from Abramoff MD, Garvin M, Sonka M. Retinal imaging and image analysis. IEEE Rev Biomed Eng 2010;3:169–208.)

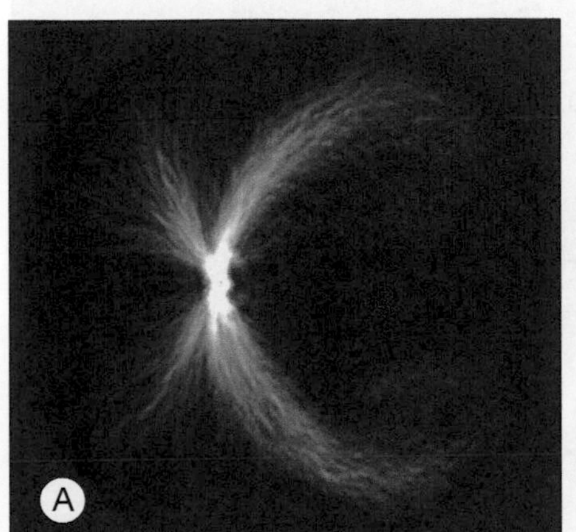

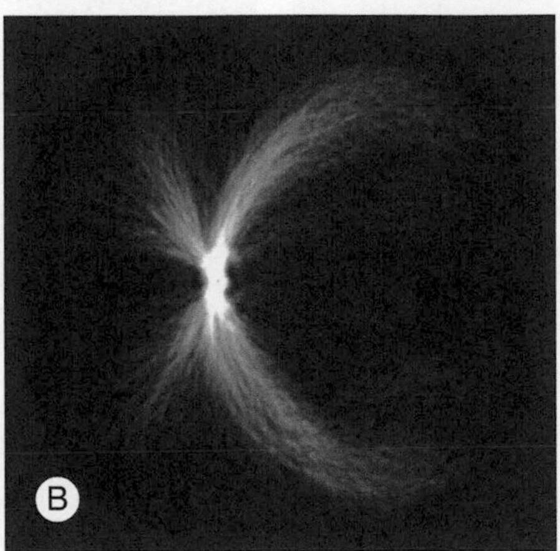

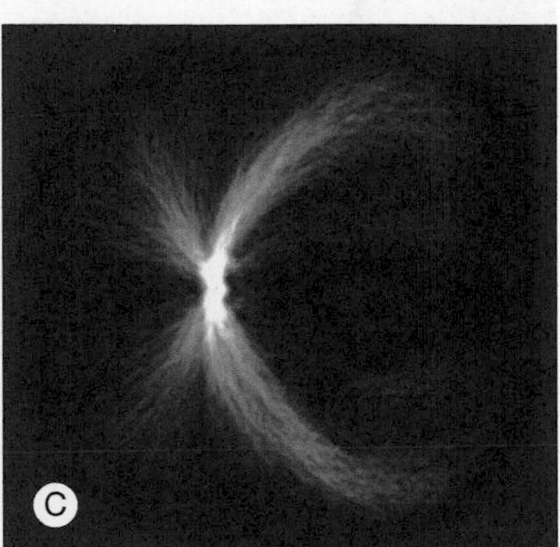

Fig. 6.11 Registration of anatomic structures according to increasing complexity of registration transform – 500 retinal vessel images are overlaid and marked with one foveal point landmark each (red spots). Rigid coordinate alignment by (A) translation, (B) translation and scale, and (C) translation, scale, and rotation. (Reproduced with permission from Abramoff MD, Garvin M, Sonka M. Retinal imaging and image analysis. IEEE Rev Biomed Eng 2010;3:169–208.)

Performance of DR detection algorithms

Several groups have studied the performance of detection algorithms in a real-world setting. The main goal of such a system is to decide whether the patient should be evaluated by a human expert or can return for routine follow-up, based solely on automated analysis of retinal images.[43,44]

DR detection algorithms appear to be mature and competitive algorithms and have now reached the human intrareader variability limit.[41,42,95] Additional validation studies on larger, well-defined, but more diverse populations of patients with diabetes are urgently needed; anticipating cost-effective early detection of DR in millions of people with diabetes to triage those patients who need further care at a time when they have early rather than advanced DR. Validation trials are currently under way in the USA, UK, and the Netherlands.

To drive the development of progressively better fundus image analysis methods, research groups have established publicly available, annotated image databases in various fields. Fundus imaging examples are represented by the STARE,[96] DRIVE,[57] REVIEW,[97] and MESSIDOR databases,[98] with large numbers of annotated retinal fundus images, with expert annotations for vessel segmentation, vessel width measurements, and DR detection. Image analysis competitions such as the Retinopathy Online Challenge[95] have also been initiated.

The Digital Retinal Images for Vessel Evaluation (DRIVE) database was established to enable comparative studies on segmentation of retinal blood vessels in retinal fundus images. It contains 40 fundus images from subjects with diabetes, both with and without retinopathy, as well as retinal vessel segmentations performed by two human observers. Starting in 2005, researchers have been invited to test their algorithms on this

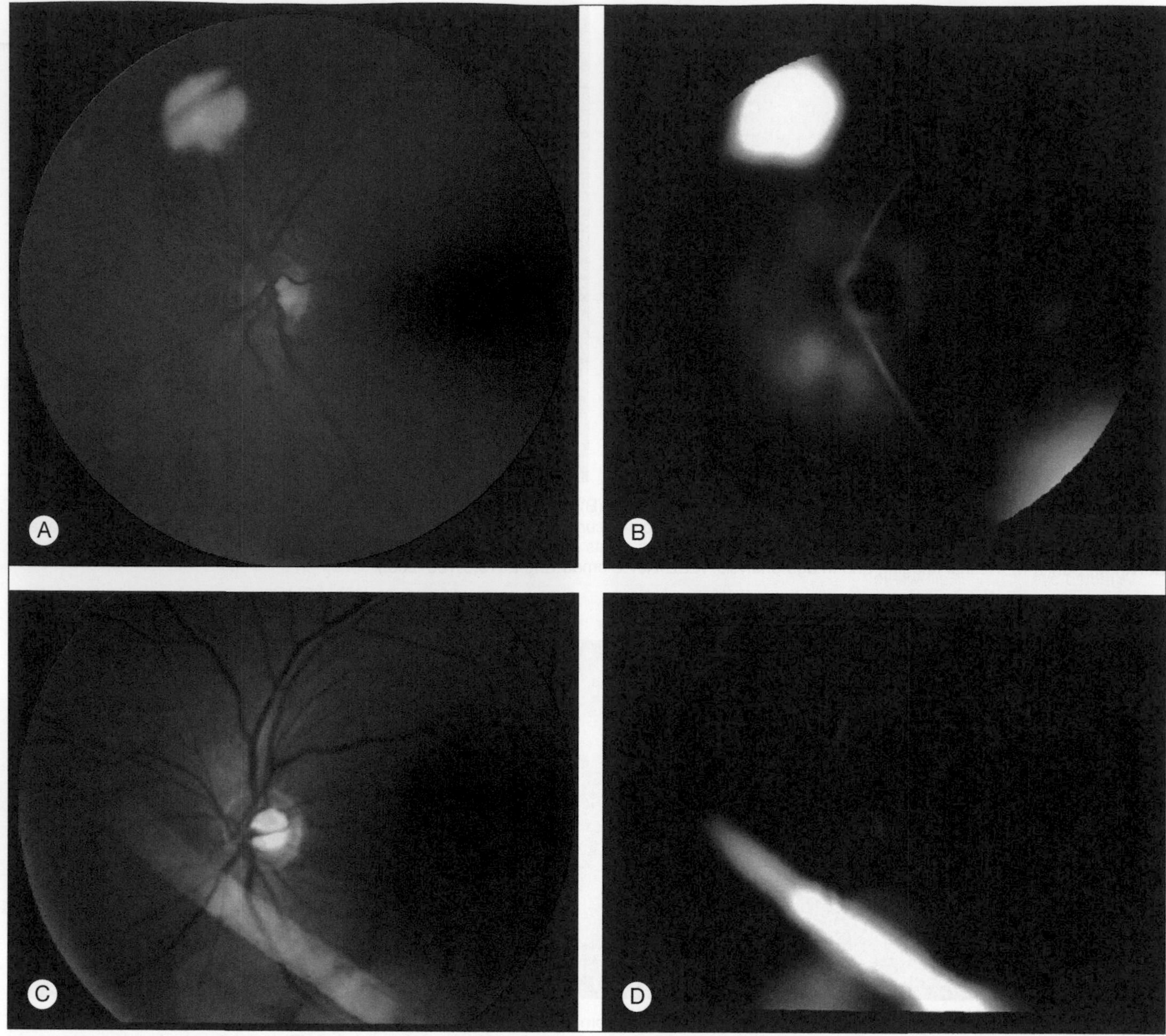

Fig. 6.12 Example application of employing retinal atlas to detect imaging artifacts. (A, C) Color fundus images with artifacts. (B, D) Euclidean distance maps in atlas space using atlas coordinate system. Note that distances are evaluated within atlas image. Consequently, field of view of distance map is not identical to that of fundus image. (Reproduced with permission from Abramoff MD, Garvin M, Sonka M. Retinal imaging and image analysis. IEEE Rev Biomed Eng 2010;3:169–208.)

database and share their results with other researchers through the DRIVE website.[89] At the same web location, results of various methods can be found and compared. Currently, retinal vessel segmentation research is primarily focusing on improved segmentation of small vessels, as well as on segmenting vessels in images with substantial abnormalities.

The DRIVE database was a great success, allowing comparisons of algorithms on a common data set. In retinal image analysis, it represented a substantial improvement over method evaluations on unknown data sets. However, different groups of researchers tend to use different metrics to compare the algorithm performance, making truly meaningful comparisons difficult or impossible. Additionally, even when using the same evaluation measures, implementation specifics of the performance metrics may influence final results. Consequently, until the advent of the Retinopathy Online Challenge competition in 2009, comparing the performance of retinal image analysis algorithms was difficult.[95] This competition focused on detection of microaneurysms. Twenty-six groups participated in the competition, out of which six groups submitted their results on time. The results from each of the methods in this competition are summarized in Table 6.1.

A logical next step was to provide publicly available annotated data sets for use in the context of online, standardized, asynchronous competitions. In an asynchronous competition, a subset of images is made available with annotations, while the remainder of the images are available with annotations withheld. This allows researchers to optimize their algorithm performance on the population from which the images were drawn (assuming the subset with annotated images is representative

Table 6.1 Sensitivities of the different methods at the average false-positive (FP) rate of the human expert (1.08 FP/image) for various categories of microaneurysm. The ranking of the methods for a particular category is given between brackets after the sensitivities

Lesion category	All	Subtle	Regular	Obvious	Close to vessel
Method 1[152]	0.31 (3)	0.03 (4)	0.33 (3)	0.66 (4)	0.22 (2)
Method 2[153]	0.21 (5)	0.03 (4)	0.21 (5)	0.51 (5)	0.22 (2)
Method 3[154]	0.40 (1)	0.13 (1)	0.41 (1)	0.80 (1)	0.30 (1)
Method 4[155]	0.36 (2)	0.10 (2)	0.38 (2)	0.69 (3)	0.19 (3)
Method 5[156]	0.29 (4)	0.05 (3)	0.28 (4)	0.71 (2)	0.30 (1)

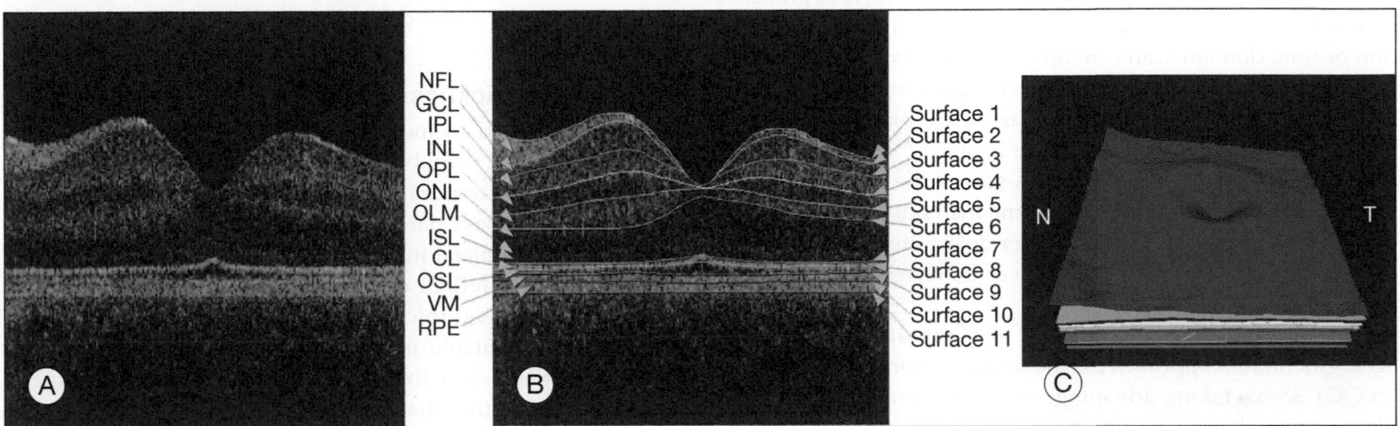

Fig. 6.13 Segmentation results of 11 retinal surfaces (10 layers). (A) X-Z image of optical coherence tomography volume. (B) Segmentation results: nerve fiber layer (NFL), ganglion cell layer (GCL), inner plexiform layer (IPL), inner nuclear layer (INL), outer plexiform layer (OPL), outer nuclear layer (ONL), outer limiting membrane (OLM), plus inner-segment layer (ISL), outer-segment layer (OSL), and retinal pigment epithelium complex (RPE). CL, Inner–outer segment interface complex surface; VM, Verhoeff's membrane. (C) Three-dimensional rendering of segmented surfaces. N, nasal; T, temporal. (Reproduced with permission from Abramoff MD, Garvin M, Sonka M. Retinal imaging and image analysis. IEEE Rev Biomed Eng 2010;3:169–208.)

of the entire population), but they are unable to test–retest on the evaluation images, because those annotations are withheld. All results are subsequently evaluated using the same evaluation software and research groups are allowed to submit results continuously over time.

Areas of active research in fundus image analysis

Major progress has been accomplished in fundus image analysis. Current challenges, on which multiple research groups worldwide are actively working, include the following areas: differentiating arteries from veins, assessing accurate vessel diameter (particularly in vessels only a few pixels in diameter) and vessel tortuosity, vessel tree analysis including tree branching patterns, detection of irregularly shaped hemorrhages, detection of lesion distribution patterns (i.e., drusen), and segmentation of atrophy. Finally, integration of fundus image-based quantification with other metrics of disease risk, such as serum glucose level or patient history, is an area of active research with immediate clinical application.

OPTICAL COHERENCE TOMOGRAPHY IMAGE ANALYSIS

Because of OCT's relatively recent presence in ophthalmic care compared to fundus photography, the use of image analysis techniques for processing OCT images has a shorter history. Nevertheless, it is a rapidly growing and important area, especially as spectral domain (SD).

SD-OCT technology has enabled true 3D volumetric scans of the retina to be acquired. Thus, the importance of developing advanced image analysis techniques to maximize the extraction of clinically relevant information is especially important. Nevertheless, the development of such advanced techniques can be challenging as OCT images are inherently noisy, thus often requiring the utilization of 3D contextual information (Fig. 6.13). Furthermore, the structure of the retina can drastically change during disease. Here, we review some of the important image analysis steps for processing OCT images. We start with the segmentation of retinal layers, one of the earliest, yet still extremely important, OCT image analysis areas. We then discuss techniques for flattening OCT images in order to correct scanning artifacts. Building upon the ability to extract layers, we discuss use of thickness information and of texture information. This is followed by the segmentation of retinal vessels, which currently has its technical basis in many of the techniques used for segmenting vessels in fundus photography, but is beginning to take advantage of the 3D information only available in SD-OCT. The use of both layer-based and texture-based properties to detect the locations of retinal lesions is then described. The ability to segment layers in the presence of lesions is described. This section is based on a review paper.[19]

Retinal layer analysis from 3D OCT

Retinal layer detection

The segmentation of retinal layers in OCT scans has been an important goal, because thickness changes in the layers are one indication of disease status. Previous-generation time domain scanning systems (such as the Stratus OCT by Carl Zeiss Meditec) offered the ability to segment and provide thickness measurements for a single layer of the retina. In particular, the retinal nerve fiber layer thickness measurements of peripapillary circular scans and total retinal thickness measurements were available and used clinically. It can be assumed that commercialized methods utilized an inherently 2D approach (i.e., if multiple 2D slices are available in a particular scanning sequence they are segmented independently). Indeed, most of the early approaches that have been reported in the literature[99–104] for the segmentation of time domain scans are also 2D in nature.

While variations to each of the early 2D approaches exist for the segmentation of retinal boundaries, a typical 2D approach proceeds as follows: preprocess the image,[99–101,103] perform a 1D peak detection (detection) on each A-scan of the processed image to find points of interest, and (in some methods) correct for possible discontinuities in the 1D border detection.[99] Other 2D time domain approaches include the use of 2D dynamic programing by Baroni et al.[105]

Haeker et al.[106–108] and Garvin et al.[109] reported the first true 3D segmentation approach for the segmentation of retinal layers on OCT scans, taking advantage of 3D contextual information. Their approach was unique in that the layers were segmented simultaneously.[110] For time domain macular scans, they segmented 6–7 surfaces (5–6 layers), obtaining an accuracy and reproducibility similar to that of retinal specialists. By extending the approach to SD-OCT volumes,[111] utilization of 3D contextual information had more of an advantage (Fig. 6.14). By employing a multiscale approach, the processing time was subsequently decreased from hours to a few minutes while enabling segmenting additional layers.[112] A similar approach for segmenting the intraretinal layers in optic nerve head-centered SD-OCT volumes was reported with an accuracy similar to that of the inter-observer variability of two human experts.[113] A preliminary layer thickness atlas was built from a small set of normal subjects. Thickness loss of the macular ganglion cell layer in people with diabetes without retinopathy was thus demonstrated, showing that diabetes also leads to retinal neuropathy.[114,115]

OCT image flattening

SD-OCT volumes frequently demonstrate motion artifacts and other artifacts may also be present, such as the tilting due to an off-axis placement of the pupil. Approaches for reducing these artifacts include 1D and 2D methods that use cross-correlation of either A-scans[100] or B-scans.[116,117] In some cases, a complete flattening of the volume is desired based on a surface segmentation to ensure a consistent shape for segmentation and visualization. Flattening the volumes makes it possible to truncate the image substantially in the axial direction (*z*-direction), thereby reducing the memory and time requirements of an intraretinal layer segmentation approach. Flattening an image involves first segmenting the retinal pigment epithelial surface in a lower resolution, fitting a thin-plate spline to this surface, and then vertically realigning the columns of the volume to make this surface completely flat.[111]

Retinal layer thickness analysis

After flattening and segmentation, the properties of the macular tissues in each layer can be extracted and analyzed. In addition to layer thickness, textural properties can also be quantified, as explained in the next paragraph. Measuring the thickening of specific layers is crucial in the management of diabetic macular edema and other retinal disorders.[118] Typically, it is useful to compare the obtained thickness values to a normative database or atlas, as is available in commercial machines for the total macular thickness and the retinal nerve fiber layer thickness. However, a normative atlas for all the layers in 3D currently only exists within individual research groups.[119] Nevertheless, work has been done to demonstrate previously unknown changes in the ganglion cell layer in patients with diabetes.[114,115]

Retinal texture analysis

Texture, defined as measures of the spatial distribution of image intensities, can be used to characterize tissue properties and tissue differences. Textural properties may be important for assessing changes in the structural or tissue composition of layers that cannot be measured by changes in thickness alone. Texture can be determined in each of the identified layers three-dimensionally.[83,120,121] 3D formulations of texture descriptors were developed for pulmonary parenchymal analysis[122] and have been directly employed for OCT texture analysis.[123] The wavelet transform, a form of feature detection, has been used in OCT analysis for de-noising and de-speckling[124–126] as well as for

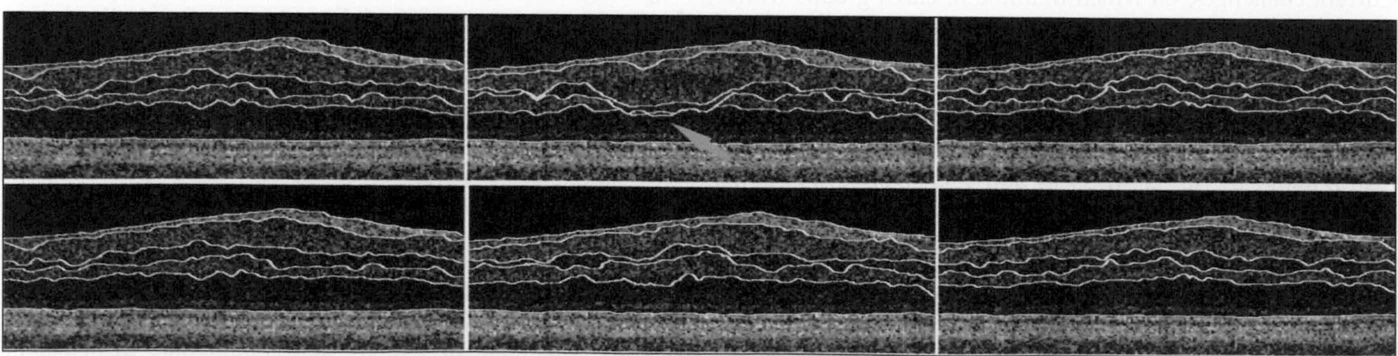

Fig. 6.14 An illustration of why using the complete three-dimensional (3D) contextual information in the intraretinal layer segmentation process is superior. (Top) Sequence of two-dimensional (2D) results on three adjacent slices within a spectral domain volume obtained using a slice-by-slice 2D graph-based approach. Note the "jump" in the segmentation result for third and fourth surfaces in middle slice. (Bottom) Sequence of 3D results on same three adjacent slices using same graph-based approach, but with the addition of 3D contextual information. 3D contextual information prevented third and fourth surface segmentation from failing.

texture analysis.[127] Early work on 3D wavelet analysis of OCT images was based on a computationally efficient yet flexible nonseparable lifting scheme in arbitrary dimensions.[123,128]

Texture characteristics can be computed for each segmented layer, several adjacent layers, or in layer combinations (Fig. 6.12).

Detection of retinal vessels from 3D OCT

Segmenting the retinal vasculature in 3D SD-OCT volumes[129,130] allows OCT-to-fundus and OCT-to-OCT image registration. The absorption of light by the blood vessel walls causes vessel silhouettes to appear below the position of vessels, which thus causes the projected vessel positions to appear dark on either a full projection image of the entire volume[130] or a projection image from a segmented layer for which the contrast between the vascular silhouettes and background is highest, as proposed by Niemeijer et al.[129,131] In particular, this approach used the layer near the retinal pigment epithelium to create the projection image. Vessels were segmented using feature detection with gaussian filter-banks and a k-NN pixel classification approach. The performance of the automated method was evaluated for both optic nerve head-centered as well as macula-centered scans. The retinal vessels were successfully identified in a set of 16 3D OCT volumes (8 optic nerve head and 8 macula-centered), with high sensitivity and specificity as determined using ROC analysis, AUC = 0.96. Xu et al. reported an approach for segmenting the projected locations of the vasculature by utilizing pixel classification of A-scans.[132] The features used in the pixel classification were based on a projection image of the entire volume in combination with features of individual A-scans. Both of these reported prior approaches focused on segmenting the vessels in the region outside the optic disc region because of difficulties in the segmentation inside this region. The neural canal opening shares similar features with vessels, thus causing false positives.[133] Hu et al.[127] proposed a modified 2D pixel classification algorithm to segment the blood vessels in SD-OCT volumes centered at the optic nerve head, with a special focus on better identifying vessels near the neural canal opening. Given an initial 2D segmentation of the projected vasculature, Lee et al. presented an approach for segmenting the 3D vasculature in the volumetric scans[134] by utilizing a graph-theoretic approach (Fig. 6.15). One of the current limitations of that approach is the inability to resolve the depth information of crossing vessels properly.

Detection of retinal lesions

Calculated texture and layer-based properties can be used to detect retinal lesions as a 2D footprint[123] or in 3D. Out of many kinds of possible retinal lesions, symptomatic exudate-associated derangements (SEADs), a general term for fluid-related abnormalities in the retina, are of great interest in assessing the severity of choroidal neovascularization, diabetic macular edema, and other diseases. Detection of drusen, cotton-wool spots, areas of pigment epithelial atrophy, or pockets of fluid under epiretinal membranes may be attempted in a similar fashion.

The deviation of local retinal tissue from normal can be computed by determining the local deviations from the normal appearance at each location $(x; y)$ in each layer and selecting the areas where the absolute deviation is greater than a predefined cutoff. More generally, in order to build an abnormality-specific detector, a classifier can be trained, the inputs of which may be the z-scores computed for relevant features. Comprehensive z-scores are appropriate since an abnormality may affect several layers in the neighborhood of a given location $(x; y)$. The classifier-determined label associated with each column may be selected on relevant features by one of the many available cross-validation and/or feature selection methods,[135-137] thus forming a SEADness or probabilistic abnormality map.

Fluid detection and segmentation

In choroidal neovascularization, diabetic macular edema, and other retinal diseases, intraretinal or subretinal fluid is reflective of disease status and changes in fluid are an indicator of disease progression or regression. With the availability of anti-VEGF therapy, assessment of the extent and morphology of fluid is expected to contribute to patient-specific therapy. While regions of fluid are inherently 3D, determining their 2D retinal footprint is highly relevant. Following the above-described analysis, fluid detection employs generalization of properties derived from expert-defined examples. Utilizing the differences between normal regional appearance of retinal layers as described by texture descriptors and other morphologic indices, a classifier can be trained to identify abnormal retinal appearance. The fluid detection starts with 3D OCT layer segmentation, resulting in 10 intraretinal layers, plus an additional artificial layer below the deepest intraretinal layer so that subretinal abnormalities can also be detected.[123] Texture-based and morphologic descriptors are calculated regionally in rectangular subvolumes, the most discriminative descriptors are identified, and these descriptors are used for training a probabilistic classifier. The performance of a (set of) feature(s) is assessed by calculating the area under the ROC of the fluid classifier. Once the probabilistic classifier is trained, fluid-related probability is determined for each retinal location. In order to obtain a binary

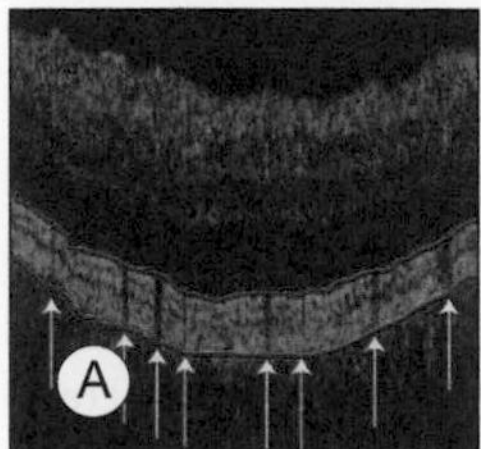

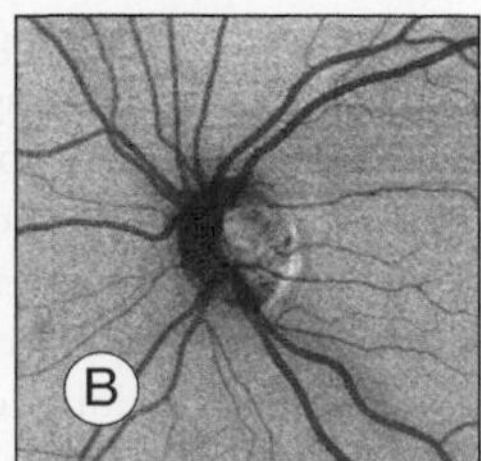

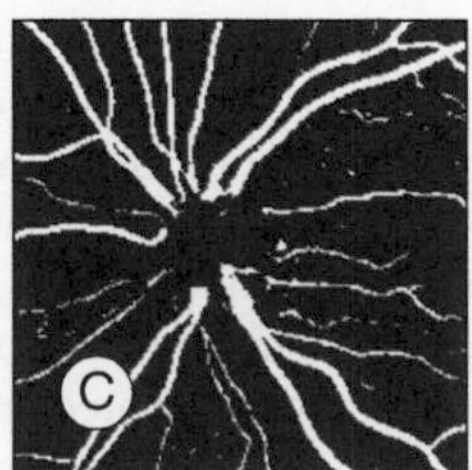

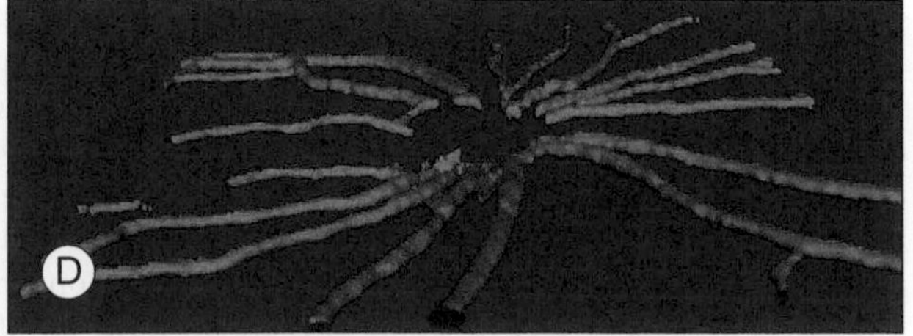

Fig. 6.15 Example of spectral three-dimensional (3D) optical coherence tomography (OCT) vessel segmentation. (A) Vessel silhouettes indicate position of vasculature. Also indicated in red are slice intersections of two surfaces that delineate the subvolume in which vessels are segmented (superficial retinal layers toward vitreous are at the bottom). (B) 2D projection image extracted from projected subvolume of spectral 3D OCT volume. (C) Automatic vessel segmentation. (D) 3D rendering of vessel around the optic nerve head. (Reproduced with permission from Lee K, Abràmoff M, Niemeijer MK, et al. 3D segmentation of retinal blood vessels in spectral-domain OCT volumes of the optic nerve head. Proc SPIE Med Imaging 2010;7626:76260 V.)

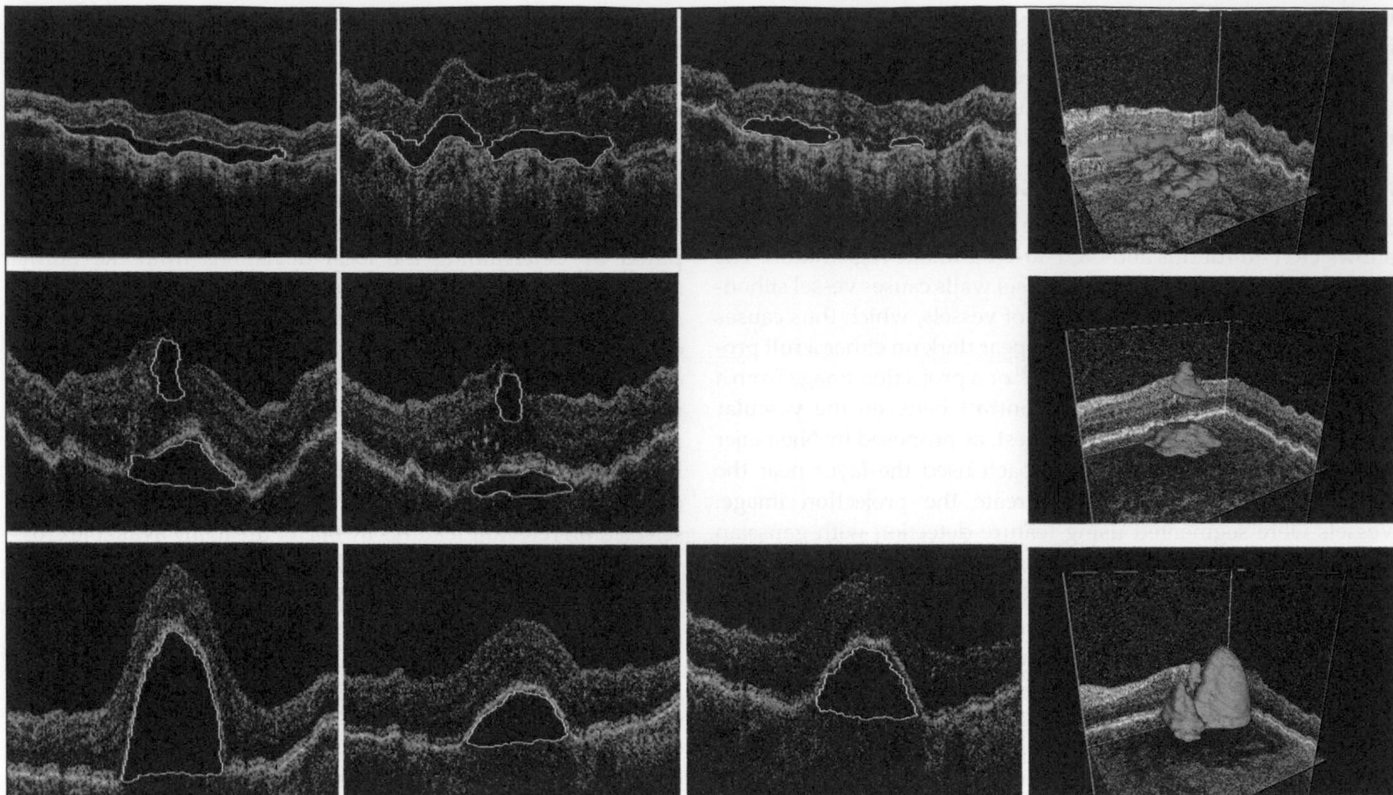

Fig. 6.16 Symptomatic exudate-associated derangement (SEAD) segmentation from three-dimensional optical coherence tomography and SEAD development over time. Top row: 0, 28, and 77 days after first imaging visit. Middle row: 0 and 42 days after first imaging visit. Bottom row: 0, 14, and 28 days after first imaging visit. Three-dimensional visualization in right column shows data from week 0. Each imaging session was associated with anti-vascular endothelial growth factor reinjection.

footprint for fluid in an image input to the system, the probabilities are thresholded and the footprint of the fluid region in this image is defined as the set of all pixels with a probability greater than a threshold. Useful 3D textural information can be extracted from SD-OCT scans and, together with an anatomical atlas of normal retinas, can be used for clinically important applications.

Fluid segmentation in 3D

Complete volumetric segmentation of fluid from 3D OCT is the subject of active research. A promising approach is based on identification of a seed point in the OCT data set that is "inside" and "outside" a fluid region. These points can be identified automatically using a 3D variant of the probabilistic classification approach outlined in the previous paragraphs. Once these two points are identified, an automated segmentation procedure that is based on regional graph-cut method[138,139] may be employed to detect the fluid volumetric region. The cost function utilized in a preliminary study was designed to identify dark 3D regions with somewhat homogeneous appearance. The desired properties of the fluid region are automatically learned from the vicinity of the identified fluid region seed point. This adaptive behavior allows the same graph-cut segmentation method driven by the same cost function to segment fluid of different appearance reliably. Figure 6.16 gives an example of 3D fluid region segmentations obtained using this approach. Note that the figure depicts the same locations in the 3D data sets imaged several times during the course of anti-VEGF treatment. The surfaces of the segmented fluid regions are represented by a 3D mesh, which can be interactively edited to maximize fluid region segmentation accuracy in difficult or ambiguous cases.

Intraretinal layer segmentation in the presence of SEADs

Another area of active research is layer segmentation in retina that contains symptomatic exudate-associated derangements (SEADs). Most likely, a two-step approach is necessary in which layers are initially segmented disregarding the SEAD presence, then SEADs are segmented, and used to constrain the second stage of layer segmentation. This process yields well-segmented retinal layers when fluid occupies a single intraretinal layer as well as in situations when the fluid resides in several adjacent retinal layers.

MULTIMODALITY RETINAL IMAGING

Multimodality imaging, defined as images from the same organ acquired using different techniques using different physical techniques, is becoming increasingly common in ophthalmology. For image information from multiple modalities to be usable in mutual context, images must be registered so that the independent information that was acquired by different methods can be concatenated and form a multimodality description vector. Thus, because of its importance in enabling multimodal analysis, retinal image registration reflects another active area of research. The several clinically used methods to image the retina were introduced above and include fundus photography, SLO, fluorescence imaging, and OCT. Additional retinal imaging techniques, such as hyperspectral imaging, oximetry, and adaptive optics SLO, will bring higher resolution and additional image information. To achieve a comprehensive description of retinal morphology and eventually function, diverse retinal images acquired by different or the same modalities at different time instants must be mutually registered to combine all available local information spatially. The following sections provide a brief overview of fundus photography and OCT registration approaches in both 2D and 3D; a more detailed review is available.[19] Registration of retinal images from other existing and future imaging devices can be performed in a similar or generally identical manner.

Registration of fundus retinal photographs

Registration of fundus photographs taken either at different regions of the retina, or of the same area of the retina but at different times, is useful to expand the effective field of view of a retinal image, determine what part of the retina is being viewed, or aid in analyzing changes over time.[140] We have previously discussed some other uses for fundus–fundus registration in regard to retinal atlases. To register 2D or planar fundus images, most existing registration approaches utilize identification and extraction of features derived from retinal vasculature segmented separately from the individual fundus images. The choice of a specific image registration algorithm to align retinal images into a montage depends on the image characteristics and the application. Images acquired with only a small overlap may be optimally aligned using feature-based registration approaches, while images acquired with larger overlaps may be satisfactorily aligned using intensity-based approaches. Examples of feature-based registration are global-to-local matching,[141] hierarchical model refinement,[142] and dual-bootstrap.[143] Local intensity features[144] are particularly useful when an insufficient number of vascular features are available. Following a step of vascular skeletonization, vascular branching points can be easily used as stable landmarks for determining image-to-image correspondence. As an example, the RADIC model[145] parameters are estimated during an optimization step that uses Powell's method[146] and is driven by the vessel centerline distance. The approach presented by Lee et al. in 2010 reported registration accuracy of 1.72 pixels (25–30 μm, depending on resolution) when tested in 462 pairs of green channel fundus images.[147] The registration accuracy was assessed as the vessel line error. The method only needed two correspondence points to be reliably identified and was therefore applicable even to cases when only a very small overlap between the retinal image pairs existed. Based on the identified vascular features, the general approach can be applied to any retinal imaging modality for which a 2D vessel segmentation is available. In registering poor-quality multimodal fundus image pairs, which may not have sufficient vessel-based features available, Chen et al. proposed the detection of corner points using a Harris detector followed by use of a partial intensity invariant feature descriptor.[148] They reported obtaining 89.9% "acceptable" registrations (defined as registrations with a median error of 1.5 pixels and a maximum error of 10 pixels when compared with ground truth correspondences) when tested on 168 pairs of multimodal retinal images.

Registration of OCT with fundus retinal photographs

Registration of 2D fundus images with inherently 3D OCT images requires that the dimensionality of OCT be reduced to 2D via *z*-axis projection. Building on the ability to obtain vascular segmentation from 3D OCT projection images, the problem of fundus–OCT registration becomes virtually identical to that of fundus–fundus registration that was described in the previous section. Using the same general method, high-quality OCT–fundus registration can be achieved. Figure 6.17 presents the main steps of the registration process and shows the registration performance achieved.

Mutual registration of 3D OCT images

Temporal changes of retinal layers leading to assessment of disease progression or regression can be accessed from longitudinal OCT images. Comparison of morphology or function over time requires that the respective OCT image data sets be registered. Since OCT is a 3D imaging modality, such registration needs to be performed in 3D. For follow-up studies, image registration is a vital tool to enable more precise, quantitative comparison of disease status. Another important aspect of OCT–OCT registration is the ability to enlarge retinal coverage by registering OCT data resulting from imaging different portions of the retina. A fully 3D scale-invariant feature transform (SIFT)-based approach was introduced in 2009.[149] The SIFT feature extractor locates minima and maxima in the difference of gaussian scale space to identify salient feature points. Using calculated histograms of local gradient directions around each found extremum in 3D, the matching points are found by comparing the distances between feature vectors. An application of this approach to rigid registration of peripapillary (ONH-centered) and macula-centered 3D OCT scans of the same patient for which the macular and peripapillary OCT scans had only a limited overlap has been

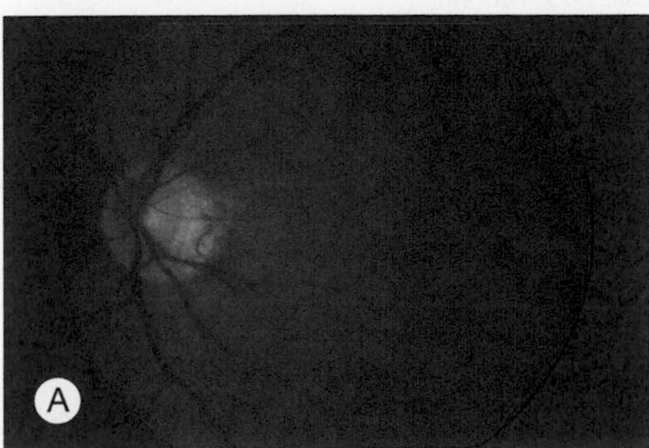

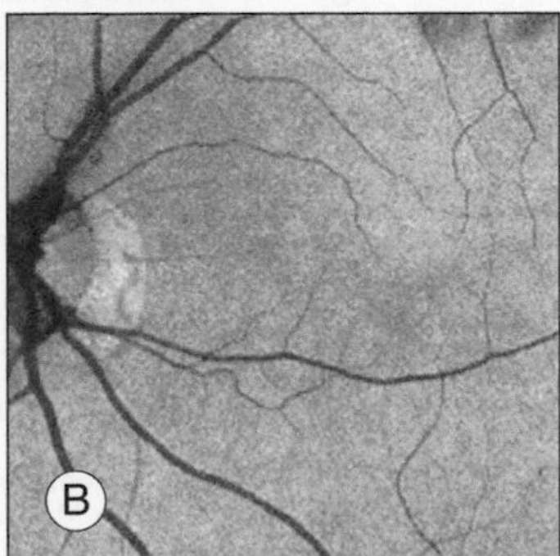

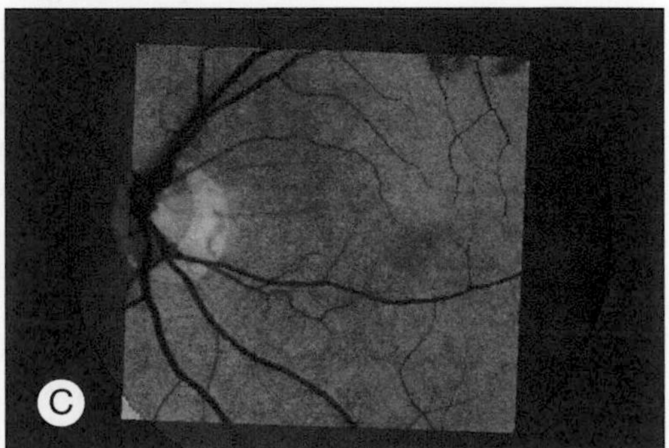

Fig. 6.17 Registration of fundus images to 2D optical coherence tomography (OCT) projection data. (A) Fundus camera image. (B) 2D projection (through depth dimension) of three-dimensional OCT data. (C) Registered and blended fundus OCT images via application of affine transformation model with three identified vascular landmarks.

reported.[148] The work built on a number of analysis steps introduced earlier, including segmentation of the main retinal layers and 3D flattening of each of the two volumes to be registered. 3D SIFT feature points were subsequently determined.[150,151] Using the customary terminology for image registration, when one of the registered images is called the "source" (say the macular image) and the other the "target" (say the peripapillary image), the feature point detection is performed in both source and target images. After feature point extraction, those which are in corresponding positions in both images are identified. In a typical pair of two OCT scans, about 70 matching pairs can be found with a high level of certainty. The primary deformations that need to be resolved are translation and limited rotation, so simple rigid or affine transform is appropriate to achieve the desired image registration. The transform parameters are estimated from the identified correspondence points. Niemeijer et al. demonstrated the functionality of such an approach to OCT–OCT registration of macular and peripapillary OCT scans.[149] 3D registration achieved 3D accuracy of 2.0 ± 3.3 voxels, assessed as an average voxel distance error in 1572 matched locations. Qualitative evaluation of performance demonstrated the utility of this approach to clinical-quality images. Temporal registration of longitudinally acquired OCT images from the same subjects can be obtained in an identical manner.

FUTURE OF RETINAL IMAGING AND IMAGE ANALYSIS

Translation of research in imaging and image analysis into the clinic has been relatively rapid in the past, and can be expected to accelerate in the future. This is partially explained by the lower capital expenditure for ophthalmic imaging devices compared to radiologic imaging devices - the latter can often be 10–100 times more expensive - and also because retinal specialists manage patients directly and are directly involved in the ordering and interpreting of images, while radiologists typically do not directly manage patients. This subtle difference in the physician–patient relationship leads to a more direct coupling between imaging innovation and clinical impact that is so visible in retinal imaging and analysis. Given the above, it can be expected that translation of fundamental research findings in retinal imaging will remain rapid in the future. The need to computerize and automate image interpretation is correspondingly high. A global push toward cost-effective imaging and image analysis for wide-scale retinal and/or systemic disease detection in a population-screening setting will mandate continued efforts in perfecting automated image analysis.[19]

We expect that retinal image analysis and interpretation will be coupled to genetic and other assessment indices, allowing truly personalized approaches to complex analyses of broad sets of patient-specific data. On the technological side, it will require development and wide utilization of highly automated techniques for combined analysis of retinal image data in 2D, 3D, and 4D (3D + time), quantification of temporal changes, including the assessment of local and/or systemic severity of the findings. On the patient management side, it will therefore lead to broad utilization of semiautomated, clinician-supervised management of retinal diseases, especially DR, and choroidal neovascularization. Overall, we envision that, in the next decade, the utilization of retinal imaging will go far beyond the direct needs of retinal disease management, and that the quantified retinal exam will become broadly used in systemic disease assessment both for patient-specific care and for population studies.

Retinal imaging and image analysis have developed rapidly over the past 10 years, and image analysis now plays a crucial role in the care of patients with retinal diseases, as well as diseases that manifest in the retina. So far, image analysis has mostly operated reactively, i.e., waiting for what the newest imaging devices have as output, and then trying to find approaches to analyze and quantify the image data. Moving forward, we expect that imaging device development and image analysis research will start to operate more in concert and become closely integrated, so that retinal image analysis successes and difficulties can directly influence device developers to focus on details that will help analyze the images reliably, and vice versa. Ultimately, research and development in retinal imaging and analysis are driven by the overarching goal of preventing visual loss and suffering from retinal and systemic disease. We expect that this integrated development, in which a number of high-profile groups participate worldwide, will recognize the needs of the developed as well as the developing world.

REFERENCES

1. Zhang X, Saaddine JB, Chou CF, et al. Prevalence of diabetic retinopathy in the United States, 2005–2008. JAMA 2010;304:649–56.
2. Flick CS. Centenary of Babbage's ophthalmoscope. Optician 1947;113:246.
3. Keeler CR. 150 years since Babbage's ophthalmoscope. Arch Ophthalmol 1997;115:1456–7.
4. von Helmholtz H. Beschreibung eines Augens-Spiegels zur Untersuchung der Netzhaut im lebenden Auge. Berlin: Foerstner; 1851.
5. Trigt AC. Dissertatio ophthalmologica inauguralis de speculo oculi. Utrecht: Universiteit van Utrecht; 1853.
6. Gerloff O. Über die Photographie des Augenhintergrundes. Klin Monbl Augenheilkd 1891;29:397ff.
7. Gullstrand A. Neue methoden der reflexlosen Ophthalmoskopie. Berichte Dtsch Ophthalmologische Gesellschaft 1910;36.
8. Novotny HR, Alvis DL. A method of photographing fluorescence in circulating blood in the human retina. Circulation 1961;24:82–6.
9. Allen L. Ocular fundus photography: suggestions for achieving consistently good pictures and instructions for stereoscopic photography. Am J Ophthalmol 1964;57:13–28.
10. Webb RH, Hughes GW. Scanning laser ophthalmoscope. IEEE Trans Biomed Eng 1981;28:488–92.
11. Youngquist RC, Carr S, Davies DE. Optical coherence-domain reflectometry: a new optical evaluation technique. Optics Lett 1987;12:158–60.
12. Youngquist RC, Wentworth RH, Fesler KA. Selective interferometric sensing by the use of coherence synthesis. Optics Lett 1987;12:944–6.
13. Huang D, Swanson EA, Lin CP, et al. Optical coherence tomography. Science 1991;254:1178–81.
14. Swanson EA, Izatt JA, Hee MR, et al. In vivo retinal imaging by optical coherence tomography. Optics Lett 1993;18:1864–6.
15. Matsui M, Tashiro T, Matsumoto K, et al. [A study on automatic and quantitative diagnosis of fundus photographs. I. Detection of contour line of retinal blood vessel images on color fundus photographs (author's transl).] Nippon Ganka Gakkai Zasshi 1973;77:907–18.
16. Baudoin CE, Lay BJ, Klein JC. Automatic detection of microaneurysms in diabetic fluorescein angiography. Rev Epidemiol Sante Publique 1984;32: 254–61.
17. Wild S, Roglic G, Green A, et al. Global prevalence of diabetes: estimates for the year 2000 and projections for 2030. Diabetes Care 2004;27:1047–53.
18. Germain N, Galusca B, Deb-Joardar N, et al. No loss of chance of diabetic retinopathy screening by endocrinologists with a digital fundus camera. Diabetes Care 2011;34:580–5.
19. Abramoff MD, Garvin M, Sonka M. Retinal imaging and image analysis. IEEE Rev Biomed Eng 2010:169–208.
20. Fujimoto JG. Optical coherence tomography for ultrahigh resolution in vivo imaging. Nat Biotechnol 2003;21:1361–7.
21. Fercher AF, Mengedoht K, Werner W. Eye-length measurement by interferometry with partially coherent light. Optics Lett 1988;13:186–8.
22. Choma M, Sarunic M, Yang C, et al. Sensitivity advantage of swept source and Fourier domain optical coherence tomography. Optics Express 2003;11:2183–9.
23. Abramoff MD, Kardon RH, Vermeer KA, et al. A portable, patient friendly scanning laser ophthalmoscope for diabetic retinopathy imaging: exudates and hemorrhages. Invest Ophthalm Vis Sci 2007;48 E-Abstract 2592.

24. Hammer DX, Ferguson RD, Ustun TE, et al. Line-scanning laser ophthalmoscope. J Biomed Opt 2006;11:041126.
25. Suansilpong A, Rawdaree P. Accuracy of single-field nonmydriatic digital fundus image in screening for diabetic retinopathy. J Med Assoc Thai 2008;91:1397–403.
26. Delori FC, Pflibsen KP. Spectral reflectance of the human ocular fundus. Appl Opt 1989;28:1061–77.
27. Abramoff MD, Kwon YH, Ts'o D, et al. Visual stimulus-induced changes in human near-infrared fundus reflectance. Invest Ophthalmol Vis Sci 2006;47: 715–21.
28. Whited JD. Accuracy and reliability of teleophthalmology for diagnosing diabetic retinopathy and macular edema: a review of the literature. Diabetes Technol Ther 2006;8:102–11.
29. Lin DY, Blumenkranz MS, Brothers R. The role of digital fundus photography in diabetic retinopathy screening. Digital Diabetic Screening Group (DDSG). Diabetes Technol Ther 1999;1:477–87.
30. Standards and Guidelines in Telehealth for Diabetic Retinopathy: American Telemedicine Association position statement. Available online at: http://www.americantelemed.org/ICOT/drpositionpaper.paper.technical.htm) (accessed 1 October, 2004).
31. Bresnick GH, Mukamel DB, Dickinson JC, et al. A screening approach to the surveillance of patients with diabetes for the presence of vision-threatening retinopathy. Ophthalmology 2000;107:19–24.
32. Kinyoun JL, Martin DC, Fujimoto WY, et al. Ophthalmoscopy versus fundus photographs for detecting and grading diabetic retinopathy. Invest Ophthalmol Vis Sci 1992;33:1888–93.
33. Preferred Practice Pattern: Diabetic Retinopathy. Available online at: www.aao.org/ppp (accessed October 10, 2006).
34. Fong DS, Aiello L, Gardner TW, et al. Diabetic retinopathy. Diabetes Care 2003;26:226–9.
35. Fong DS, Sharza M, Chen W, et al. Vision loss among diabetics in a group model Health Maintenance Organization (HMO). Am J Ophthalmol 2002;133: 236–41.
36. Wilson C, Horton M, Cavallerano J, et al. Addition of primary care-based retinal imaging technology to an existing eye care professional referral program increased the rate of surveillance and treatment of diabetic retinopathy. Diabetes Care 2005;28:318–22.
37. Klonoff DC, Schwartz DM. An economic analysis of interventions for diabetes. Diabetes Care 2000;23:390–404.
38. Lin DY, Blumenkranz MS, Brothers RJ, et al. The sensitivity and specificity of single-field nonmydriatic monochromatic digital fundus photography with remote image interpretation for diabetic retinopathy screening: a comparison with ophthalmoscopy and standardized mydriatic color photography. Am J Ophthalmol 2002;134:204–13.
39. Williams GA, Scott IU, Haller JA, et al. Single-field fundus photography for diabetic retinopathy screening: a report by the American Academy of Ophthalmology. Ophthalmology 2004;111:1055–62.
40. Lawrence MG. The accuracy of digital-video retinal imaging to screen for diabetic retinopathy: an analysis of two digital-video retinal imaging systems using standard stereoscopic seven-field photography and dilated clinical examination as reference standards. Trans Am Ophthalmol Soc 2004;102: 321–40.
41. Abramoff MD, Suttorp-Schulten MS. Web-based screening for diabetic retinopathy in a primary care population: the EyeCheck project. Telemed J E Health 2005;11:668–74.
42. Abramoff MD, Reinhardt JM, Russell SR, et al. Automated early detection of diabetic retinopathy. Ophthalmology 2010;117:1147–54.
43. Abramoff MD, Niemeijer M, Suttorp-Schulten MS, et al. Evaluation of a system for automatic detection of diabetic retinopathy from color fundus photographs in a large population of patients with diabetes. Diabetes Care 2008;31:193–8.
44. Philip S, Fleming AD, Goatman KA, et al. The efficacy of automated "disease/no disease" grading for diabetic retinopathy in a systematic screening programme. Br J Ophthalmol 2007;91:1512–7.
45. Cheung N, Rogers S, Couper DJ, et al. Is diabetic retinopathy an independent risk factor for ischemic stroke? Stroke 2007;38:398–401.
46. Photocoagulation treatment of proliferative diabetic retinopathy: the second report of diabetic retinopathy study findings. Ophthalmology 1978;85:82–106.
47. Rosenfeld PJ, Moshfeghi AA, Puliafito CA. Optical coherence tomography findings after an intravitreal injection of bevacizumab (Avastin) for neovascular age-related macular degeneration. Ophthalm Surg Lasers Imaging 2005;36:331–5.
48. Heier JS, Antoszyk AN, Pavan PR, et al. Ranibizumab for treatment of neovascular age-related macular degeneration: a phase I/II multicenter, controlled, multidose study. Ophthalmology 2006;113:633.e1–4.
49. Preliminary report on effects of photocoagulation therapy. The Diabetic Retinopathy Study Research Group. Am J Ophthalmol 1976;81:383–96.
50. Grading diabetic retinopathy from stereoscopic color fundus photographs – an extension of the modified Airlie House classification. ETDRS report number 10. Early Treatment Diabetic Retinopathy Study Research Group. Ophthalmology 1991;98:786–806.
51. Harvey JN, Craney L, Nagendran S, et al. Towards comprehensive population-based screening for diabetic retinopathy: operation of the North Wales diabetic retinopathy screening programme using a central patient register and various screening methods. J Med Screen 2006;13:87–92.
52. Sonka M, Fitzpatrick JM. Handbook of medical imaging, vol. 2. Medical image processing and analysis. Wellingham, WA: International Society for Optical Engineering Press; 2000.
53. Supplement 91: Ophthalmic Photography Image SOP Classes. Available online at: ftp://medical.nema.org/medical/dicom/final/sup91_ft2.pdf.
54. DICOM. Supplement 110: Ophthalmic Tomography Image Storage SOP Class. Available online at: ftp://medical.nema.org/medical/dicom/final/sup110_ft4.pdf.
55. Abramoff MD, Alward WL, Greenlee EC, et al. Automated segmentation of the optic nerve head from stereo color photographs using physiologically plausible feature detectors. Invest Ophthalm Vis Sci 2007;48:1665–73.
56. Tobin KW, Abramoff MD, Chaum E, et al. Using a patient image archive to diagnose retinopathy. Conf Proc IEEE Eng Med Biol Soc 2008;2008:5441–4.
57. Niemeijer M, Staal JS, van Ginneken B, et al. Comparative study of retinal vessel segmentation on a new publicly available database. Proc SPIE 2004: 5370–9.
58. Soares JV, Leandro JJ, Cesar Junior RM, et al. Retinal vessel segmentation using the 2-D Gabor wavelet and supervised classification. IEEE Trans Med Imaging 2006;25:1214–22.
59. Staal J, Abramoff MD, Niemeijer M, et al. Ridge-based vessel segmentation in color images of the retina. IEEE Trans Med Imaging 2004;23:501–9.
60. Hubbard LD, Brothers RJ, King WN, et al. Methods for evaluation of retinal microvascular abnormalities associated with hypertension/sclerosis in the Atherosclerosis Risk in Communities Study. Ophthalmology 1999;106: 2269–80.
61. Owens DR, Gibbins RL, Lewis PA, et al. Screening for diabetic retinopathy by general practitioners: ophthalmoscopy or retinal photography as 35 mm colour transparencies? Diabet Med 1998;15:170–5.
62. Niemeijer M, Xu X, Dumitrescu AV, et al. Automated measurement of the arteriolar-to-venular width ratio in digital color fundus photographs. IEEE Trans Med Imaging 2011;30:1941–50
63. Lalonde M, Gagnon L, Boucher M-C. Non-recursive paired tracking for vessel extraction from retinal images. Proc Conf Vis Interface. 2000:61–8.
64. Gang L, Chutatape O, Krishnan SM. Detection and measurement of retinal vessels in fundus images using amplitude modified second-order Gaussian filter. IEEE Trans BioMed Eng 2002;49:168–72.
65. Hoover A, Goldbaum M. Locating the optic nerve in a retinal image using the fuzzy convergence of the blood vessels. IEEE Trans Med Imaging 2003;22: 951–8.
66. Foracchia M, Grisan E, Ruggeri A. Detection of optic disc in retinal images by means of a geometrical model of vessel structure. IEEE Trans Med Imaging 2004;23:1189–95.
67. Lowell J, Hunter A, Steel D, et al. Optic nerve head segmentation. IEEE Trans Med Imaging 2004;23:256–64.
68. Fleming AD, Goatman KA, Philip S, et al. Automatic detection of retinal anatomy to assist diabetic retinopathy screening. Phys Med Biol 2007;52: 331–45.
69. Li H, Chutatape O. Automated feature extraction in color retinal images by a model based approach. IEEE Trans Biomed Eng 2004;51:246–54.
70. Sinthanayothin C, Boyce JF, Cook HL, et al. Automated localisation of the optic disc, fovea, and retinal blood vessels from digital colour fundus images. Br J Ophthalmol 1999;83:902–10.
71. Tobin KW, Chaum E, Govindasamy VP, et al. Detection of anatomic structures in human retinal imagery. IEEE Trans Med Imaging 2007;26:1729–39.
72. Abramoff MD, Niemeijer M. The automatic detection of the optic disc location in retinal images using optic disc location regression. Conf Proc IEEE Eng Med Biol Soc 2006;1:4432–5.
73. Niemeijer M, Abramoff MD, van Ginneken B. Segmentation of the optic disc, macula and vascular arch in fundus photographs. IEEE Trans Med Imaging 2007;26:116–27.
74. Walter T, Klein JC, Massin P, et al. A contribution of image processing to the diagnosis of diabetic retinopathy – detection of exudates in color fundus images of the human retina. IEEE Trans Med Imaging 2002;21:1236–43.
75. Spencer T, Olson JA, McHardy KC, et al. An image-processing strategy for the segmentation and quantification of microaneurysms in fluorescein angiograms of the ocular fundus. Comput Biomed Res 1996;29:284–302.
76. Frame AJ, Undrill PE, Cree MJ, et al. A comparison of computer based classification methods applied to the detection of microaneurysms in ophthalmic fluorescein angiograms. Comput Biol Med 1998;28:225–38.
77. Hipwell JH, Strachan F, Olson JA, et al. Automated detection of microaneurysms in digital red-free photographs: a diabetic retinopathy screening tool. Diabet Med 2000;17:588–94.
78. Niemeijer M, van Ginneken B, Staal J, et al. Automatic detection of red lesions in digital color fundus photographs. IEEE Trans Med Imaging 2005;24:584–92.
79. Niemeijer M, van Ginneken B, Russell SR, et al. Automated detection and differentiation of drusen, exudates, and cotton-wool spots in digital color fundus photographs for diabetic retinopathy diagnosis. Invest Ophthalmol Vis Sci 2007;48:2260–7.
80. Cree MJ, Olson JA, McHardy KC, et al. A fully automated comparative microaneurysm digital detection system. Eye (Lond) 1997;11:622–8.
81. Gardner GG, Keating D, Williamson TH, et al. Automatic detection of diabetic retinopathy using an artificial neural network: a screening tool [see comments]. Br J Ophthalmol 1996;80:940–4.
82. Sinthanayothin C, Boyce JF, Williamson TH, et al. Automated detection of diabetic retinopathy on digital fundus images. Diabet Med 2002;19:105–12.
83. Quellec G, Lamard M, Cazuguel G, et al. Adaptive nonseparable wavelet transform via lifting and its application to content-based image retrieval. IEEE Trans Image Process 2010;19:25–35
84. Osareh A, Mirmehdi M, Thomas B, et al. Automated identification of diabetic retinal exudates in digital colour images. Br J Ophthalmol 2003;87: 1220–3.

85. Al-Diri B, Hunter A, Steel D. An active contour model for segmenting and measuring retinal vessels. IEEE Trans Med Imaging 2009;28:1488–97.
86. Brinchmann-Hansen O. The light reflex on retinal arteries and veins. A theoretical study and a new technique for measuring width and intensity profiles across retinal vessels. Acta Ophthalmol Suppl 1986;179:1–53.
87. Brinchmann-Hansen O, Sandvik L. The intensity of the light reflex on retinal arteries and veins. Acta Ophthalmol 1986;64:547–52.
88. Brinchmann-Hansen O, Sandvik L. The width of the light reflex on retinal arteries and veins. Acta Ophthalmol 1986;64:433–8.
89. Xu X, Niemeijer M, Song Q, et al. Vessel boundary delineation on fundus images using graph-based approach. IEEE Trans Med Imaging 2011;30:1184–91.
90. Niemeijer M, Xu X, Dumitrescu A, et al. Automated measurement of the arteriolar-to-venular width ratio in digital color fundus photographs. IEEE Trans Med Imaging 2011.
91. Lee S, Reinhardt JM, Cattin PC, et al. Objective and expert-independent validation of retinal image registration algorithms by a projective imaging distortion model. Med Image Anal 2010;14:539–49.
92. Lee S, Abràmoff MD, Reinhardt JM. Retinal image mosaicing using the radial distortion correction model. In: Reinhardt JM, Pluim JP, editors. Medical imaging 2008: image processing. Proc SPIE 2008;6914:691435–9.
93. Karnowski TP, Aykac D, Chaum E, et al. Practical considerations for optic nerve location in telemedicine. Conf Proc IEEE Eng Med Biol Soc 2009;2009:6205–9.
94. Lamard M, Cazuguel G, Quellec G, et al. Content based image retrieval based on wavelet transform coefficients distribution. Conf Proc IEEE Eng Med Biol Soc 2007;2007:4532–5.
95. Niemeijer M, van Ginneken B, Cree MJ, et al. Retinopathy online challenge: automatic detection of microaneurysms in digital color fundus photographs. IEEE Trans Med Imaging 2010;29:185–95.
96. Hoover A, Kouznetsova V, Goldbaum M. Locating blood vessels in retinal images by piecewise threshold probing of a matched filter response. IEEE Trans Med Imaging 2000;19:203–10.
97. Giancardo L, Abramoff MD, Chaum E, et al. Elliptical local vessel density: a fast and robust quality metric for retinal images. Conf Proc IEEE Eng Med Biol Soc 2008;2008:3534–7.
98. Messidor. 2005. Available online at: http://latim.univ-brest.fr/index.php?option=com_content&view=article&id=61&Itemid=100034&lang=en)
99. Tang L, Niemeijer M, Abramoff MD. Splat feature classification: detection of large retinal hemorrhages. 2011 IEEE International Symposium on Biomedical Imaging: From Nano to Macro. Chicago, IL.
100. Lee K, Garvin MK, Russell S, et al. Automated intraretinal layer segmentation of 3-D macular OCT scans using a multiscale graph search. ARVO Meeting Abstracts 2010;51:1767.
101. Tang L, Kwon YH, Alward WLM, et al. Automated measurement of optic nerve head shape from stereo color photographs of the optic disc: validation with SD-OCT. ARVO Meeting Abstracts 2010;51:1774.
102. Antony BJ, Tang L, Abramoff M, et al. Automated method for the flattening of optical coherence tomography images. ARVO Meeting Abstracts 2010;51:1781.
103. Mahajan VB, Folk JC, Russell SR, et al. Iowa membrane maps: SD OCT guided therapy for epiretinal membrane. ARVO Meeting Abstracts 2010;51:3604.
104. Verbraak FD, Van Dijk HW, Kok PH, et al. Reduced retinal thickness in patients with type 2 diabetes mellitus. ARVO Meeting Abstracts 2010;51:4671.
105. Baroni M, Barletta G. Contour definition and tracking in cardiac imaging through the integration of knowledge and image evidence. Ann Biomed Eng 2004;32:688–95.
106. Haeker M, Abràmoff MD, Kardon R, et al. Segmentation of the surfaces of the retinal layer from OCT images. Lecture Notes Computer Sci 2006;4190:800–7.
107. Haeker M, Abramoff MD, Wu X, et al. Use of varying constraints in optimal 3-D graph search for segmentation of macular optical coherence tomography images. Med Image Comput Comput Assist Interv 2007;10:244–51.
108. Haeker M, Wu X, Abramoff M, et al. Incorporation of regional information in optimal 3-D graph search with application for intraretinal layer segmentation of optical coherence tomography images. Inf Process Med Imaging 2007;20:607–18.
109. Garvin MK, Abramoff MD, Kardon R, et al. Intraretinal layer segmentation of macular optical coherence tomography images using optimal 3-D graph search. IEEE Trans Med Imaging 2008;27:1495–505.
110. Galler KE, Folk JC, Russell SR, et al. Patient preference and safety of bilateral intravitreal injection of anti-VEGF therapy. ARVO Meeting Abstracts 2009;50:247.
111. Garvin MK, Abramoff MD, Wu X, et al. Automated 3-D intraretinal layer segmentation of macular spectral-domain optical coherence tomography images. IEEE Trans Med Imaging 2009;28:1436–47.
112. Reinhardt JM, Lee S, Xu X, et al. Retina atlas mapping from color fundus images. ARVO Meeting Abstracts 2009;50:3811.
113. Antony BJ, Abramoff MD, Lee K, et al. Automated 3D segmentation of intraretinal layers from optic nerve head optical coherence tomography images. In: Molthen RC, Weaver JB, editors. Medical Imaging 2010: Biomedical Applications in Molecular, Structural, and Functional Imaging. Proc SPIE 2010;7626:76260U.
114. Van Dijk HW, Kok PH, Garvin M, et al. Selective loss of inner retinal layer thickness in type 1 diabetic patients with minimal diabetic retinopathy. Invest Ophthalmol Vis Sci 2009;50:3404–9.
115. van Dijk HW, Verbraak FD, Kok PH, et al. Decreased retinal ganglion cell layer thickness in patients with type 1 diabetes. Invest Ophthalmol Vis Sci 2010;51:3660–5.
116. Longmuir SQ, Longmuir R, Matthews K, et al. Retinal arterial but not venous tortuosity correlates with facioscapulohumeral muscular dystrophy (FSHD) severity. ARVO Meeting Abstracts 2009;50:5419.
117. Quellec G, Lamard M, Cazuguel G, et al. Multimodal information retrieval to assist diabetic retinopathy diagnosis. ARVO Meeting Abstracts 2009;50:1363.
118. Agurto Rios C, Pattichis MS, Murillo S, et al. Detection of structures in the retina using AM-FM for diabetic retinopathy classification. ARVO Meeting Abstracts 2009;50:313.
119. Tso DY, Schallek JB, Kardon R, et al. Hemodynamic components contribute to intrinsic signals of the retina and optic disc. ARVO Meeting Abstracts 2009;50:4322.
120. Garvin MK, Niemeijer M, Kardon RH, et al. automatically correcting for the presence of retinal vessels on spectral-domain optical coherence tomography images decreases variability of the segmented retinal layers. ARVO Meeting Abstracts 2009;50:1099.
121. Lee K, Niemeijer M, Garvin MK, et al. Automated optic disc segmentation from 3D SD-OCT of the optic nerve head (ONH). ARVO Meeting Abstracts 2009;50:1102.
122. Xu Y, Sonka M, McLennan G, et al. MDCT-based 3-D texture classification of emphysema and early smoking related lung pathologies. IEEE Trans Med Imaging 2006;25:464–75.
123. Quellec G, Lee K, Dolejsi M, et al. Three-dimensional analysis of retinal layer texture: identification of fluid-filled regions in SD-OCT of the macula. IEEE Trans Med Imaging 2010;29:1321–30.
124. Van Dijk HW, Kok PHB, Garvin M, et al. Selective loss of inner retinal layer thickness in type 1 diabetic patients with minimal diabetic retinopathy. ARVO Meeting Abstracts 2009;50:3244.
125. Abramoff MD, Russell SR, Mahajan V, et al. Performance of automated detection of diabetic retinopathy does not improve by using the distance of each lesion to the fovea. ARVO Meeting Abstracts 2009;50:3268.
126. Barriga ES, Russell SR, Pattichis MS, et al. Relationship between visual features and analytically derived features in non-exudated AMD phenotypes: closing the sematic gap. ARVO Meeting Abstracts 2009;50:3274.
127. Hu Z, Niemeijer M, Lee K, et al. Automated segmentation of the optic canal in 3D spectral-domain OCT of the optic nerve head (ONH) using retinal vessel suppression. ARVO Meeting Abstracts 2009;50:3334.
128. Niemeijer M, Garvin MK, Lee K, et al. Automated segmentation of the retinal vasculature silhouettes in isotropic 3D optical coherence tomography scans. ARVO Meeting Abstracts 2009;50:1103.
129. Niemeijer M, Garvin MK, van Ginneken B, et al. Vessel segmentation in 3D spectral OCT scans of the retina. Medical Imaging 2008: Image Processing 2008;6914:69141R–8.
130. Niemeijer M, Sonka M, Garvin MK, et al. Automated segmentation of the retinal vasculature in 3D optical coherence tomography images. ARVO Meeting Abstracts 2008;49:1832.
131. Davis B, Russell SR, Abramoff MD, et al. Application of independent component analysis to classify non-exudative amd phenotypes quantitatively from vision-based derived features in retinal images. ARVO Meeting Abstracts 2008;49:887.
132. Xu J, Ishikawa H, Wollstein G, et al. Retinal vessel segmentation on SLO image. Conf Proc IEEE Eng Med Biol Soc 2008;2008:2258–61.
133. Nelson D, Abramoff MD, Kwon YH, et al. Correlation of progression between structure and function in ocular hypertensive patients from the SAFE study. ARVO Meeting Abstracts 2008;49:738.
134. Lee K, Abramoff MD, Niemeijer M, et al. 3-D segmentation of retinal blood vessels in spectral-domain OCT volumes of the optic nerve head. In: Molthen RC, Weaver JB, editors. Medical Imaging 2010: Biomedical Applications in Molecular, Structural, and Functional Imaging. Proc SPIE 2010;7626:76260V.
135. Duda RA, Hart PE, Stork DG. Pattern classification. New York: Wiley-Interscience; 2001.
136. Lee S, Reinhardt JM, Niemeijer M, et al. Comparing the performance of retinal image registration algorithms using the centerline error measurement metric. ARVO Meeting Abstracts 2008;49:1833.
137. Garvin MK, Sonka M, Kardon RH, et al. Three-dimensional analysis of SD OCT: thickness assessment of six macular layers in normal subjects. ARVO Meeting Abstracts 2008;49:1879.
138. Boykov Y, Kolmogorov V. An experimental comparison of min-cut/max-flow algorithms for energy minimization in vision. IEEE Trans Pattern Anal Mach Intell 2004;26:1124–37.
139. Yang EB, Jin Jones Y, Alward WLM, et al. Comparing resident and fellow performance on evaluation of stereoscopic optic disc images. ARVO Meeting Abstracts 2008;49:3626.
140. Tobin KW, Chaum E, Abramoff MD, et al. Automated diagnosis of retinal disease in a large diabetic population. ARVO Meeting Abstracts 2008;49:3225.
141. Graff JM, Abramoff MD, Russell SR. Stereo video indirect ophthalmoscopy: a novel educational and research tool. ARVO Meeting Abstracts 2008;49:3228.
142. Abramoff MD, Kardon RH, Vermeer KA, et al. A portable, patient friendly scanning laser ophthalmoscope for diabetic retinopathy imaging: exudates and hemorrhages. ARVO Meeting Abstracts 2007;48 E-Abstract:2592.
143. Russell SR, Abramoff MD, Radosevich MD, et al. Quantitative assessment of retinal image quality compared to subjective determination. ARVO Meeting Abstracts 2007;48:2607.

144. Piette SD, Adix ML, Abramoff MD, et al. Comparison of computer aided planimetry between simultaneous and non-simultaneous stereo optic disc photographs. ARVO Meeting Abstracts 2007;48:1184.
145. Lee S, Abramoff MD, Reinhardt J. Feature-based pairwise retinal image registration by radial distortion correction. Med Imaging: Image Anal Proc SPIE Med Imaging 2007;6512.
146. Tso DY, Schallek J, Kwon Y, et al. Blood flow dynamics contribute to functional intrinsic optical signals in the cat retina in vivo. ARVO Meeting Abstracts 2007;48:1951.
147. Lee S, Abramoff MD, Reinhardt JM. Retinal atlas statistics from color fundus images. In: Dawant BM, Haynor DR, editors. Medical Imaging 2010: Image Processing. Proc SPIE 2010;7623:762310–9.
148. Vermeer KA, Mensink MH, Kardon RH, et al. Super resolution in retinal imaging. ARVO Meeting Abstracts 2007;48:2766.
149. Niemeijer M, Garvin MK, Lee K, et al. Registration of 3D spectral OCT volumes using 3D SIFT feature point matching. Med Imaging 2009: Image Processing 2009;7259:72591I–8.
150. Lowe DG. Distinctive image features from scale-invariant keypoints. Int J Comput Vision 2004;60:91–110.
151. Klein R, Chou CF, Klein BE, et al. Prevalence of age-related macular degeneration in the US population. Arch Ophthalmol 2011;129:75–80.
152. Sánchez CI, Hornero R, Mayo A, et al. Mixture model-based clustering and logistic regression for automatic detection of microaneurysms in retinal images. In: Karssemeijer N, Giger ML, editors. Medical Imaging 2009: Computer-Aided Diagnosis. Proc SPIE 2009;7260:72601M.
153. Cree MJ. The Waikato Microaneurysm Detector Univ. Waikato, Tech. Rep., 2008. Available online at: http://roc.healthcare.uiowa.edu/results/documentation/waikato.pdf
154. Quellec G, Lamard M, Josselin PM, et al. Optimal wavelet transform for the detection of microaneurysms in retina photographs. IEEE Trans Med Imag 2008;27:1230–41.
155. Zhang B, Wu X, You J, et al. Hierarchical detection of red lesions in retinal images by multiscale correlation filtering. In: Karssemeijer N, Giger ML, editors. Medical Imaging 2009: Computer-Aided Diagnosis. Proc SPIE 2009;7260:72601L.
156. Mizutani A, Muramatsu C, Hatanaka Y, et al. Automated microaneurysm detection method based on double ring filter in retinal fundus images. In: Karssemeijer N, Giger ML, editors. Medical Imaging 2009: Computer-Aided Diagnosis. Proc SPIE 2009;7260:72601N.

Section 2 Retinal Diagnostics

Chapter 7

Electrogenesis of the Electroretinogram

Laura J. Frishman

INTRODUCTION

The electroretinogram (ERG) is an electrical potential generated by the retina in response to a change in illumination. It is an excellent tool for evaluating retinal function in both the clinic and the laboratory because it can be recorded noninvasively from the corneal surface in vivo under physiological or nearly physiological (anesthetized) conditions. However, the ERG response to a flash of light is complex. It is the summed activity of all retinal cells, and consists of overlapping positive and negative component potentials that originate from different stages of retinal processing. For the ERG to be an effective tool in assessing normal and pathologic retinal activity, it is important that the contributions of the various retinal cell types be distinguished and characterized.

This chapter will review current knowledge of the cellular origins and mechanisms of generation of the various ERG component waves, progressing from distal retina to proximal retina. As will be described, the ERG is generated by radial currents arising either directly from retinal neurons, or as a result of the effect on retinal glia of changes in extracellular potassium concentration ($[K^+]_o$) brought about by retinal neuronal activity. Our understanding of the electrogenesis of the ERG was initially based on studies in a variety of cold-blooded vertebrate and as well as some mammalian species, described in more detail in previous reviews.[1,2] Studies in a nonhuman primate model (macaque monkey) whose retina and ERG are very similar to that of humans (Fig. 7.1),[3] and particularly those over the past two decades, have improved our understanding of the electrogenesis of the ERG in humans. This work will be highlighted wherever possible in this chapter. Clinical applications of the ERG will be described in the following chapter (Chapter 8, Clinical electrophysiology). Another recent review has examined the electrogenesis of a common animal model for retinal disease, the mouse.[3]

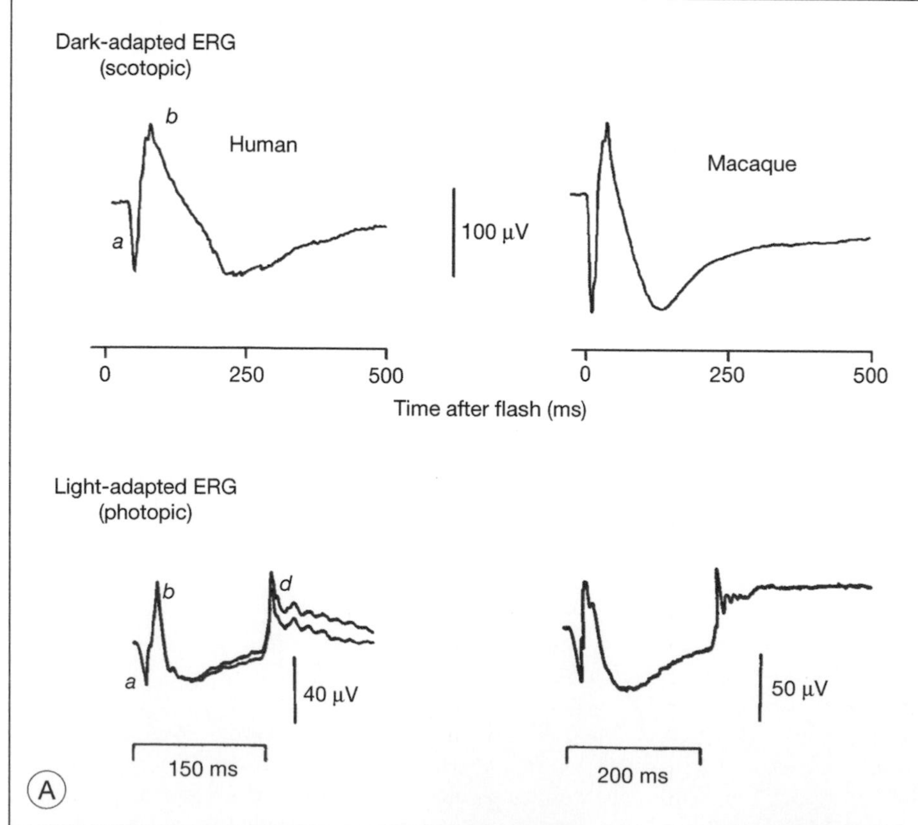

Fig. 7.1 Dark- and light-adapted full-field flash electroretinograms (ERGs) of human subjects and macaque monkeys. (A) Top: Dark-adapted (scotopic) ERGs in response to brief high-energy flashes from darkness occurring at time zero for a normal human subject (left) and an anesthetized macaque monkey (right). The stimulus energy was ~400 sc td/s. Bottom: Light-adapted (photopic) flash ERGs in response to longer-duration flashes on a rod-saturating background for a normal human subject (left) and a macaque monkey (right). For the human subject the stimulus was a 150-ms white full-field flash of 4.0 log ph td presented on a steady background of 3.3 log sc td. For the macaque, the same stimulus was used, but the flashes were 200 ms in duration. (Adapted from Sieving PA, Murayama K, Naarendorp F. Push–pull model of the primate photopic electroretinogram: a role for hyperpolarizing neurons in shaping the b-wave. Vis Neurosci 1994;11:519–32.)

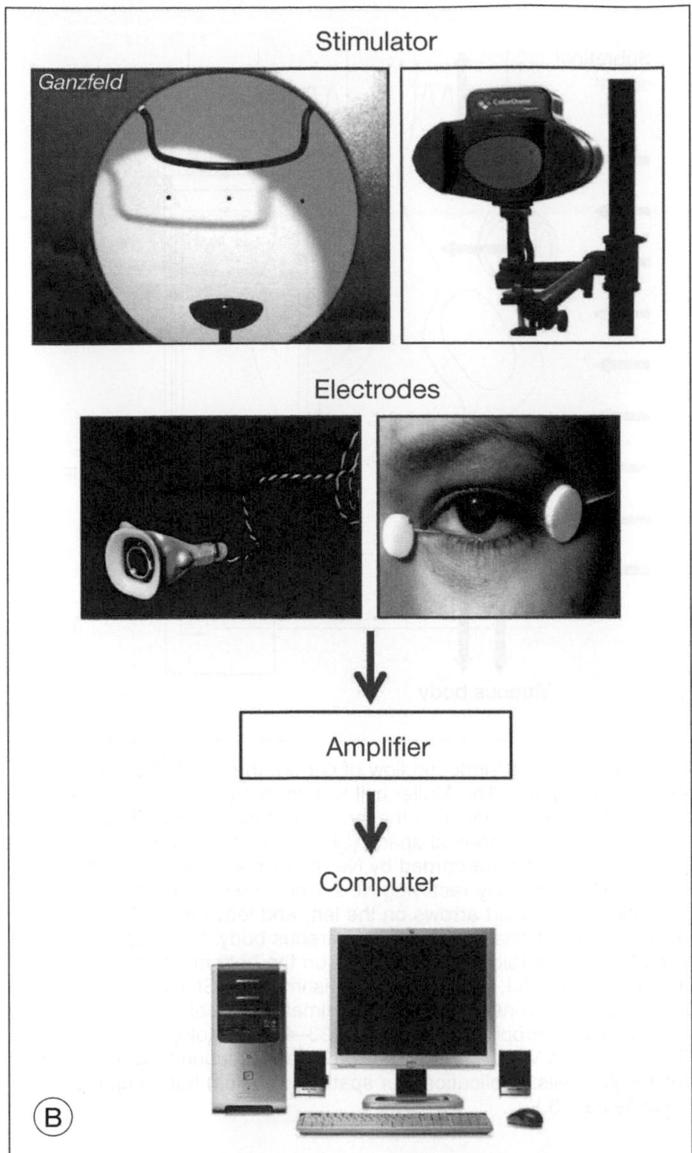

Fig. 7.1 Cont'd (B) ERG recording setup: recordings are made using a traditional ganzfeld bowl (left) or more modern light-emitting diode-based full-field stimulator. Burian-Allen and DTL fiber electrodes[4] are illustrated. ERG recordings are amplified and sent to a computer for averaging, display, and analysis.

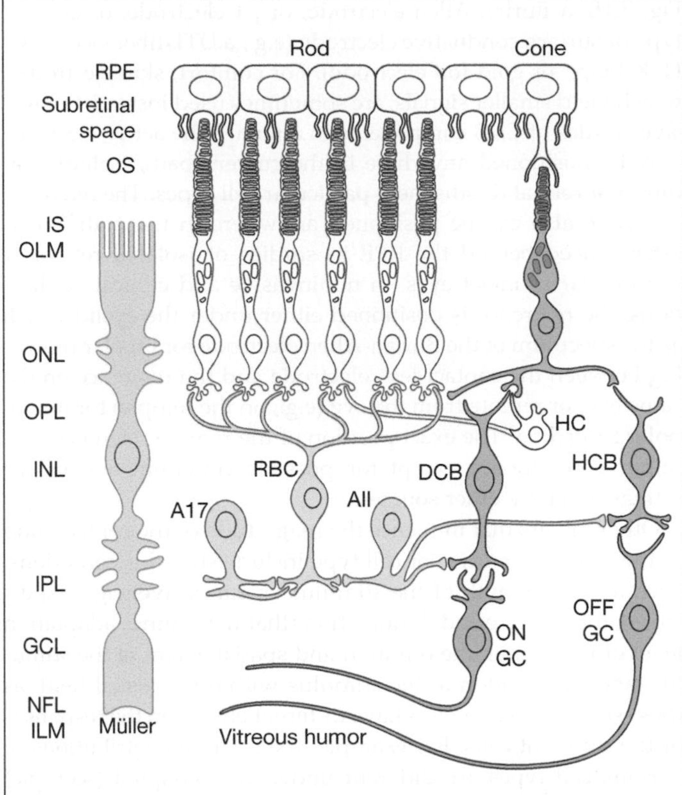

Fig. 7.2 Schematic of rod and cone pathways of the mammalian retina. The blue-filled cells indicate the cone pathways; the yellow-filled cells indicate the primary rod pathway. RPE, retinal pigment epithelium; OS, outer segment; IS, inner segment; HC, horizontal cell; RBC, rod bipolar cell; DCB, depolarizing (ON) cone bipolar cell; HCB, hyperpolarizing (OFF) bipolar cell; A, amacrine cell; GC, ganglion cell; OLM, outer limiting membrane; ONL, outer nuclear layer; OPL, outer plexiform layer; INL, inner nuclear layer; IPL, inner plexiform layer; GCL, ganglion cell layer; NFL, nerve fiber layer; ILM, inner limiting membrane. Scale bar = 20 µm.

GENERATION OF EXTRACELLULAR POTENTIALS: GENERAL CONCEPTS

Extracellular potentials that can be recorded noninvasively, such as the ERG (and visual evoked potential of the cortex), are the result of localized conductance changes in the membranes of activated cells that give rise to inward or outward currents. These currents also flow in the extracellular space (ECS) and create extracellular potentials. The current flowing through the conductive fluid surrounding a cell whose activation has given rise to a local current is directed mainly toward the relatively less activated parts of the cell. Thus, when neurons are arranged so that the extracellular currents of many synchronously activated cells all flow in the same direction, the resulting extracellular potential change, called a "field potential," may be large enough to be recorded at a distance, e.g., at the cornea in the case of the ERG. In the retina, because all neurons generate light-evoked currents, in principle they should all contribute to the retinal field potentials. However, depending upon various factors, considered below, the contribution from any particular cell type could be quite large, or not discernible in the response.

An important factor affecting a given cell's contribution to the ERG is its orientation in the retina. Radially oriented neurons in the retina (photoreceptors and bipolar cells) and glial cells (Müller cells and retinal pigment epithelial (RPE) cells) make larger contributions to the ERG than cells that are oriented more irregularly or laterally (e.g., horizontal and amacrine cells) (Fig. 7.2). The currents around cells that underlie the ERG enter the ECS at one retinal depth (the current source), and return into the cell at another depth (the current sink), creating a current dipole. Although most of the extracellular current flowing from source to sink traverses the ECS within the retina, some travels extraretinally - through the vitreous humor, extraocular tissues, sclera, choroid, the high resistance of the RPE (R-membrane), and back into the neural retina.

The polarity and amplitude of the recorded ERG will depend upon the location of the active and reference electrodes. In noninvasive studies, a common location for the active electrode is on the cornea via a contact lens electrode, e.g., as illustrated in

Fig. 7.1B, a Burian-Allen electrode, or jet electrode, or another type of surface conductive electrode (e.g., a DTL fiber electrode,[4] H–K loop,[5] or gold foil electrode). For comfort, skin electrodes, which yield smaller signals, are sometimes used instead. In invasive studies of ERG components in animals, the active electrode may be positioned anywhere in the current path, including at different retinal depths, near particular cell types. The reference electrode also can be positioned anywhere in the path, but is often placed behind the RPE in studies of isolated retina, or retrobulbar in intact eyes. In noninvasive and clinical applications, the reference is positioned either under the eyelids, such as the speculum of the Burian-Allen electrode for bipolar recording between the contact lens electrode and the reference on the same eye, or remote from the eye (e.g., on the temple) for monopolar recording. The exact position of the remote reference is of minor consequence except for possible contamination of the retinal signal by other sources.

Other factors that influence the magnitude of the contribution to the ERG of a particular cell type include stimulus conditions, such as the strength of the stimulus and its wavelength (spectrum), the background illumination (that determines adaptation level of the retina), the duration and spatial extent of the stimulus, and the location of the stimulus within the visual field, as these stimulus parameters have different effects on the responses of the different cells. For example, the relative contributions of various cell types are different under dark-adapted (scotopic) and light-adapted (photopic) conditions when rod and cone pathways, respectively, are involved in generating responses. Spatially extended diffuse stimuli, i.e., full-field (ganzfeld) flashes that fill the retina evenly, using stimulators such as those illustrated in Fig. 7.1B, are commonly used to elicit the major ERG waves (a-, b-, and d-waves) from photoreceptors and bipolar cells. Contributions from these cells generally increase with the area of the retina stimulated as the number of cells, and hence the total extracellular current, is increased. In contrast, contributions of retinal ganglion cells (and other cells with antagonistic regions within their receptive fields) to the full-field flash ERG will be limited by the strength of surround antagonism. For photopic ERGs, particularly from subjects with trichromatic color vision, such as the macaque and human, stimulus wavelength also affects contributions from cells whose responses are dependent upon spectral antagonism.[6,7]

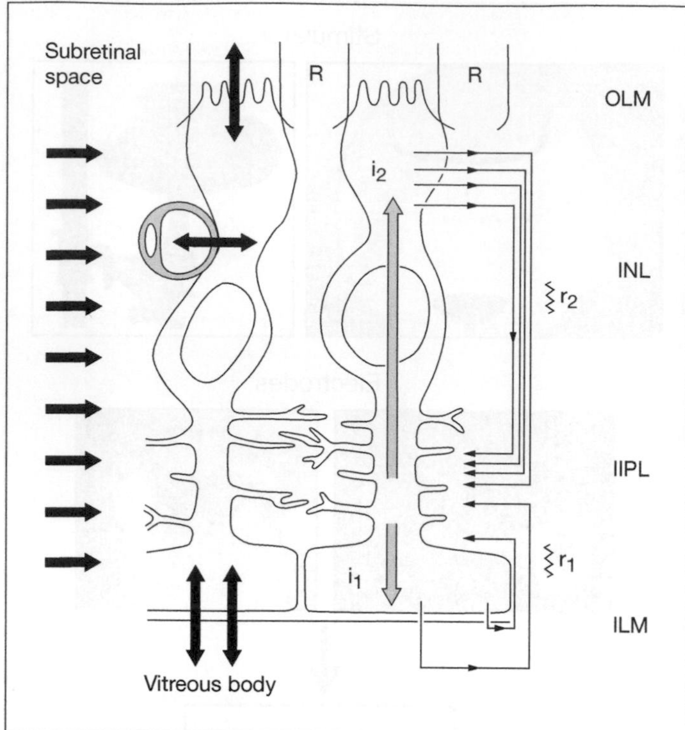

Fig. 7.3 Model of K^+-induced flow of current through Müller cells and extracellular space. The Müller cell K^+ currents (grey arrows) are induced by $[K^+]_o$ increases in the inner plexiform layer or $[K^+]_o$ decreases in the subretinal space (SRS); the return currents in the extracellular space are carried by Na^+ and Cl^- ions. K^+ enters the Müller cell via strongly rectifying Kir 2.1 channels in and around the synaptic layers (short arrows on the left) and leave the cell via weakly rectifying Kir 4.1 channels near the vitreous body, blood vessels, and subretinal space (bidirectional arrows on the bottom). The I_2 current generates slow PIII. (Adapted from Frishman LJ, Steinberg RH. Light-evoked increases in $[K^+]_o$ in proximal portion of the dark-adapted cat retina. J Neurophysiol 1989;61:1233–43 and Kofuji P, Biedermann B, Siddharthan V, et al. Kir potassium channel subunit expression in retinal glial cells: implications for spatial potassium buffering. Glia 2002;39:292–3.)

Spatial buffering by glial cells

Spatial buffering of $[K^+]_o$ by radially oriented Müller cells, RPE cells, and perhaps astrocytes in the optic nerve head is an important mechanism for generating the currents underlying several ERG components, to be described later in this chapter, e.g., c-wave, slow PIII, tail of the b-wave, scotopic threshold response (STR), M-wave, and photopic negative response (PhNR). Due to its importance in generating ERGs, an overview of $[K^+]_o$ spatial buffering in Müller cells will be presented here.

$[K^+]_o$ spatial buffering is important for maintaining the electrochemical gradients across cell membranes necessary for normal neuronal activity and for minimizing the changes in local $[K^+]_o$ that occur as a consequence of neuronal activation. Membrane depolarization leads to the leak of K^+ from neurons, causing $[K^+]_o$ to be elevated, particularly in synaptic layers of the retina (Fig. 7.3); membrane hyperpolarization leads to reduced $[K^+]_o$ as the leak conductance is reduced, but the Na^+–K^+ ATPase in the membranes continues to pump K^+ into (and Na^+ out of) cells. K^+ from the ECS enters the Müller cells via inwardly rectifying K^+ channels and is carried radially as an intracellular (spatial buffer) current to regions of lower $[K^+]_o$. Thus a current loop is set up: the current inside the Müller cell is carried by K^+ and, to complete the circuit, the dominant extracellular ions, Na^+ and Cl^-, carry the extracellular return current. Because the magnitude of the $[K^+]_o$ changes depends upon the integral of K^+ flow rate into the ECS, ERG components that reflect this glial current will be slower than components that reflect the currents around neurons. This "slowing" would be equivalent to low-pass filtering of the neuronal signal.

The electrical properties of the Müller cell membrane are important for the creation of spatial buffer currents. The membrane is selectively permeable to K^+,[8,9] but the K^+ conductance is not distributed evenly over the cell surface. Instead, it is concentrated in the vicinity of extracellular sinks (i.e., the vitreous body, subretinal space, and blood vessels). This regional distribution facilitates "K^+ siphoning" from synaptic areas where $[K^+]_o$ is high, to those regions of high K^+ conductance where $[K^+]_o$ is lower.[10,11] In mouse retina, as indicated in Fig. 7.3, strongly inward rectifying Kir 2.1 channels have been localized to synaptic layers (small arrows on the left) where K^+ moves from the ECS into Müller cells, whereas less strongly rectifying Kir 4.1 channels at the extracellular sinks allow K^+ to leave the Müller cell.[12]

APPROACHES FOR DETERMINING THE ORIGINS OF THE ELECTRORETINOGRAM

Historically, several different approaches have been used to determine the neuronal origins and cellular mechanisms of generation of the ERG.

Intraretinal depth recordings

A microelectrode positioned at some locus in the retinal ECS records a field potential called the "local" or "intraretinal" ERG.[13] The recorded potential reflects electrical activity of the cells located near the microelectrode tip, and when a local stimulus, such as a small spot of light, is used, the local activity will be the entire signal. However, when full-field diffuse flashes are used, currents can be sufficiently large to produce a corneal ERG simultaneously with the local ERG. Local potentials with a similar timecourse to that of the corneal ERG components can be helpful in locating the cells of origin. However, this type of analysis has some complications:

1. Field potentials that spread over long distances will superimpose in space and time, making it difficult to locate the cells of origin with certainty.
2. Retinal resistivity varies between and within retinal layers,[14,15] which causes currents passing through layers of different resistance to set up complex voltages.

Both of these problems occur in the intact eye when a scleral reference is used, and the local signal recorded with a microelectrode is contaminated by the diffuse ERG, due to the high resistance of the RPE and sclera. Some of this contamination can be eliminated by using a vitreal reference.[16]

Current source density (CSD) or "source-sink" analysis can provide a solution to these problems. Local field potentials are measured and analyzed, but in addition, radial resistance is taken into account to obtain direct estimates of radial current.[17] The result is a spatiotemporal profile of relatively well-localized current sources and sinks that can be compared with the retinal structure (layers) and physiology. CSD analysis has elucidated the origins of particular ERG components (e.g., for the bipolar cell origin of the b-wave).[18,19]

For ERG components believed to depend specifically on glial K^+ spatial buffer currents, intraretinal depth recordings with ion-selective microelectrodes have been used to locate the retinal layer(s) where neurally induced changes of $[K^+]_o$ were largest and most similar in timecourse to a particular component.[20–25] Application of barium (Ba^{2+}) to block Kir channels in glial cell membranes,[26,27] and the ERG components dependent upon the spatial buffer currents, or genetic inactivation of Kir4.1 channels in mice,[28] have been used to provide evidence for the role of Müller cells in generating certain slow waves of the ERG.

Correlation of ERG with single-cell recordings

Correlations of the ERG with single-cell electrophysiology are most useful when the light-evoked currents from a particular cell type are the primary determinant of an ERG component, as is the case for rod photoreceptors and the currents around the photoreceptor that generate the scotopic a-wave,[29] or rod bipolar cells and the scotopic b-wave in mammals.[30,31] Correlation also may be useful for identifying the origin of a response property, such as oscillatory potentials (OPs) in the ERG, and the light-evoked oscillatory behavior in amacrine cells as a possible source for the potentials. However, if currents from several cell types contribute to a local field potential, the relationship between field potential and local cellular responses may be difficult to determine without using other tools, such as pharmacologic agents.

Pharmacologic dissection

The use of pharmacologic agents that have specific effects on cellular functions has been very helpful in determining origins of ERG components. In Granit's classical pharmacologic study of the dark-adapted ERG of the cat, he observed that components disappeared sequentially during induction of ether anesthesia.[32] He called the components "processes" and numbered them in the order of disappearance: PI, the positive c-wave, was first to leave, then PII, the positive b-wave, disappeared, and finally, PIII, the negative a-wave. We now know that these processes correspond roughly to RPE, bipolar, and photoreceptor cell contributions to the ERG respectively. The terms PII and PIII are still used.

In recent years, much has been learned about retinal microcircuitry and biophysics, including information at cellular and molecular levels about retinal neurotransmitters (their identity, release mechanisms, and receptors), signal transduction cascades, ion channels, and other cellular proteins. This knowledge has allowed better use of pharmacologic tools in isolating ERG components and in interpreting experimental observations. For example, specific knowledge about glutamatergic neurotransmission in the retina and appropriate agonists and antagonists for specific receptors has improved our understanding of the major waves of the ERG, including the ERG in primates.[33–35] Use of the voltage-gated Na^+ channel blocker tetrodotoxin (TTX) has made it possible to identify ERG components resulting from the Na^+-dependent spiking activity of inner retinal cells.

Site-specific lesions/pathology or targeted mutations

Removal of a cell type or types or circuits allows assessment of their role in the electrogenesis of the ERG. A specific cell type can be lesioned selectively (e.g., retinal ganglion cells as a consequence of optic nerve section) or lost due to pathologic changes (e.g., ganglion cells in glaucoma), or inherited degenerations (e.g., rod and/or cone dystrophy). Cellular functions, such as light responses or synaptic transmission, can be abnormal or eliminated due to inherited or acquired conditions, or targeted genetic manipulation, most commonly done in mice.

Modeling of cellular responses and ERG components

As our understanding of the function of retinal cell types has improved, it has been possible to develop quantitative models that predict the light responses of those cells, and to apply the models to the analysis of the ERG. Models based on suction electrode recordings from single photoreceptor outer segments have been used to predict the leading edge of the a-wave,[36–38] although more proximal portions of the photoreceptor cell will

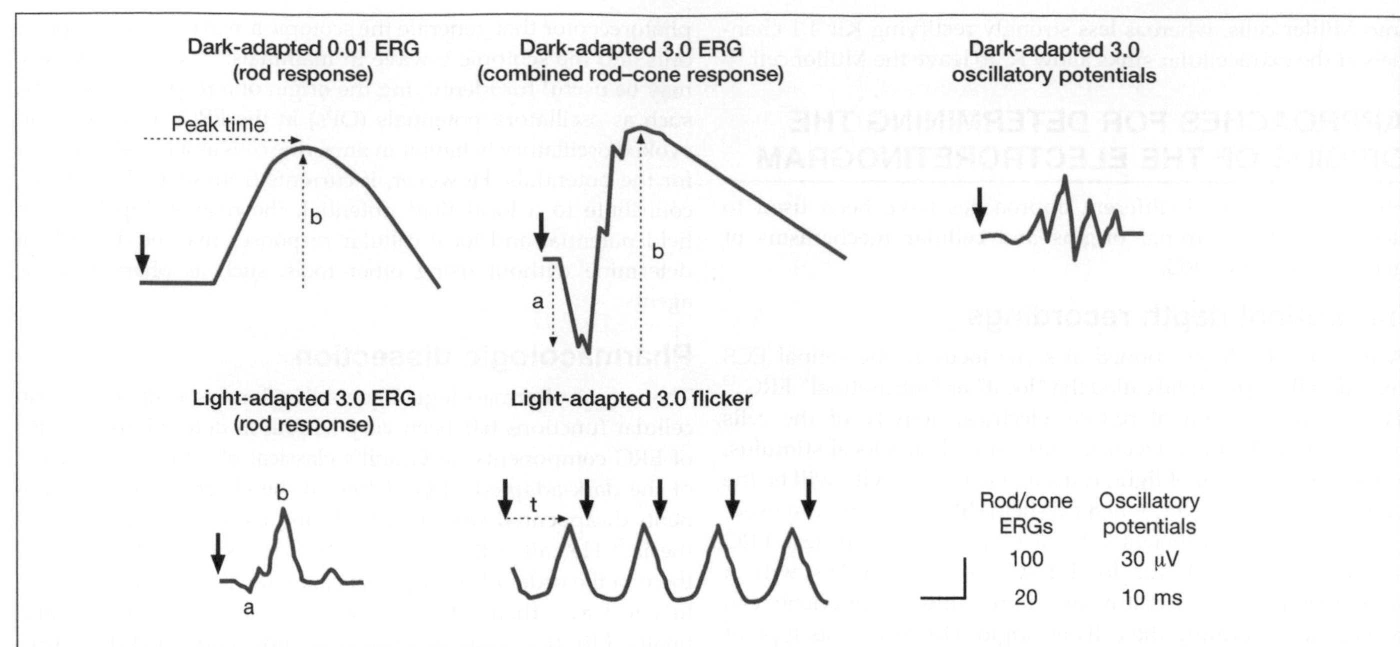

Fig. 7.4 Five standard electroretinogram (ERG) tests with full-field stimulation recommended by the International Society for the Clinical Electrophysiology of Vision (ISCEV) for use worldwide in clinical electrodiagnostic facilities. This figure shows examples, but not norms, of ERG responses in the recommended tests in normal humans. Light calibrations in candela seconds per meter squared (cd s/m^2) for each test are indicated above the ERGs. Large arrowheads indicate time at which the stimulus flash occurred. Dotted arrows show common ways to measure the time-to-peak (t, implicit time), and a- and b-wave amplitude. (Reproduced with permission from Marmor MF, Fulton AB, Holder GE, et al. ISCEV standard for full-field clinical electroretinography (2008 update). Doc Ophthalmol 2009;118:69–77.)

also participate in its generation.[39] The models have been extended to predict the leading edge of the scotopic b-wave.[30] Models of stimulus–response relations of specific retinal cells can be used to analyze amplitude versus energy curves obtained from ERG measurements into components related to the different cell types.[40,41]

STANDARD ERG TESTS IN THE CLINIC

Standard and more specialized tests for use in the clinic that examine key aspects of light- and dark-adapted retinal (and more central visual) function have been described in various publications by the International Society for the Clinical Electrophysiology of Vision (ISCEV), with the most recent update for the flash and flicker ERG in 2008.[42] The "standard" tests advocated by ISCEV for basic ERG testing are listed in Box 7.1, and typical responses to these tests are illustrated in Fig. 7.4. The standards were developed so that ERGs recorded in clinics around the world would be comparable. The ISCEV publications, which now cover several other ERG tests as well, i.e., the ones with an asterisk in Box 7.1, describe basic technology and clinical protocols.

Box 7.1 Standard and more specialized electroretinogram (ERG) tests

Standard ERG tests described by ISCEV standard for full-field clinical electroretinography (2008 update);[42] all numbers are stimulus calibrations in cd/s/m^2

- Dark-adapted 0.01 ERG ("rod response")
- Dark-adapted 3.0 ERG ("maximal or standard combined rod–cone response")
- Dark-adapted 3.0 oscillatory potentials ("oscillatory potentials")
- Light-adapted 3.0 ERG ("single-flash cone response")
- Light-adapted 3.0 flicker ERG ("30-Hz flicker")
- Recommended additional response: either dark-adapted 10.0 ERG or dark-adapted 30.0 ERG

Specialized types of ERG and recording procedures

- Macular or focal ERG
- Multifocal ERG*
- Pattern ERG*
- Early receptor potential (ERP)
- Scotopic threshold response (STR), negative and positive
- Photopic negative response (PhNR)
- Direct-current (dc) ERG
- Electro-oculogram*
- Long-duration light-adapted ERG (ON–OFF responses)
- Paired-flash ERG
- Chromatic stimulus ERG (including S-cone ERG)
- Dark and light adaptation of the ERG
- Dark-adapted and light-adapted luminance response analyses
- Saturated a-wave slope analysis
- Specialized procedures for young and premature infants*

**See relevant standard or guideline published by International Society for the Clinical Electrophysiology of Vision (ISCEV).*

DISTAL RETINAL COMPONENTS: SLOW PIII, C-WAVE, FAST OSCILLATION TROUGH, AND LIGHT PEAK

After the onset of a step of light, the early waves of the dark-adapted ERG, the a- and b-waves, are followed by the c-wave and then by a succession of slower responses that include the fast oscillation trough (FOT), which is a negative deflection, and the light peak, which is a large slow positive deflection (Fig. 7.5A). Because these responses are so slow, lasting seconds to minutes, patients cannot keep their eyes steady long enough for them to develop. Therefore, in the clinic, these slower responses are generally recorded by using electro-oculography.

The electro-oculogram (EOG) is an eye movement-dependent voltage recorded between electrodes placed near the eye at the inner and outer canthus. The patient is asked to look back and forth between a pair of fixation lights separated by 30° of visual angle, situated in a ganzfeld bowl. The source of the voltage is a corneofundal potential, also called the "standing potential" that renders the cornea positive with respect to the back of the eye. Light-evoked changes in the EOG reflect changes in the transepithelial potential (TEP) of the RPE. These changes have been studied experimentally in human and animal preparations using direct current electroretinography (dc-ERG[43]), and these studies will be reviewed briefly here.

Electrogenesis of the c-wave, FOT, and light peak of the dc-ERG involves ion concentration changes in the subretinal space between photoreceptors and the RPE that in turn produce slow membrane responses in the Müller and RPE cells that face the space. The Müller and/or RPE component voltages overlap in time and sum to produce the recorded dc-ERG components. The (sub)component voltages from Müller cells and RPE have been recorded in anesthetized animals by placing a microelectrode in the subretinal space, and simultaneously recording the potentials across neural retina and the RPE, as illustrated in the schematic in Fig. 7.5B. Such experiments have provided a good understanding of the origins and mechanisms of generation of the c-wave and other slow potentials from distal retina.

c-Wave

The cornea-positive c-wave that follows the b-wave is the sum of two major (sub)component voltages: a cornea-negative voltage, generated by the neural retina, and a cornea-positive voltage of similar latency and timecourse, generated by the RPE (Figs 7.5 and 7.6). The c-wave is cornea-positive when the RPE component is larger than the neural retinal component. If the two components are equal in amplitude, the c-wave will be absent, as observed in some monkeys.[44]

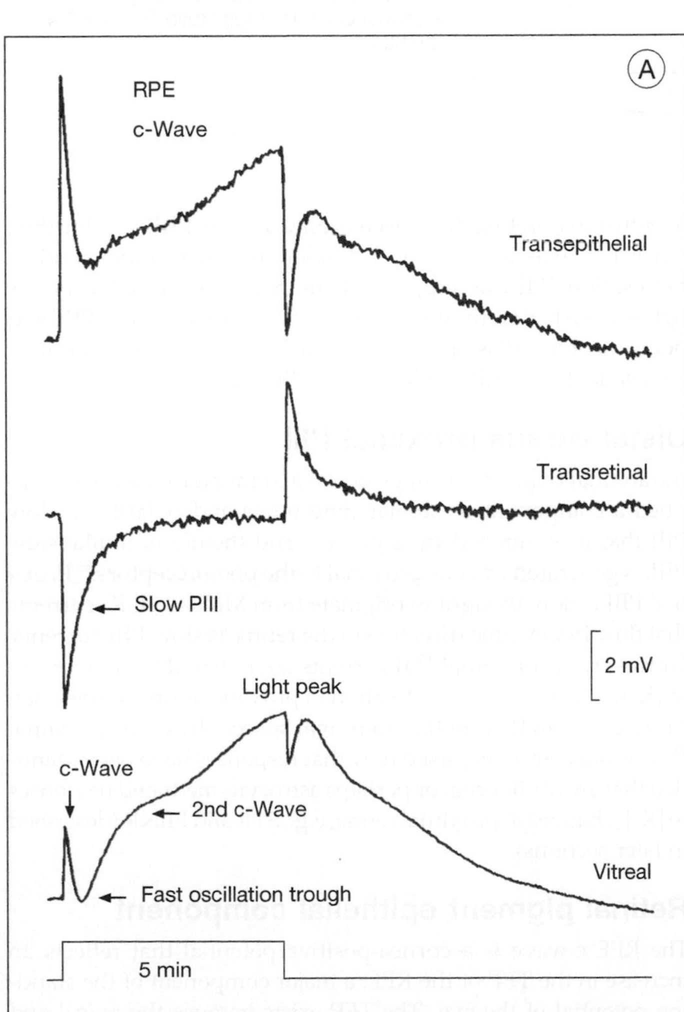

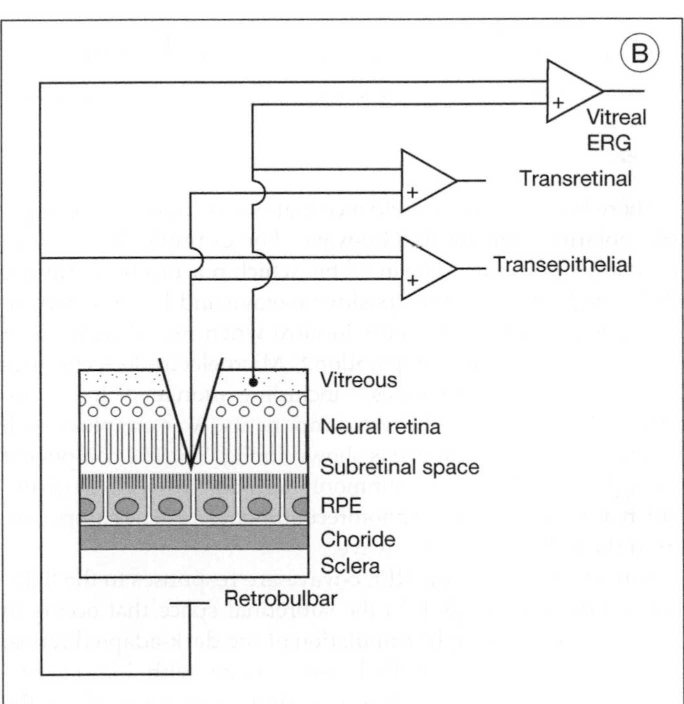

Fig. 7.5 Subretinal recordings from the intact cat eye. (A) The vitreal, transretinal, and transepithelial potentials were recorded simultaneously in response to a 5-minute period of illumination. The a- and b-waves cannot be seen using this compressed timescale. In the vitreal electroretinogram (ERG), the c-wave is followed by the fast oscillation trough (FOT) and then the light peak. The intraretinal recordings show that the c-wave is composed of two (sub)components: the larger cornea-positive retinal pigment epithelial (RPE) transepithelial response, and the slightly smaller cornea-negative transretinal component, the Müller cell-generated slow PIII response. For the light peak, only an RPE component is present. (Reproduced with permission from Steinberg RH, Linsenmeier RA, Griff ER. Retinal pigment epithelial cell contributions to the electroretinogram and electrooculogram. Prog Retin Res 1985;4:33–66.) (B) Schematic showing the recording arrangement for transretinal and transepithelial recordings in the intact eye. The transretinal ERG is recorded between a vitreal reference and a retrobulbar reference. The microelectrode is referenced to the vitreal reference for the transretinal recording and to the retrobulbar reference for the transepithelial recording. Double-barreled microelectrodes were used to measure field potentials and changes in $[K^+]_o$. (Reproduced with permission from Frishman LJ, Steinberg RH. Light-evoked increases in $[K^+]_o$ in proximal portion of the dark-adapted cat retina. J Neurophysiol 1989;61:1233–43.)

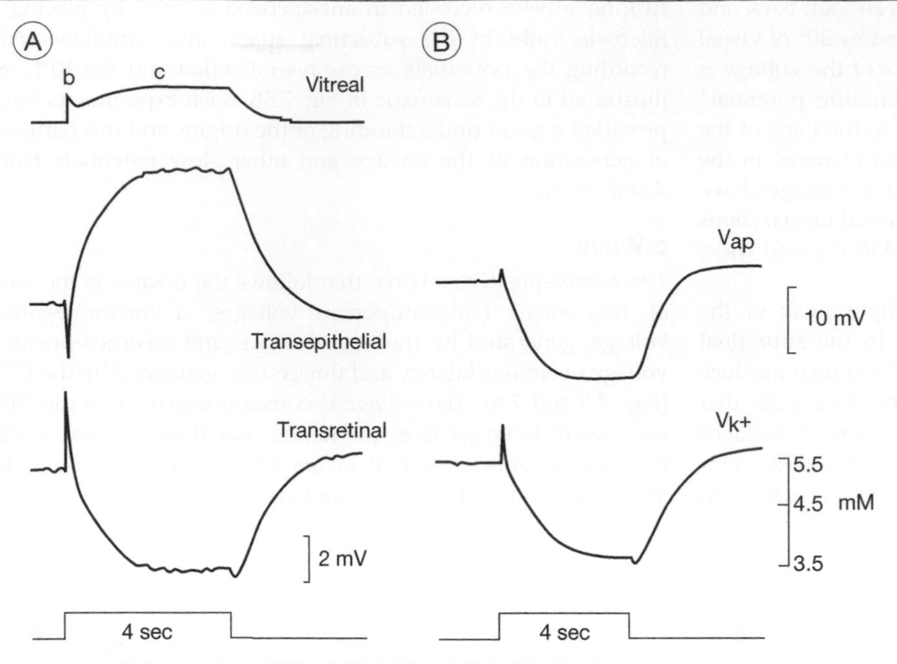

Fig. 7.6 The components of c-wave of the dark-adapted cat (DC) electroretinogram (ERG): the (sub)components, and correlation of recorded $[K^+]_o$ and the retinal pigment epithelial (RPE) apical membrane hyperpolarization. Stimuli were 4-second flashes at 8.3 log q deg^2/s^2. (A) The vitreal c-wave consists of a transepithelial component (TEP c-wave) and a transretinal component (slow PIII). B-wave deflections can be seen in both recordings; the b-wave current generated in neural retina creates a passive voltage drop across the large resistance of the RPE and sclera. (B) RPE apical membrane and subretinal $[K^+]_o$ in response to the same stimulus as in part A, recorded in a separate experiment. The apical membrane potential was derived by subtracting an intracellular recording of the basal membrane potential from the transepithelial potential. (Reproduced with permission from Steinberg RH, Linsenmeier RA, Griff ER. Retinal pigment epithelial cell contributions to the electroretinogram and electrooculogram. Prog Retin Res 1985;4: 33–66.)

There is long-standing evidence that two components of opposite polarity form the ERG c-wave. For example, intravenous injection of sodium iodate in rabbit, which poisons primarily the RPE, abolishes the cornea-positive c-wave and leaves a cornea-negative potential,[45] as occurs in vitro when recording from an isolated neural retina preparation.[46] Microelectrode recordings in retinas of several species,[43] including monkey,[47] have confirmed the presence of the two components. An example of such recordings in intact cat eye is shown in Fig. 7.6. The component from the neural retina is commonly termed slow PIII, to distinguish it from fast PIII, the photoreceptor current. The component from the RPE is the RPE c-wave.

Both slow PIII and the RPE c-wave are responses to the light-evoked decrease in $[K^+]_o$ in the subretinal space that occurs in response to intense light stimulation of the dark-adapted retina. When measurements of $[K^+]_o$ were made with ion-selective microelectrodes, either in intact eyes or in vitro preparations, the timecourse of the $[K^+]_o$ decrease was found to predict that of the ERG c-wave and its component parts (Fig. 7.6). Blocking K^+ conductance (via Kir channels) with various agents eliminated both the slow PIII[48] and the RPE c-wave.[49]

Müller cell contribution (slow PIII)

Intraretinal recording at various depths[50] have shown that slow PIII is generated by a radially oriented current across the neural retina. A Müller cell generator, rather than a neuronal generator, was suggested because slow PIII persisted after treatment with aspartate, a nonselective glutamate agonist, to suppress all responses of postreceptoral neurons.[51]

Studies in amphibia and mammals have shown that slow PIII is initiated when the distal ends of the Müller cells are passively hyperpolarized by a photoreceptor-dependent decrease in subretinal $[K^+]_o$. This sets up a transretinal "K^+ spatial buffer" current,[25] and the current drop across the extracellular resistance produces the slow PIII voltage.[50,52,53] The slow hyperpolarization recorded in Müller cells was observed to be similar in timecourse to both the subretinal $[K^+]_o$ decrease and to slow PIII.[20,21,53] Further, when Ba^{2+} was used to block Müller cell Kir channel conductances, slow PIII was suppressed but there was little effect on the light-evoked subretinal K^+ decrease.[22,27,54] Finally, slow PIII was not present in ERGs of mice with Kir 4.1 channels, the dominant Kir channels in Müller cells, genetically inactivated.[28]

Distal versus proximal PIII

Intraretinal depth recordings in isolated rabbit retina have identified a component of similar timecourse and polarity to slow PIII that is eliminated by aspartate, and therefore, unlike slow PIII, is generated by cells proximal to the photoreceptors.[55] Proximal PIII is now thought to originate from Müller cell K^+ currents that flow in the same direction in the retina as slow PIII currents. However, the proximal PIII currents are initiated by an increase in $[K^+]_o$ due to neuronal activation in proximal retina, rather than the decrease in $[K^+]_o$ in the subretinal space. The term "proximal PIII" is not commonly used now that responses have been identified that are Müller cell, or perhaps astrocyte-mediated responses to $[K^+]_o$ changes in proximal retina, e.g., STR and PhNR (described in later sections).

Retinal pigment epithelial component

The RPE c-wave is a cornea-positive potential that reflects an increase in the TEP of the RPE, a major component of the standing potential of the eye. The TEP exists because the apical and basal membranes of RPE cells are electrically separated by high-resistance tight junctions that encircle the monolayer of cells (the "R membrane"). The TEP is equal to the difference between the apical (V_{ap}) and basal (V_{ba}) membrane potentials.[43] V_{ap} is generally more hyperpolarized than V_{ba}, making the TEP cornea-positive. During c-wave generation in response to an increase in light, the TEP increases (becomes even more positive). This is initiated by a hyperpolarization of the apical membrane, and passive shunting of current to the basal membrane, resulting in a (smaller) hyperpolarization of basal membrane, and a greater difference in potential between the two membranes.[43]

As was observed for Müller cells, the slow hyperpolarization of the apical membrane, with its large K^+ conductance,[56] and the RPE c-wave have a timecourse that is very similar to the subretinal $[K^+]_o$ decrease, as illustrated in Fig. 7.6. In an isolated RPE preparation (where only the apical bath $[K^+]$ was altered), Oakley et al.[57] demonstrated that the RPE c-wave was due solely to the $[K^+]_o$ decrease.

The fast oscillation trough

The FOT (usually measured by EOG) is a change in the corneoretinal potential - it decreases and increases in synchrony with an alternating light/dark stimulus. The response in the dc-ERG that corresponds to the EOG decrease (trough) also is termed the FOT. The FOT response to maintained illumination follows the c-wave peak, and, when a light peak occurs, it appears as a dip between the c-wave and the light peak (Fig. 7.5A).

The FOT originates from both neural retina and RPE. It involves recovery of Müller and RPE cells from their peak polarizations as subretinal K^+ reaccumulates following the reduction in concentration caused by light. This recovery may be greater than predicted by the reaccumulation, particularly for the RPE component. Light initially elicits a hyperpolarization of the apical membrane that increases the TEP and then produces a delayed basal hyperpolarization that decreases the TEP. This extra decrease in TEP underlies most of the cornea-negative potential of the FOT.[43]

The ionic mechanisms of the basal membrane hyperpolarization involve Cl^- conductances.[58] In intact sheets of RPE/choroid from human fetal eyes, the Miller lab distinguished two types of basal membrane Cl^- channels: a 4,4′-diisothiocyanostilbene-2, 2′-disulfonate (DIDS)-inhibitable Ca^{2+}-sensitive Cl^- channel, and a cyclic AMP-dependent channel that is inhibited by DIDS as well as by 5-nitro-2-(3phenylpropylamino) benzoate (NPPB), which identifies it as a cystic fibrosis transmembrane regulator (CFTR) channel.[59] In CF patients, the FOT, but not the light peak (see below) is reduced, implicating CFTR in generation of the FOT.

The light peak

Maintained illumination causes a slow increase in the standing potential in the dc-ERG called the light peak that can be recorded as a slow oscillation of the EOG (Fig. 7.6). Intraretinal recordings in several species,[43,58] including monkey,[47] have shown that this cornea-positive potential originates solely from an increase in the TEP (Fig. 7.5A). Intracellular RPE recordings localized the origin of the increase to a slow depolarization of the basal membrane caused by an increase in basal Cl^- conductance. In both chick RPE and human RPE cell sheets the Cl^- conductance increase was suppressed by DIDS.[58,59] In mouse, the light peak is also dependent on a Cl^- conductance, and it is regulated by voltage-dependent Ca^{2+} channel CaV1.3 subunits.[60]

Although the light peak voltage originates from the RPE basal membrane, it is then initiated in neural retina via the photoreceptors.[61] Light stimulation leads to a change in concentration of a "light peak substance" which then affects the basal membrane via a second-messenger system. The identities of the "light peak substance" and the second messenger(s) involved in producing the light peak are unresolved. Although dopamine affected the light peak in the perfused cat eye,[62] studies in chick did not support its being the "light peak substance."[61] Epinephrine also has been proposed as a candidate, and a role for ligands binding to adrenergic alpha-1 receptors on the apical membrane is likely.[59] Cyclic AMP has been investigated as a second messenger in light peak generation but, as described above, it may be involved in generation of the FOT, rather than the light peak.[59]

ORIGIN OF THE A-WAVE

Fig. 7.7 shows the dark- and light-adapted flash ERG of macaque monkey, a good animal model for studying the origins of the human response, as illustrated in Fig. 7.1. The a-wave in the dark-adapted ERG is the initial negative wave that occurs in response to strong stimuli from darkness (Fig. 7.7, top left column) and it is primarily rod-driven (scotopic), but contains a cone contribution when flashes are very strong. When the background is rod-saturating the a-wave is cone-driven (photopic; right column). Under both dark- and light-adapted conditions, the a-wave is truncated by the rise of the positive-going b-wave that originates primarily from ON bipolar cells,[30] as reviewed below. The slow negative wave in the dark-adapted ERG in response to the weakest stimuli, called the STR, is not the a-wave, but instead is initiated by amacrine and/or ganglion cell activity. This is known because STR is eliminated when postreceptoral activity is blocked pharmacologically.[63,64]

The a-wave as a reflection of rod and cone receptor photocurrent

Early intraretinal depth studies in intact cat eyes[13,65] found that the signal at the timecourse of the a-wave was largest in the vicinity of the photoreceptors. The case for a receptoral origin for PIII was strengthened by microelectrode recordings in macaque monkey retina, with the inner retinal circulation clamped to suppress retinal activity proximal to the photoreceptors.[66]

Penn and Hagins[67] in CSD analyses of the isolated rat retina demonstrated that light suppressed the circulating (dark) current of the photoreceptors, and proposed that this suppression was seen in the ERG as the a-wave. Figure 7.8 provides a schematic of the photoreceptor layer current from a review by Pugh et al.[68] The figure shows that, in the dark, cation channels (Na^+, Ca^{2+}, and Mg^{2+}) in the receptor outer segment (ROS) are open, current flows into the ROS (a current sink with respect to the ECS), and K^+ leaks out of the inner segment (a current source), creating dipole current. This dipole current produces a corneal (and vitreal) potential that is positive with respect to the scleral side of the retina. Suppression of the dark current reduces the cornea-positive potential, creating the negative-going a-wave. Consistent with this view, as illustrated in Fig. 7.9, intraretinal recordings and CSD analyses in the intact macaque retina have localized current sources and sinks for a local potential, corresponding to the a-wave, to the distal third of the retina.[18]

Hood and Birch[38] sought to relate the timecourse of the leading edge of the ERG a-wave directly to the leading edge of the photoreceptor outer-segment response to light. They demonstrated that both the linear and the nonlinear (i.e., saturating) behavior of the leading edge of the a-wave in the human ERG could be predicted by a model of photoreceptor function derived from in vitro suction electrode recordings of currents around the outer segments of primate rod photoreceptors.[69] Subsequently a simplified kinetic model of the leading edge of the photoreceptor response (in vitro current recordings) that took into account the

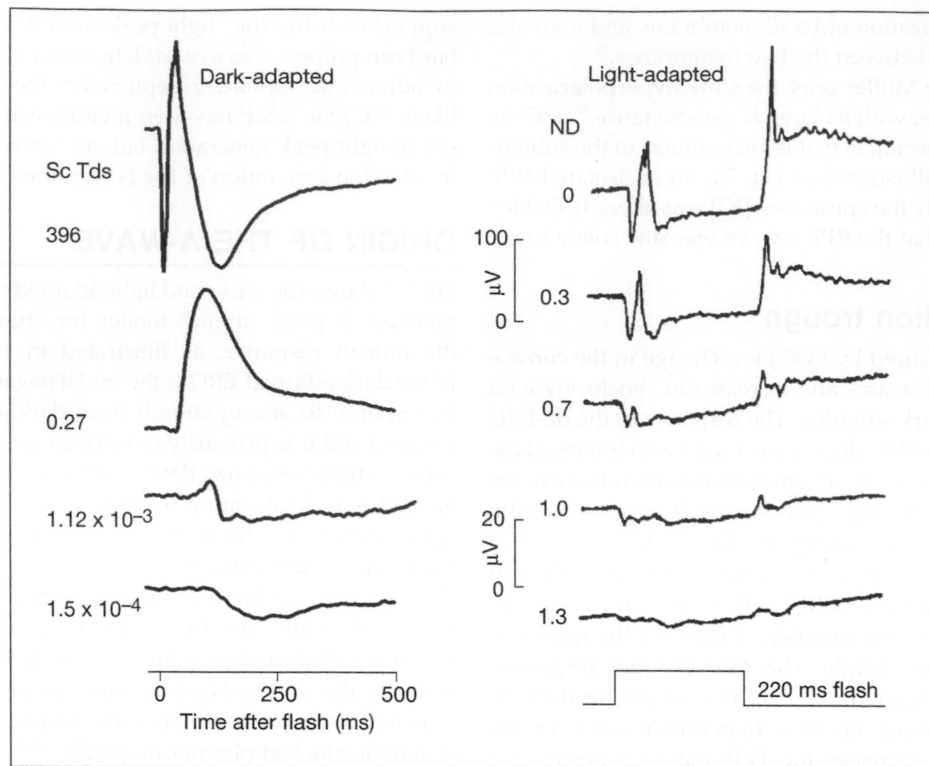

Fig. 7.7 Dark- and light-adapted electroretinograms (ERGs) of the macaque retina. (Left) Dark-adapted full-field ERGs of anesthetized macaque monkeys were measured in response to brief (<5 ms) flashes from darkness generated by computer-controlled light-emitting diodes (LEDs). Responses were recorded differentially between DTL fibers on the two eyes. Flash strength was increased over a 6-log-unit range. Responses to the weakest stimuli were rod-driven (scotopic), whereas for the strongest stimuli there were mixed rod–cone responses. (Reproduced with permission from Robson JG, Frishman LJ. Dissecting the dark-adapted electroretinogram. Doc Ophthalmol 1998;95:187–215.) (Right) Light-adapted full-field ERGs of anesthetized macaques were measured using Burian-Allen electrodes. Stimulus strength was controlled with neutral-density (ND) filters. Stimulus strength increased over a 1.3-log-unit range to a maximum at 0 ND of 4.0 log ph td for 220-ms flashes. Stimuli were presented on a steady rod-saturating background of 3.3 log sc td. The 20 µV calibration bar applies both to the dark-adapted ERG responses to weak stimuli and to the light-adapted ERGs. (Reproduced with permission from Sieving PA, Murayama K, Naarendorp F. Push–pull model of the primate photopic electroretinogram: a role for hyperpolarizing neurons in shaping the b-wave. Vis Neurosci 1994;11:519–32.)

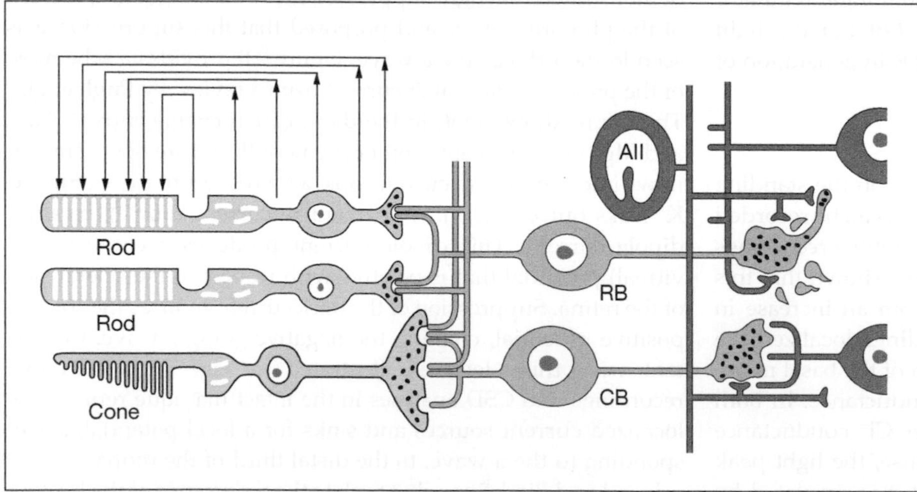

Fig. 7.8 Schematic of a longitudinal section of the mammalian retina illustrating how circulating currents in the photoreceptor layer create an extracellular field potential, in which the vitreal side of the retina has a more positive potential than the scleral side. A very bright flash will suppress the circulating current around the photoreceptor, leading to a vitreal or corneal response which is negative relative to the resting preflash baseline. (Reproduced with permission from Pugh EN Jr, Falsini B, Lyubarsky A. The origin of the major rod- and cone-driven components of the rodent electroretinogram and the effects of age and light-rearing history on the magnitude of these components. Photostasis and related phenomena. New York: Plenum Press; 1998. p 93–128.)

stages of the biochemical phototransduction cascade was developed by Lamb and Pugh.[70] This model could be fit to the leading edge of the human a-wave generated by strong stimuli and it has been used in noninvasive studies of human rod[36,71] and cone photoreceptor[72] function. Recent analyses suggest that the a-wave generated in response to strong stimuli includes additional currents associated with more proximal regions of the photoreceptor cell that form a sharp "nose" on the leading edge of the response that quickly relaxes to the level of the photocurrent.[39]

Postreceptoral contributions to the a-wave

The receptoral origins of the a-wave (Granit's PIII),[32] as well as postreceptoral contributions of similar timecourse, have been

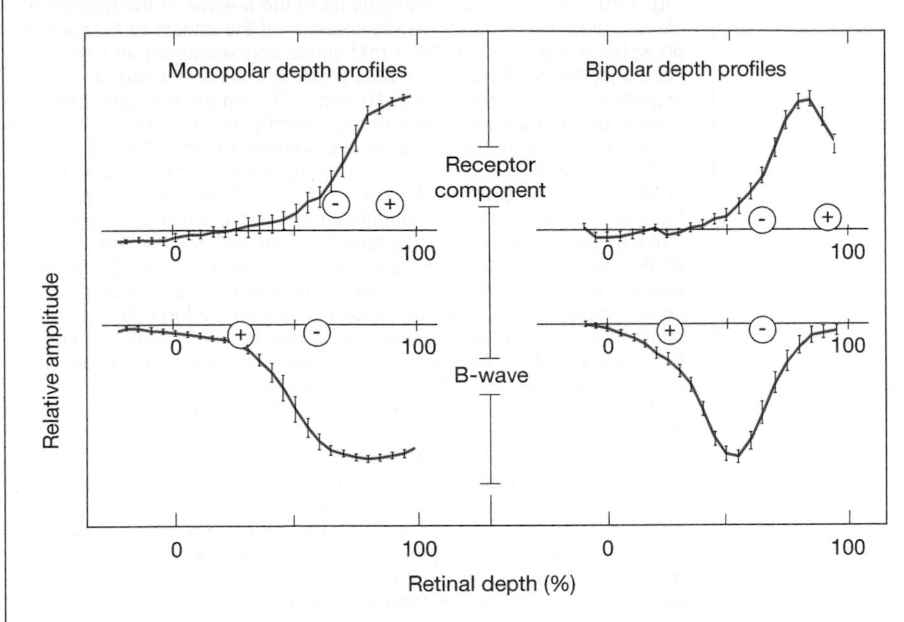

Fig. 7.9 Depth profiles and current source density results in anesthetized macaque monkey retina for the a-wave and the b-wave. Left: Monopolar depth profiles using an intraretinal microelectrode referenced to the forehead. Right: bipolar depth profiles using a coaxial electrode with a distance of 25 μm between the tips to measure field potential amplitudes at the peak time of the receptor component, the b-wave and the dc component of the macaque light-adapted electroretinogram. The pluses and minuses indicate the current sources (+) and sinks (–) for the components, as calculated from current source density analyses based on the coaxial electrode recordings and resistance measurements. The a-wave source and sink are in the distal quarter of the retina. The b-wave has a large sink near the outer nuclear layer and a distributed source extending to the vitreal surface of the retina. Plots represent means of 26 penetrations. (Adapted from Heynen H, van Norren D. Origin of the electroretinogram in the intact macaque eye – II. Current source-density analysis. Vision Res 1985;25:709–15.)

clarified in pharmacological studies. In early in vitro studies of the isolated retina (amphibian and human), the nonspecific glutamate agonist aspartate in the perfusate suppressed all postreceptoral responses, and isolated the a-wave, revealing its presence under the b-wave.[51,73] Our understanding of the receptoral and postreceptoral contributions to the light-adapted a-wave, as well as other waves of the macaque monkey photopic ERG, was greatly advanced by studies of Sieving and colleagues in which they utilized more specific glutamate analogs than aspartate to dissect retinal circuits, and particularly ON versus OFF circuits set up by depolarizing and hyperpolarizing bipolar cells, respectively (Fig. 7.2).[33,35] They made intravitreal injections in anesthetized macaques of an mGluR6 receptor agonist, 2-amino-4-phosphonobutyric acid (APB, L isomer, also called L-AP4) to block metabotropic glutamatergic neurotransmission to depolarizing (ON) bipolar cells. This eliminated light-evoked responses of ON bipolar cells as well as contributions from more proximal cells of the retinal ON pathway. Alternatively, they injected *cis*-2,3-piperidine dicarboxylic acid (PDA) (or kynurenic acid) to block major ionotropic glutamate receptors in the retina (α-amino-3-hydroxy-5-methyl-4-isoxazolepropionic acid (AMPA) and kainate receptors).[74] These ionotropic receptors, blocked by PDA, mediate signal transmission to hyperpolarizing (OFF) bipolar cells and horizontal (Hz) cells, as well as to amacrine and ganglion cells of both OFF and ON pathways. Results of such experiments are illustrated in Fig. 7.10A for responses to fairly weak stimuli presented on a rod-suppressing background; functions relating a-wave amplitude and stimulus strength over a wider range of stimuli in the same study are shown in Fig. 7.10B. The a-wave was reduced in amplitude by PDA (or kynurenic acid, not shown), but not by APB. Fig. 7.10 also shows that PDA had a similar effect to that of aspartate, or to cobalt (Co^{2+}), which was used to block the voltage-gated Ca^{2+} channels which are essential for vesicular release of glutamate.

When the effects of PDA versus APB on the photopic a-wave amplitude were evaluated over a wider range of stimuli, PDA-sensitive postreceptoral neurons, rather than photoreceptors, or APB-sensitive contributions from ON pathway, were found to generate the leading edge for the first 1.5 log units of flash strengths that elicited a measurable a-wave (Fig. 7.10B). Postreceptoral cells in the OFF pathway and inner retina continued to contribute 10–15 μV to the total a-wave amplitude when photoreceptoral contributions also were present. Postreceptoral contributions to the a-wave in alert humans have also been demonstrated, by analysis of ERGs.[75]

Postreceptoral contributions to the dark-adapted a-wave have been observed as well in the monkey.[34,76] For weak to moderate stimuli from darkness, a-waves are dominated by rod signals, but a strong flash elicits a mixed rod–cone ERG like the macaque ERG illustrated in Fig. 7.11. To study purely rod-driven responses it is therefore necessary to separate the rod- and cone-driven responses to strong stimuli when investigating their relative contributions to the ERG.

The rod-driven response can be extracted by subtracting the isolated cone-driven response to the same stimulus from the mixed rod–cone response. Isolated cone-driven responses in Fig. 7.11 (triangles) were obtained by briefly suppressing the rod response with an adapting flash, and then measuring the response to the original test stimulus presented a few hundred milliseconds (300 ms) after offset of the adapting flash. Cone-driven responses in primates recover to full amplitude within about 300 ms whereas rod-driven responses take at least a second, making it possible to isolate the cone-driven response.[34]

The effect of PDA on the rod-isolated a-wave of the macaque is shown in Fig. 7.12 for a range of stimulus strengths.[34] Most of the leading edge of the a-wave in response to the weakest stimulus was eliminated (Fig. 7.12A), and much of the leading edge that occurred later than 15 ms after the flash was removed in response to stronger stimuli (Fig. 7.12B), and even for stimuli that saturated the response (not shown). When APB was injected along with PDA, to eliminate remaining ON bipolar cell contributions as well (Fig. 7.13B), the shape of the early portion of PIII could be seen to form a nose, generally obscured by

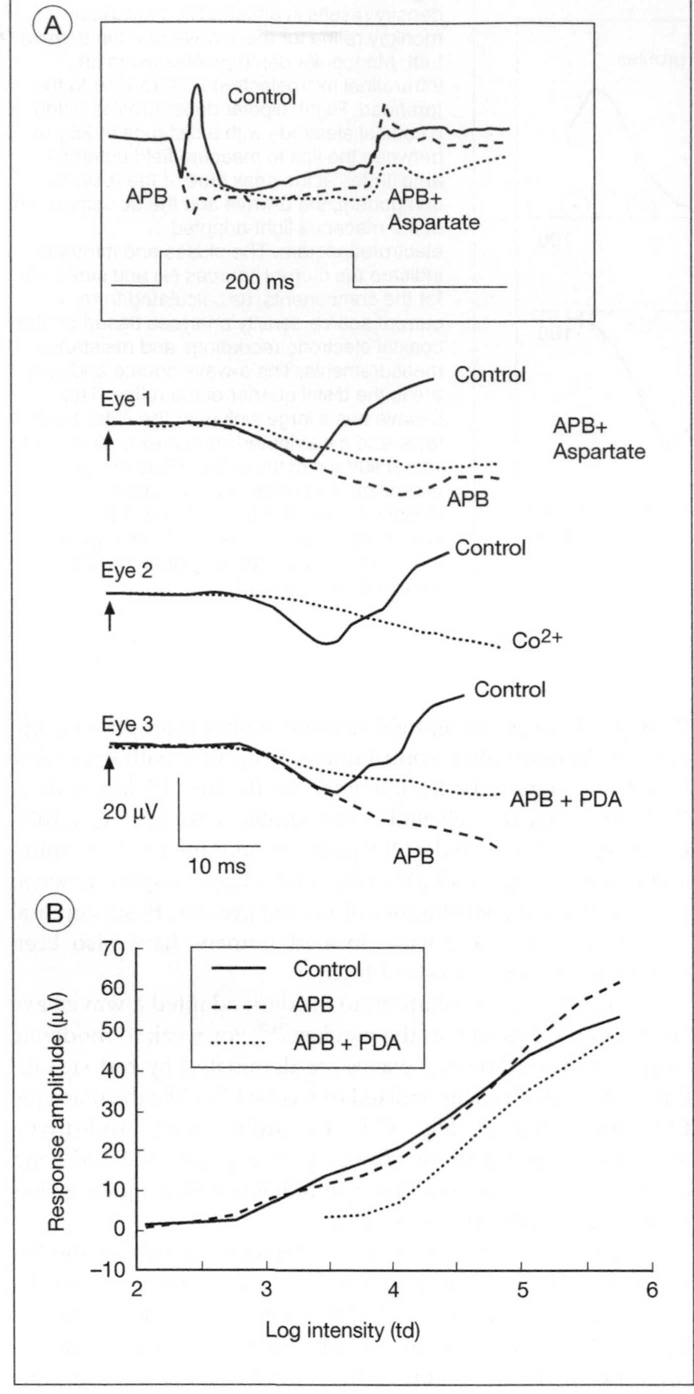

Fig. 7.10 Postreceptoral contributions to the a-wave of the macaque electroretinogram (ERG). (A) Comparison of the effects of 2-amino-4-phosphonobutyric acid (APB:1 mM vitreal concentration) and APB + *cis*-2,3-piperidine dicarboxylic acid (PDA: 5 mM) with those of aspartate (50 mM) and cobalt (10 mm, CO^{2+}) on the photopic ERG a-wave of three different eyes of two anesthetized monkeys. The inset at the top shows the response of eye number 1 to the 200-ms stimulus of 3.76 log td (2.01 log cd/m^2) on a steady background of 3.3 log td (1.55 cd/m^2). The a-waves for eyes 1, 2, and 3 were all in response to the same stimulus. For this stimulus, most of the small a-wave (10 µV) that was elicited was postreceptoral in origin. In the clinic the a-wave elicited by brief flashes often is larger, 20 µV or more, and therefore also will include several microvolts of photoreceptor contribution, as shown in part B. (B) Stimulus response function (V log I plot) of the photopic a-wave of the macaque measured at times corresponding to the a-wave peak in the control responses (solid line). Amplitudes after APB (broken line) and after APB + PDA (dotted line) were measured at the same latency as the trough of the control a-waves measured at the same stimulus intensity. The points are connected by solid lines. In this figure, as in part A, APB had no effect on the a-wave amplitude. In contrast, PDA reduced the amplitude, and the postreceptoral contribution was maximally between 10 and 15 µV, about 50% of a 20 µV a-wave, but less than 25% of a saturated a-wave of about 65 µV. (Reproduced with permission from Bush RA, Sieving PA. A proximal retinal component in the primate photopic ERG a-wave. Invest Ophthalmol Vis Sci 1994;35:635–45.)

negative-going signals removed by PDA, and the b-wave removed by APB (Fig. 7.12C).

PDA blocks signal transmission not only to hyperpolarizing bipolar and horizontal cells, but also to amacrine and ganglion cells of the inner retina. In order to test whether the effect of PDA on the a-wave was due to OFF bipolar cells or more proximal cells, it was necessary selectively to suppress amacrine and ganglion cell activity. This was done using *N*-methyl-D-aspartate (NMDA), as only the proximal retinal neurons have functional NMDA (ionotropic glutamate) receptors. Results (not shown) were similar in the dark-adapted ERG to those after PDA alone, indicating a proximal retinal origin for most of the rod-driven postreceptoral contributions to the dark-adapted a-wave, rather than a contribution from OFF bipolar cells.[77]

The timecourse of the photoreceptor response

The leading edge of the a-wave is the only visible portion of the photoreceptor response in the normal ERG. In order to see the entire timecourse of the photoreceptor response it is necessary to remove postreceptoral contributions, as was done pharmacologically for the ERGs in Figs 7.11 and 7.12. However, such a manipulation is invasive, and does not eliminate slow PIII and the c-wave, should they be present. Another approach is to use

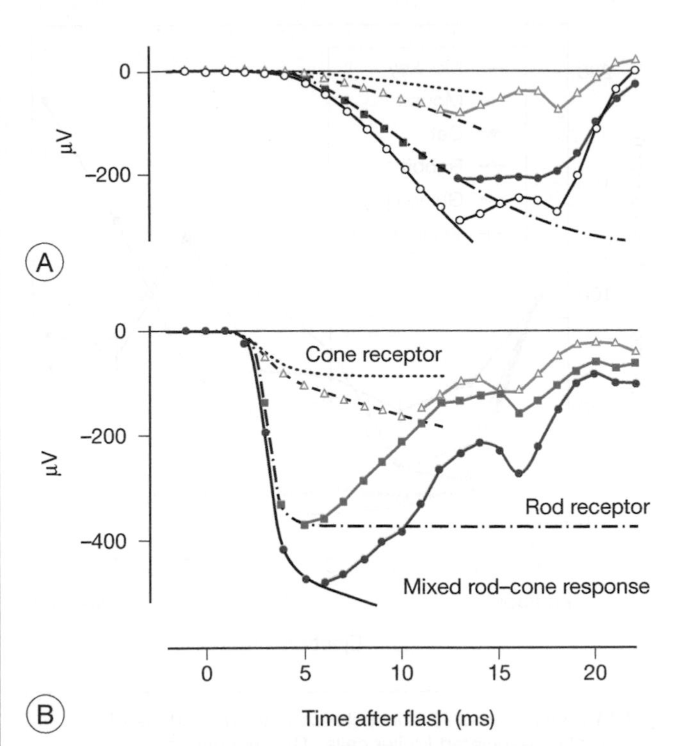

Fig. 7.11 Dark-adapted electroretinogram (ERG) of a macaque showing the mixed rod–cone a-wave and separate components measured (symbols) and modeled (solid lines fit to the leading edge of the a-wave) for two stimulus strengths. (A) Responses of an anesthetized macaque to a brief blue light-emitting diode (LED) flash of 188 sc td/s (57 ph td/s) and (B) responses to a xenon white flash of 59000 sc td/s, (34000 ph td/s). In both parts, the largest response (open circles) is the entire mixed rod–cone a-wave; the green solid line restricted to the leading edge shows the modeled mixed rod–cone response. The second largest response is the (isolated) rod-driven response (filled circles); the red solid line through the leading edge is the modeled rod photoreceptor contribution. The second to smallest response (open triangles) is the (isolated) cone-driven response, including the postreceptoral contribution; the cyan solid line through the leading edge shows the modeled cone-driven response. The smallest response is the modeled cone photoreceptor contribution, based on post *cis*-2,3-piperidine dicarboxylic acid (PDA) findings for the cone-driven response. Given the animal's 8.5-mm pupil, the stimulus for part A was about 1 cd s/m^2, i.e., about three times less intense (for cones) than the International Society for the Clinical Electrophysiology of Vision (ISCEV) standard flash of 3 cd s/m^2, whereas the stimulus for part B is about 2000 times stronger. ISCEV also suggests flashes of 10 and 30 cd s/m^2 for mixed rod–cone ERG. (Adapted from Robson JG, Saszik SM, Ahmed J, et al. Rod and cone contributions to the a-wave of the electroretinogram of the macaque. J Physiol 2003;547:509–30.)

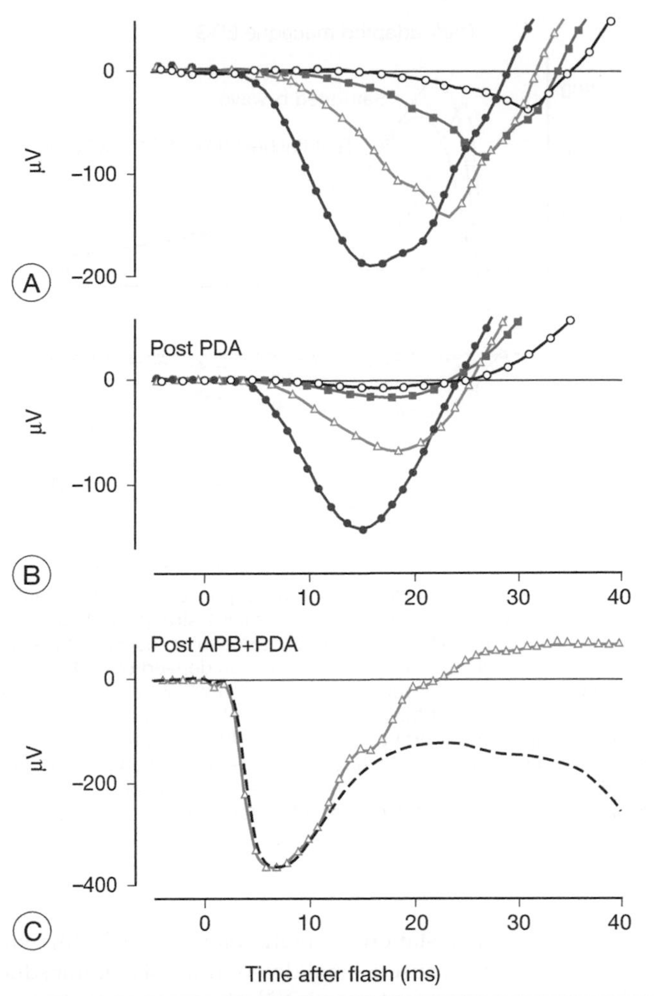

Fig. 7.12 Postreceptoral contribution to rod-driven dark-adapted macaque electroretinogram (ERG). Rod-driven responses from an anesthetized macaque were obtained after subtracting isolated cone-driven response from the mixed rod–cone ERG. Rod-driven responses are shown to a range of stimulus energies (15.8–509 sc td/s) before (A) and after (B) intravitreal injection of *cis*-2,3-piperidine dicarboxylic acid (PDA) (4 mM). For comparison, the ERG remaining after adding PDA and 2-amino-4-phosphonobutyric acid (APB) is shown in part C. The stimulus was a xenon white flash of 59000 sc td/s, and cone signals were not removed in this recording. The control response is shown by the green line, the post PDA+APB by the dashed black line. (A and B, adapted from Robson JG, Saszik SM, Ahmed J, et al. Rod and cone contributions to the a-wave of the electroretinogram of the macaque. J Physiol 2003;547:509–30; C, from unpublished data.)

the paired-flash technique developed by Pepperberg and colleagues[78] to derive, in vivo, the photoreceptor response. The derived photoreceptor response (underneath) and the full ERG responses to three stimuli of the same strength are shown for a macaque monkey in Fig. 7.13. The timecourse of the derived response is similar to that of current recordings in vitro from individual rod photoreceptor outer segments in the macaque, although it reaches its peak a little earlier in vivo in the ERG than in vitro. However, the amplitude of the derived response is rather large, perhaps twice that expected for the photocurrent. The large amplitude of the derived response may occur because the method for deriving responses uses measurements in the "nose" portion of saturated a-wave (Fig. 7.12C), which reflects currents from more proximal regions of the photoreceptor in addition to outer-segment currents.[39]

ORIGIN OF THE B-WAVE

The cornea-positive b-wave, Granit's PII, is the largest component of the dark-adapted diffuse-flash ERG. There is general consensus that the neuronal generator of the b-wave is primarily the depolarizing (ON) bipolar cells.[30,31,79,80] APB (L-AP4), which binds to mGluR6 receptors of ON bipolar cells and removed the cone b-wave in experiments of Sieving et al., also removed the dark-adapted b-wave in several species, including primates.[30,80] The b-wave is also absent, causing a negative ERG (Fig. 7.12C). Negative ERGs also occur in patients and murine models with

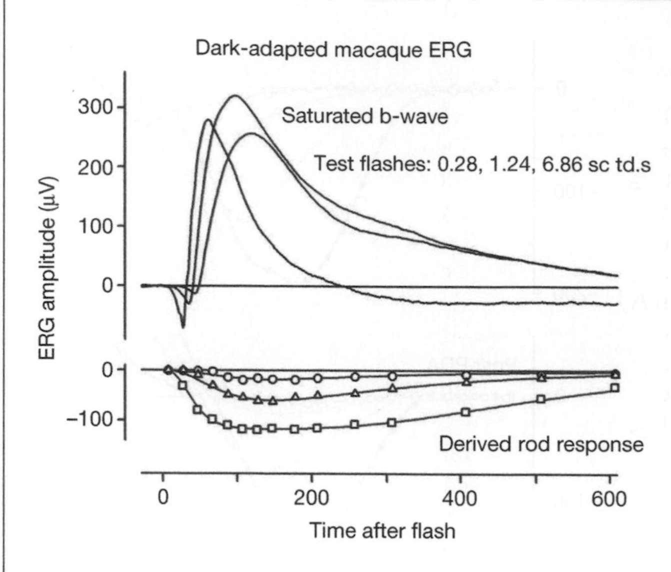

Fig. 7.13 Dark-adapted electroretinogram response of the anesthetized macaque monkey to three different test stimulus strengths (0.28, 1.24, and 6.86 sc td/s) and the derived rod photoreceptor response for each test stimulus. The photoreceptor response was derived using the paired-flash approach of Pepperberg et al.,[78] in which a rod-saturating probe flash follows a test flash at fixed intervals after its onset, and the residual response of the probe is subtracted from the probe alone to derive the rod receptor response at each time point (data points). The model lines used modifications of equations from Robson et al.[34] (Frishman LJ, Robson JG, unpublished observations.)

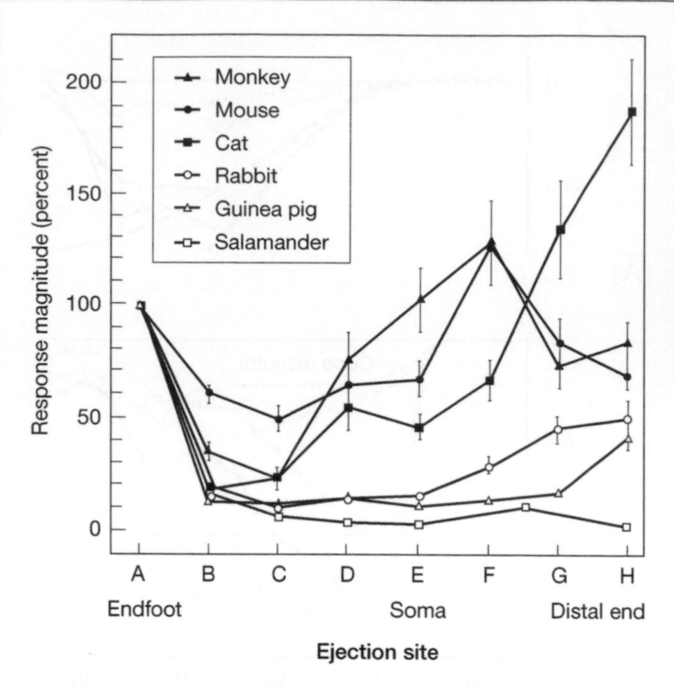

Fig. 7.14 Distribution of K^+ conductance over the surface of enzymatically dissociated Müller cells. The magnitude of depolarizations in response to focal K^+ ejections is plotted as a function of ejection location along the Müller cell surface. Responses are normalized to response magnitude at the endfoot. In species with avascular retinas (salamander, rabbit, guinea pig), K^+ conductance is largest at the endfoot. In vascularized species, conductance is largest near the cell soma (mouse, monkey) or at the distal end of the cell (cat). (Reproduced with permission from Newman EA. Distribution of potassium conductance in mammalian Müller (glial) cells: a comparative study. J Neurosci 1987;7:2423–32.)

complete congenital stationary night blindness (CSNB) who have mutations that cause a breakdown in the signal transduction cascade in ON bipolar cells.[81,82] However, experimental support also exists for a Müller cell contribution, likely due to K^+ currents as a consequence of bipolar cell depolarization, particularly at times past the leading edge of the response, as described below.

Resolving the role of bipolar cells and Müller cells in generating the b-wave has been difficult. Early intraretinal depth recordings demonstrated a negative-going intraretinal b-wave with a (negative) peak amplitude in distal retina, near the outer plexiform layer (OPL), and the largest change in amplitude across the inner nuclear layer (INL).[13,65] These results suggested that the b-wave was generated by current flowing through a radially oriented cell that acted as a dipole. Bipolar cells, the only radially oriented neurons that span the INL, and Müller cells, the radially oriented glial cells, were implicated.

Müller cell hypothesis

CSD profiles for the b-wave from intraretinal recordings in frog retina[83] showed an OPL current sink and a current source extending from the OPL almost all the way to the vitreal surface, and this also was found in monkey retina (Fig. 7.9).[18] Due to the extensive radial spread of sinks and sources, it was hypothesized that Müller cells generate b-wave currents, and supporting this, Miller and Dowling[84] found that intracellularly recorded Müller cell responses in amphibian resemble b-wave responses to the same stimuli. However studies of local changes in $[K^+]_o$ and Müller K^+ conductances were not fully consistent with the Müller cell hypothesis.

Measurements using intraretinal K^+-selective microelectrodes of local changes in light-evoked $[K^+]_o$ skate,[85] amphibian,[20,86] and rabbit[21] retinas demonstrated only small transient $[K^+]_o$ increases in the OPL at light onset, presumably from dendrites of ON bipolar cells. The Müller cell hypothesis required a large sink activity in the OPL. In contrast, a large sustained inner plexiform layer (IPL) $[K^+]_o$ increase was recorded in the proximal retina of several species at the onset, or at onset and offset of a light stimulus.[87] The large proximal $[K^+]_o$ increase reflected activation of amacrine and ganglion cells as well, and is now understood to contribute strongly to Müller cell or astrocyte-mediated ERG components of proximal retinal origin, e.g., M-wave, STR, or PhNR.

As described in the section on spatial buffering, above, the selective permeability of the Müller cell membrane to K^+ and the nonuniform distribution of K^+ conductances (Fig. 7.3) provide the opportunity for K^+ siphoning from synaptic layers where $[K^+]_o$ is high to regions of lower $[K^+]_o$. In species with avascular retinas, e.g., amphibian and rabbit, the Müller cell endfoot adjacent to the vitreous humor has more than 90% of the K^+ conductance in the cell, as shown in the Newman lab study of enzymatically isolated Müller cells subjected to puffs of K^+ (Fig. 7.14). K^+ entering the Müller cell via strongly inward rectifying Kir channels in synaptic regions will exit predominantly from the vitreal endfoot where the K^+ conductance is only weakly rectifying (Fig. 7.3).[28] The OPL $[K^+]_o$ increase could establish a current loop that extends all the way to the vitreal surface. The IPL $[K^+]_o$ increase would contribute to the same current loop, creating a vitreal positive proximally generated potential in addition to the bipolar cell-dependent b-wave. However, as noted above, the OPL increases in $[K^+]_o$ were small, and because of this, did not predict the large b-wave recorded in the ERG.

In contrast, in species with vascularized retinas such as mouse and monkey, K^+ conductance, although high at the endfoot, is greatest in the INL, near capillaries. In cat, K^+ conductance is greatest near the subretinal space (Fig. 7.14). In these species with vascularized retinas the Müller cell current that arises as a consequence of the proximal $[K^+]_o$ increase contributes to a distally directed current loop (like slow PIII), thereby producing a cornea-negative potential (e.g., m-wave or negative STR), rather than positive b-wave.

ON bipolar cells as the generator of the b-wave

Experiments using Ba^{2+} to block Kir channels have not supported the Müller cell hypothesis for generation of the b-wave. Although Ba^{2+} blocks slow PIII[48] as well other responses associated with Müller cell K^+ currents, it is far less effective in blocking the b-wave.[23,54,88,89] In CSD studies in frog[88] and rabbit,[89] only the proximal sink source activity associated with the inner retinal M-wave was removed by Ba^{2+}. At least two-thirds of the OPL sink was retained, and the IPL source involved in generating the b-wave was enhanced. These results indicated that the major b-wave generator is the bipolar cell itself.

Scotopic b-wave (PII) in mammals

In the mammalian retina, the scotopic ERG response to weak stimuli reflects activity of the sensitive primary rod circuit, including rods, the main interneuron, rod bipolar cells, AII amacrine cells, cone bipolar cell terminals, and ganglion cells (Fig. 7.2). Given the simplicity of the circuit, with contributions from amacrine and ganglion cells pharmacologically suppressed, the isolated b-wave (Granit's PII) should reflect the rod bipolar cell response, either directly as the bipolar cell current, or via Müller cell K^+ currents resulting from K^+ outflow from bipolar cells. Only for strong stimuli would the underlying photoreceptor PIII be a significant factor in the ERG. Figure 7.15A shows pharmacologically isolated PII from ERGs, recorded in vivo, of four normal C57BL/6 mice, in response to a weak stimulus. An intravitreal injection of the inhibitory neurotransmitter γ-aminobutyric acid (GABA) was used to suppress inner retinal activity.[31,90] Also included in the figure is PII isolated from human ERG using weak adapting backgrounds to suppress the very sensitive STRs.[91] The isolated PII responses have been superimposed on an average of several patch electrode current recordings in a mouse retinal slice preparation of rod bipolar cell responses to a stimulus of similar effect on the rods. The timecourse of the ERG and the single cell currents is very similar, supporting the

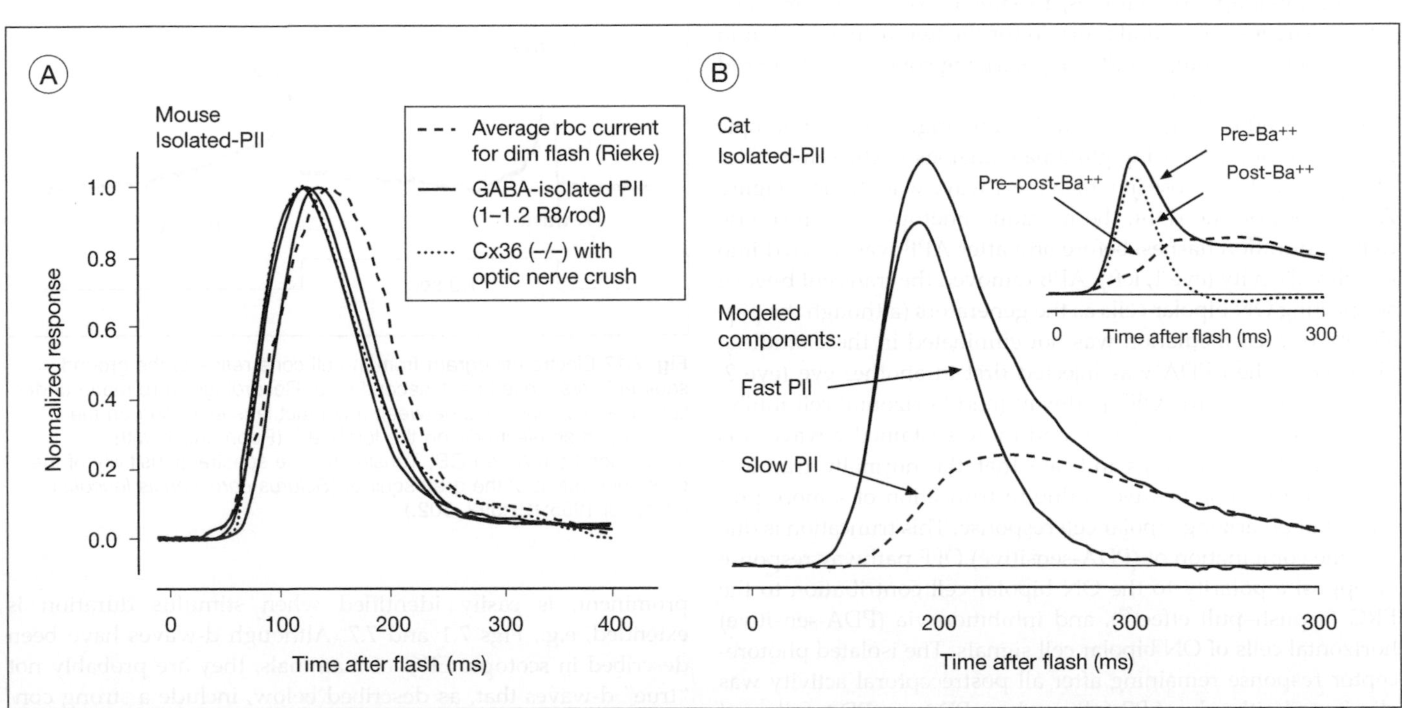

Fig. 7.15 Rod bipolar cell component (PII) of the dark-adapted electroretinogram (ERG) of mouse, cat, and human. (A) (left) Comparison of rod bipolar cell current from patch recordings in mouse retinal slice (courtesy of F. Rieke) with isolated PII (by weak light adaptation) from humans, isolated PII from ERGs of six C57BL/6 mice by intravitreal injection of γ-aminobutyric acid (GABA: 32–46 mM) and additionally from a Cx36$^{(-/-)}$ mouse lacking ganglion cells that lacked scotopic threshold responses. (Reproduced with permission from Cameron AM, Mahroo OA, Lamb TD. Dark adaptation of human rod bipolar cells measured from the b-wave of the scotopic electroretinogram. J Physiol 2006;575:507–26, with permission.) (B) (right) Pharmacologically isolated cat PII (by inner retinal blockade). The response has been analyzed into a fast component, proposed to be a direct reflection of the postsynaptic current, and a slow component, that is a low-pass filtered version of the faster component, believed to be the Müller cell response, contributing mainly to the tail of the response. Identification of the Müller cell component is supported by the observation (shown in the inset) that intravitreal injection of Ba^{2+}, used to block Kir channels in Müller cells removed a similar portion of the total PII response. For stronger stimuli, in order to isolate the bipolar cell response, it would be necessary also to remove the underlying negative (photoreceptor) PIII signal. (Reproduced with permission from Robson JG, Frishman LJ. Dissecting the dark-adapted electroretinogram. Doc Ophthalmol 1998;95:187–215, and from LJ Frishman, JG Robson, unpublished observations.)

view that isolated PII reflects rod bipolar cell activity. If Müller cell currents had generated PII, the signal would have been delayed relative to the bipolar cell responses recorded in the slice, due to the time necessary for accumulation of K^+ ions in the ECS.

Pharmacologically isolated PII of cat (Fig. 7.15B) revealed a response similar to that in mouse in its rising phase, but recovered more slowly to baseline. The cat PII response to a brief flash can be analyzed into a fast component and a slow component that is a low-pass filtered version of the fast component, as indicated by the lines in Fig. 7.15B. The inset to Fig. 7.15B shows that intravitreal Ba^{2+} eliminated a slow portion of the response that was very similar in timecourse to the modeled slow component, but did not alter the fast component, suggesting that bipolar cell current provides the leading edge of PII in the cat, and the Müller cell current contributes at later times. Although the slow component (in response to a brief flash) was lower in amplitude than the fast component, the area under the two curves was similar. With longer stimulus durations such as those used in early studies of the b-wave origins, the contribution to the ERG of the two sources would be about equal.[85] Pharmacologic isolation of macaque PII showed a similar waveform to that in cat.[3]

Cone-driven b-wave

The photopic ERG is commonly measured in the presence of a rod-suppressing background. Depth profiles of the rod b-wave measured under dark-adapted conditions and the cone b-wave, under light-adapted conditions, are similar in cat[92,93] and monkey retinas, suggesting a similar origin for the two responses, but in the case of the photopic ERG, depolarizing cone rather than rod bipolar cells are involved.

Sieving and colleagues[33,35] studied the origins of the photopic b-wave in monkeys using glutamate analogs in the same series of experiments as those in which the a-wave was studied. Figure 7.16 shows, on the right, the macaque photopic ERG response to long-duration flashes, before and after APB was injected into the vitreal cavity (eye 1, left). APB removed the transient b-wave supporting ON bipolar cells as the generators (although the possibility of glial mediation was not eliminated in these studies). However, when PDA was injected first in another eye (eye 2, right), to remove the OFF pathway (and horizontal cell inhibitory feedback), a much larger and more sustained b-wave was revealed. These findings indicate that the normally transient nature of the cone b-wave is due to truncation of a more prolonged depolarizing bipolar cell response. This truncation is due to some combination of (PDA-sensitive) OFF pathway response of opposite polarity to the ON bipolar cell contribution to the ERG (a push-pull effect[28]), and inhibition via (PDA-sensitive) horizontal cells of ON bipolar cell signals. The isolated photoreceptor response remaining after all postreceptoral activity was eliminated either by APB followed by PDA, or PDA followed by APB, was similar.

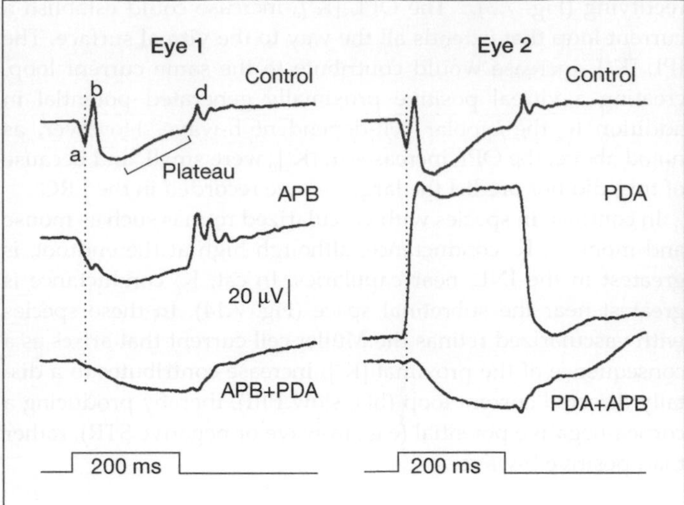

Fig. 7.16 Effects of 2-amino-4-phosphonobutyric acid (APB) and *cis*-2,3-piperidine dicarboxylic acid (PDA) on the light-adapted photopic electroretinogram of two monkey eyes. Drugs were given sequentially, APB followed by PDA for eye 1, and PDA followed by APB for eye 2. The vertical line shows the time of the a-wave trough in the control response. The 200-ms stimulus was 3.76 log td (2.01 log cd/m²) on a steady rod-saturating background of 3.3 log td (1.55 cd/m²). (Reproduced with permission from Bush RA, Sieving PA. A proximal retinal component in the primate photopic ERG a-wave. Invest. Ophthalmol Vis Sci 1994;35:635–45.)

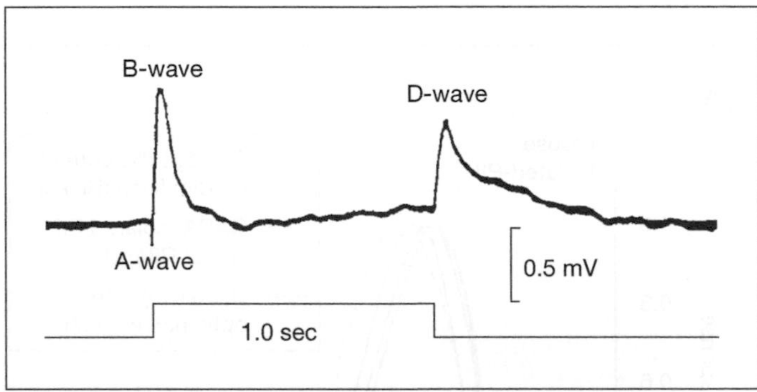

Fig. 7.17 Electroretinogram from the all-cone retina of the ground squirrel in response to a 1-second step. Recordings were made under light-adapted conditions between a contact lens electrode on the cornea and an electrode on the forehead. (Reproduced with permission from Arden GB, Tansley K. The spectral sensitivity of the pure-cone retina of the grey squirrel (*Sciurus carolinensis leucotis*). J Physiol 1955;127:592–602.)

ORIGIN OF THE D-WAVE

The d-wave is a positive-going deflection at light offset that occurs in the photopic ERG. It is best seen when the light step is prolonged. In mammals, the d-wave is very prominent in the all-cone retina of the ground squirrel, as seen in the response to a long-duration stimulus in Fig. 7.17, and in the monkey retina, with its mixture of rods and cones, the d-wave, although less prominent, is easily identified when stimulus duration is extended, e.g., Figs 7.1 and 7.7. Although d-waves have been described in scotopic ERG of mammals, they are probably not "true" d-waves that, as described below, include a strong contribution from the offset of the cone photoreceptor, and the depolarization at light offset of OFF cone bipolar cells. In the predominantly rod-driven cat ERG, the small positive deflection that Granit[32] called a "d-wave" occurred only in response to offset of very intense and long-duration stimuli for which the decay of the rod receptor potential appeared as a small positive deflection that followed, at light offset, the negative-going offset of PII.

Intraretinal analysis in monkey retina indicated that the corneal d-wave represents a combination of the rapid positive-going offset of the cone receptor potential followed by the negative-going offset of the b-wave.[16,66] Although the early work on primate ERG cited above did not identify OFF bipolar cells as major contributors to the d-wave, more recent studies using intravitreal injection of glutamate analogs have demonstrated that these cells provide a significant portion of the response.[35,94] Figs 7.10 and 7.16 both show that PDA, which blocks OFF bipolar cell responses, reduced the d-wave, eliminating it entirely when a large b-wave was present. The effect of PDA was not replicated by NMDA blockade of inner retinal cells, that also would have been affected by PDA, confirming a role of the OFF bipolar cells themselves. PDA, but not the blockade of inner retinal cells, also eliminated a small positive wave that occurs in the falling phase of the b-wave, or just after it, in the brief flash ERG in monkeys and humans, called the "i-wave."[95]

Photopic hill

The stimulus response function acquired by measuring b-wave peak amplitudes in response to brief flashes over a range of increasing stimulus strengths has a characteristic inverted "U" shape. More specifically, Peachey et al.[96] observed that the b-wave amplitude increased with increasing stimulus strength until it reached a peak and then decreased for stronger stimuli. This function was later named the "photopic hill" by Wali and Leguire.[97] A model of the stimulus response function has indicated that the positive peak of the function is formed by addition of a saturating b-wave from ON pathway,[98] and an early d-wave from OFF pathway, and this has been confirmed in experiments using glutamate analogs in macaques.[99]

ORIGIN OF THE PHOTOPIC FAST-FLICKER ERG

The fast-flicker ERG (nominally 30 Hz flicker) is used to examine cone-driven responses in humans because rod-driven responses generally do not respond to fast flicker. For many years the human (or macaque) photopic ERG response to fast-flickering stimuli was believed to reflect primarily the response of cone photoreceptors. However pharmacologic dissection studies have shown that most of the fast-flicker response seen clinically with a full-field stimulus (or focal stimulus) is generated postreceptorally.

Bush and Sieving[100] used glutamate analogs to remove selectively postreceptoral ON and OFF pathway responses, as was done in studies of a-, b-, and d-waves. Intravitreal injection of APB to remove the b-wave left a delayed flicker response, reflecting OFF bipolar contribution. When both APB and PDA were used, the flicker response was practically eliminated. From experiments of this type they concluded that postreceptoral cells that normally produce the b- and d-waves are strong contributors to the fast-flicker response. Further experiments in macaques have more thoroughly investigated the interaction of the ON and OFF pathways over a wide range of temporal frequencies and stimulus conditions.[101] The amplitude in both humans and macaques dips around 12 Hz, as ON and OFF inputs cancel, and it reaches a peak around 50 Hz. Other studies have demonstrated a small inner retinal contribution to the flicker response, and particularly to the second harmonic component of the response, which has a strong input from TTX-sensitive sodium-dependent spiking activity of ganglion and perhaps amacrine cells.[102]

ORIGIN OF THE MULTIFOCAL ERG

Multifocal electroretinography (mfERG) was developed by Sutter and Tran[103] as a means of recording many focal retinal responses simultaneously in a brief time period (e.g., 7 minutes) to achieve a topographical array of little ERGs. Recording ERGs from many different focal regions of the retina otherwise would be impractical, due to the time involved in averaging of the small signals. The common mfERG stimulus is an array of hexagons (e.g., 64 or 103 hexagons over 30–40° of central visual field). In the standard mode for stimulation each hexagon reverses in contrast, according to a predetermined random "m-sequence," at the frame rate of the visual display monitor, often 75 Hz for CRTs and 60 Hz for LCD displays. At any given time, each hexagon has a 50% chance of being light or dark. The m-sequence for all hexagons is the same, except for a specific and unique lag (number of frames) in initiation of the sequence for each hexagon, to allow extraction of the locally generated response by a correlation approach. The resulting "first-order" focal ERGs to the rapidly changing stimulation look similar but not identical to full-field flash ERGs that integrate responses over a longer period of time. The mfERG is generally recorded under photopic conditions, for which the foveal response is large, and is useful for detecting local changes in function that may not be detected in a full-field ERG, such as those that occur in macular dystrophies.

Experiments using intravitreal injections of glutamate analogs, APB, and PDA in macaques showed that, despite differences in the mfERG and full-field flash ERG, the cellular origins of the major negative and positive waves are essentially the same in two types of ERG.[104] The outcome of such experiments is shown in Fig. 7.18, where the findings from the experiments on macaque mfERG were applied to the human response. When blank frames were interposed so that flashes occurred every 100 or 200 ms, a complete ERG including OPs could form before the next m-frame. For this slow-sequence ERG, experiments in macaques again yielded origins similar to full-field flash ERG, and provided some evidence for spike-dependent oscillatory activity related to the optic nerve head component in the mfERG, proposed by Sutter and Bearse.[105–107]

ERG WAVES FROM PROXIMAL RETINA

Origin of the proximal negative response and the M-wave

The proximal negative response (PNR) is a light-evoked field potential recorded intraretinally in proximal retina, named and most fully described by Burkhardt.[108] The PNR consists of a sharp, negative-going transient at onset and again at offset of a small light spot centered on the microelectrode tip placed in the IPL. It can be recorded in a range of vertebrate retinas, including the cat[109] and primate.[110] A PNR contribution to the transretinal ERG is necessarily small because the intraretinal response, which is largest in response to small spots, will be shunted through adjacent low-resistance retinal regions that are not activated by the light.

The M-wave, like the PNR, is a light-evoked field potential, recorded in proximal retina with microelectrodes in response to the onset and offset of a small well-centered spot, but it has a

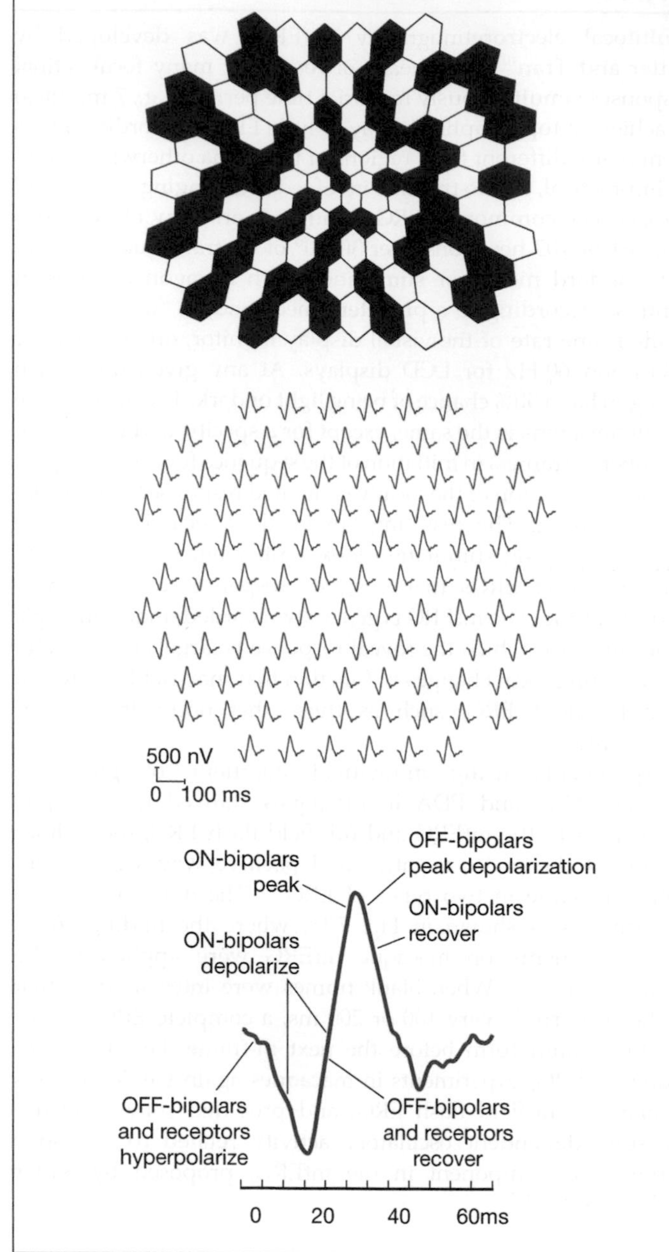

Fig. 7.18 Major components of the multifocal electroretinogram (mfERG). (A) mfERG trace array (field view) using 103 hexagons scaled with eccentricity and covering about 35° of visual angle, as illustrated above the traces. (B) Model for the retinal contributions to the human mfERG based on results from the macular region of a macaque after pharmacological separation of components. (Reproduced with permission from Hood DC, Frishman LJ, Saszik S, et al. Retinal origins of the primate multifocal ERG: implications for the human response. Invest Ophthalmol Vis Sci 2002;43:1673–85.)

slower timecourse than the PNR. The M-wave was initially described in studies of amphibians,[87] but also has been identified in the cat,[23,92] as illustrated in Fig. 7.19.

In retinas in which both an M-wave and a PNR can be recorded (amphibia and cats), the PNR is thought to be the transient neuronally generated portion of the proximal retinal response, while the slower M-wave reflects spatial buffer currents in Müller cells, generated as a consequence of K^+ release from the same proximal neurons.[23,87] As illustrated in Fig. 7.19, for cat, changes in $[K^+]_o$ recorded in proximal retina show a similar timecourse to the simultaneously recorded field potentials. In isolated amphibian retina it was shown that the Kir channel blocker Ba^{2+} had only minor effects on light-evoked neural activity (PNR) and the proximal retinal $[K^+]_o$ increase, but it blocked the M-wave and K^+ spatial buffer currents.[25] Similar findings in intact cat retina are illustrated in Fig. 7.19. Note that after intravitreal Ba^{2+} injection, the proximal $[K^+]_o$ increase was larger, but the more distal increase seen in control records was absent. This is consistent with blockade by Ba^{2+} of spatial buffer currents that normally would carry the K^+ away from proximal retina to the distal extracellular sinks where $[K^+]_o$ was lower.

The local M-wave's contribution to the transretinal ERG would be small. The contribution of the M-wave may be greater when periodic stimuli such as grating patterns that stimulate large regions of retina are used. Sieving and Steinberg[111] showed that the M-wave is tuned to a spot diameter similar to the bar width of the optimal spatial frequency for the intraretinal pattern ERG (PERG) in the cat. The contribution of the proximal retina to the ERG can also be enhanced by using full-field stimulation.

Origin of the photopic negative response

In contrast to the PNR and M-wave, which provide small contributions at most to the transretinal ERG, negative-going responses from proximal retina to full-field stimulation are present in the corneal ERGs of several species, including cats, monkeys, and humans.[40,63,92,93,112–114] These responses, called the PhNR, and STR are generated by mechanisms similar to those documented above for the M-wave.

The PhNR is a negative-going wave in the photopic ERG that occurs after the b-wave in response to a brief flash, and again after the d-wave in response to a long flash. It is more prominent in primates than in rodents. In humans and monkeys, the PhNR is thought to reflect spiking activity of retinal ganglion cells.[113,114] As shown in Fig. 7.20, the PhNR is reduced in macaque eyes with experimental glaucoma (also after TTX injection)[113] and in humans with primary open angle glaucoma. It is reduced in several other disorders affecting inner retina and optic nerve head as well. The slow timecourse of the PhNR suggests glial involvement, perhaps via K^+ currents in astrocytes in the optic nerve head or Müller cells set up by increased $[K^+]_o$ due to spiking of ganglion cells. In intraretinal microelectrode recordings in cats, local signals of the same timecourse as the PhNR were largest in and around the optic nerve head and the PhNR was disrupted in cats by Ba^{2+}, indicating glial involvement in generation of the response (Viswanathan and Frishman, unpublished observations).

PhNRs can be evoked using white flashes on a white background, if the flash is strong enough. However a red LED flash on a blue background, as was used for ERGs shown in Fig. 7.20, elicits PhNRs over a wider range of stimulus strengths. The red flash may minimize spectral opponency that would reduce ganglion cell responses, and use of a blue background suppresses rods while minimizing light adaptation of L-cone signals.[7] Blue stimuli on a yellow background which minimize spectral antagonism are good stimuli as well. The PhNR can be enhanced relative to other major ERG components, and can dominate the ERG when using focal stimuli in the region of the macula.[115–117]

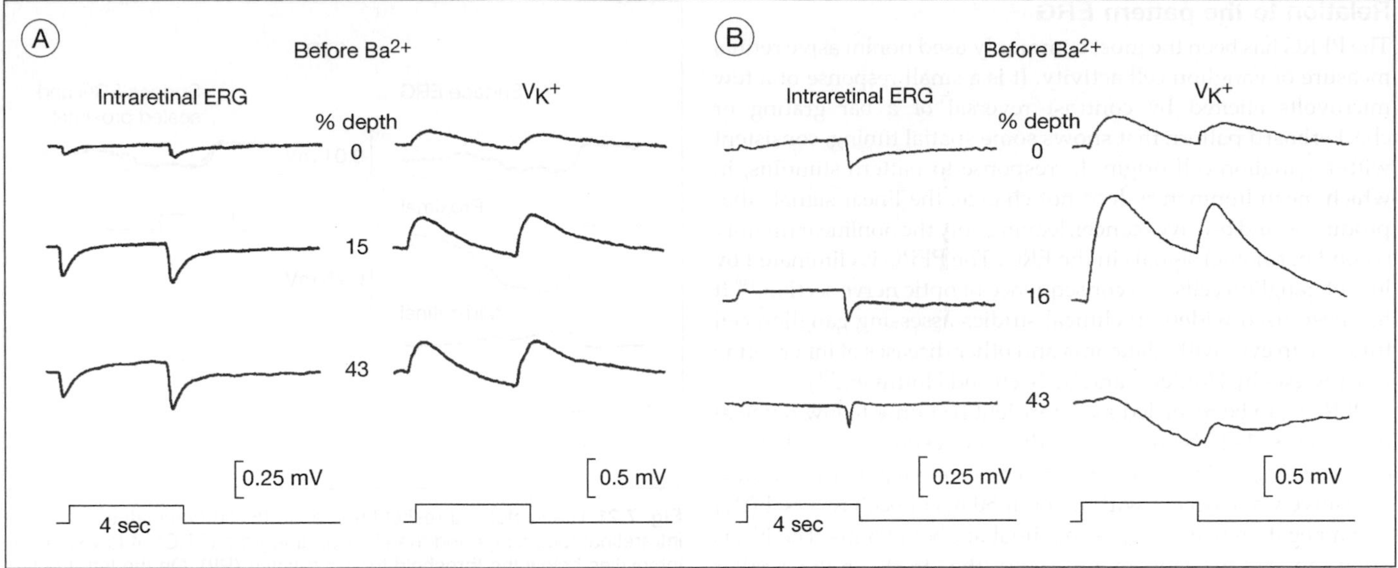

Fig. 7.19 Effect of Ba^{2+} on the M-wave of the light-adapted cat retina. Effect of intravitreal barium chloride ($BaCl^{2+}$, 3 mM vitreal concentration) on the depth distribution of field potentials and $[K^+]_o$ changes in light-adapted retina. Recordings were made before (A) and 30–60 minutes after (B) $BaCl^{2+}$ was injected. The stimulus was a small spot (0.8° in diameter); steady background illumination was 10.5 log q deg²/s; flash illumination was 11.6 log q deg²/s. (Adapted from Frishman LJ, Yamamoto F, Bogucka J, et al. Light-evoked changes in $[K^+]_o$ in proximal portion of light-adapted cat retina. J Neurophysiol 1992;67:1201–12.)

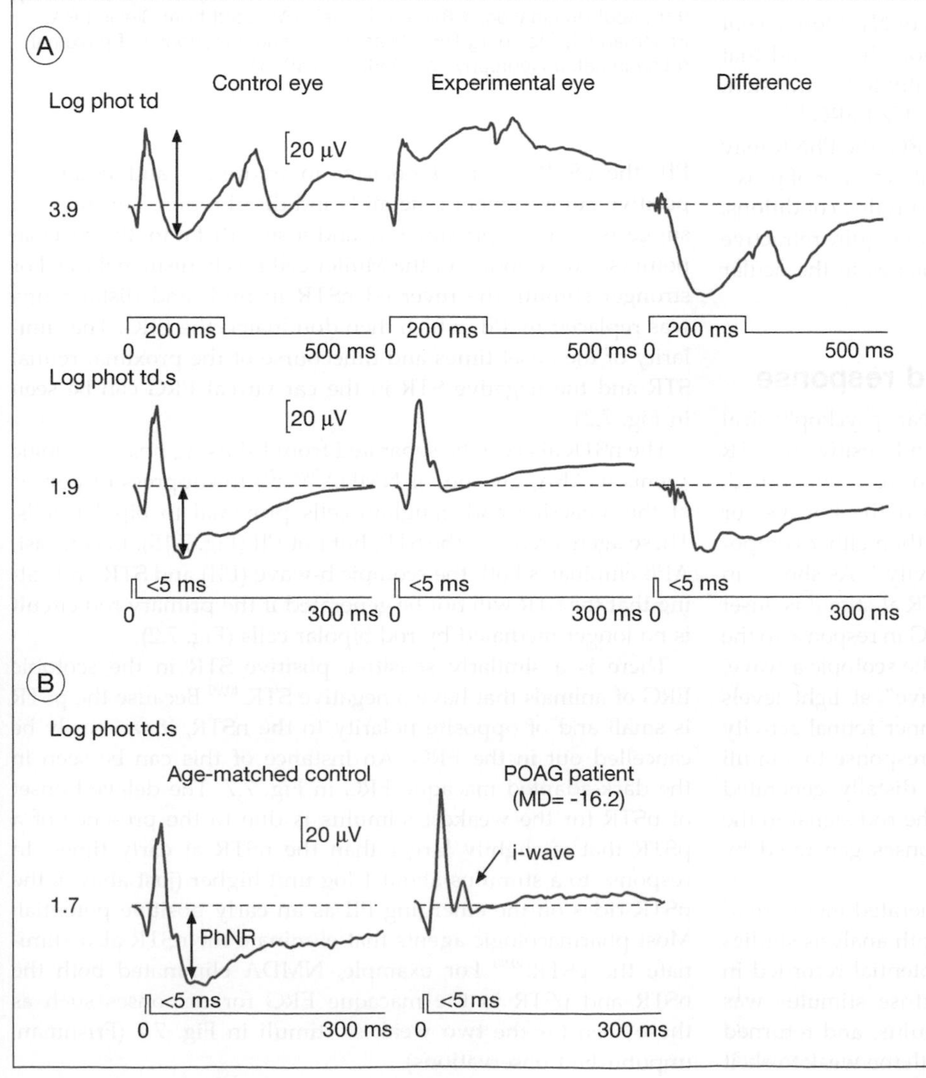

Fig. 7.20 Photopic negative response (PhNR) in macaque monkey and human in normal and glaucomatous eyes. (A) Full-field flash electroretinogram (ERG) showing the PhNR of a macaque in response to long (top) and brief (middle) red light-emitting diode (LED) flashes on a rod-saturating blue background (3.7 log sc td) from the control (left) and "experimental" (middle) fellow eye with laser-induced glaucoma, and the difference between control and experimental records (right). Arrows mark the amplitude of the PhNR. The mean deviation (MD, static perimetry, C24–2 full threshold program) for the experimental eye was –2.65 dB. (Adapted from Viswanathan S, Frishman LJ, Robson JG, et al. The photopic negative response of the macaque electroretinogram: reduction by experimental glaucoma. Invest Ophthalmol Vis Sci 1999;40:1124-36, with permission.) (B) Full-field flash ERGs of an age-matched 63-year-old normal human subject and a patient with primary open angle glaucoma (POAG) under similar stimulus conditions to those used above for monkeys. The MD (static perimetry, C24–2 full threshold program) for the patient's eye was –16.2 dB. (Adapted from Viswanathan S, Frishman LJ, Robson JG, et al. The photopic negative response of the flash electroretinogram in primary open angle glaucoma. Invest Ophthalmol Vis Sci 2001;42:514–22.)

Relation to the pattern ERG

The PERG has been the most commonly used noninvasive retinal measure of ganglion cell activity. It is a small response of a few microvolts elicited by contrast reversal of a bar grating or checkerboard pattern that shows some spatial tuning, consistent with a ganglion cell origin. In response to pattern stimulus, in which mean luminance does not change, the linear signals that produce a- and b-waves cancel, leaving only the nonlinear (mainly second harmonic) signals in the ERG. The PERG is eliminated by loss of ganglion cells as a consequence of optic nerve section.[118] It has been used widely in clinical studies assessing ganglion cell function in eyes with glaucoma and other diseases of inner retina (see reviews by Holder[117] and by Bach and Hoffmann[116]).

PERGs can be recorded as a transient response to low reversal frequencies (1–2 Hz) or as a steady-state response to higher frequencies, i.e., 8 Hz. For 1–2-Hz reversals of the pattern stimulus, a positive wave occurs within about 50 ms of each reversal (P_{50}) and a negative wave, N_{95}, is maximal at about 95 ms. The N_{95} is often reduced in glaucomatous eyes (the effects on the smaller P_{50} response are less consistent). Because the PhNR has a similar implicit time to the N_{95}, Viswanathan et al.[119] compared effects of experimental glaucoma and of TTX on the two responses in macaques, and found similar effects on both, indicating common retinal origins. Furthermore, the PERG waveform for a given stimulation frequency (2 or 8 Hz) could be simulated by adding together the ERGs at onset and offset of a uniform field, with strong contributions of PhNRs in generation of N_{95}. More recent work using glutamate analogs and simulations has found that both ON and OFF pathways contribute equally to the transient PERG, but the ON pathway dominates the 8 Hz PERG.[120]

Given the similar origins of PhNR and PERG, the PhNR may have some advantages over PERG as a clinical indicator of proximal retinal dysfunction. With appropriate stimulus conditions, the PhNR is a much larger response, it does not require refractive correction, and will be less affected by opacities in the ocular media than the PERG.

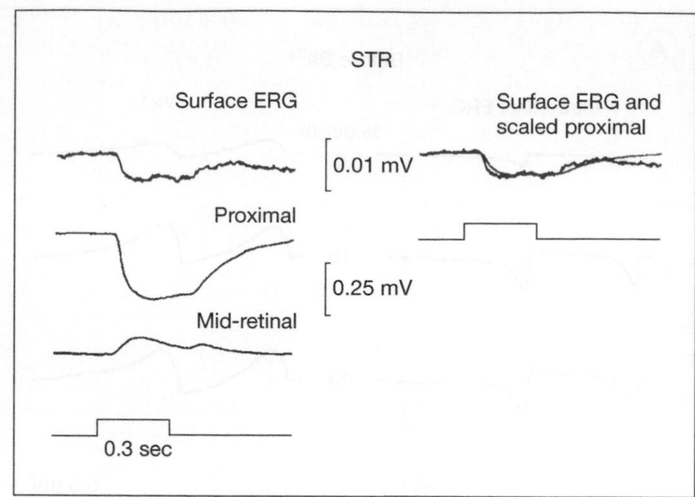

Fig. 7.21 The scotopic threshold response (STR) dominates intraretinal recordings and the electroretinogram (ERG) at low stimulus intensities below the threshold for the b-wave (PII). On the left, the top trace is the surface ERG recorded about 25 μm from the retinal surface, and the bottom two traces are recordings of the STR in the proximal retina (about 6% retinal depth) and the inverted STR around 50% retinal depth. On the right, the scaled STR recorded in the proximal retina is superimposed on the surface ERG to show the similarity of the responses. For the surface ERG, a microelectrode was referenced to a wire in the vitreous in order to reduce the effects of stray light. This minimized contributions to the ERG of retinal regions distant from the recording site of the intraretinal signals (spot diameter, 9.9°; spot illumination, 4.8 log q deg^2/s). (Adapted from Sieving PA, Frishman LJ, Steinberg RH. Scotopic threshold response of proximal retina in cat. J Neurophysiol 1986;56:1049–61.)

Origin of the scotopic threshold response

For very weak flashes from darkness, near psychophysical threshold in humans,[33,90] small negative (n) and positive (p) STR dominate the ERG of most mammals that have been studied. This response, which is more sensitive than the b-wave (or a-wave) and saturates at a lower light level than either component, was thus named because of its sensitivity.[63] As shown in Fig. 7.7, for the monkey and human, the nSTR at stimulus onset dominates the dark-adapted diffuse flash ERG in response to the weakest stimuli. The nSTR is distinct from the scotopic a-wave, although it can appear as a "pseudo a-wave" at light levels where it can be removed by suppressing inner retinal activity pharmacologically.[121,122] The STRs occur in response to stimuli much weaker than those that elicit more distally generated waves of the ERG because convergence of the rod signal in the retinal circuitry increases the gain of responses generated by inner retinal neurons.

The nSTR was initially observed to be generated more proximally (IPL) than PII (INL) in intraretinal depth analysis studies in cats.[63] As shown in Fig. 7.21, the field potential recorded in proximal retina in response to a weak diffuse stimulus was negative-going for the duration of the stimulus, and returned slowly to baseline after light offset. For stimuli too weak to elicit PII, the nSTR reversed polarity in midretina and became a positive-going signal in the mid- and distal retina. This reversal suggests a source proximal to, and a sink distal to, the reversal point (see description of the Müller cell mechanism, below). For stronger stimuli, the reversed nSTR in mid- and distal retina was replaced by PII, which then dominated the ERG. The similarity of the onset times and timecourse of the proximal retinal STR and the negative STR in the cat vitreal ERG can be seen in Fig. 7.21.

The nSTR also can be separated from PII using pharmacologic agents (GABA, glycine, or NMDA[30,90,121]) to suppress responses of the amacrine and ganglion cells proximal to bipolar cells. These agents remove the STR, but not PII (Fig. 7.15). In contrast, APB eliminates both the scotopic b-wave (PII) and STR, indicating that the STR will not be generated if the primary rod circuit is no longer mediated by rod bipolar cells (Fig. 7.2).

There is a similarly sensitive positive STR in the scotopic ERG of animals that have a negative STR.[40,90] Because the pSTR is small and of opposite polarity to the nSTR, it can easily be cancelled out in the ERG. An instance of this can be seen in the dark-adapted macaque ERG in Fig. 7.7. The delayed onset of nSTR for the weakest stimulus is due to the presence of a pSTR that is slightly larger than the nSTR at early times. In response to a stimulus about 1 log unit higher (just above), the pSTR rides on the emerging PII as an early positive potential. Most pharmacologic agents that eliminate the nSTR also eliminate the pSTR.[40,90] For example, NMDA eliminated both the nSTR and pSTR in the macaque ERG for responses such as those seen for the two weakest stimuli in Fig. 7.7 (Frishman, unpublished observations).

A linear model of the contributions of pSTR, nSTR, and PII to the dark-adapted cat ERG is shown in Fig. 7.22. The model assumes that each ERG component initially rises in proportion to stimulus strength, and then saturates in a characteristic manner, as has been demonstrated in single-cell recordings in mammalian retinas, as well as for ERG a- and b-waves in numerous studies. Only with the inclusion of a small pSTR does the model accurately predict the whole ERG at a given "fixed" time in response to a weak stimulus. The model was fit in Fig. 7.22 to responses measured at 140 ms after a brief full-field flash (<5 ms), which was the peak of the nSTR in the cat scotopic ERG. Similar models have been applied to mouse[90] and human ERG.[40]

K^+ Müller cell mechanism for generation of the STR

The STR, like the M-wave, is associated with Müller cell responses to $[K^+]_o$ released by proximal retinal neurons. In intraretinal studies in cat, a proximal increase in $[K^+]_o$ was observed that had clear similarities to the local STR that was simultaneously recorded: the dynamic range from "threshold" to saturation of

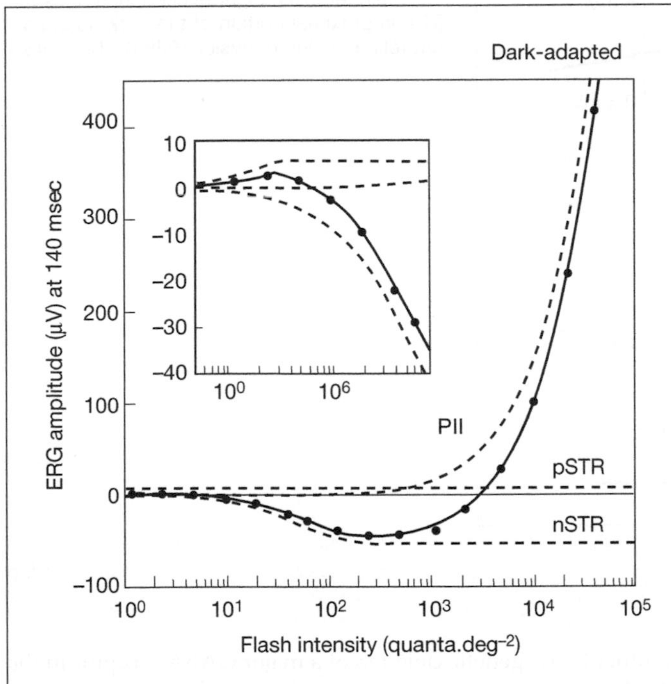

Fig. 7.22 Amplitude of cat dark-adapted electroretinogram responses measured 140 ms after a brief flash at the maximum negativity of the negative scotopic threshold response (nSTR). Dashed lines show model curves for the positive scotopic threshold response (pSTR), nSTR, and PII. Explicitly, the pSTR rises as a linear function that saturates abruptly at V_{max}, while the exponential saturation of the nSTR is defined by:

$$V = V_{max}(1 - \exp(-I/I_o))$$

where V_{max} is the maximum saturated amplitude, and I_o is the intensity for an amplitude of $(1 - 1/e)V_{max}$, while the hyperbolic relation used for PII is defined by:

$$V = V_{max} I/(I + I_o)$$

where V_{max} has the same meaning but I_o is the intensity at which the amplitude is $V_{max}/2$. The inset shows the pSTR and nSTR at the lowest light levels that were used. (1 q deg^2 is equivalent to ~−7.5 log sc cd m^2/s). (Adapted from Frishman LJ, Robson JG. Processing, adaptation to environmental light. In: Archer SN, Djamgoz MBA, Loew ER, et al., editors. Adaptive mechanisms in the ecology of vision. Dordrecht: Kluwer Academic.; 1999. p. 383–412, with permission.)

the light-evoked proximal $[K^+]_o$ increase was similar to that of the field potentials, and the retinal depth maxima for the two responses were the same.[22,54] A causative role for the $[K^+]_o$ increase in generating the nSTR (and a slow negative response in the vitreal ERG following the initial STR) was supported by the finding (Fig. 7.23) that Ba^{2+} removed the proximal retinal field potential and the nSTR in the ERG but did not, initially, eliminate the light-evoked increase in $[K^+]_o$. The cornea-negative polarity of the nSTR suggests a distally directed Müller cell K^+ current (similar to M-wave and PIII currents in the vascularized cat retina). As noted above for the light-adapted M-wave, in the dark-adapted retina Ba^{2+} also appears to block K^+ siphoning by the Müller cells. Whereas the proximal $[K^+]_o$ increase remained intact when related field potentials were abolished, the distal $[K^+]_o$ increase was eliminated by Ba^{2+}.

Neuronal origins of the STR

Whether the neurons involved in the genesis of the nSTR and pSTR are amacrine or ganglion cells is species-dependent. In monkeys it is likely that the nSTR arises predominantly from ganglion cells. It was absent in eyes in which the ganglion cells were eliminated as a consequence of experimental glaucoma[112] and by intravitreal injection of TTX to block Na^+-dependent spiking activity of those neurons; the pSTR remained intact. In contrast, in cats and humans[122] as well as in rodents,[3] the nSTR is not eliminated by ganglion cell loss, and thus may be more amacrine cell-based. In rodents the pSTR relies upon the integrity of ganglion cells. A characteristic of Müller/glial cell-mediated ERG components is their slow timecourse. Glial cell mediation of the nSTR was demonstrated most directly in cat, but the timecourse of the nSTR is slow in all species. Glial mediation may explain the similarity in timecourse of nSTR across species regardless of the particular type of neuron producing the local changes in proximal $[K^+]_o$ that generate the response.

Origin of oscillatory potentials

The OPs of the ERG consist of a series of high-frequency, low-amplitude wavelets, mainly superimposed on the b-wave, that occur in response to strong stimulation. OPs are present under light- and dark-adapted conditions, with contributions from both rod- and cone-driven signals.[123] The mixed rod–cone ERG in humans in the ISCEV standards in Fig. 7.4 shows at least four OPs that can be extracted with a filter with a low-frequency cutoff of 75 Hz. OPs are of postreceptoral origin, and occur in isolated retinas in the absence of the RPE.[73] The number of OPs induced by a flash of light varies between about 4 and 10 depending upon species and stimulus conditions; the temporal frequency of the OPs varies as well. Figure 7.24 shows the photopic flash ERG of a macaque monkey (top); at least five OPs at frequency of about 150 Hz can be seen by filtering the response to extract the high-frequency signals.

There is consensus that OPs are generated in proximal retina. Three important and unresolved questions regarding their origins are: (1) Do all the OPs have the same origin? (2) Which cells generate the OPs? (3) What mechanisms are involved in generating OPs?

Do all the OPs have the same origin?

In amphibia, where early studies were done, the various OPs do not all have the same origin. Depth profiles from isolated frog retina showed that the earliest OPs in the response arose near the IPL whereas the later OPs arose more distally, perhaps in the

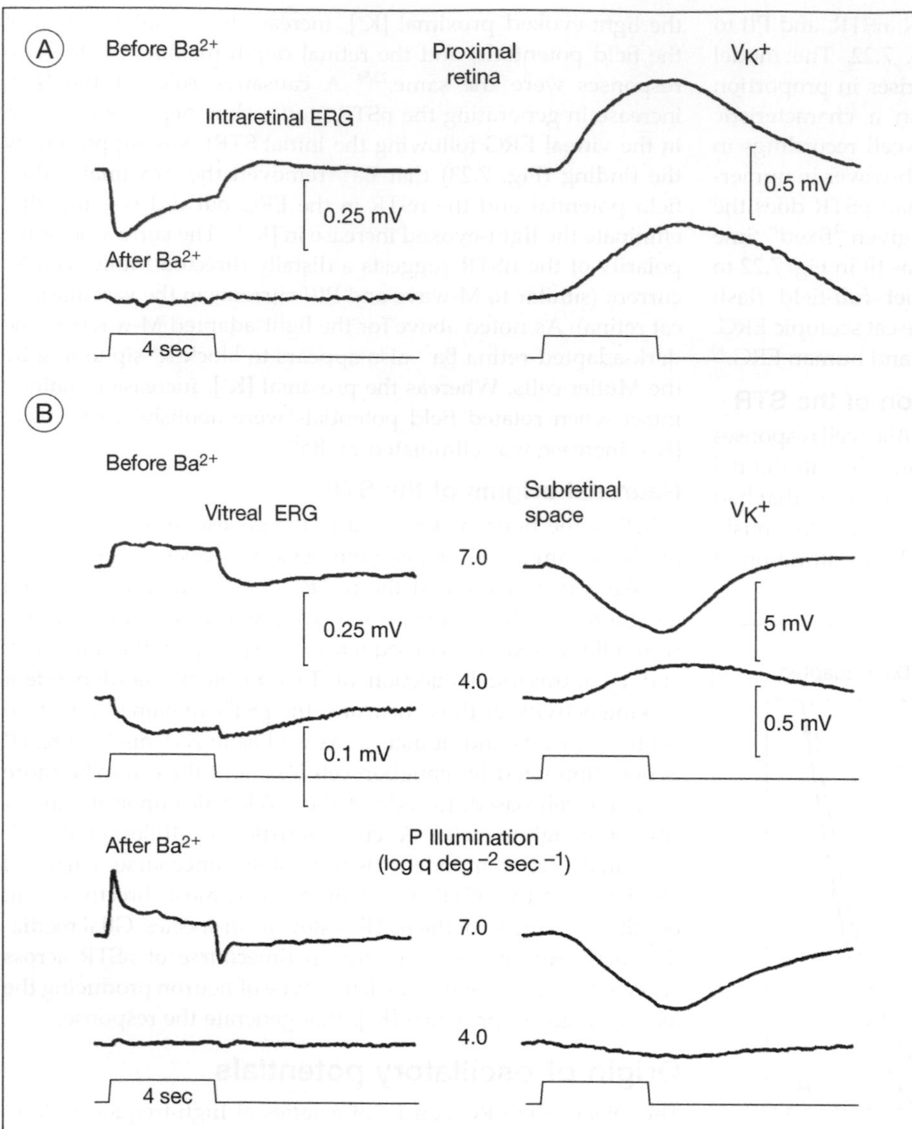

Fig. 7.23 Effect of Ba^{2+} on the scotopic threshold response (STR) and b-wave (PII) in scotopic electroretinogram (ERG) of the cat. (A) Effect of intravitreal Ba^{2+} ($BaCl_2$, 3.9 mM vitreal concentration) on the intraretinal STR and slower K^+-related negative response in response to a 4-second stimulus and the simultaneously recorded light-evoked decrease in $[K^+]_o$ (V_{K+}) in the proximal retina measured at 10% retinal depth, proximal to the peak K^+ change at 17% depth. Top response was measured before Ba^{2+} and the bottom response 56 minutes after Ba^{2+} injection. (B) Effect of intravitreal $BaCl_2$ (3.9 mM vitreal concentration) on the STR and slow negative response in the vitreal ERG (left) and the simultaneously recorded change in $[K^+]_o$ in the subretinal space. Measurements of the amplitude of dark-adapted responses in the proximal retina and the light-evoked increase in $[K^+]_o$ in proximal and distal retina before and after intravitreal injection of Ba^{2+} were made with double-barreled K^+-sensitive microelectrodes. (Reproduced with permission from Frishman LJ, Steinberg RH. Light-evoked increases in $[K^+]_o$ in proximal portion of the dark-adapted cat retina. J Neurophysiol 1989;61:1233–43.)

INL. Studies of Wachmeister[124] in amphibian retina also found that earlier OPs were depressed by GABA antagonists, the dopamine antagonist haloperidol, β-alanine, and substance P, whereas later OPs were depressed by the glycine antagonist strychnine and by ethanol.

In primates, intraretinal studies using stimuli that would elicit responses from both rod and cone systems did not find differences in the depth profiles of the different OPs.[44,125] Considering the complexity of inner retinal circuitry, the similarity in depth profiles does not necessarily mean that the same neurons were involved in all cases. For example, in the photopic flash ERG response to brief stimuli, the major OPs are APB-sensitive in primates and other mammals, indicating an origin in the ON pathways, but later OPs and at light offset originate in the OFF pathway.[105,126] Such a difference could lead to differences in the depth distribution in the IPL which is stratified in outer OFF sublamina and inner ON sublamina.

Pharmacologic agents that block inner retinal activity, such as glycine and GABA, remove OPs in mammals, as does PDA,[105] but the effects were not reported to be specific for given OPs. On the other hand, genetic deletion of a major GABA receptor in the IPL, the $GABA_C$ receptor, enhances the OPs.[127]

Which cells generate the OPs?

The observations described above indicate that amacrine or perhaps, in some instances, retinal ganglion cells are involved in generating OPs. A study of rabbit ERG indicates a distal to proximal progression in origin, with the late but not early OPs having input from spiking cells.[126] The role of ganglion cells in the generation of OPs has been controversial, with inconsistent reports on the effects of ganglion cell loss on OPs. In Ogden's studies in primates, optic nerve section resulted in ganglion cell degeneration and disappearance of the OPs, and antidromic stimulation of the optic nerve reduced OP amplitudes.[125] Further, in the primate photopic ERG elicited using a multifocal paradigm with a slow sequence to allow formation of OPs, both TTX and experimental glaucoma removed or reduced a high-frequency band of OPs, while affecting a lower-frequency band less.[105,106] It is possible in primates that high-frequency OPs (centered around 150 Hz, compared to >100 Hz for the

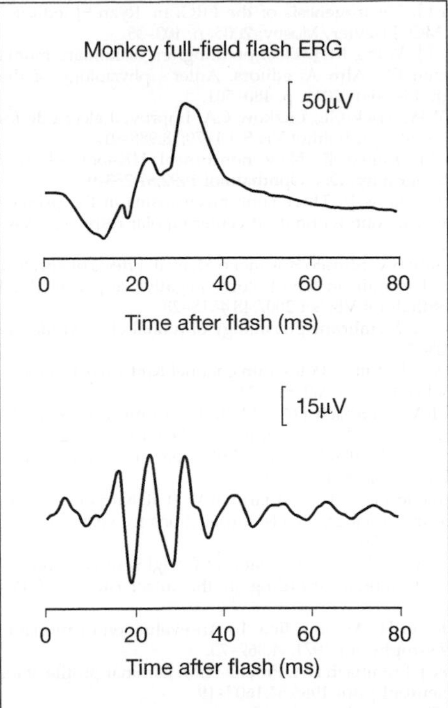

Fig. 7.24 Full-field flash photopic electroretinogram of a macaque monkey (top) and the oscillatory potentials (OPs) extracted from these records. Filtering was between 90 and 300 Hz for OPs that occurred between 100 and 200 Hz. The stimulus was a xenon flash presented on a rod-saturating blue background. (Adapted from Rangaswamy NV, Hood DC, Frishman LJ. Regional variations in local contributions to the primate photopic flash ERG: revealed using the slow-sequence mfERG. Invest Ophthalmol Vis Sci 2003;44:3233–47).

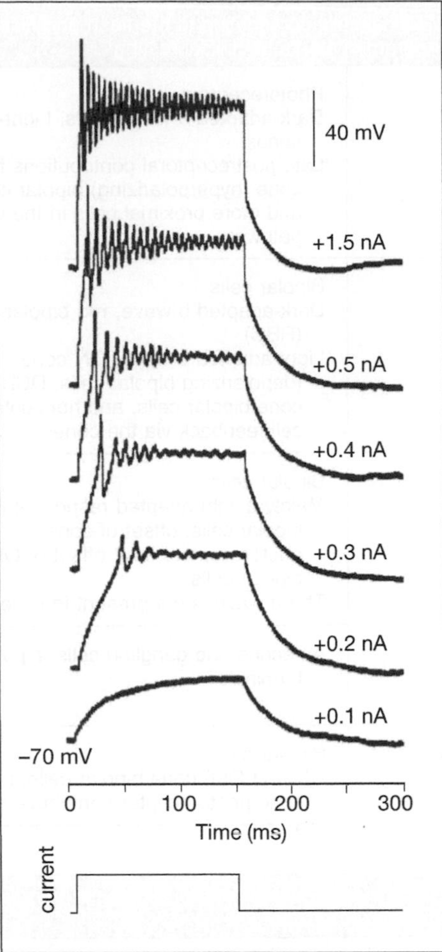

Fig. 7.25 Oscillatory potentials of isolated wide-field amacrine cells in the white perch retina. Oscillatory membrane potentials (OMPs) were elicited by depolarizing current steps of increasing amplitude obtained in whole-cell recordings from isolated amacrine cells that were maintained in culture. The duration and frequency of the OMPs increased with depolarization. Voltage traces are shifted vertically for visibility. Bottom: application of depolarizing pulse. The magnitude of depolarizing current is indicated with each trace. Holding potential was –70 mV. (Reproduced with permission from Vigh J, Solessio E, Morgans CW, et al. Ionic mechanisms mediating oscillatory membrane potentials in wide-field retinal amacrine cells. J Neurophysiol 2003;90:431–43.)

lower-frequency band) under fully photopic conditions reflect activity in ganglion cell axons, and the manifestation of an optic nerve head component of the ERG. Under conditions where rod signals are also involved, the ganglion cell contribution may be less prominent. In other mammals, TTX-sensitive OPs may be among the late ones.

What mechanisms are involved in generating OPs?

Neuronal interaction; inhibitory feedback circuits

Two mechanisms are commonly proposed for generating OPs: neuronal interactions/feedback circuits, and the intrinsic membrane properties of cells, both of which implicate amacrine cells. The case for an inhibitory feedback mechanism is supported by involvement of receptors for GABA and glycine, which are prominent in feedback circuits in the inner retina. Gap junctions between inner retinal neurons can also be involved in feedforward mechanism.

OPs in intracellular responses from neurons

In retinal intracellular recordings from many different species, high-frequency oscillations have rarely been observed in responses of photoreceptors, horizontal, or bipolar cells. In contrast, membrane oscillations have been observed in recordings from amacrine cells, especially in turtle and fish retina. For example, GABAergic wide-field ACs isolated from white bass retina generated oscillatory membrane potentials in response to extrinsic depolarization, as illustrated in Fig. 7.25, that reached more than 100 Hz for strong depolarization. Analysis of the mechanism of generation of the oscillatory membrane potentials in these isolated cells indicated that they arose from "a complex interplay between voltage-dependent Ca^{2+} currents and voltage- and Ca^{2+}-dependent K^{+} currents."[128]

In summary, there is consensus that high-frequency OPs originate from the inner retina. The exact cellular origins may depend upon species and stimulus conditions. The mechanisms by which they are generated are unresolved, with evidence for both involvement of feedback circuitry, and for intrinsic membrane mechanisms in amacrine cells.

CLOSING REMARKS

This chapter has reviewed the increasingly specific information about the electrogenesis of the ERG that has become available as our understanding of retinal microcircuitry and cellular and synaptic mechanisms has increased. Due to the extensive research on ERG, it has become feasible to use it to assess retinal function at every level, from the RPE to the optic nerve head; also see other recent reviews on this subject.[3,129–131] Tables 7.1 and 7.2

Table 7.1 Retinal cells contributing to the flash and flicker electroretinogram in standard clinical testing

a-wave	Photoreceptors Dark-adapted a-wave: rods. Light-adapted: cones Late postreceptoral contributions from OFF cone (hyperpolarizing) bipolar cells (HCB) and more proximal cells in the OFF pathway
b-wave	Bipolar cells Dark-adapted b-wave, rod bipolar cells (RBC) Light-adapted b-wave, ON cone (depolarizing bipolar cells: DCB), OFF cone bipolar cells, and horizontal (Hz) cell feedback via the cones
d-wave	Bipolar cells Mainly a light-adapted response: OFF cone bipolar cells, offset of cone photoreceptors, and offset of ON cone bipolar cells The d-wave is not present in mice and rats
Oscillatory potentials (OPs)	Amacrine and ganglion cells, bipolar cell terminals?
"30 Hz" fast flicker	Bipolar cells ON and OFF cone bipolar cells, and a small cone photoreceptor contribution

Table 7.2 Retinal cells contributing to the electroretinogram (ERG) in specialized testing

Scotopic threshold response	Inner retinal neurons
pSTR	Amacrine cells (monkey) Retinal ganglion cells (rodents)
nSTR	Retinal ganglion cells (monkey) Partially retinal ganglion cells (rats, human?) Amacrine cells (AII) (mice) Partially amacrine cells (rats, human) Glial currents
Photopic negative response (PhNR)	Retinal ganglion cells (human, monkey) Amacrine cells (rodents) Glial currents
Pattern ERG (PERG)	Retinal ganglion cells (human, monkey, rodent) Glial currents (transient PERG: N95, N2?)
Multifocal ERG	Initial negative and positive waves have similar origins to a- and b-waves in photopic ERG (monkey, and presumably human)

summarize our current understanding of the origins of ERGs recorded in standard and specialized tests. Continued refinement of stimuli, protocols, and analysis will further enhance the power of this noninvasive tool in the laboratory and the clinic.

REFERENCES

1. Frishman LJ. Origins of the ERG. In: Heckenlively J, Arden GB, editors. Principles and practice of clinical electrophysiology of vision. 2nd ed. Cambridge, MA: MIT Press; 2006. p. 139–83.
2. Frishman LJ. Electrogenesis of the ERG. In: Ryan SJ, editor. Retina. 4th ed. St Louis, MO: Elsevier/Mosby; 2005. p. 103–35.
3. Frishman LJ, Wang MH. Electroretinogram of human, monkey and mouse. In: Kaufman PL, Alm A, editors. Adler's physiology of the eye. 11th ed. Edinburgh: Elsevier; 2011. p. 480–501.
4. Dawson WW, Trick GL, Litzkow CA. Improved electrode for electroretinography. Invest Ophthalmol Vis Sci 1979;18:988–91.
5. Hawlina M, Konec B. New noncorneal HK-loop electrode for clinical electroretinography. Doc Ophthalmol 1992;81:253–9.
6. Evers HU, Gouras P. Three cone mechanisms in the primate electroretinogram: two with, one without off-center bipolar responses. Vision res 1986;26:245–54.
7. Rangaswamy NV, Shirato S, Kaneko M, et al. Effects of spectral characteristics of Ganzfeld stimuli on the photopic negative response (PhNR) of the ERG. Invest Ophthalmol Vis Sci 2007;48:4818–28.
8. Newman EA. Membrane physiology of retinal glial (Müller) cells. J Neurosci 1985;5:2225–39.
9. Connors NC, Kofuji P. Potassium channel Kir4.1 macromolecular complex in retinal glial cells. Glia 2006;53:124–31.
10. Newman EA, Frambach DA, Odette LL. Control of extracellular potassium levels by retinal glial cell K^+ siphoning. Science 1984;225:1174–5.
11. Newman E, Reichenbach A. The Müller cell: a functional element of the retina. Trends Neurosci 1996;19:307–12.
12. Kofuji P, Biedermann B, Siddharthan V, et al. Kir potassium channel subunit expression in retinal glial cells: implications for spatial potassium buffering. Glia 2002;39:292–303.
13. Brown KT, Wiesel TN. Localization of origins of electroretinogram components by intraretinal recording in the intact cat eye. J Physiol 1961;158:257–80.
14. Ogden TE, Ito H. Avian retina. II. An evaluation of retinal electrical anisotropy. J Neurophysiol 1971;34:367–73.
15. Karwoski CJ, Frambach DA, Proenza LM. Laminar profile of resistivity in frog retina. J Neurophysiol 1985;54:1607–19.
16. Brown KT. The electroretinogram: its components and their origins. Vision res 1968;8:633–77.
17. Freeman JA, Nicholson C. Experimental optimization of current source-density technique for anuran cerebellum. J Neurophysiol 1975;38:369–82.
18. Heynen H, van Norren D. Origin of the electroretinogram in the intact macaque eye–II. Current source-density analysis. Vision Res 1985;25:709–15.
19. Xu X, Karwoski CJ. Current source density (CSD) analysis of retinal field potentials. I. Methodological considerations and depth profiles. J Neurophysiol 1994;72:84–95.
20. Dick E, Miller RF. Extracellular K^+ activity changes related to electroretinogram components. I. Amphibian (I-type) retinas. J Gen Physiol 1985;85:885–909.
21. Dick E, Miller RF, Bloomfield S. Extracellular K^+ activity changes related to electroretinogram components. II. Rabbit (E-type) retinas. J Gen Physiol 1985;85:911–31.
22. Frishman LJ, Steinberg RH. Light-evoked increases in $[K^+]o$ in proximal portion of the dark-adapted cat retina. J Neurophysiol 1989;61:1233–43.
23. Frishman LJ, Yamamoto F, Bogucka J, et al. Light-evoked changes in $[K^+]o$ in proximal portion of light-adapted cat retina. J Neurophysiol 1992;67:1201–12.
24. Oakley 2nd B, Green DG. Correlation of light-induced changes in retinal extracellular potassium concentration with c-wave of the electroretinogram. J Neurophysiol 1976;39:1117–33.
25. Karwoski CJ, Lu HK, Newman EA. Spatial buffering of light-evoked potassium increases by retinal Müller (glial) cells. Science 1989;244:578–80.
26. Halgrimson CG, Wilson CB, Dixon FJ, et al. Goodpasture's syndrome. Treatment with nephrectomy and renal transplantation. Arch Surg 1971;103:283–9.
27. Newman EA. Potassium conductance block by barium in amphibian Müller cells. Brain Res 1989;498:308–14.
28. Kofuji P, Ceelen P, Zahs KR, et al. Genetic inactivation of an inwardly rectifying potassium channel (Kir4.1 subunit) in mice: phenotypic impact in retina. J Neurosci 2000 ;20:5733–40.
29. Penn RD, Hagins WA. Signal transmission along retinal rods and the origin of the electroretinographic a-wave. Nature 1969;223:201–4.
30. Robson JG, Frishman LJ. Response linearity and kinetics of the cat retina: the bipolar cell component of the dark-adapted electroretinogram. Vis Neurosci 1995;12:837–50.
31. Robson JG, Maeda H, Saszik SM, et al. In vivo studies of signaling in rod pathways of the mouse using the electroretinogram. Vision Res 2004;44:3253–68.
32. Granit R. The components of the retinal action potential in mammals and their relation to the discharge in the optic nerve. J Physiol 1933;77:207–39.
33. Bush RA, Sieving PA. A proximal retinal component in the primate photopic ERG a-wave. Invest Ophthalmol Vis Sci 1994;35:635–45.
34. Robson JG, Saszik SM, Ahmed J, et al. Rod and cone contributions to the a-wave of the electroretinogram of the macaque. J Physiol 2003;547:509–30.
35. Sieving PA, Murayama K, Naarendorp F. Push-pull model of the primate photopic electroretinogram: a role for hyperpolarizing neurons in shaping the b-wave. Vis Neurosci 1994;11:519–32.
36. Breton ME, Schueller AW, Lamb TD, et al. Analysis of ERG a-wave amplification and kinetics in terms of the G-protein cascade of phototransduction. Invest Ophthalmol Vis Sci 1994;35:295–309.

37. Hood DC, Birch DG. A quantitative measure of the electrical activity of human rod photoreceptors using electroretinography. Vis Neurosci 1990;5: 379–87.
38. Hood DC, Birch DG. The A-wave of the human electroretinogram and rod receptor function. Invest Ophthalmol Vis Sci 1990;31:2070–81.
39. Robson JG, Frishman LJ. The a-wave of the electroretinogram: importance of axonal currents. ARVO E-abstracts 2011:692.
40. Frishman LJ, Reddy MG, Robson JG. Effects of background light on the human dark-adapted electroretinogram and psychophysical threshold. J Opt Soc Am A Opt Image Sci Vis 1996;13:601–12.
41. Saszik S, Alexander A, Lawrence T, et al. APB differentially affects the cone contributions to the zebrafish ERG. Vis Neurosci 2002;19:521–9.
42. Marmor MF, Fulton AB, Holder GE, et al. ISCEV standard for full-field clinical electroretinography (2008 update). Doc Ophthalmol 2009;118:69–77.
43. Steinberg RH, Linsenmeier RA, Griff ER. Retinal pigment epithelial cell contributions to the electroretinogram and electrooculogram. Prog Retin Res 1985;4:33–66.
44. Heynen H, Wachtmeister L, van Norren D. Origin of the oscillatory potentials in the primate retina. Vision Res 1985;25:1365–73.
45. Noell W. Studies on the electrophysiology and the metabolism of the retina. USAF SAM project no 21-2101-004. United States Airforce: Randolph Field, TX; 1953. p. 1–122.
46. Sillman AJ, Ito H, Tomita T. Studies on the mass receptor potential of the isolated frog retina. I. General properties of the response. Vision Res 1969;9:1435–42.
47. Valeton JM, van Norren D. Intraretinal recordings of slow electrical responses to steady illumination in monkey: isolation of receptor responses and the origin of the light peak. Vision Res 1982;22:393–9.
48. Bolnick DA, Walter AE, Sillman AJ. Barium suppresses slow PIII in perfused bullfrog retina. Vision Res 1979;19:1117–9.
49. Hu KG, Marmor MF. Selective actions of barium on the c-wave and slow negative potential of the rabbit eye. Vision Res 1984;24:1153–6.
50. Witkovsky P, Dudek FE, Ripps H. Slow PIII component of the carp electroretinogram. J Gen Physiol 1975;65:119–34.
51. Sillman AJ, Ito H, Tomita T. Studies on the mass receptor potential of the isolated frog retina. II. On the basis of the ionic mechanism. Vision Res 1969;9:1443–51.
52. Faber D. Analysis of slow transretinal potentials in response to light. PhD thesis. Buffalo: University of New York; 1969.
53. Karwoski CJ, Proenza LM. Relationship between Müller cell responses, a local transretinal potential, and potassium flux. J Neurophysiol 1977;40:244–59.
54. Frishman LJ, Steinberg RH. Intraretinal analysis of the threshold dark-adapted ERG of cat retina. J Neurophysiol 1989;61:1221–32.
55. Hanitzsch R. Intraretinal isolation of P3 subcomponents in the isolated rabbit retina after treatment with sodium aspartate. Vision Res 1973;13:2093–102.
56. Miller SS, Steinberg RH. Passive ionic properties of frog retinal pigment epithelium. J Membr Biol 1977;36:337–72.
57. Oakley 2nd B, Steinberg RH, Miller SS, et al. The in vitro frog pigment epithelial cell hyperpolarization in response to light. Invest Ophthalmol Vis Sci 1977;16:771–4.
58. Gallemore RP, Steinberg RH. Light-evoked modulation of basolateral membrane Cl^- conductance in chick retinal pigment epithelium: the light peak and fast oscillation. J Neurophysiol 1993;70:1669–80.
59. Quinn RH, Quong JN, Miller SS. Adrenergic receptor activated ion transport in human fetal retinal pigment epithelium. Invest Ophthalmol Vis Sci 2001;42:255–64.
60. Wu J, Marmorstein AD, Striessnig J, et al. Voltage-dependent calcium channel CaV1.3 subunits regulate the light peak of the electroretinogram. J Neurophysiol 2007;97:3731–5.
61. Gallemore RP, Hughes BA, Miller SS, editors. Light-induced responses of the retinal pigment epithelium. New York: Oxford University Press; 1998.
62. Dawis SM, Niemeyer G. Dopamine influences the light peak in the perfused mammalian eye. Invest Ophthalmol Vis Sci 1986;27:330–5.
63. Sieving PA, Frishman LJ, Steinberg RH. Scotopic threshold response of proximal retina in cat. J Neurophysiol 1986;56:1049–61.
64. Wakabayashi K, Gieser J, Sieving PA. Aspartate separation of the scotopic threshold response (STR) from the photoreceptor a-wave of the cat and monkey ERG. Invest Ophthalmol Vis Sci 1988;29:1615–22.
65. Brown KT, Wiesel TN. Analysis of the intraretinal electroretinogram in the intact cat eye. J Physiol 1961;158:229–56.
66. Brown KT, Watanabe K, Murakami M. The early and late receptor potentials of monkey cones and rods. Cold Spring Harbor Symposia Quant Biol 1965;30:457–82.
67. Penn RD, Hagins WA. Kinetics of the photocurrent of retinal rods. Biophys J 1972;12:1073–94.
68. Pugh Jr EN, Falsini B, Lyubarsky A. The origin of the major rod- and cone-driven components of the rodent electroretinogram and the effects of age and light-rearing history on the magnitude of these components. Photostasis and related phenomena. New York: Plenum Press; 1998. p. 93–128.
69. Baylor DA, Nunn BJ, Schnapf JL. The photocurrent, noise and spectral sensitivity of rods of the monkey *Macaca fascicularis*. J Physiol 1984;357:575–607.
70. Lamb TD, Pugh Jr EN. A quantitative account of the activation steps involved in phototransduction in amphibian photoreceptors. J Physiol 1992;449: 719–58.
71. Hood DC, Birch DG. Light adaptation of human rod receptors: the leading edge of the human a-wave and models of rod receptor activity. Vision Res 1993;33:1605–18.
72. Hood DC, Birch DG. Human cone receptor activity: the leading edge of the a-wave and models of receptor activity. Vis Neurosci 1993;10:857–71.
73. Yonemura D, Kawasaki K, Shibata N. The electroretinographic PIII component of the human excised retina. Jpn J Ophthalmol 1974;18:322–33.
74. Slaughter MM, Miller RF. An excitatory amino acid antagonist blocks cone input to sign-conserving second-order retinal neurons. Science 1983; 219:1230–2.
75. Friedburg C, Allen CP, Mason PJ, et al. Contribution of cone photoreceptors and post-receptoral mechanisms to the human photopic electroretinogram. J Physiol 2004;556:819–34.
76. Jamison JA, Bush RA, Lei B, et al. Characterization of the rod photoresponse isolated from the dark-adapted primate ERG. Vis Neurosci 2001;18: 445–55.
77. Robson JG, Frishman LJ. Dissecting the dark-adapted electroretinogram. Doc Ophthalmol 1998;95:187–215.
78. Pepperberg DR, Birch DG, Hood DC. Photoresponses of human rods in vivo derived from paired-flash electroretinograms. Vis Neurosci 1997;14: 73–82.
79. Stockton RA, Slaughter MM. B-wave of the electroretinogram. A reflection of ON bipolar cell activity. J Gen Physiol 1989;93:101–22.
80. Knapp AG, Schiller PH. The contribution of on-bipolar cells to the electroretinogram of rabbits and monkeys. A study using 2-amino-4-phosphonobutyrate (APB). Vision Res 1984;24:1841–6.
81. Bech-Hansen NT, Naylor MJ, Maybaum TA, et al. Mutations in NYX, encoding the leucine-rich proteoglycan nyctalopin, cause X-linked complete congenital stationary night blindness. Nature genet 2000;26:319–23.
82. McCall MA, Gregg RG. Comparisons of structural and functional abnormalities in mouse b-wave mutants. J Physiol 2008;586:4385–92.
83. Newman EA, Odette LL. Model of electroretinogram b-wave generation: a test of the K^+ hypothesis. J Neurophysiol 1984;51:164–82.
84. Miller RF, Dowling JE. Intracellular responses of the Müller (glial) cells of mudpuppy retina: their relation to b-wave of the electroretinogram. J Neurophysiol 1970;33:323–41.
85. Kline RP, Ripps H, Dowling JE. Light-induced potassium fluxes in the skate retina. Neuroscience 1985;14:225–35.
86. Wen R, Oakley B, 2nd. K(+)-evoked Müller cell depolarization generates b-wave of electroretinogram in toad retina. Proc Natl Acad Sci USA 1990;87: 2117–21.
87. Karwoski CJ, Proenza LM. Neurons, potassium, and glia in proximal retina of *Necturus*. J Gen Physiol 1980;75:141–62.
88. Xu X, Karwoski CJ. Current source density analysis of retinal field potentials. II. Pharmacological analysis of the b-wave and M-wave. J Neurophysiol 1994;72:96–105.
89. Karwoski CJ, Xu X. Current source-density analysis of light-evoked field potentials in rabbit retina. Vis Neurosci 1999;16:369–77.
90. Saszik SM, Robson JG, Frishman LJ. The scotopic threshold response of the dark-adapted electroretinogram of the mouse. J Physiol 2002;543: 899–916.
91. Cameron AM, Mahroo OA, Lamb TD. Dark adaptation of human rod bipolar cells measured from the b-wave of the scotopic electroretinogram. J Physiol 2006;575:507–26.
92. Sieving PA, Frishman LJ, Steinberg RH. M-wave of proximal retina in cat. J Neurophysiol 1986;56:1039–48.
93. Sieving PA, Nino C. Scotopic threshold response (STR) of the human electroretinogram. Invest Ophthalmol Vis Sci 1988;29:1608–14.
94. Ueno S, Kondo M, Ueno M, et al. Contribution of retinal neurons to d-wave of primate photopic electroretinograms. Vision Res 2006;46:658–64.
95. Rangaswamy NV, Frishman LJ, Dorotheo EU, et al. Photopic ERGs in patients with optic neuropathies: comparison with primate ERGs after pharmacologic blockade of inner retina. Invest Ophthalmol Vis Sci 2004;45:3827–37.
96. Peachey NS, Alexander KR, Fishman GA, et al. Properties of the human cone system electroretinogram during light adaptation. Appl Opt 1989;28: 1145–50.
97. Wali N, Leguire LE. The photopic hill: a new phenomenon of the light adapted electroretinogram. Doc Ophthalmol 1992;80:335–45.
98. Hamilton R, Bees MA, Chaplin CA, et al. The luminance-response function of the human photopic electroretinogram: a mathematical model. Vision Res 2007;47:2968–72.
99. Ueno S, Kondo M, Niwa Y, et al. Luminance dependence of neural components that underlies the primate photopic electroretinogram. Invest Ophthalmol Vis Sci 2004;45:1033–40.
100. Bush RA, Sieving PA. Inner retinal contributions to the primate photopic fast flicker electroretinogram. J Opt Soc Am A Opt Image Sci Vis 1996;13:557–65.
101. Kondo M, Sieving PA. Primate photopic sine-wave flicker ERG: vector modeling analysis of component origins using glutamate analogs. Invest Ophthalmol Vis Sci 2001;42:305–12.
102. Viswanathan S, Frishman LJ, Robson JG. Inner-retinal contributions to the photopic sinusoidal flicker electroretinogram of macaques. Macaque photopic sinusoidal flicker ERG. Doc Ophthalmol 2002;105:223–42.
103. Sutter EE, Tran D. The field topography of ERG components in man–I. The photopic luminance response. Vision Res 1992;32:433–46.
104. Hood DC, Frishman LJ, Saszik S, et al. Retinal origins of the primate multifocal ERG: implications for the human response. Invest Ophthalmol Vis Sci 2002; 43:1673–85.
105. Rangaswamy NV, Hood DC, Frishman LJ. Regional variations in local contributions to the primate photopic flash ERG: revealed using the slow-sequence mfERG. Invest Ophthalmol Vis Sci 2003;44:3233–47.

106. Rangaswamy NV, Zhou W, Harwerth RS, et al. Effect of experimental glaucoma in primates on oscillatory potentials of the slow-sequence mfERG. Invest Ophthalmol Vis Sci 2006;47:753–67.
107. Sutter EE, Bearse MA, Jr. The optic nerve head component of the human ERG. Vision Res 1999;39:419–36.
108. Burkhardt DA. Proximal negative response of frog retina. J Neurophysiol 1970;33:405–20.
109. Frishman LJ, Steinberg RH. Origin of negative potentials in the light-adapted ERG of cat retina. J Neurophysiol 1990;63:1333–46.
110. Ogden TE. The proximal negative response of the primate retina. Vision Res 1973;13:797–807.
111. Sieving PA, Steinberg RH. Proximal retinal contribution to the intraretinal 8-Hz pattern ERG of cat. J Neurophysiol 1987;57:104–20.
112. Frishman LJ, Shen FF, Du L, et al. The scotopic electroretinogram of macaque after retinal ganglion cell loss from experimental glaucoma. Invest Ophthalmol Vis Sci 1996;37:125–41.
113. Viswanathan S, Frishman LJ, Robson JG, et al. The photopic negative response of the macaque electroretinogram: reduction by experimental glaucoma. Invest Ophthalmol Vis Sci 1999;40:1124–36.
114. Viswanathan S, Frishman LJ, Robson JG, et al. The photopic negative response of the flash electroretinogram in primary open angle glaucoma. Invest Ophthalmol Vis Sci 2001;42:514–22.
115. Kondo M, Kurimoto Y, Sakai T, et al. Recording focal macular photopic negative response (PhNR) from monkeys. Invest Ophthalmol Vis Sci 2008;49:3544–50.
116. Bach M, Hoffmann MB. Update on the pattern electroretinogram in glaucoma. Optom Vis Sci 2008;85:386–95.
117. Holder GE. Pattern electroretinography (PERG) and an integrated approach to visual pathway diagnosis. Prog Retin Eye Res 2001;20:531–61.
118. Maffei L, Fiorentini A, Bisti S, et al. Pattern ERG in the monkey after section of the optic nerve. Exp Brain Res 1985;59:423–5.
119. Viswanathan S, Frishman LJ, Robson JG. The uniform field and pattern ERG in macaques with experimental glaucoma: removal of spiking activity. Invest Ophthalmol Vis Sci 2000;41:2797–810.
120. Luo X, Frishman LJ. Retinal pathway origins of the pattern electroretinogram (PERG). Invest Ophthalmol Vis Sci 2011;52:8571–84.
121. Naarendorp F, Sieving PA. The scotopic threshold response of the cat ERG is suppressed selectively by GABA and glycine. Vision Res 1991;31:1–15.
122. Sieving PA. Retinal ganglion cell loss does not abolish the scotopic threshold response (STR) of the cat and human ERG. Clin Vis Sci 1991;2:149–58.
123. Peachey NS, Alexander KR, Fishman GA. Rod and cone system contributions to oscillatory potentials: an explanation for the conditioning flash effect. Vision Res 1987;27:859–66.
124. Wachtmeister L. Oscillatory potentials in the retina: what do they reveal. Prog retinal eye res 1998;17:485–521.
125. Ogden TE. The oscillatory waves of the primate electroretinogram. Vision Res 1973;13:1059–74.
126. Dong CJ, Agey P, Hare WA. Origins of the electroretinogram oscillatory potentials in the rabbit retina. Vis Neurosci 2004;21:533–43.
127. McCall MA, Lukasiewicz PD, Gregg RG, et al. Elimination of the rho1 subunit abolishes GABA(C) receptor expression and alters visual processing in the mouse retina. J Neurosci 2002;22:4163–74.
128. Vigh J, Solessio E, Morgans CW, et al. Ionic mechanisms mediating oscillatory membrane potentials in wide-field retinal amacrine cells. J Neurophysiol 2003;90:431–43.
129. Heckenlively J, Arden GB. Principles and practice of clinical electrophysiology of vision. 2nd ed. Cambridge, MA: MIT Press; 2006.
130. Fishman GA, Birch DG, Holder GE, et al. Electrophysiological testing in disorders of the retina, optic nerve, and visual pathways. 2nd ed. Singapore: American Academy of Ophthalmology; 2001.
131. Lam BL. Electrophysiology of vision; clinical testing and applications. Boca Raton, FL: Taylor and Francis Group; 2005.

Chapter 8

Clinical Electrophysiology

Yozo Miyake, Kei Shinoda

In this chapter, we describe the method and value of various clinical electrophysiological tests and how they play a role in the diagnosis, analysis of pathogenesis, prognostic evaluation, and understanding of the underlying genetics of retinal disorders, using several examples of clinical cases. We also demonstrate the role of the focal macular electroretinogram (ERG) and multifocal ERG (mfERG) for particular diseases where the affected region is limited to a certain region of the retina. During the recent history of clinical electrophysiology, several new clinical entities have been defined by analyzing electrophysiological results. These new entities will also be discussed in this chapter.

STANDARD FULL-FIELD ERG

Stimulus and recording devices

The human ERG recorded at the cornea and elicited by a full-field stimulus is a mass response generated by cells across the entire retina. To obtain reproducible amplitudes and implicit times in the response, the stimulus and background light should be homogeneous and cover the entire retina, so all of the receptors are stimulated or adapted in a relatively homogeneous manner. The full-field, or Ganzfeld, stimulator represents such a stimulus. It consists of a large-diameter (40-cm) hemispheric dome (see Chapter 7, Electrogenesis of the electroretinogram) with a xenon stroboscopic light bulb placed at the top of the dome. This stimulus system has been recommended by the International Society of Clinical Electrophysiology for Vision (ISCEV) Standards Committee[1] for use when obtaining clinical ERG recordings internationally.

The ERG is recorded using corneal electrodes, usually referred to surface reference electrodes at the ipsilateral outer canthi or zygomatic fossae. Electrodes in common use[2] include the Burian–Allen and the ERG jet, both of which are contact lens electrodes, the gold foil, Dawson–Trick–Litzkow (DTL), and H-K loop electrodes, which are noncontact lens. The representative electrodes are shown in Fig. 8.1.

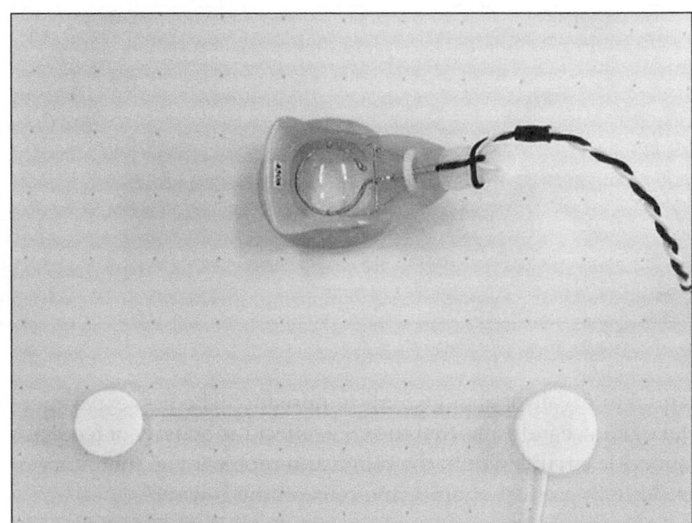

Fig. 8.1 Representative electroretinogram recording electrodes. Top, Burian–Allen electrode. A contact lens-type electrode with a lid speculum to minimize the effect of blinking and eyelid closure. Bottom, Dawson–Trick–Litzkow (DTL) electrode – a conductive Mylar thread usually placed in the lower fornix, it contacts the inferior bulbar conjunctiva or the corneal limbus. Dots show 10-mm distance.

Stimulus intensity versus ERG responses and components

Scotopic condition

Figure 8.2 shows the full-field ERGs elicited by increasing stimulus intensities from a normal subject after 1 hour of dark adaptation. The ERGs elicited by relatively weak stimulus intensities are shown at the left and those by stronger stimulus are shown at the right. The calibrations for the amplitude and time are different for the weak and strong stimulus ERGs. The maximum stimulus luminance (0 log unit) is 44.2 cd/m^2/s.

At the left, the scotopic threshold response (STR),[3] a cornea-negative wave, is first recorded at −8.2 log units, approximately 0.6 log units higher than psychophysical threshold. The maximum amplitude of STR is approximately 20 μV before it is masked by the developing b-wave. The implicit time of the STR near threshold is approximately 160 ms, and the implicit time decreases as the stimulus intensity increases. The STR originates from retinal neurons that are postsynaptic to the photoreceptors (see Chapter 7, Electrogenesis of the electroretinogram).

The b-wave is first seen at an intensity of −5.8 log units; the amplitude increases and the implicit time shortens as the stimulus intensity increases. The amplitude of b-wave essentially saturates at −3.4 log units; and at intensities higher than −0.8 log unit, the oscillatory potentials (OPs) become clearly visible on the ascending limb of the b-wave. The a-wave is first seen at −1.7 log units and increases progressively as the stimulus intensity increases.

As shown fully in Chapter 7, Electrogenesis of the ERG, many studies have shown that the a-wave of the full-field ERGs recorded in the dark is the leading edge of the photoreceptor potential.[4] The b-wave originates indirectly from bipolar and Müller cells in the middle layers of the retina.[5] The OPs are seen as a series of three or four rhythmic wavelets having almost

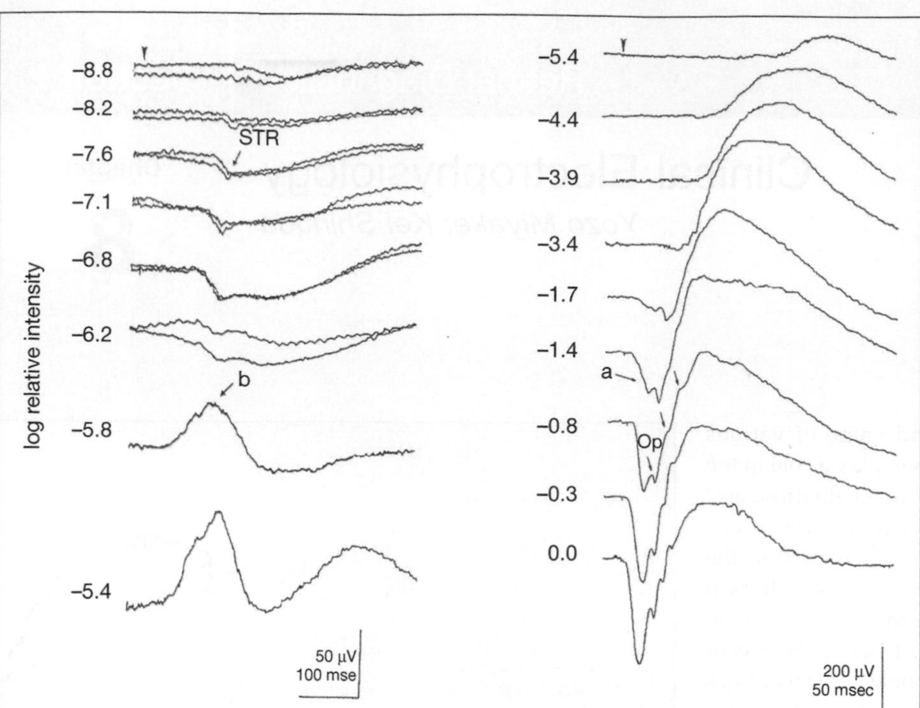

Fig. 8.2 The full-field electroretinogram (ERG) elicited by increasing stimulus intensities recorded from a normal subject after 1 hour of dark adaptation. The left column shows responses elicited by relative low intensity and the right by relative high intensity. Note that the calibration differs for the ERGs in the two columns. Arrowheads indicate the stimulus onset. STR, scotopic threshold response; b, b-wave; a, a-wave; Op, oscillatory potentials. (Reproduced with permission from Miyake Y, Horiguchi M, Terasaki H, et al. Invest Ophthalmol Vis Sci 1994;35:3770–5.)

equal intervals of about 6.5 ms in humans.[6] The best experimental evidence indicates that the OPs reflect the activity of feedback synaptic circuits within the retina and represent an inhibitory or modulating effect of amacrine cells on the b-wave.[7]

Photopic condition

The photopic, short-flash ERGs elicited by increasing stimulus intensities in a normal subject are shown in Fig. 8.3.[8] At lower stimulus intensities, the amplitude of the b-wave increases with increasing stimulus until it reaches a maximum at a stimulus intensity of 3.0 log cd/m^2. Further increases in the stimulus intensity result in a progressive decrease in the amplitude of the b-wave. Because a plot of the b-wave amplitude as a function of the stimulus intensity has an inverted U shape, this phenomenon has been termed the photopic hill phenomenon.[9]

Bright flash mixed rod–cone ERG

ERG recorded with a bright flash of light after dark adaptation for 30 minutes or longer (0 log unit in Fig. 8.2) shows mixed rod–cone response, which can provide variable information about retinal pathology and is of significant diagnostic value. We have an impression that about 70% of ERG information can be obtained by the evaluation of only the mixed rod–cone ERG. The five different types of mixed rod–cone ERG are shown in Fig. 8.4.

Normal

The normal type shows a-wave, b-wave, and OPs. The amplitude of b-wave is always larger than that of a-wave in the regular stimulus intensity range. The normal ERG can be seen in patients with localized macular dysfunction, optic nerve diseases, and central nervous system disease such as amblyopia. Even when the entire retina is ophthalmoscopically abnormal, such as rubella retinopathy or female carrier of ocular albino and choroideremia (Fig. 8.5), the ERG can be essentially normal.

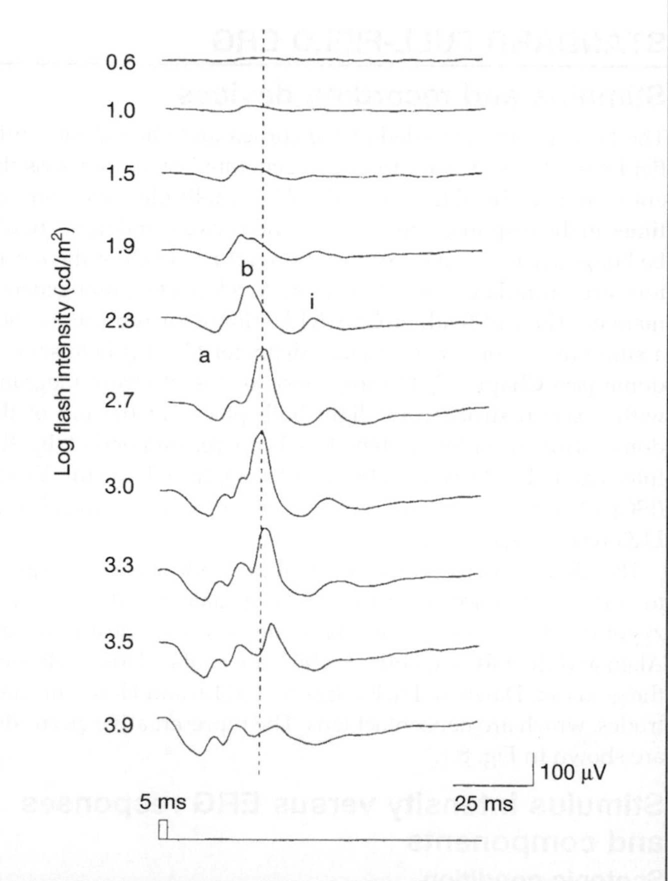

Fig. 8.3 Photopic short-flash electroretinograms elicited by various stimulus intensities from a normal subject. Stimulus duration is 5 ms and the constant background illumination is 40 cd/m^2. The vertical dashed line indicates 30 ms. The b-wave amplitude increases with increasing stimulus intensity until 3.0 log cd/m^2. It decreases with further increases in stimulus intensity. When the b-wave amplitude is plotted against stimulus intensity, it shows an inverted U shape; this phenomenon has been termed the photopic hill phenomenon. (Reproduced with permission from Kondo M, Piao CH, Tanikawa A, et al. Japanese Journal of Ophthalmology 2000;44:20–8.)

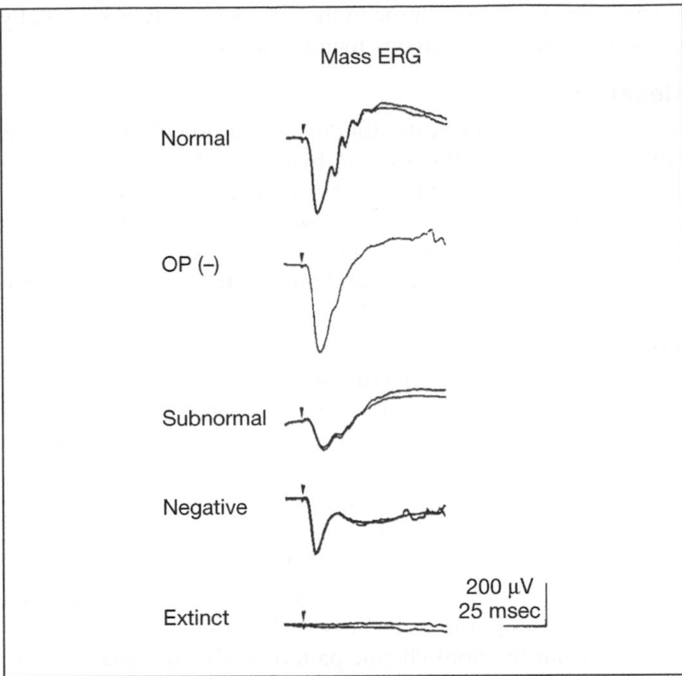

Fig. 8.4 The five different types of mixed rod–cone electroretinogram (ERG). OP(–), selective reduction of oscillatory potentials; subnormal, both a- and b-waves are attenuated approximately to the same degree; negative, the amplitude of the b-wave is smaller than that of the a-wave; extinct, no discernible a- or b-wave.

Selectively abnormal oscillatory potentials

An OP abnormality means either reduction of amplitude or delay of implicit time, or both. A selective OP abnormality is observed in the early stage of diabetic retinopathy[10,11] (Fig. 8.6) or mild circulatory disturbance of retina such as central retinal vein occlusion.

Subnormal

The amplitudes of all components are reduced approximately to the same degree. A reduced a-wave indicates abnormal photoreceptor function. This pattern is seen in patients with localized damage of the photoreceptors, such as partial retinal detachment or sectoral retinal degeneration. The amplitude of the full-field ERG is proportional to the area of functioning retina. This rule is shown when the extent of retinal detachment is compared with the ERG (Fig. 8.7).

This rule is also shown in eyes with panretinal photocoagulation (PRP) in diabetic retinopathy. Following PRP, the amplitudes of ERG components are reduced by 40–45%, but the b-wave: a-wave (b/a) ratio is not changed significantly.[11] When the media is hazy due to vitreous hemorrhage and the fundus is invisible, the presence or absence of retinal detachment is an important evaluation preoperatively. By combining ERG and ultrasonography, the differentiation between totally detached retina and dense vitreous membrane may be possible, as shown in Fig. 8.8. When the ERG is recordable, even if the amplitude

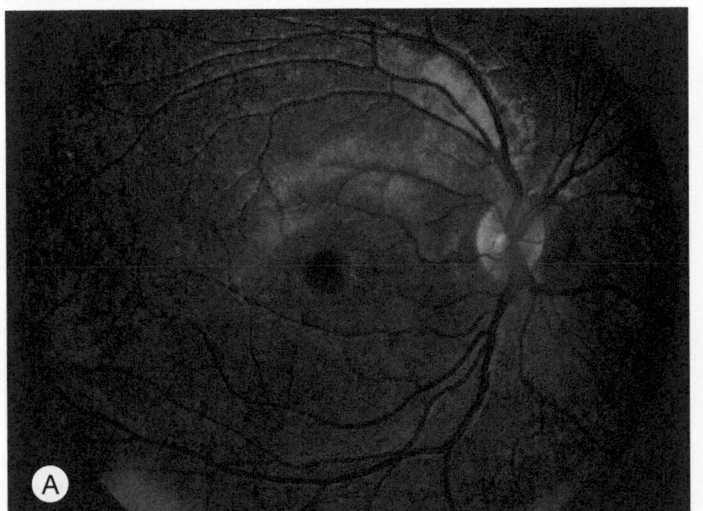

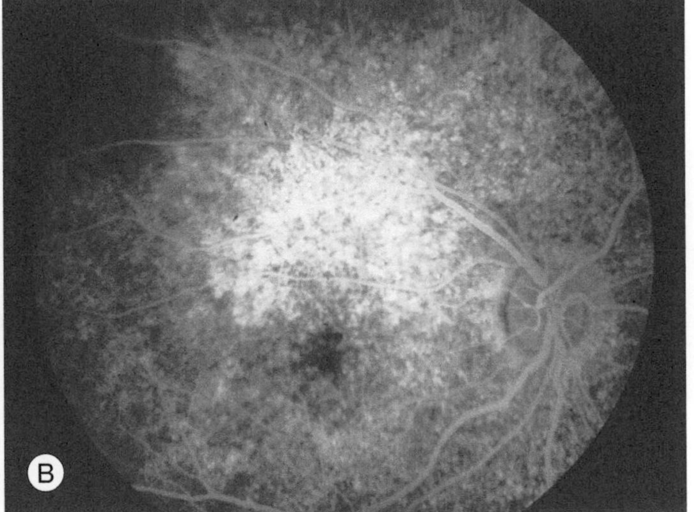

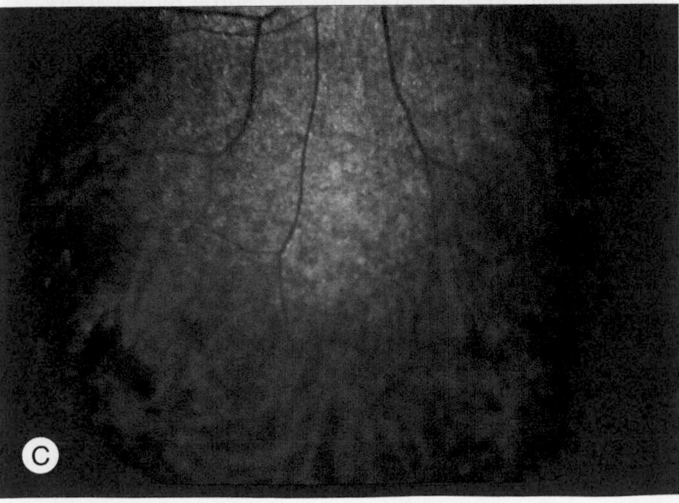

Fig. 8.5 Fundus photograph (A) and fluorescein angiogram (B) obtained from a 20-year-old man with rubella retinitis. Fundus photograph from a 60-year-old female carrier of choroideremia (C). The electroretinograms in these two patients were normal. (Reproduced with permission from Miyake Y. Electrodiagnosis of retinal diseases. Tokyo: Springer-Verlag; 2006.)

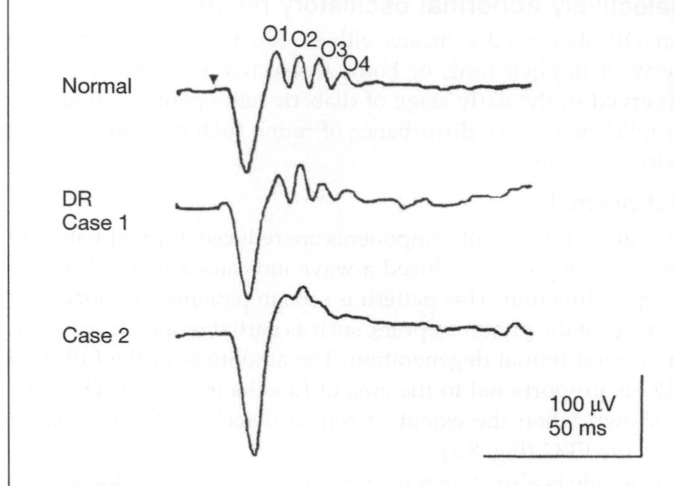

Fig. 8.6 Oscillatory potentials (OPs) of full-field electroretinograms recorded from a normal subject (top) and two patients with diabetic retinopathy (cases 1 and 2). The oscillatory potentials were found to have delayed implicit time (case 1) or reduced amplitude (case 2). DR, diabetic retinopathy. (Reproduced with permission from Miyake Y. Electrodiagnosis of retinal diseases. Tokyo: Springer-Verlag; 2006.)

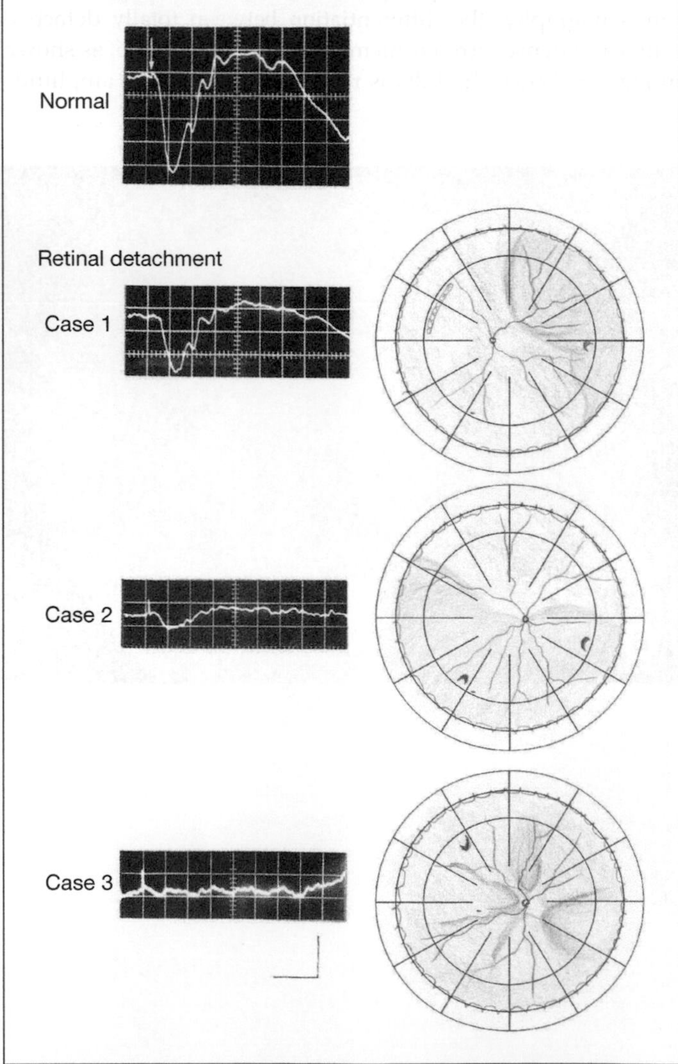

Fig. 8.7 Mixed rod–cone (bright flash) electroretinograms (left) and fundus drawings of three patients with rhegmatogenous retinal detachment (right). The reduction of the electroretinogram amplitude corresponds proportionally to the extent of retinal detachment.

is small, the thick membrane in the vitreous cavity is not totally detached retina, but vitreous membrane.

Negative

The negative ERG indicates that the amplitude of the b-wave is smaller than that of the a-wave (b/a ratio <1.0). As mentioned above, the amplitude of the b-wave is always larger than that of the a-wave in normal subjects. A normal a-wave with a reduced b-wave localizes the defect to postphototransduction processes. The negative ERG can be of useful prognostic or diagnostic value in retinal diseases.

Prognostic value

Among the acquired retinal diseases, the negative ERG may be seen in severe retinal circulatory disturbance such as central retinal arterial occlusion or proliferative diabetic retinopathy. In central retinal vein occlusion, the ischemic type shows negative ERG more frequently than nonischemic type, indicating that the b/a ratio can be an important index for evaluating the prognosis of central retinal vein occlusion.[12,13] Figure 8.9 shows a patient with an initially normal, but later lower, b/a ratio which resulted in negative configuration in ERG.[11] The fluorescein angiogram changed from the nonischemic pattern to the ischemic pattern, showing an extensive nonperfusion area accordingly.

When massive vitreous hemorrhage prevents ophthalmoscopic examination of the fundus in patients with proliferative diabetic retinopathy, it makes it difficult to predict the surgical and visual outcome after vitrectomy. In these eyes, the amplitudes of the ERGs may be markedly reduced by various factors: pathological changes induced by the diabetic retinopathy, earlier PRP, and vitreous hemorrhage. As mentioned above, the PRP reduces the ERG amplitude without changing the b/a ratio.[11] Because most diabetic patients with vitreous hemorrhage have undergone PRP, it is difficult to arrive at a prognosis of the outcome after vitrectomy using only the amplitudes. The b/a ratio provides more useful information about the visual prognosis after vitrectomy.[14] The preoperative mixed rod-cone ERGs were classified into three groups in patients with diabetic retinopathy associated with significant vitreous hemorrhage (Fig. 8.10, left). Group A indicates those with a b/a ratio>1.0 and the OPs are clearly recordable. Group B includes those with a b/a ratio >1.0 but the OPs are absent. Group C comprises those with a b/a ratio <1.0 with absent OPs. Thick proliferative tissues were found at the disc (Fig. 8.11) intraoperatively in 36% of the eyes in group A, 67% in group B, and 90% in group C.[14] It was suggested that the fibrous proliferation at the disc may restrict retinal circulation by compressing the central retinal artery.

The distribution of the postoperative visual acuity for each group is shown in Fig. 8.10, right.[14] The postoperative visual acuity for group C was significantly worse than for group A or group B. The low b/a ratio may indicate more severe ischemic retina, which in turn may account for the relatively good correlation with visual acuity. However, among the patients in group C, there were some whose postoperative visual acuity was good, indicating that a b/a ratio <1.0 is not necessarily a contraindication for vitrectomy. Another important finding is that most patients who have distinct OPs preoperatively have favorable visual acuity after vitrectomy. This observation is important when we discuss the visual prognosis with patients before surgery. The light-filtering effect of a dense vitreous hemorrhage should also be considered when evaluating the preoperative ERG in diabetic patients. Severe vitreous hemorrhage reduces

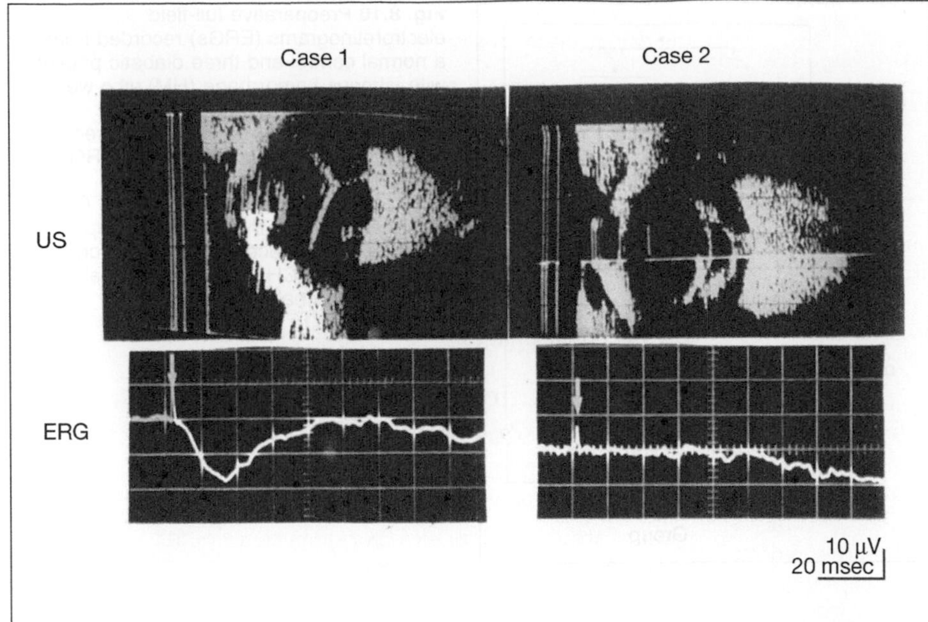

Fig. 8.8 Ultrasonographic (US) image (top) and mixed rod–cone electroretinogram (ERG) (bottom) from eyes with vitreous hemorrhage. Ultrasonography shows thick membrane-like reflex in the vitreous cavity in both eyes. When the ERG is recordable, even if the amplitude is small, the thick membrane in the vitreous cavity is not totally detached retina, but vitreous membrane (case 1). In contrast, when the ERG is unrecordable, the thick membrane is most likely totally detached retina (case 2).

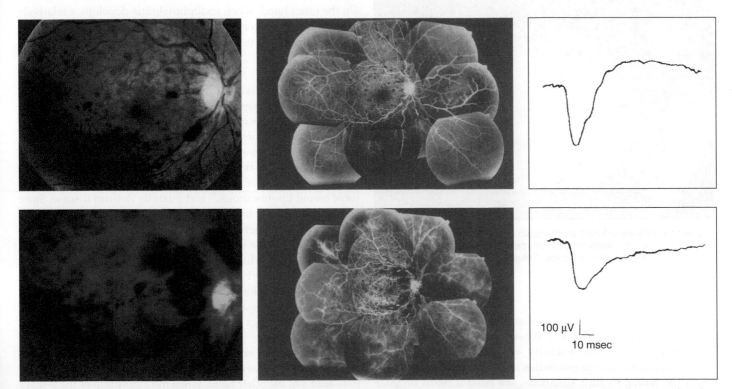

Fig. 8.9 Top panel, a 39-year-old woman had a central retinal vein occlusion in the right eye (top left). Fluorescein angiogram (top center) and electroretinogram (ERG) (top right) showed nonischemic pattern at her initial visit. Bottom panel, one month later, the retinal hemorrhage increased (bottom left), the fluorescein angiogram showed extensive areas of nonperfusion (bottom center), and the waveform of the ERG became negative (right). (Reproduced with permission from Miyake Y. Electrodiagnosis of retinal diseases. Tokyo: Springer-Verlag; 2006.)

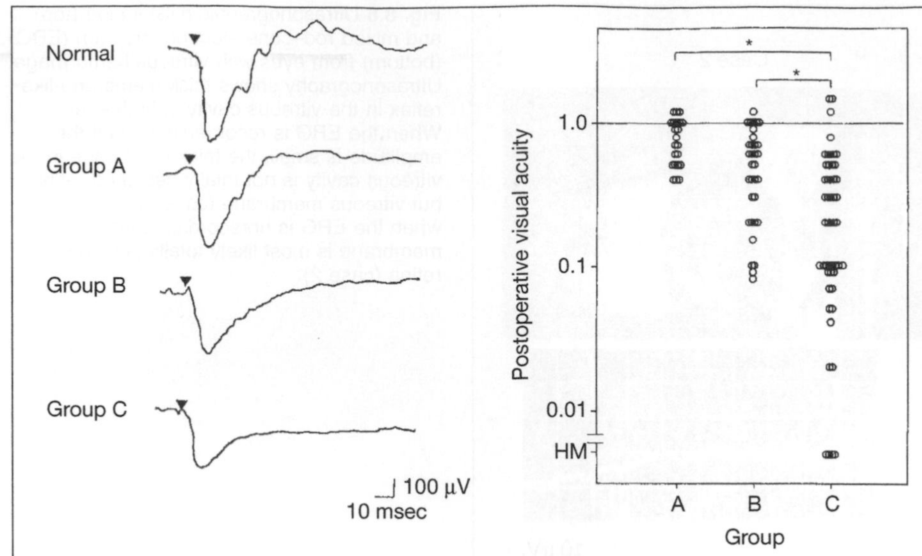

Fig. 8.10 Preoperative full-field electroretinograms (ERGs) recorded from a normal control and three diabetic patients with vitreous hemorrhage (HM) who were classified into three groups (left). Postoperative visual acuity in the three groups classified according to the ERG waveform (right), showing that the postoperative visual acuity for group C was significantly worse than that for group A or group B. (Reproduced with permission from Kondo M, Piao CH, Tanikawa A, et al. Japanese Journal of Ophthalmology 2000;44:20–8.)

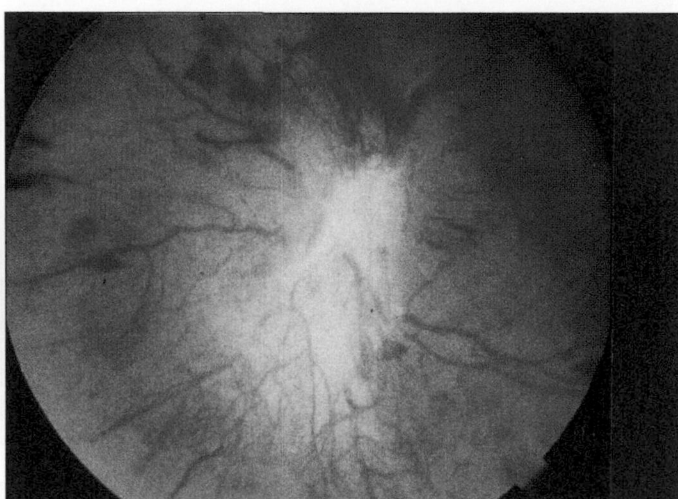

Fig. 8.11 Proliferative tissue on the optic disc in a patient with diabetic retinopathy. (Reproduced with permission from Miyake Y. Electrodiagnosis of retinal diseases. Tokyo: Springer-Verlag; 2006.)

the intensity of the stimulus light reaching the retina, which can increase the b/a ratio (Fig. 8.2). When the vitreous hemorrhage is extremely dense, the intensity of stimulus light may be decreased and the effective stimulus light to evoke ERG may not reach the retina. In such situations, we need a much brighter stimulus than the regular maximum stimulus to evoke ERG. Such an example is shown in Fig. 8.12. In such cases, we have an impression that ERG often has a negative configuration, as shown in this patient.

In the prognostic evaluation of eyes that develop endophthalmitis after intraocular lens implantation, the b/a ratio is also valuable.[15] Eyes with early (within 1 week) endophthalmitis associated with a b/a ratio of <1.0 have a worse postoperative prognosis than eyes with late-onset endophthalmitis and/or a b/a ratio of >1.0. These observations are quite important when deciding on the appropriate time to perform vitrectomy for treatment. For example, a patient with endophthalmitis that was detected within 1 week of intraocular lens implantation and with an ERG b/a ratio of <1.0 should undergo vitrectomy urgently. On the other hand, when endophthalmitis develops a relatively long time after surgery and the ERG b/a ratio is >1.0, the timing of the vitrectomy is not as critical. Representative examples[15] are shown in Fig. 8.13.

Diagnostic value

The negative ERG is seen in some hereditary retinal diseases, which provides diagnostic information, particularly when the a-wave amplitude is normal. The representative diseases, where the negative ERG shows the diagnostic value, include complete-type congenital stationary night blindness[16] (CSNB: see Fig. 8.20, below), incomplete-type CSNB[16] (see Fig. 8.20, below), X-linked juvenile retinoschisis[11] (XLRS: see Fig. 8.20), juvenile-onset neuronal ceroid lipofuscinosis,[17] and infantile Refsum disease. Since both complete and incomplete CSNB show essentially normal fundi and most patients with CSNB have moderately low visual acuity,[16] the negative ERG finding is extremely important to pick up these disorders, differentiating them from other diseases with normal fundi, low visual acuity, and normal ERG, such as psychological eye problems, amblyopia, optic nerve disease, central nervous system disease, or occult macular dystrophy (OMD). The detailed findings separating rod and cone components will be treated later.

When the a-wave amplitude is normal and the b/a ratio is less than 1.0, the selective abnormality of the second-order neuron is indicated. On the other hand, when the amplitude of the a-wave is smaller than normal with the b/a ratio <1.0, there are two interpretations. One is the combined dysfunction of photoreceptor and middle retinal layer. This situation is often observed in patients with retinitis pigmentosa. The other is the ERG showing the photopic hill phenomenon[8] (see above). When the rod function is completely gone and the cone function is well preserved, the ERG shows cone ERG even in the dark. In this condition, when the stimulus light intensity is strong, the ERG reveals the photopic hill phenomenon (Fig. 8.3), showing negative configuration with a small a-wave. Such examples are seen in bright flash mixed rod–cone ERG in the dark in Oguchi disease or fundus albipunctatus (FA) (Fig. 8.16).

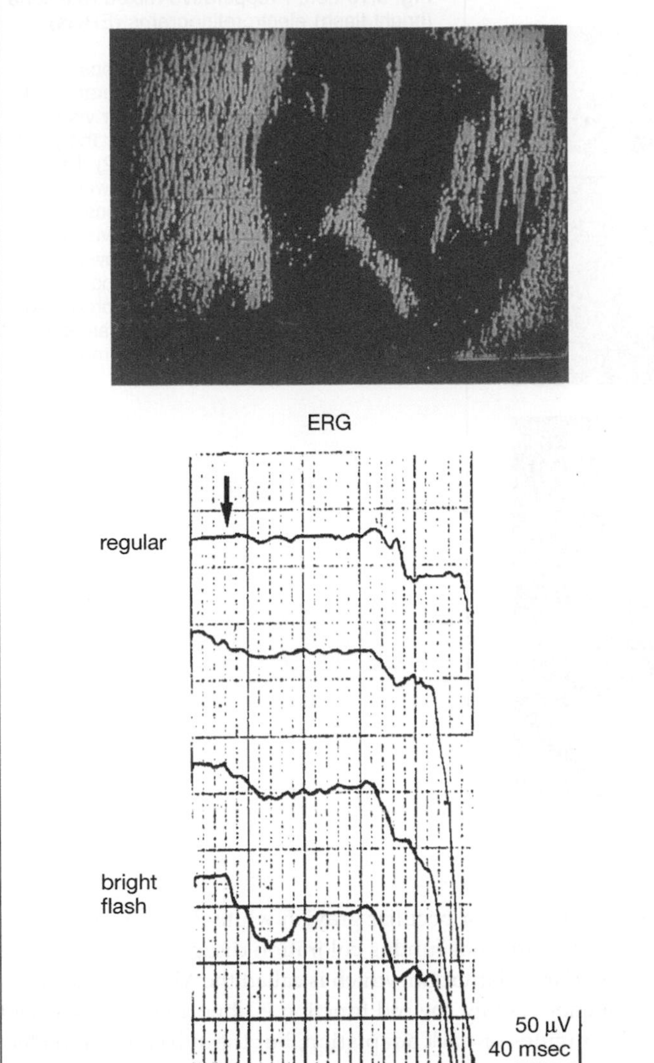

Fig. 8.12 Ultrasonographic image (top) and mixed rod–cone electroretinograms (ERGs) (bottom) with various stimulus intensities from eyes with extremely dense vitreous hemorrhage. As the intensity of the stimulus light is decreased, a sufficiently bright stimulus to evoke the ERG may not reach the retina. In this situation, a much brighter stimulus than the regular maximum stimulus may evoke the ERG response. In such cases, it appears that the ERG frequently shows negative configuration.

In acquired diseases, negative ERG may be seen in melanoma-associated retinopathy,[18,19] birdshot choroidopathy,[20] ocular siderosis, quinine retinopathy, and methanol toxicity. The negative configuration of ERG provides the diagnostic value in these disorders.

Extinct

The extinct ERG is often seen in the advanced stage of rod–cone dystrophy, including retinitis pigmentosa, gyrate atrophy or choroideremia, and total retinal detachment. In retinitis pigmentosa, gyrate atrophy, or choroideremia, even when the macular area is preserved, ERG may become undetectable. Cancer-associated retinopathy,[19] an autoimmune retinopathy, may often show extinct ERG and should be differentiated from retinitis pigmentosa.

Isolation of rod and cone components in standardized ERG

Although the rods outnumber the cones 13 to 1 in the normal human retina, the cone ERG response accounts for 20–25% of the ERG response amplitude. For the purposes of diagnosis, it often becomes necessary for the examiner to evaluate rod and cone activity separately. The full-field ERGs using the ISCEV Standard (see Chapter 7, Electrogenesis of the electroretinogram) in a normal subject are shown in Fig. 8.14.

After 30 minutes of dark adaptation, a rod (scotopic) ERG is recorded with a dim flash of light at approximately -3.9 log units in Fig. 8.2. A bright flash (mixed rod–cone) ERG is elicited by a single flash of white light at maximum intensity of log 0 units in Fig. 8.2. Cone and 30-Hz flicker ERG are recorded with a stimulus intensity of 3.3 log units in Fig. 8.3 under the background illumination of 40 cd/m^2, which is sufficient to suppress all rod activity. The photopic recordings (cone and 30-Hz flicker ERG) are made after 10 minutes of light adaptation to 40 cd/m^2, because the maximum photopic ERG can be obtained when recorded after light adaptation.[11] In addition to the conventional ERG components, the photopic negative response (PhNR) was introduced[21]: this originates from retinal ganglion cells and will be treated more fully later.

The representative patients diagnosed by the isolation of rod and cone components of full-field ERG are shown below in relation to the abnormal cells of the retina.

Cone photoreceptor dysfunction

The congenital stationary disorder of cone dysfunction is represented by rod monochromacy which is inherited in an autosomal recessive mode. This disorder is characterized in the complete form by complete absence or severely depressed color vision, reduced visual acuity, nystagmus, and photophobia[11]. There is also an incomplete form of this disorder, where color vision and/or visual acuity is not severely affected.[11] In both forms, the fundus and fluorescein angiograms are normal, and the most characteristic feature in terms of the diagnosis is selective reduction or absence of the photopic components while preserving normal scotopic components of the full-field ERG even in incomplete form (Fig. 8.15). Molecular genetic studies have shown that mutations in the *CNGB3* gene encoding the β-subunit of the cone photoreceptor cGMP-gated channel are responsible for rod monochromacy.[22]

Blue cone monochromacy shares many characteristics with rod monochromacy, except that the hereditary mode is X-linked recessive[11]. The visual acuity is approximately 0.2–0.3, which is slightly better than that of the complete form of rod monochromacy. Unlike rod monochromacy, the blue cone function is selectively preserved. Panel D-15 test shows several crossing lines perpendicular to the tritan axis (Fig. 8.15). The fundus is essentially normal, although in the late stage some atrophic changes may develop in the macula. The molecular genetics study indicated that mutations exist in the red and green opsin in the blue cone monochromacy. The full-field ERGs are similar to those of rod monochromacy, showing nearly normal rod ERGs with absence of the photopic ERG (Fig. 8.15). Although the blue cone ERG is normally present, the amplitude of the normal blue cone ERG is too small to be detected in the regular full-field cone ERG, and the implicit time is too long to follow 30-Hz flicker ERG stimuli (see section on S-cone ERG, below).

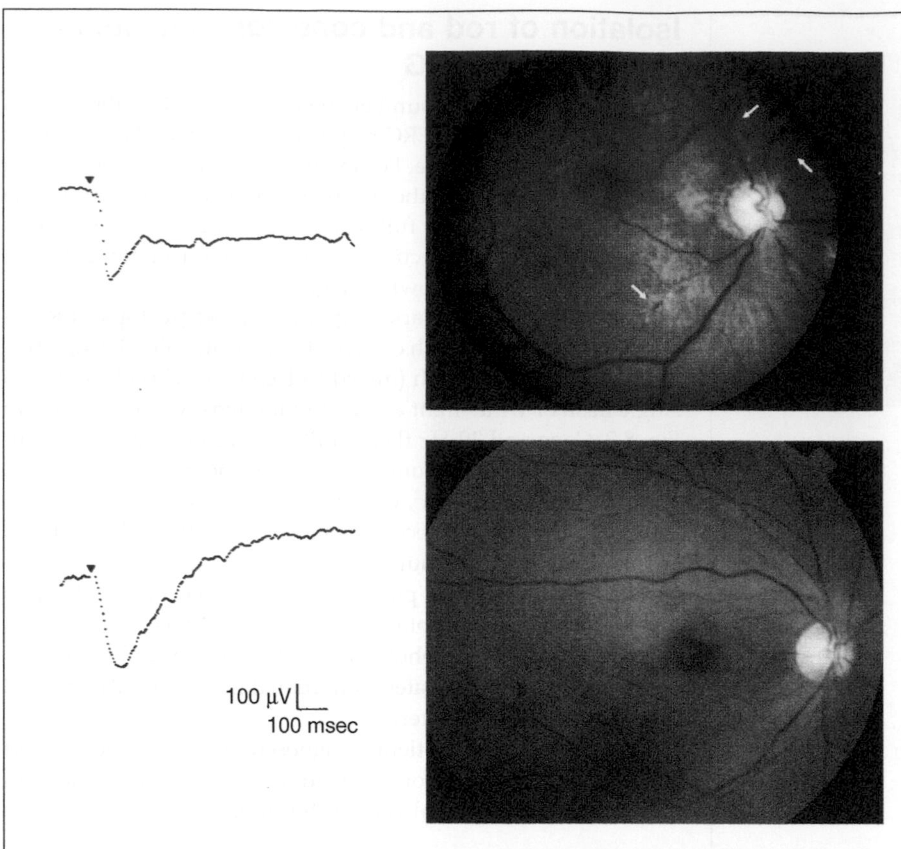

Fig. 8.13 Left, Preoperative mixed rod–cone (bright flash) electroretinograms (ERGs) recorded from two patients with endophthalmitis after intraocular lens implantation. The negative configuration of the ERG (case 1) suggests poorer visual prognosis after vitrectomy than for the patient with normal-shaped ERGs (case 2). Right, postoperative fundus. Case 1 showed extensive retinal vascular occlusions (arrows), with poor postoperative visual function, as expected. Case 2 showed an essentially normal fundus with good postoperative visual function. (Reproduced with permission from Horio N, Terasaki H, Yamamoto E, et al. Am J Ophthalmol 2001;132:258–9.)

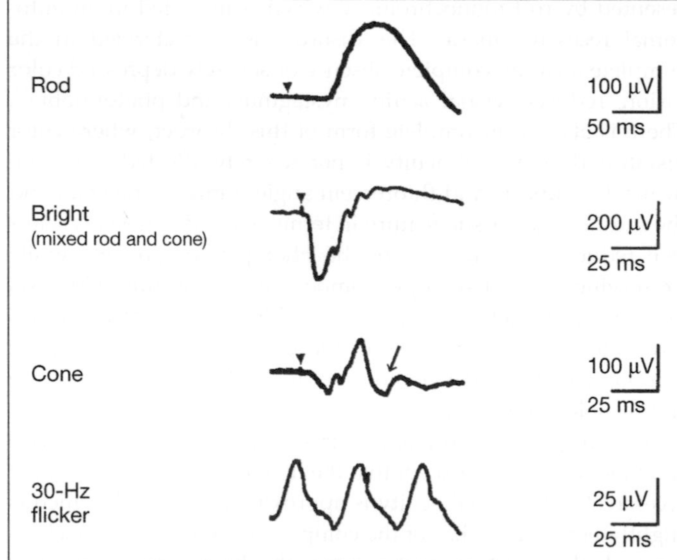

Fig. 8.14 Standard full-field electroretinograms with isolation of the rod and cone components. Arrowheads indicate the stimulus onset. The arrow indicates photopic negative response.

Rod photoreceptor dysfunction

The model diseases with congenital rod photoreceptor dysfunction include Oguchi disease and FA, both of which are categorized as CSNB.

Oguchi disease, first reported by Oguchi[23] in 1907, is an unusual form of CSNB with autosomal recessive inheritance. It is characterized by a peculiar grayish white discoloration of the fundus. This unusual fundus coloration disappears after a long period of dark adaptation, which is called the Mizuo–Nakamura phenomenon[24]. Only the rod function is abnormal and is absent after 30 minutes of dark adaptation, but the subjective and electroretinographic rod function may increase after 2–3 hours of dark adaptation.[25] Mutations in the gene of arrestin[26] or the rhodopsin kinase,[27] both of which are rod phototransduction, cause the recessive form of Oguchi disease.

Full-field ERGs (Fig. 8.16) recorded after 30 minutes of dark adaptation show absent rod ERG and essentially normal cone-mediated ERG.[25] The mixed rod–cone ERG has a negative configuration with relatively well-preserved OPs. The a-wave amplitude in Oguchi disease is reduced compared to that of normal controls. As mentioned above, this ERG indicates the cone ERG in spite of the fact that the ERG is recorded in the dark and after 30 minutes of dark adaptation, because rod function is absent even under this condition. When the cone ERG is recorded with a bright flash of light, it shows the photopic hill phenomenon, and the ERG configuration is negative with a small a-wave. After 3 hours of dark adaptation, the amplitudes of the a-wave and b-wave of the mixed rod–cone ERGs are larger, but they are still negative in configuration. As the mutated genes indicate, the pathogenesis that only the rod itself is impaired in Oguchi disease is comparable to the normal photopic ERG and negative configuration with small a-wave in mixed rod–cone ERG, but the negative configuration with normal a-wave after a long time of dark adaptation may suggest some additional abnormalities of the bipolar cell function. Electro-oculogram (EOG) is abnormal with low light to dark ratio in most patients with Oguchi disease.[25]

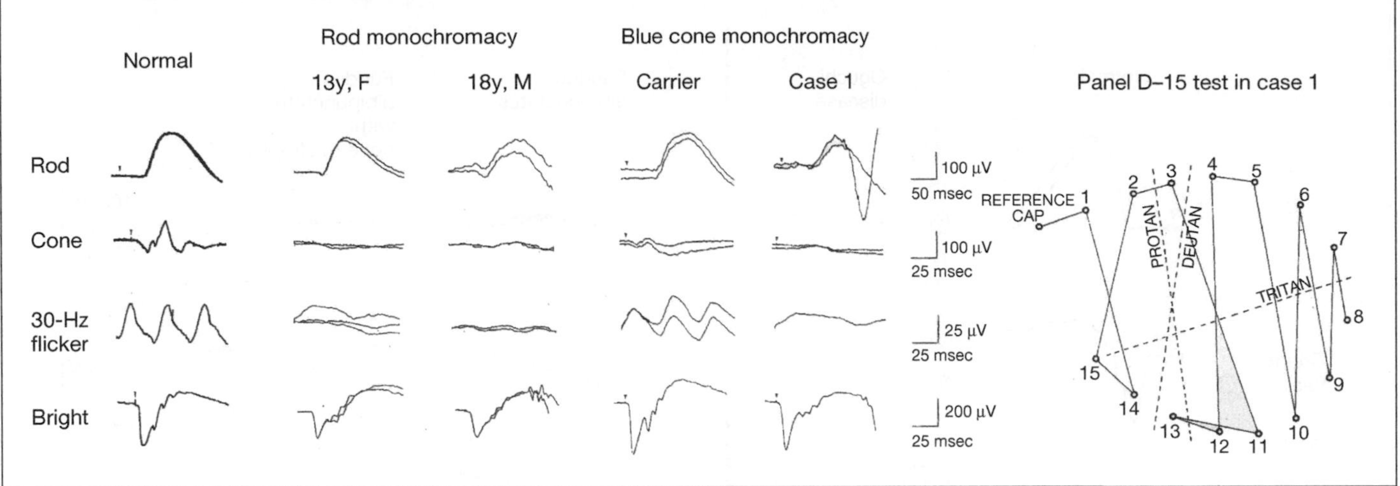

Fig. 8.15 Full-field electroretinograms (ERGs) and Farnsworth dischromous panel D-15 test from patients with cone photoreceptor dysfunction. Second and third columns (from left), full-field ERGs recorded from two siblings with rod monochromacy showing selective absence of the photopic components. During 10-year follow-up, their visual function remained stable and their fundi remained normal. Visual acuity was 0.1/0.4 in a 13-year-old sister and 1.0/1.0 in an 18-year-old brother. The sister showed mild acquired red–green deficiency and the brother had normal color vision due to functional cones preserved only in the fovea.

Fourth and fifth (columns from left), full-field ERGs recorded from a family with blue cone monochromacy (carrier mother and son) showing normal rod components and nearly absent cone components. Although the blue cone ERG is normally present, the amplitude of the normal blue cone ERG is too small to be detected in the regular full-field cone ERG, and the implicit time is too long to follow 30-Hz flicker ERG stimuli.

Rightmost column, Farnsworth dischromous panel D-15 test from case 1 showing that several crossing lines were perpendicular to the tritan axis. (Revised and reproduced with permission from Kondo M, Piao CH, Tanikawa A, et al. Japanese Journal of Ophthalmology 2000;44:20–8, with permission.)

The pathogenesis of Oguchi disease has long been believed to exist in the rod bipolar function, as seen in complete CSNB, because reports published a long time ago[28] indicated normal a-wave with reduced b-wave (negative ERG) as well as normal EOG. In addition, normal rhodopsin kinetics were shown by rhodopsin densitometry.[29] We demonstrated that many patients with Oguchi disease show smaller a-wave than normal and abnormal EOG, suggesting that there is a dysfunction of phototransduction.[25] Our hypothesis, obtained from electrophysiological results, was proven true by mutated gene of Oguchi disease.[26,27]

FA has been considered to be a type of CSNB with autosomal recessive inheritance. The fundus has a characteristic appearance of a large number of discrete, small, round or elliptical yellowish white regions at the level of the retinal pigment epithelium. The most characteristic property of their visual function is a delay in dark adaptation, which can be detected by the psychologically determined dark adaptation curve, ERGs and EOGs. It requires 2–3 hours to attain the final dark adaptation threshold, the maximum scotopic ERG response, and the normal EOG light rise.[11,29–31] Examples of full-field ERGs after 30 minutes of dark adaptation and after 3 hours of dark adaptation in a typical patient with FA are shown in Fig. 8.16. The scotopic (rod) ERG is absent after 30 minutes of dark adaptation but becomes normal after 3 hours of dark adaptation. The mixed rod–cone ERG after 30 minutes of dark adaptation shows a negative configuration with a small a-wave, just as is seen in Oguchi disease. However, unlike Oguchi disease, it becomes normal after 3 hours of dark adaptation. EOG is abnormal when measured in the regular method of 15 minutes of dark adaptation; however, it becomes normal when the dark adaptation is prolonged.[31] Mutations in the gene encoding 11-*cis* retinol dehydrogenase (*RDH5)* cause delayed dark adaptation and FA.[32]

Although FA has been believed to be a stationary condition, our study indicated that about one-third of patients with FA are progressive, and associated with cone dystrophy.[33] Such patients often have bull's-eye maculopathy (Fig. 8.17). In addition to the characteristic ERG findings of FA, the photopic ERGs are extremely abnormal (Fig. 8.16). All of these patients also showed *RDH5* gene mutation.[34] The ERG results have changed the disease concept of FA, which had been believed to be a subtype of CSNB.

Rod–cone or cone–rod photoreceptor dystrophy

Patients with cone–rod or rod–cone dystrophy belong clinically and genetically to a heterogeneous group of patients with inherited retinal dystrophies and the disease process is progressive. They are characterized by widespread degeneration of predominantly the cone (cone dystrophy) or the rod (rod dystrophy) photoreceptors in the early stage and, at the advanced stage, patients also have remaining rod (cone–rod dystrophy) or cone (rod–cone dystrophy) degeneration. The fundus in patients with cone or cone–rod dystrophy may be within normal limits or may have subtle changes in the early stage. In such cases, patients may be misdiagnosed as having optic nerve disease, central nervous system disease, amblyopia, or OMD (see below). These changes may progress to bull's-eye maculopathy and diffuse atrophy of the RPE in the far-advanced stage. Patients with rod–cone dystrophy show abnormal scotopic vision first, followed by abnormal photopic vision. The diseases include retinitis pigmentosa, choroideremia, gyrate atrophy, and others. Full-field ERG is important to differentiate between cone–rod and rod–cone dystrophy, particularly in their early stage.

Full-field ERGs in a typical patient with cone dystrophy and rod–cone dystrophy are shown in Fig. 8.18. Selective abnormalities of the photopic components (cone and 30-Hz flicker ERG) are seen in cone dystrophy and a more severe abnormality in rod

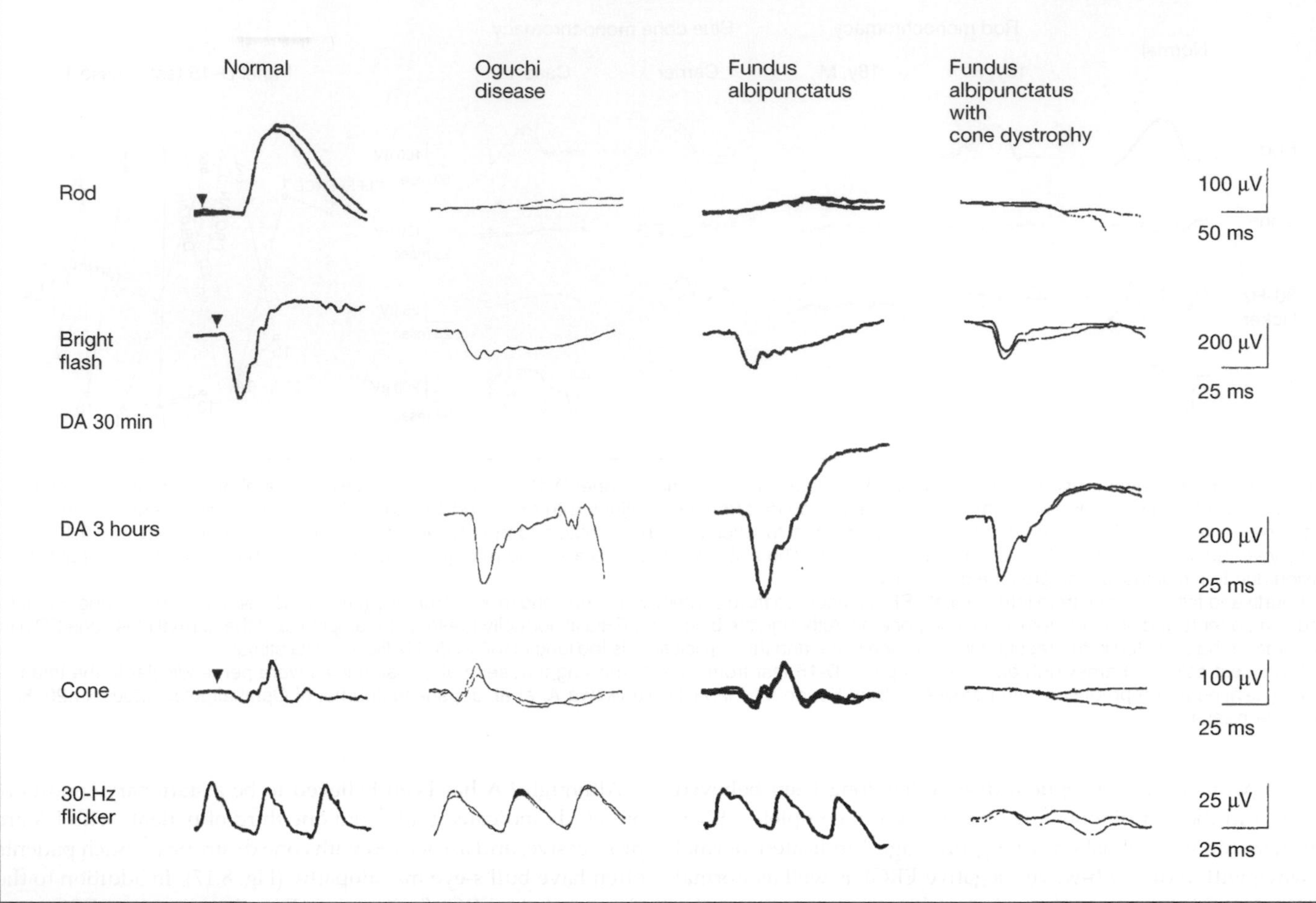

Fig. 8.16 Full-field electroretinograms (ERGs) recorded from normal control, patients with Oguchi disease, fundus albipunctatus (FA), and FA with cone dystrophy. Bright flash ERGs were recorded after 30 minutes and after 3 hours' dark adaptation.

In Oguchi disease, full-field ERGs recorded after 30 minutes of dark adaptation show absent rod ERG and essentially normal cone-mediated ERG. The mixed rod–cone ERG has a negative configuration with relatively well-preserved oscillatory potentials. Because the rod function is absent, it shows photopic hill phenomenon, and the ERG configuration is negative with a small a-wave. But the negative configuration with normal a-wave after 3 hours' dark adaptation may suggest some additional abnormalities of the bipolar cell function.

In FA, the rod ERG is absent after 30 minutes of dark adaptation but becomes normal after 3 hours of dark adaptation. The mixed rod–cone ERG after 30 minutes of dark adaptation shows a negative configuration with a small a-wave, just as is seen in the photopic phenomenon of Oguchi disease. However, unlike Oguchi disease, it becomes normal after 3 hours of dark adaptation. About one-third of patients with FA have associated cone dystrophy, often showing bull's-eye maculopathy (Fig. 8.17). Such patients show extremely abnormal photopic ERGs in addition to the characteristic ERG findings of FA. (Revised and reproduced with permission from Kondo M, Piao CH, Tanikawa A, et al. Japanese Journal of Ophthalmology 2000;44:20–8.)

than cone function is shown in retinitis pigmentosa as a representative disease of rod–cone dystrophy. At the advanced stage, most patients with cone dystrophy also have abnormal scotopic vision (cone–rod dystrophy) and may sometimes be difficult to differentiate from rod–cone dystrophy, such as retinitis pigmentosa.

Second-order neuron dysfunction

The fundamental differences between rod and cone connections to the bipolar cells are shown in Fig. 8.19.[35] The photoreceptors transmit visual information to the bipolar cells, which are the second-order neurons. Rods contact only depolarizing (ON) bipolar cells (DBCs), creating ON visual pathways. On the other hand, cones have more extensive postsynaptic connections. They synapse on to depolarizing DBCs and hyperpolarizing OFF bipolar cells.

Complete and incomplete CSNB were classified as independent clinical entities based mainly on the analysis of full-field ERGs.[36] Unlike Oguchi disease and FA, where the responsible pathology lies mainly in the rod itself, complete and incomplete CSNB are caused by the dysfunction of ON or ON–OFF bipolar cells, respectively.[35,37] They are the model disorders of bipolar cell dysfunction. EOGs in both diseases are normal.[36] It should be noted that all this new information in terms of the classification and pathology of both complete and incomplete CSNB was obtained from detailed analysis of ERG,[36,37] and molecular genetics confirmed these ERG findings later.

The hereditary mode of complete CSNB is X-linked recessive or autosomal recessive.[36] X-linked complete CSNB has a mutation of the leucine-rich repeat proteoglycan (*NYX*) gene,[38] and autosomal recessive complete CSNB has a mutation of *GRM6* gene[39] encoding the metabotropic glutamate receptor mGluR6 and transient receptor potential cation channel subfamily member 1 (*TRPM1*).[40] All these proteins are distributed on the postsynaptic ON bipolar cells and are required for the depolarization of the cell. The visual functions and ERGs are essentially the same in patients with these three different gene mutations, which have an almost complete block of ON synaptic

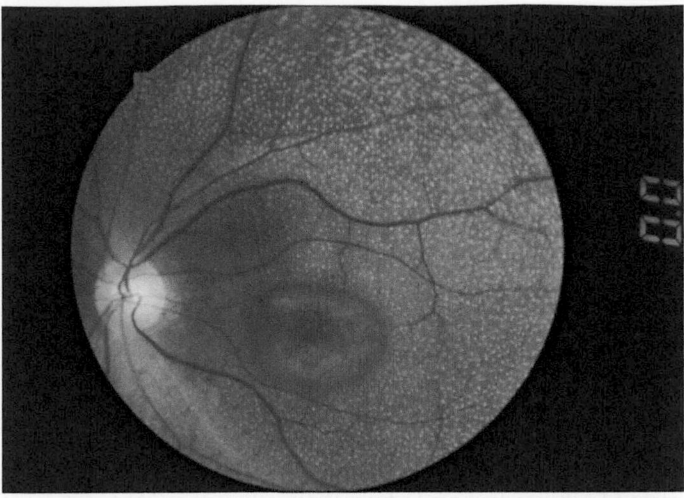

Fig. 8.17 Fundus of a patient with fundus albipunctatus associated with bull's-eye maculopathy. (Reproduced with permission from Miyake Y, Shiroyama N, Sugita S, et al. Fundus albipunctatus associated with cone dystrophy. Br J Ophthalmol 1992;76:375–9, with permission from BMJ Publishing Group.)

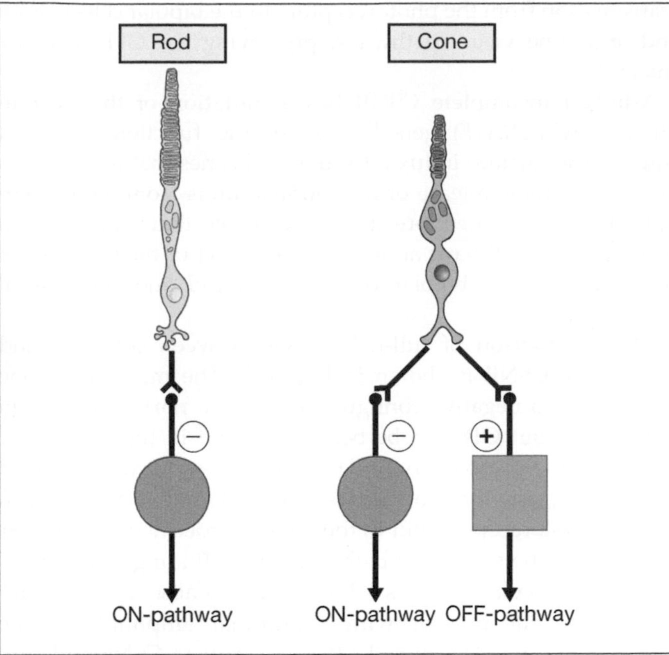

Fig. 8.19 Simplified schema showing retinal wiring of the rod and cone pathway. The photoreceptors transmit visual information to the bipolar cells, which are the second-order neurons. Rods contact only depolarizing bipolar cells (DBCs: ●), creating ON visual pathways. On the other hand, cones have more extensive postsynaptic connections. They synapse on to depolarizing DBCs and hyperpolarizing OFF bipolar cells (HBCs: ■).

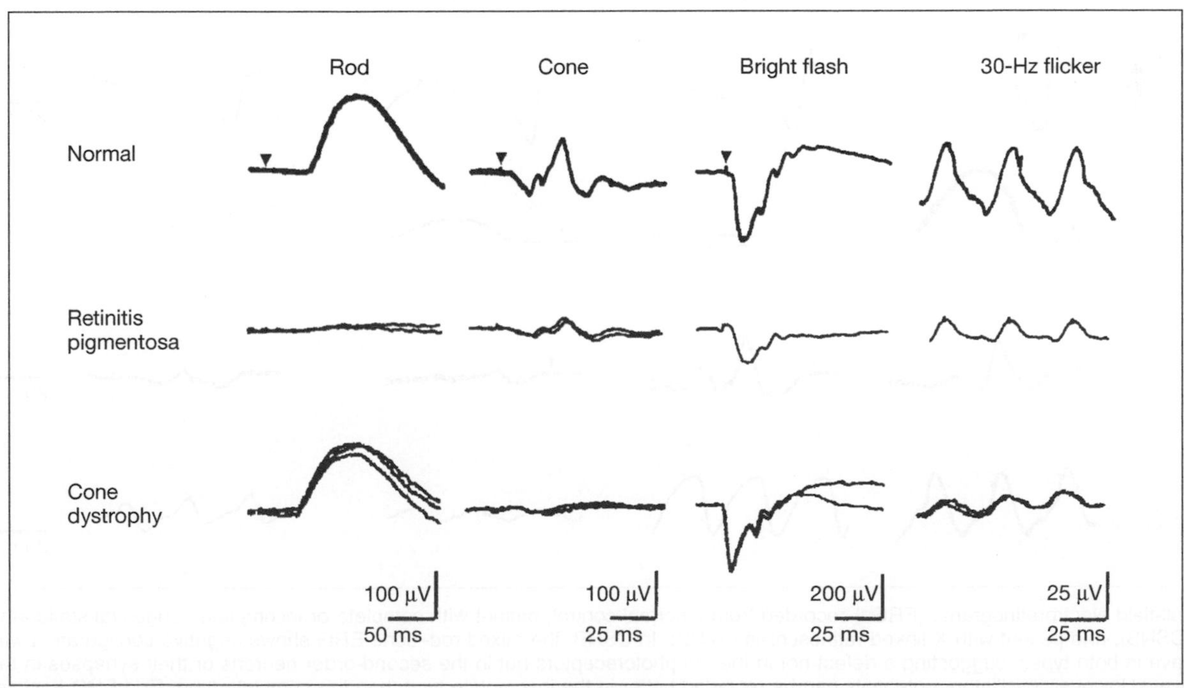

Fig. 8.18 Full-field electroretinograms (ERGs) recorded from a normal control (top) and a patient with retinitis pigmentosa at an early stage (middle) and a patient with cone dystrophy (bottom). The more severe abnormality in rod than cone function is shown in retinitis pigmentosa as a representative disease of rod–cone dystrophy and selective abnormalities of the photopic components (cone and 30-Hz flicker ERG) are seen in cone dystrophy. At the advanced stage, most patients with cone dystrophy also have abnormal scotopic vision (cone–rod dystrophy) and it may sometimes be difficult to differentiate from a rod–cone dystrophy, such as retinitis pigmentosa. (Reproduced with permission from Miyake Y. Electrodiagnosis of retinal diseases. Tokyo: Springer-Verlag; 2006.)

transmission from the photoreceptors to the bipolar cells in both rod and cone visual pathways, preserving the OFF pathway intact.[11]

X-linked incomplete CSNB has a mutation of the calcium channel (*CACNA1F*) gene.[41] Loss of the functional channel impairs the calcium influx into rods and cones that is needed to sustain the tonic release of neurotransmitters from the presynaptic terminals. Therefore it is conceivable that patients with incomplete CSNB have an incomplete defect of the synapses in the ON and OFF bipolar cells in both rod and cone visual pathways.[11]

The comparison of full-field ERGs between complete and incomplete CSNB is shown in Fig. 8.20. The mixed rod–cone ERG shows a negative configuration with a normal a-wave in both types, but OPs can be better recorded in the incomplete type than the complete type. The normal a-wave with reduced b-wave suggests that both types of CSNB have a defect not in the rod photoreceptors but in the second-order neurons or their synapses in the rod visual pathway. These findings are comparable to molecular genetics.[36–41] Rod ERG is absent in the complete type but present with subnormal amplitude in the incomplete type. Absent rod ERG in complete CSNB and subnormal rod ERG in incomplete CSNB are comparable to the pathology of complete defect (complete CSNB) and incomplete defect (incomplete CSNB) of rod bipolar cell transmission. On the other hand, cone and 30-Hz flicker ERGs appear nearly normal in the complete type except that the a-wave of the cone ERG has a plateau-like bottom (Fig. 8.20). In contrast, the cone and 30-Hz flicker ERGs are extremely reduced in incomplete CSNB, which is highly characteristic and extremely important for the differential diagnosis.

In spite of the complete defect of ON visual pathway, cone and 30-Hz flicker ERG of complete CSNB appear nearly normal. This mechanism can be explained by the analysis of photopic long-flash ERG[35,37] as shown in Fig. 8.21. Using photopic ERGs elicited by long-duration square-wave stimuli, the cone ON response generated by depolarizing ON bipolar cells is selectively and severely depressed in patients with complete CSNB; moreover, the waveform is similar to that of monkeys after 2-amino-4-phosphonobutyric acid (APB) is injected into the vitreous to block the synapse between photoreceptors and ON bipolar cells.[35] The OFF response, on the other hand, which is generated by hyperpolarizing bipolar cells, is intact in patients with complete CSNB, leading us to hypothesize that the ON function of both the rod and cone visual pathway is completely blocked in eyes with complete CSNB.[35,37] The mechanism as to why normal-looking brief-flash cone ERG can be obtained under this condition is shown in Figure 8.22. With long-duration stimuli, the a-waves, b-waves, and d-waves are clearly separated. As the stimulus duration is shortened (brief-flash stimuli), the positive component of the photopic ERG consists mainly of the d-wave. Therefore even when the b-wave, a component of the ON response, is absent (as in complete CSNB), the d-wave replaces the b-wave, and a positive wave is recorded with brief-flash

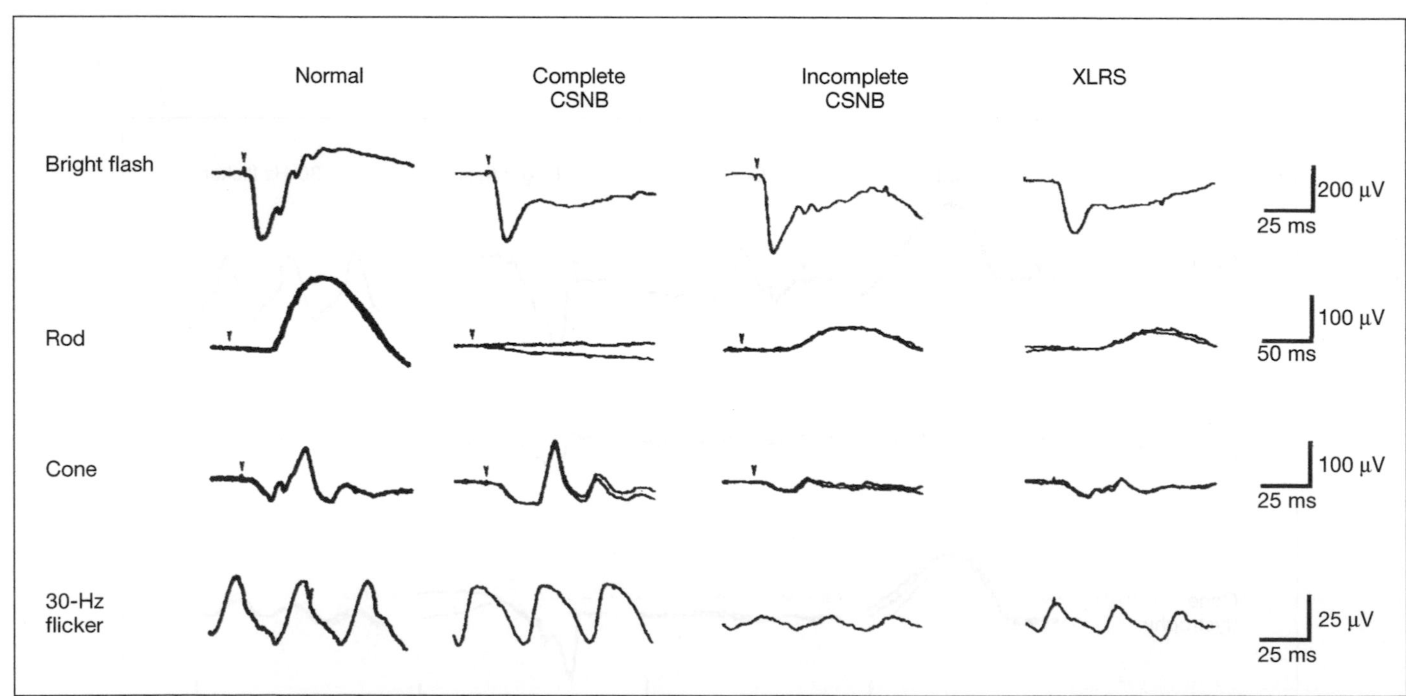

Fig. 8.20 Full-field electroretinograms (ERGs) recorded from a normal control, patient with complete or incomplete congenital stationary night blindness (CSNB), and patient with X-linked retinoschisis (XLRS). In CSNB, the mixed rod–cone ERG shows negative configuration with a normal a-wave in both types, suggesting a defect not in the rod photoreceptors but in the second-order neurons or their synapses in the rod visual pathway. However, oscillatory potentials can be recorded better in the incomplete type than the complete type. Rod ERG is absent in the complete type but present with subnormal amplitude in the incomplete type. On the other hand, cone and 30-Hz flicker ERGs appear nearly normal in the complete type except that the a-wave of the cone ERG has a plateau-like bottom. In contrast, the cone and 30-Hz flicker ERGs are extremely reduced in incomplete CSNB, which is highly characteristic and extremely important for the differential diagnosis. In XLRS, the mixed rod–cone ERG shows a negative configuration, which is observed even when the retinoschisis is confined to the fovea ophthalmoscopically. The full-field ERG findings similar to those of incomplete CSNB suggest that both ON and OFF bipolar cell function is mainly impaired in the rod and cone visual pathways. (Reproduced with permission from Miyake Y. Electrodiagnosis of retinal diseases. Tokyo: Springer-Verlag; 2006.)

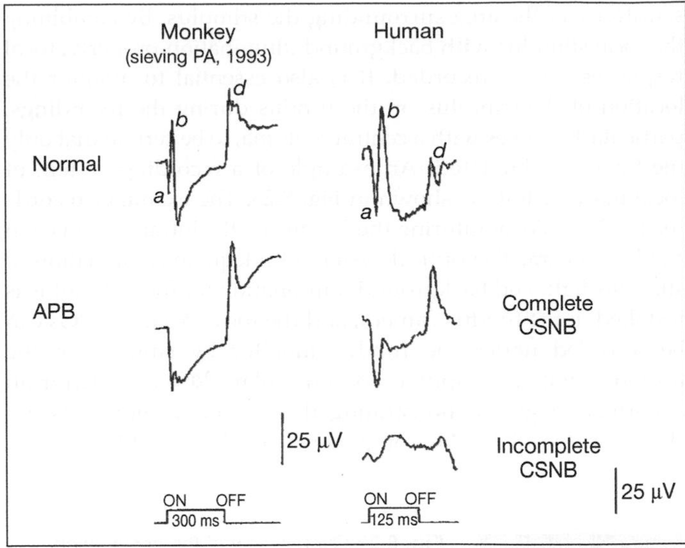

Fig. 8.21 Comparison of photopic long-duration electroretinograms (ERGs) recorded from a monkey and a human. Left, normal control ERG for the monkey eye and after being treated by 2-amino-4-phosphonobutyric acid (APB). Right, ERGs recorded from a normal human control, from a patient with complete congenital stationary night blindness (CSNB), and from a patient with incomplete CSNB. The cone ON response generated by depolarizing ON bipolar cells is selectively depressed whereas the OFF response, which is generated by hyperpolarizing bipolar cells, is intact in patients with complete CSNB; moreover, the waveform is similar to that of monkeys treated with APB. (Reproduced with permission from Kondo M, Piao CH, Tanikawa A, et al. Japanese Journal of Ophthalmology 2000;44:20–8, with permission.)

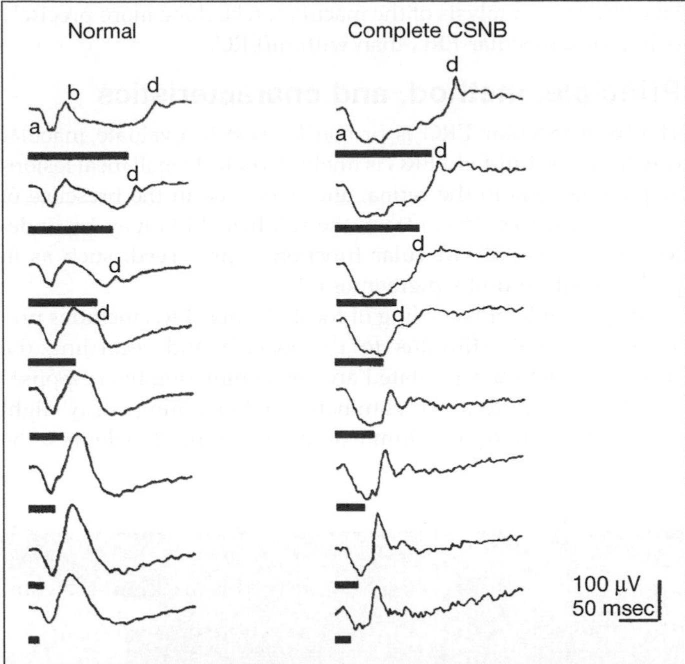

Fig. 8.22 Photopic electroretinograms (ERGs) elicited by square-wave stimuli of various durations from a normal control and a patient with complete congenital stationary night blindness (CSNB), explaining why complete CSNB shows normal-looking brief-flash cone ERG. With long-duration stimuli, the a-waves, b-waves, and d-waves are clearly separated. As the stimulus duration is shortened (brief-flash stimuli), the positive component of the photopic ERG consists mainly of the d-wave. Therefore even when the b-wave, a component of the ON response, is absent (as in complete CSNB), the d-wave replaces the b-wave, and a positive wave is recorded with brief-flash stimuli. Thick lines underneath the responses represent the stimulus duration. (Reproduced with permission from Miyake Y. Nippon Ganka Gakkai Zasshi 2002;106:737–56.)

stimuli.[11] With incomplete CSNB, on the other hand, the ON and OFF response are both subnormal, suggesting that the ON and OFF systems are incompletely disturbed at the level of the bipolar cells.[11,37]

XLRS is a vitreoretinal dystrophy that manifests early in life. XLRS is one of the more common causes of juvenile macular degeneration in males. Intraretinal cysts form in the macula and splitting of the retinal layers occurs in the peripheral retina. Most patients, including young ones, show moderately poor visual acuity that gradually decreases with increasing age. Hypermetropia has been shown to be a frequent accompaniment of this disorder.[42] In fact, many patients with XLRS are first diagnosed with hypermetropic amblyopia or heterotropia during infancy.

As mentioned above, mixed rod–cone ERG is of significant diagnostic value because of the negative configuration. The negative ERG is observed even when the retinoschisis is confined to the fovea ophthalmoscopically. The full-field ERG findings (Fig. 8.20) are similar to those of incomplete CSNB, suggesting that both ON and OFF bipolar cell function is mainly impaired in the rod and cone visual pathways. EOG in XLRS is normal.

The schisis occurs in the plane of the nerve fiber and ganglion cell layers of the retina. It has long been suggested that degenerating Müller cells or inner retinal cells may be the primary cause of the pathological changes in XLRS. The XLRS gene was cloned in 1997 and was designated *RS1*.[43] However, the *RS1* protein is heavily expressed in inner segments of both rod and cone photoreceptors and is also seen in cells of the inner nuclear layer. There is some discrepancy between the results of full-field ERG and genetic findings. Although the expression of *RS1* protein is heavily concentrated in the inner segments of both rods and cones, electroretinographic studies suggest that it does not inherently affect the photoreceptor function of either cell type. And from the above ERG and EOG results, it currently is reasonable to propose that both ON and OFF pathways are defective, although precise subcellular localization has not yet determined whether both depolarizing and hyperpolarizing bipolar cells are involved.[44]

FOCAL ERG

In order to record the ERG responses with focal stimuli, there are two methods which have been reported in the past. The conventional focal macular ERG can show a similar waveform as a conventional photopic ERG from the limited area of macula.[45] The advantage of this method is that the analysis of ERG components can be done using the same concept as that of full-field photopic ERG. By analyzing several components, layer-by-layer macular function can be evaluated.

Another method is the mfERG technique, which was developed in 1992.[46] With this method, focal ERGs can be recorded simultaneously from multiple retinal locations during a single recording session using cross-correlation techniques. Unlike conventional focal macular ERGs, there are still questions about how this method works and what it measures because the technique is relatively new. We have an impression that the layer-by-layer analysis of the macula can be done more precisely using focal macular ERG than with mfERG.

Principle, method, and characteristics

The focal macular ERG is primarily used to evaluate macular function. The full-field ERG is unable to detect small focal lesions or pathogenesis in the retina, and is normal in the presence of macular diseases. In contrast, the full-field ERG may be undetectable when only macular function is preserved, such as in patients with retinitis pigmentosa.[11]

The principle of recording of focal macular ERG includes presenting a small stimulus to the macula and recording the response from the stimulated area by summating the responses using a computer. To eliminate contaminating stray light responses, background illumination must be used to depress the sensitivity of the area surrounding the stimulus. By combining the focal stimulus with background illumination properly, focal responses can be recorded. It is also essential to monitor the location of the stimulus on the fundus during the recordings, particularly in eyes with a central scotoma, to be certain that only the fovea is stimulated. An example of a recording system of focal macular ERG is shown in Fig. 8.23. The examiner records the ERGs while monitoring the fundus by the infrared television fundus camera. The optical system of adequate combination of stimulus light and background illumination for focal stimulus is installed in the fundus camera, and the focal macular ERGs can be recorded under the fundus monitor by summating the responses with a computer. Focal macular ERGs recorded from a normal subject demonstrating the various components are shown in Fig. 8.24. All components of photopic ERG can be

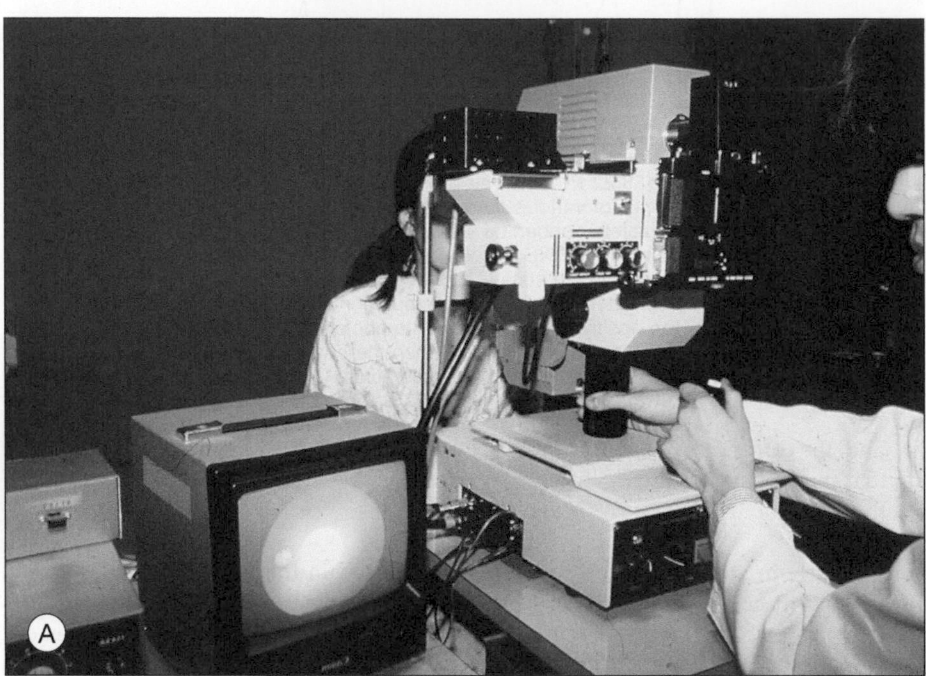

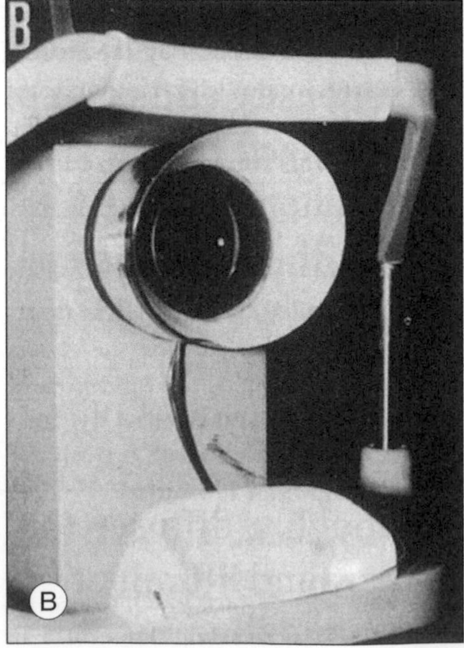

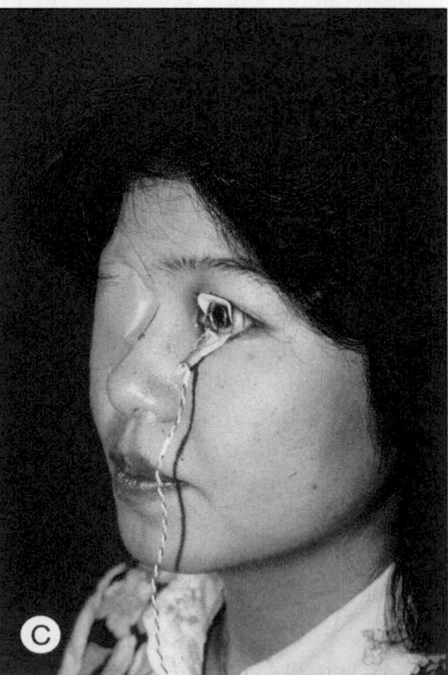

Fig. 8.23 Overall view of the observation and stimulation systems for focal macular electroretinogram (ERG) and visually evoked response (VER) recordings. The examiner records the ERGs while monitoring the stimulus on the fundus by the infrared television fundus camera (A). A plastic hemisphere with miniature lamps is attached to the top of the camera to obtain background illumination for the peripheral retina (B). A Burian-Allen bipolar contact lens is used to record the ERGs (C). (Revised with permission from Miyake Y, Yanagida K, Kondo T, et al. Nippon Ganka Gakkai Zasshi 1981;85:1521–33.)

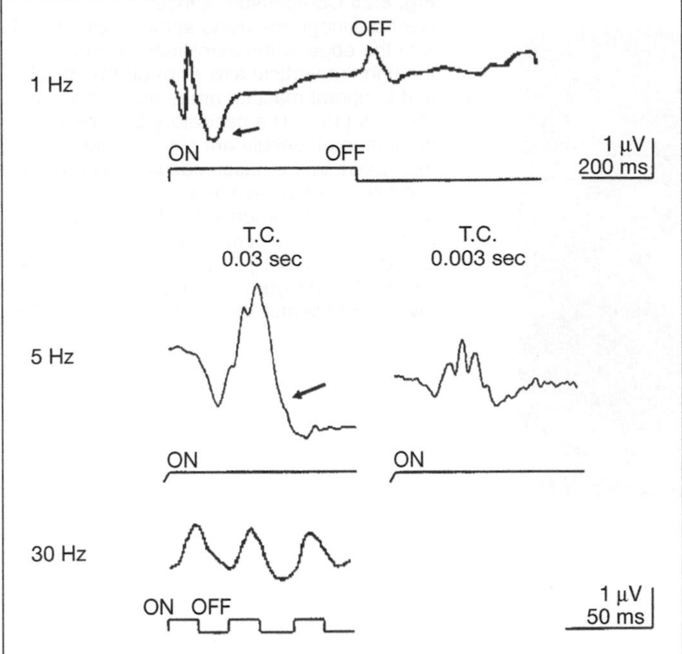

Fig. 8.24 Components of the focal macular electroretinogram recorded from a normal subject. ON and OFF responses recorded with 1-Hz stimulus frequency (top); a-wave, b-wave, and oscillatory potentials recorded with 5-Hz stimulus frequency (middle); and 30-Hz flicker responses (bottom) are shown. Arrows indicate photopic negative response. (Reproduced with permission from Miyake Y. Electrodiagnosis of retinal diseases. Tokyo: Springer-Verlag; 2006.)

recorded: they are a-waves, b-waves, OPs, PhNR, ON and OFF components, and 30-Hz flicker responses.[11]

Several important characteristics of focal macular ERG in human were detected, particularly in macular OPs.[45] An example is shown in Fig. 8.25, demonstrating nasotemporal asymmetry.[47] Semicircular stimuli were used to compare the ERGs elicited by stimulating the temporal and nasal macula. The amplitudes and implicit times of the a-waves and b-waves in the nasal retina are almost identical to those from the temporal retina, whereas the amplitudes of OPs are much larger in the temporal retina than those in the nasal retina. The amplitude of the focal ERGs recorded with circular stimulus is approximately the same sum as the amplitudes of the temporal and nasal ERGs.

The principle, recording method, and clinical applications of mfERG are described in an ISCEV guideline.[48] Readers are also referred to Chapter 7, Electrogenesis of the ERG, where the origin of the mfERG is described in detail.

Clinical applications

The examples of value of focal ERG are shown here. In focal macular ERG, the macular OPs are the most sensitive indicator in variable macular diseases. The selective reduction of macular OP amplitude is observed in the early stage of macular edema,[49] epimacular membrane,[50] and convalescent stage of central serous chorioretinopathy.[51] The fluorescein angiograms and focal macular ERGs in an eye with pseudophakic cystoid macular edema (CME) and after resolution of CME are illustrated in Fig. 8.26. The OPs of the focal macular ERGs are selectively reduced compared with that of a normal fellow eye. The visual acuity of eye with CME was 0.6. Six months later, the CME resolved spontaneously, and fluorescein angiogram disclosed a normal pattern; the visual acuity improved to 1.2. The focal macular ERGs returned to normal levels, with the amplitude of the OPs comparable to those from the normal fellow eye.[51]

Occult macular dystrophy (OMD) is one of the most representative disorders where the focal macular ERG or multifocal ERG is a key for diagnosis. OMD was discovered by focal macular ERG in 1989.[52] The clinical findings of OMD are progressive decrease of visual acuity, normal fundus and fluorescein angiograms, normal full-field ERGs, but abnormal focal macular ERG and multifocal ERG (Fig. 8.27). Although the fundus appearance and fluorescein angiogram show normal findings in OMD, optical coherence tomography (OCT) may reveal some mild abnormality from its early stage. Whether focal macular ERG or OCT is more sensitive to detect early abnormality is an interesting point of argument. The point is that OMD may not be a rare disease and that many patients with OMD may be misdiagnosed as having several other diseases, such as a psychological eye problem, optic nerve problem, central nervous system problem, or amblyopia.[53]

The hereditary mode of OMD is autosomal dominant, although some patients show sporadic mode.[52,53] Our genetic studies have detected mutations in retinitis pigmentosa 1-like 1 (*RP1L1*) gene in autosomal dominant OMD.[54] It was demonstrated that *RP1L1* plays an essential role in cone function in humans and that disruption of *RP1L1* function leads to OMD.

Acute zonal occult outer retinopathy is characterized by an acute zonal loss of one or more large zones of central retinal function in one or both eyes, predominantly in young women.[55] Other ocular findings include initially minimum ophthalmoscopic changes, photophobia, and permanent visual field loss, often associated with late development of retinal pigmentary changes and narrowing of the retinal vessels in the affected zones. Since the full-field ERG may be normal or only slightly abnormal, it is not informative. The responses of mfERG become abnormal in the limited area where visual field loss is present[11] (Fig. 8.28).

OTHER SPECIAL RESPONSES OR TECHNIQUES IN ERG

Pattern ERG

Pattern ERG (PERG) is the retinal response to a structured stimulus, such as a reversing black-and-white checkerboard or grating. The standard for PERG recording has been established by the ISCEV.[56] While the luminance ERG is evoked by changes in stimulus luminance, the PERG is evoked by changes of stimulus contrast. The PERG is therefore a retinal response that is absent of a net change of stimulus luminance. The generators of the responses are mainly the retinal ganglion cells.[57] Thus ganglion cell function can be evaluated by PERG.

The waveform consists of an initial cornea-positive response, referred to as P50, followed by a cornea-negative response, referred to as N95 (Fig. 8.29). Holder[58] reported in his review on PERG in 520 eyes that P50 was reduced with preganglion cell dysfunction but usually spared with optic nerve diseases. On the other hand, N95 loss was the most common abnormality and was reliably associated with optic nerve diseases.

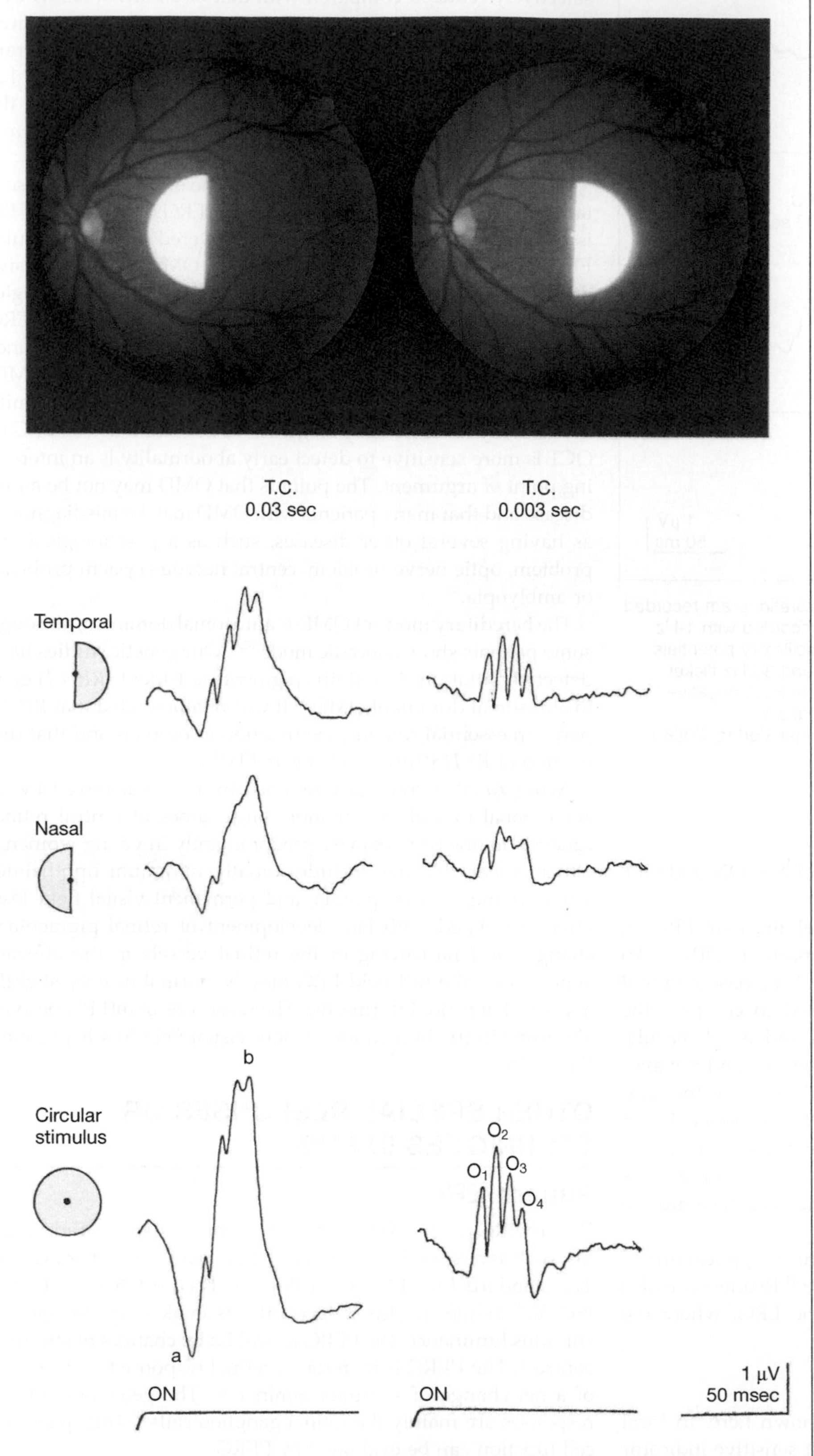

Fig. 8.25 Comparison of focal electroretinograms using semicircular stimuli with the edge of the semicircle passing through the vertical axis (top) on the nasal and temporal macular areas and a circular stimulus (15°). The oscillatory potentials in the temporal macula are significantly larger than those in the nasal macula, and only the oscillatory potentials show this significant asymmetry. (Reproduced with permission from Miyake Y. Electrodiagnosis of retinal diseases. Tokyo: Springer-Verlag; 2006, and Miyake Y, Shiroyama N, Hiroguchi M, et al. Invest Ophthalmol Vis Sci 1989;30:1743–9.)

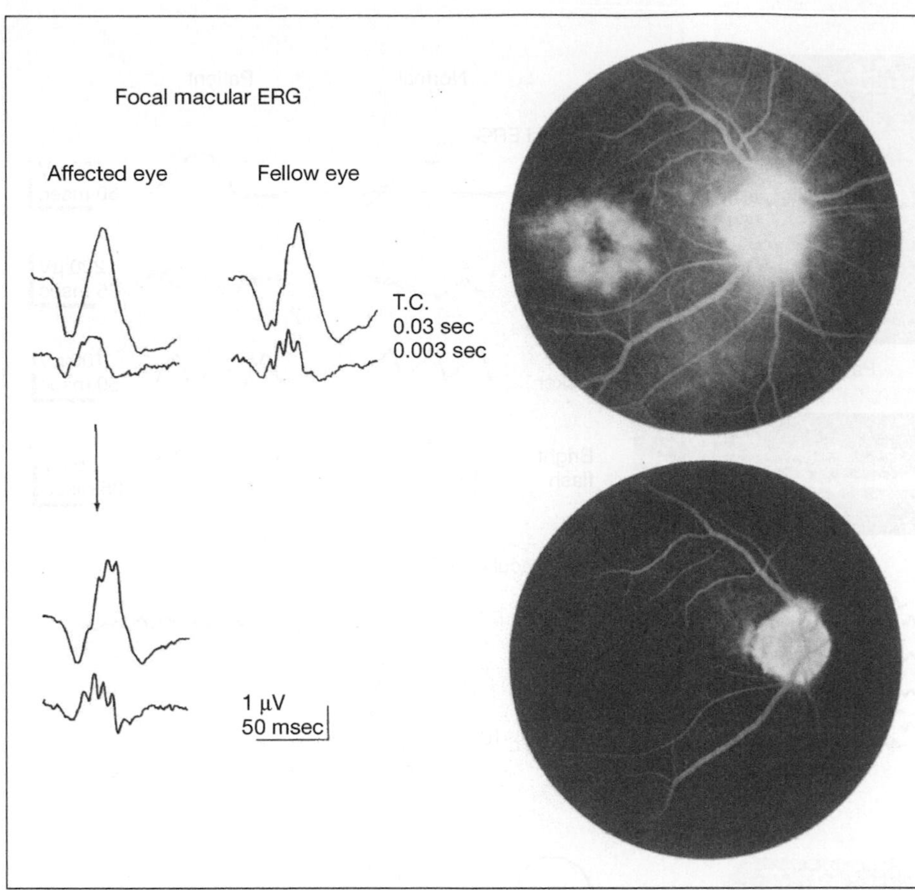

Fig. 8.26 Focal macular electroretinograms (ERGs) (left) and fluorescein angiograms (right) in a 51-year-old man with pseudophakic cystoid macular edema (CME: top) and after the resolution of CME (bottom). The oscillatory potentials of the focal macular ERGs are selectively reduced compared with that of a normal fellow eye. The visual acuity of the eye with CME was 0.6 (20/30). After spontaneous resolution of the CME, the focal macular ERGs returned to normal levels, with the amplitude of the oscillatory potentials comparable to those from the normal fellow eye. The visual acuity improved to 1.2. (Reproduced with permission from Miyake Y, Miyake K, Shiroyama N, et al. Am J Ophthalmol 1993;116:576–83.)

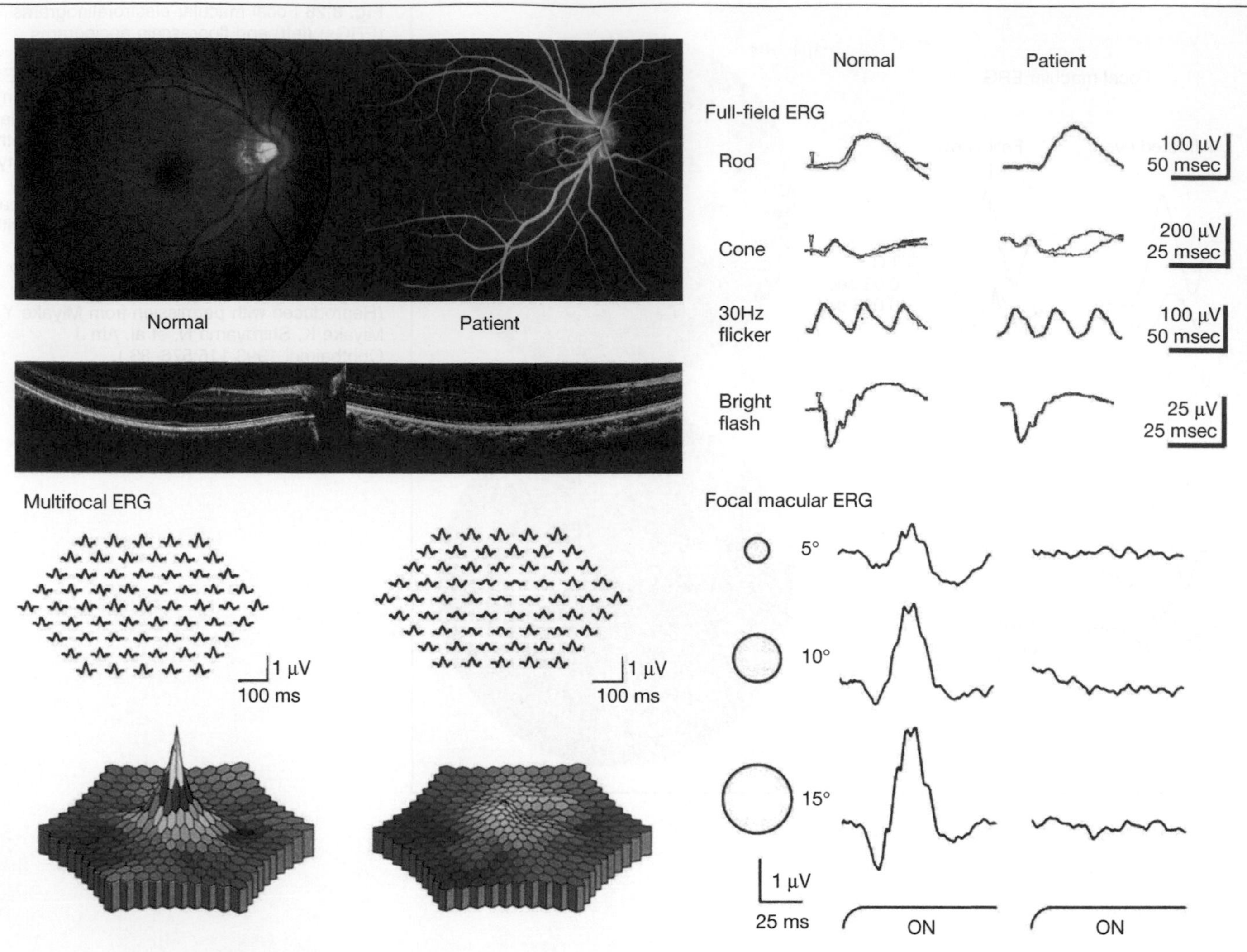

Fig. 8.27 The clinical findings of occult macular dystrophy. Left top, normal fundus and fluorescein angiograms; left middle, optical coherence tomography images from a normal person and a patient with occult macular dystrophy. The horizontal section through the foveal center demonstrates an abnormality, especially in the outer retinal bands at the fovea in the patient. Left bottom, wave three-dimensional topography and multifocal electroretinogram (ERG) trace array from a normal person and a patient, showing markedly reduced response density in the central 7° of the retina. Right top, full-field ERGs showing normal responses; right bottom, focal macular ERG showing abnormal responses in the patient.

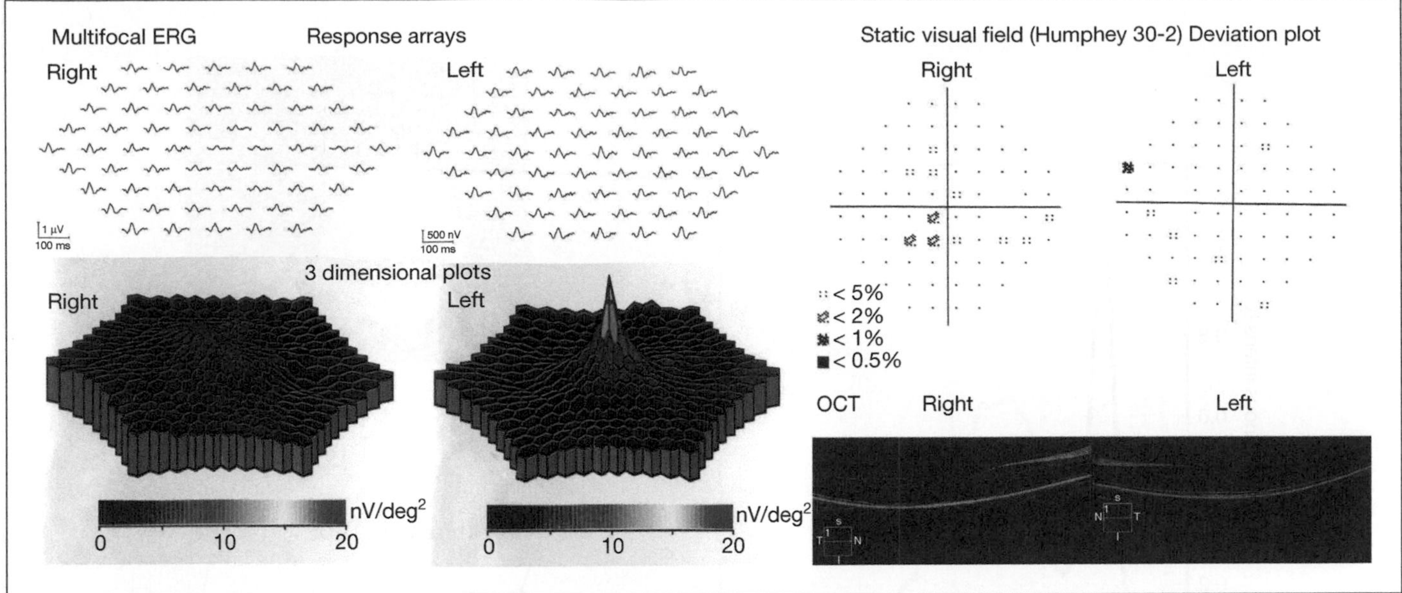

Fig. 8.28 Clinical findings of a patient with acute zonal occult outer retinopathy. A 22-year-old female developed acute central visual loss in the right eye. Visual acuity was 0.5 (20/40) OD and 1.2 (25/20) OS. The top and bottom left panels are 61 response arrays and three-dimensional plots of the multifocal electroretinograms, respectively, showing abnormal responses in the limited area, where visual field loss is present in the right eye. The top right panels are the deviation plot of the static visual field, showing reduced sensitivity in the central area in the right eye. The bottom right panels are Fourier-domain optical coherence tomographic (FD-OCT) images from the affected right eye and intact left eye, respectively, showing that both the border of the photoreceptor inner- and outer-segment line (IS/OS line) and the cone outer-segment tip (COST) line between the IS/OS line and the retinal pigment epithelium (RPE) are absent in the macular area of the right eye. The IS/OS line, COST line, and RPE/Bruch membrane are intact in the left eye.

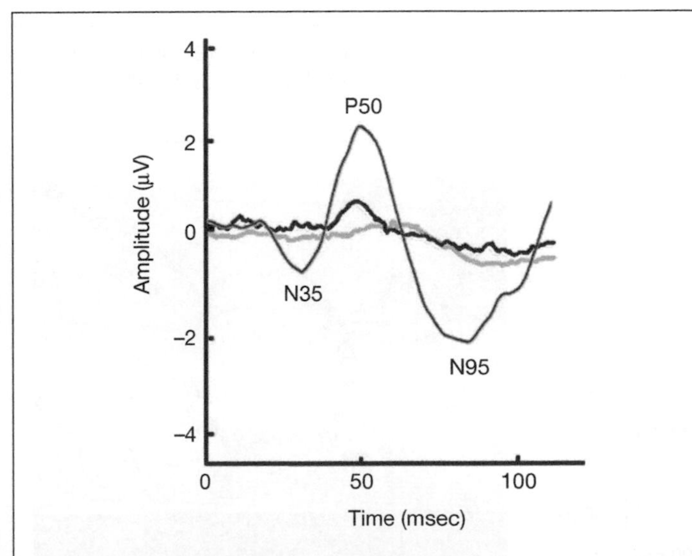

Fig. 8.29 Pattern electroretinogram responses recorded from a normal control (gray), patient with macular dysfunction (green), and patient with optic nerve dysfunction (blue).

Photopic negative response

PhNR has already been described and is a negative wave in photopic ERG that is evoked following the b-wave (Figs 8.14 and 8.24). The origin of the PhNR is the retinal ganglion cells,[21] and this is fully described in Chapter 7, Electrogenesis of the ERG. Significant reduction in PhNR was reported in patients with open angle glaucoma and several other optic neuropathies.[21] Moreover, recent analysis of PhNR recorded in focal macular ERG (Fig. 8.24) and mfERG has enabled objective assessment of retinal ganglion cell damage in glaucoma, optic nerve disease, and retinal vascular diseases.[59,60] Other studies showed that PhNR can be correlated with retinal sensitivity as well as retinal microstructure such as nerve fiber thickness.[61]

ERG recordings by LED

Light-emitting diodes (LEDs) (Fig. 8.30) have been in the limelight recently as light sources to elicit and record full-field ERG.[62] The LEDs are small and inexpensive, and they require low currents to drive them. They can be controlled by a simple electronic circuit to give either a continuous light output or extremely brief flashes over a large range of intensities. The stimulus and recording system using LED can provide not only routine full-field ERG but also some other special usages for clinical ERG, as shown below.

ERG recording under general anesthesia[11]

ERG recordings with LED are useful for recording standard ERGs from pediatric patients under general anesthesia. The equipment needed to obtain recordings that correspond to ISCEV standard ERGs is compact and easily portable.[63] The ERGs recorded using an LED system on a 3-month-old baby under general anesthesia and a normal adult are compared in Fig. 8.31.

ERG monitoring during eye surgery

As vitreoretinal surgery continues to advance, close monitoring of retinal function during these procedures has become important. Although ERGs directly reflect retinal function, monitoring during surgery has proven difficult. Each recording must be made quickly under aseptic conditions, and the instruments and electrodes must be such that they do not cause interference for

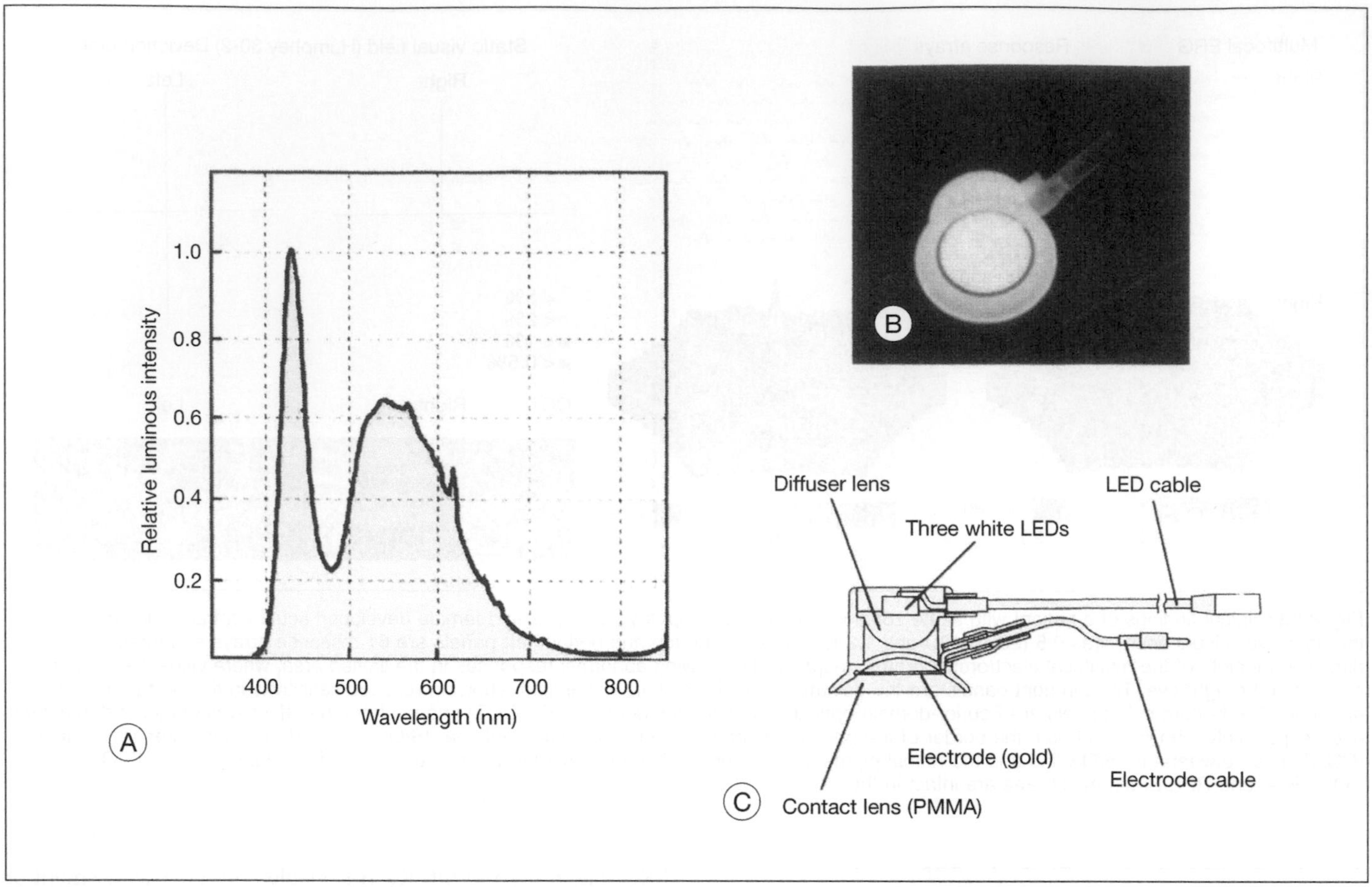

Fig. 8.30 Structure of the white light-emitting diode (LED) contact lens electrode. (A) Relative spectral emission of the LED. (B) Output that appears as visible white. (C) Structure of the contact lens electrode with three built-in white LEDs. PMMA, polymethylmethacrylate. (Reproduced with permission from Kondo M, Piao CH, Tanikawa A, et al. Doc Ophthalmol 2001;102:1–9.)

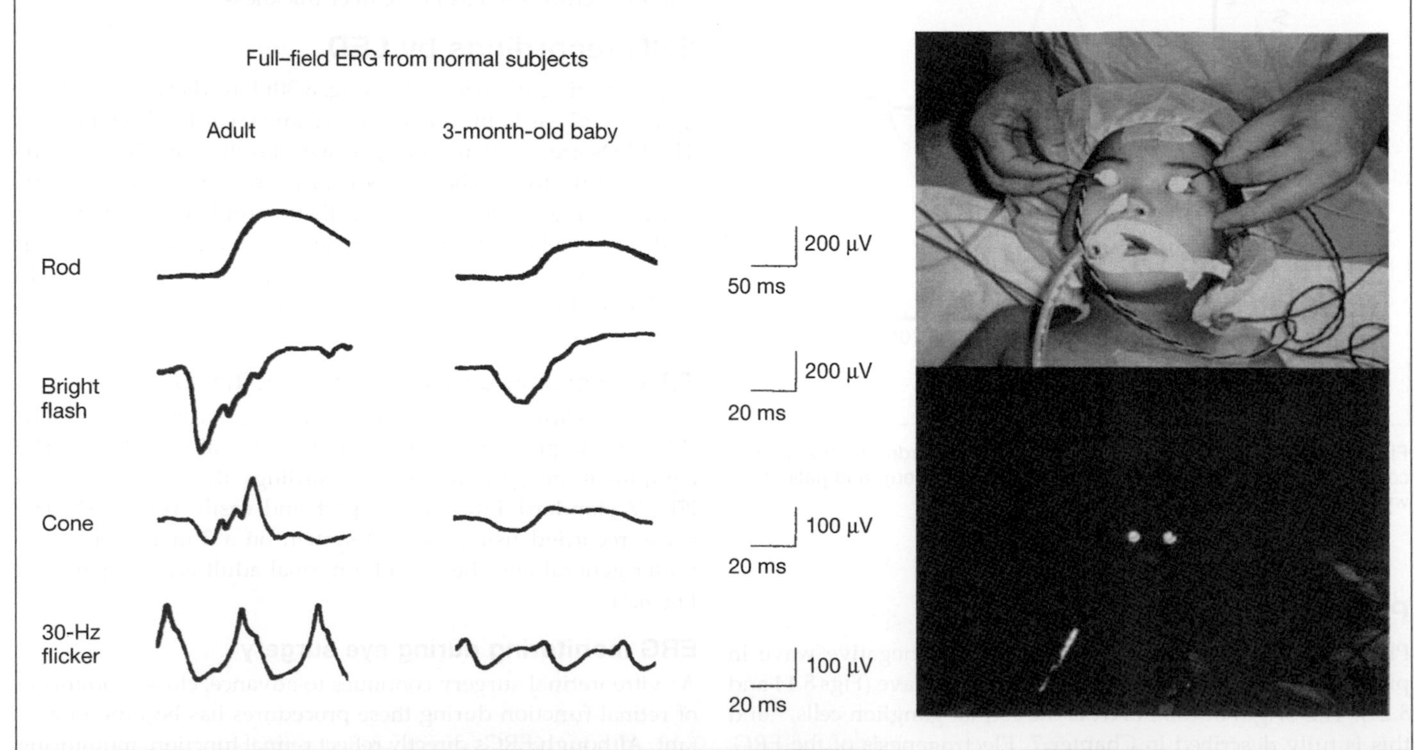

Fig. 8.31 Full-field electroretinograms (ERGs) recorded with white light-emitting diode (LED) contact lens electrodes from a normal adult subject (left) and a normal 3-month-old baby (right). The pictures show standard full-field ERG recording from a baby using this system. Top, LED contact lenses are placed in both eyes under general anesthesia. Bottom, Background illumination from the contact lens is used during the recording of the photopic ERGs in the dark. (Reproduced with permission from Miyake Y. Electrodiagnosis of retinal diseases. Tokyo: Springer-Verlag; 2006.)

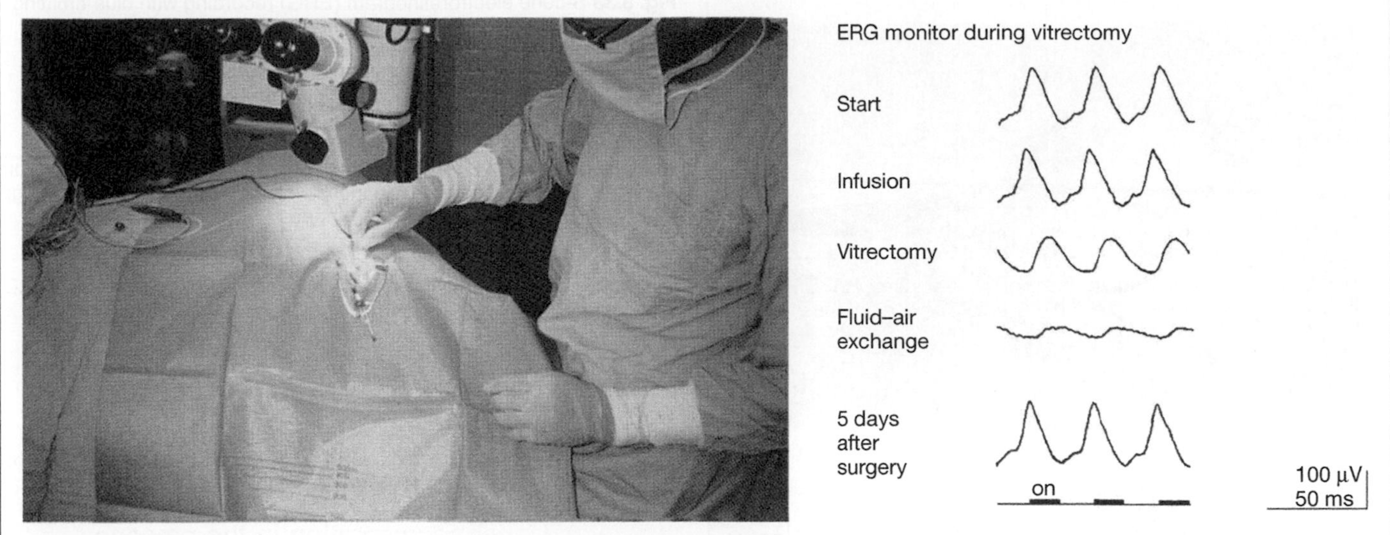

Fig. 8.32 Full-field electroretinogram (ERG) recording during vitrectomy. Left, a light-emitting diode (LED) electrode is sterilized and placed on the cornea undergoing surgery. Right, 30-Hz flicker ERGs recorded during vitrectomy in a patient with epimacular membrane. Start indicates the time when local anesthesia was completed and Infusion denotes the time the infusion needle was introduced into the vitreous cavity. (Reproduced with permission from Miyake Y. Electrodiagnosis of retinal diseases. Tokyo: Springer-Verlag; 2006, and Horiguchi M, Miyake Y. Arch Ophthalmol 1991;109:1127–9.)

the retinal surgeon. Furthermore, the eye undergoing surgery is intensively light-adapted.

The LED contact lens electrode has been found to be highly suitable for this purpose.[64] It is easily sterilized and is used as both a stimulus source and a recording electrode for 30-Hz flicker ERGs during vitreoretinal surgery (Fig. 8.32). An example of ERG monitor during vitrectomy from a patient with epimacular membrane is shown in Fig. 8.32. The ERGs recorded after local anesthesia (start), and after the introduction of the infusion needle into the vitreous cavity (infusion) were not significantly different in regard to amplitude and peak time. However, after vitrectomy, which required 10 minutes, the peak time was delayed and the amplitude decreased (vitrectomy). Additional studies have demonstrated that lowering the intravitreal temperature by applying an infusion solution kept at room temperature can alter the ERG during vitrectomy. Filling the whole vitreous cavity with air after the epimacular membrane was peeled off resulted in a markedly reduced amplitude and delayed peak time (fluid–air exchange). This extreme reduction of ERG following fluid–air or fluid–silicon oil exchange in the vitreous cavity results from reduced electrical conductivity in the vitreous cavity. Five days after surgery, when the air was resolved from the vitreous cavity, the ERG recovered to the postoperative amplitude and peak time.

S-Cone ERG

Recording short-wavelength cone (S-cone) ERGs is valuable clinically because it allows us to evaluate the S-cone visual system. S-cone ERGs have been recorded using stimulation with strong blue stimuli on a bright yellow background, which suppresses the middle- and long-wavelength (LM) cone system.[65] LEDs emitting blue light can be used in the LED built-in contact lens electrode[66] (Fig. 8.33). By using bright yellow background illumination, the S-cone ERGs are recordable and are compared with LM cone ERGs (Fig. 8.33). The amplitude is much smaller and the implicit time is longer than those of the LM cone ERG. The components that reflect the "OFF" visual system (a-waves and d-waves) are essentially absent in S-cone ERGs because, unlike the LM cone system, the S-cone is mainly connected to the "ON" visual system.[67]

ELECTRO-OCULOGRAM

In 1849, Du Bois Reymond[68] reported that in the normal eye there is a flow of electrical current, because the cornea is positive with respect to the back of the eye. The source of the voltage is the corneofundal potential. This potential difference is referred to as the standing potential or resting potential of the eye. The EOG is an indirect measure of the amplitude of the standing potential, which changes during dark and light adaptation. To obtain an EOG in humans, electrodes are placed at the inner and outer canthi of the eyes and the patient is asked to look back and forth between a pair of fixation lights (Fig. 8.34). When the cornea moves closer to one of the electrodes, it becomes more positive and the other electrode becomes more negative. The opposite happens when the eyes move to the other side.

The principle and practical use of EOG are described in the ISCEV standard.[69] The changes in the amplitude of the EOG in the dark-adapted and light-adapted state of a normal subject are shown in Fig. 8.35. The smaller amplitudes are recorded when the eyes make the saccadic eye movements in the dark (dark trough); the peak amplitude is recorded against a steady light background (light peak). The light peak/dark trough (L/D) ratio is an index (Arden index)[70] used to assess retinal function. Generally, a ratio of 1.80 is the lower limit of normal.

The origin of the retinal standing potential is thought to be in the retinal pigment epithelium. However, the light rise is generated by light stimulation of the photoreceptor–retinal pigment epithelium complex; and it is not detected when certain structures of the middle retinal layer is affected, such as in central retinal arterial occlusion.[71]

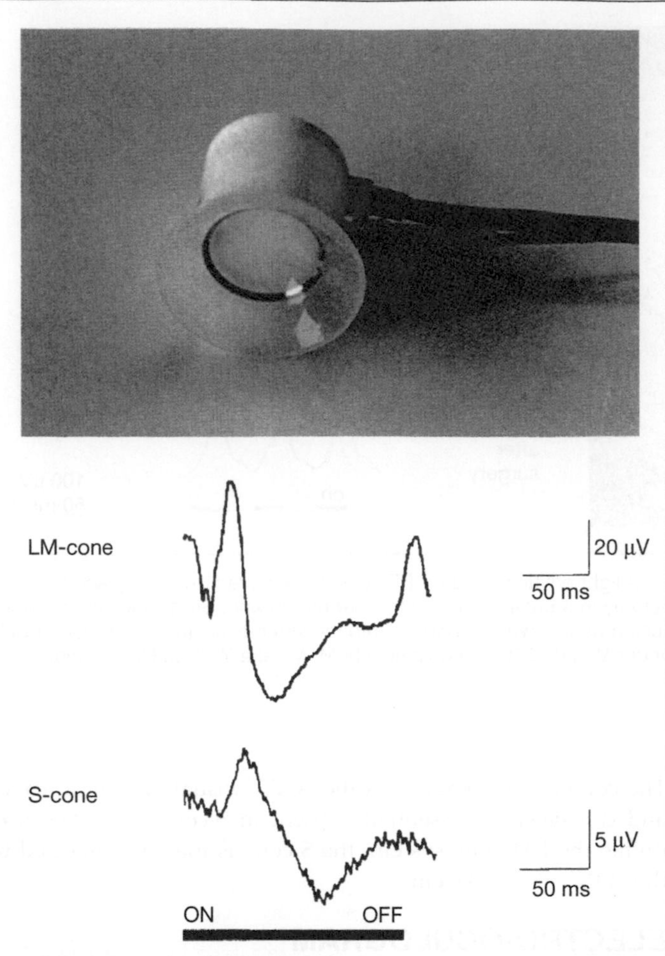

Fig. 8.33 S-cone electroretinogram (ERG) recording with blue-emitting light-emitting diode (LED) built-in contact lens electrode. Top, LED built-in contact lens electrode with blue-emitting LEDs. Bottom, comparison of long-wavelength (LM) cone and S-cone ERGs with long-duration stimuli in a normal subject. The a-wave and d-wave that reflect the "OFF" visual system are essentially absent in the S-cone ERGs, because, unlike the LM cone system, the S-cone is mainly connected to the "ON" visual system. (Reproduced with permission from Miyake Y. Electrodiagnosis of retinal diseases. Tokyo: Springer-Verlag; 2006, and Horiguchi M, Miyake Y, Kondo M, et al. Invest Ophthalmol Vis Sci 1995;36:1730–2.)

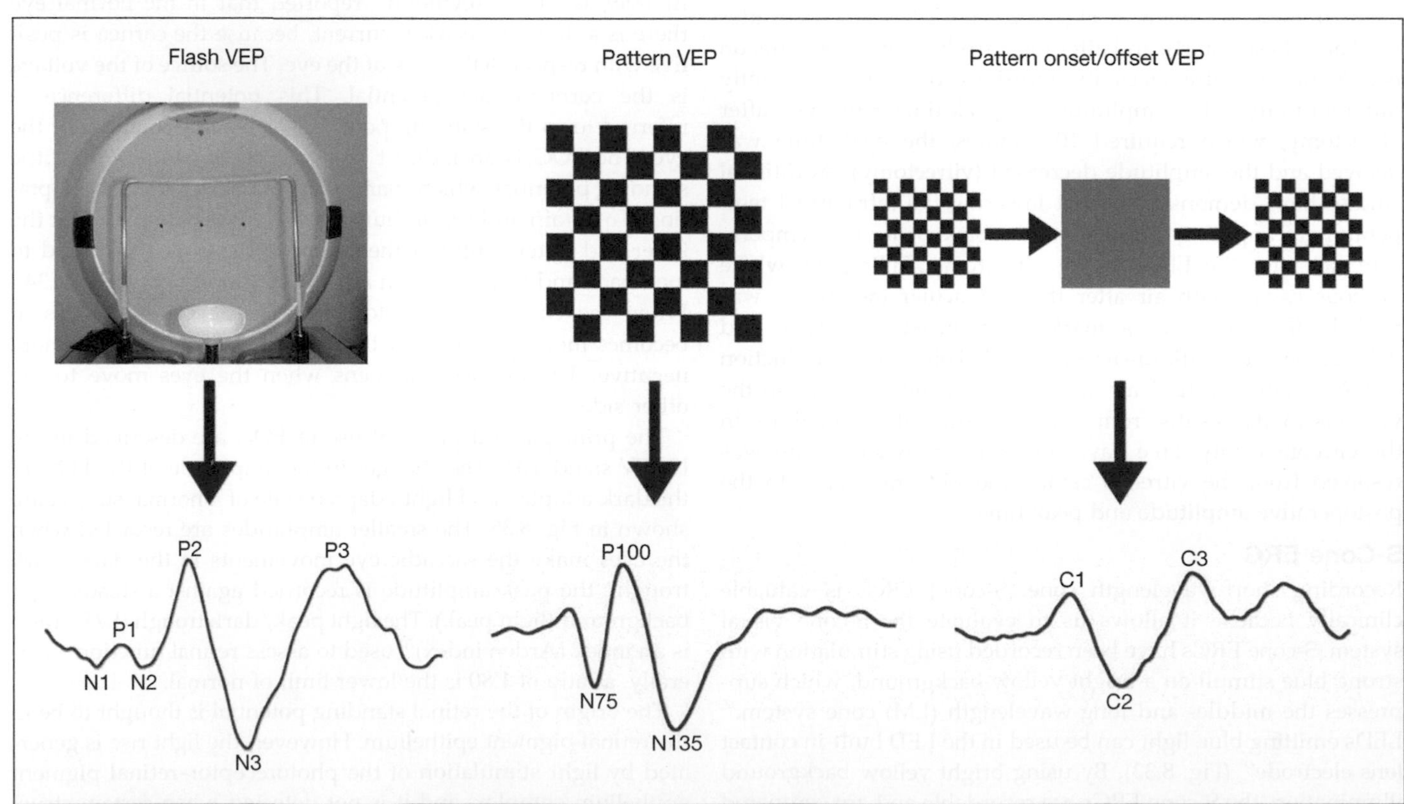

Fig. 8.34 Three standard responses in a clinical visual evoked potential (VEP) test. Top, VEP stimulation. Left, flash stimulus is delivered with monitor or full-field dome. Such a dome is used for recording full-field electroretinogram as well and a pair of fixation lights in the dome is used for an electro-oculogram test. Middle, reversing black-and-white checkerboard stimulus provided using cathode ray tube or light-emitting diode (LED) monitor. Right, reversing black-and-white checkerboard stimulus with diffuse blank screen at regular intervals is presented.

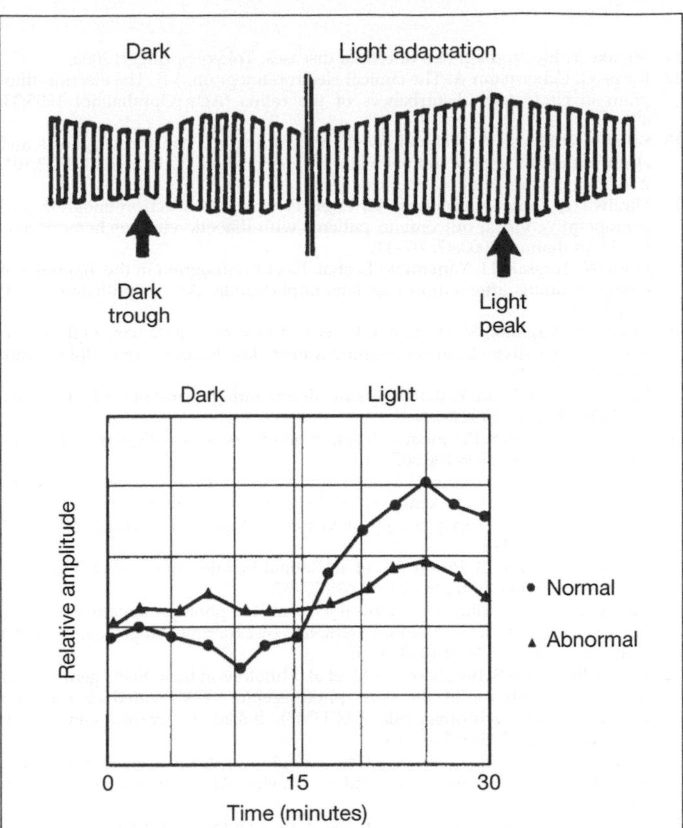

Fig. 8.35 Electro-oculogram (EOG) recordings. Top, diagram illustrating the EOG test and the determination of the light peak/dark trough (L/D) ratio (Arden ratio), which is 2.0 in this case. The smaller amplitudes are recorded when the eyes make saccadic eye movements in the dark (dark trough); the peak amplitude is recorded against a steady light background (light peak). Bottom, plottings of the amplitude of EOG in a normal subject and a patient with Best disease. The Arden ratio is 2.0 for the normal subject and 1.3 for the patient.

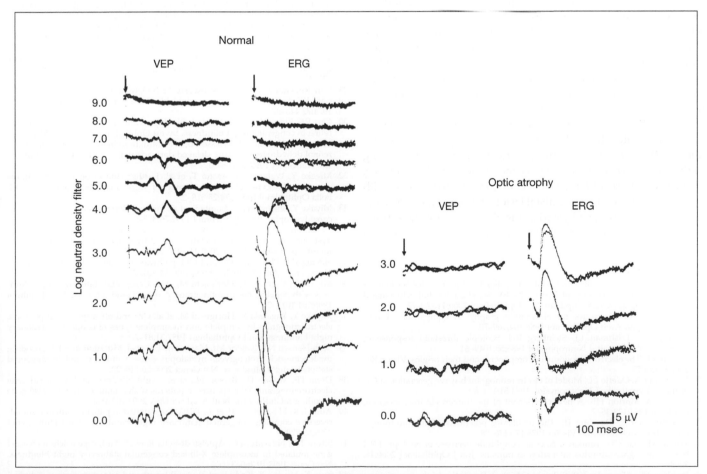

Fig. 8.36 Simultaneous recording of flash visual evoked potential (VEP) and full-field electroretinogram (ERG) with different stimulus intensities in a normal subject and in a patient with optic atrophy. For the recording, a silver disc electrode was placed on the scalp over the visual cortex at Oz according to the International 10/20 system[74] for VEP and a Beckman's electrode was attached to the center of the inferior eyelid. In a normal subject, stimulus threshold for VEP is much lower than that for ERG. In contrast, the stimulus threshold for VEP is higher than that for ERG in a patient with optic atrophy. This can be used to differentiate whether retina or optic nerve is the pathological site in eyes with opaque media. The arrow indicates stimulus onset.

The EOG is generally abnormal in any condition in which the flash ERG is abnormal, except complete or incomplete CSNB.[36] The reverse, however, is not true. An abnormal EOG with a normal ERG may be seen in Best disease, pattern dystrophy of the RPE, and dominant drusen.

VISUAL EVOKED POTENTIAL

The visual evoked potential (VEP) is the signal of the brain evoked by the visual stimulus. It is recorded, like the electroencephalogram (EEG), at the scalp in the occipital region by surface electrodes. The principle and practical use of clinical VEP are shown in the ISCEV standard.[72]

The cellular sources of the VEP are poorly understood. VEPs can be recorded under either transient or steady-state stimulus conditions. The transient VEP includes flash VEP, pattern reversal VEP, and pattern onset/offset VEP (Fig. 8.34).

Several important features of the VEP can be stated:

1. The VEP is dominated by the central 20° of retina owing to "cortical magnification."
2. The VEP is highly variable among individuals, but varies less than 10% bilaterally when responses from the two eyes of a single person are compared.
3. VEP abnormality can result from abnormality in the retina, optic nerve, optic tracts, optic radiations, or visual cortex.

Flash VEP is easy to record, so is performed for evaluation of gross visual function in infants, small children, or in persons who are unable to perform PERG because of poor fixation due to poor visual function, nystagmus, or incorporation. Since flash VEP may still be recordable in patients with undetectable ERG, such as retinitis pigmentosa or dense vitreous hemorrhage, simultaneous recordings of flash VEP and ERG may provide useful information[73] (Fig. 8.36).

Pattern VEP is elicited by a checkerboard pattern of alternating black-and-white checks that reverse in a regular phase frequency. It is a robust response and relatively consistent among individuals and in most cases is the clinical study of choice. Clinically, pattern VEP is a test of choice mainly for patients with optic nerve disease or more distal lesion and nonorganic disease, such as malingering or hysteria. It is also useful for the estimation of visual acuity and monitoring developmental changes in small children.

REFERENCES

1. Marmor MF, Fulton AB, Holder GE, et al. For the International Society for Clinical Electrophysiology of Vision. ISCEV Standard for full-field clinical electroretinography (2008 update). Doc Ophthalmol 2009;118:69–77.
2. Gjötterberg M. Electrodes for electroretinography: A comparison of four different types. Arch Ophthalmol 1986;104:569–70.
3. Sieving PA, Frishman LJ, Steinberg RH. Scotopic threshold response of proximal retina in cat. J Neurophysiol 1986;56:1049–61.
4. Brown KT. The electroretinogram: its components and their origins. Vision Res 1968;8:633–77.
5. Newman EA, Odette LL. Model of electroretinogram b-wave generation: a test of the K^+ hypothesis. J Neurophysiol. 1984;51:164–82.
6. Cobb WA, Morton HB. A new component of the human electroretinogram. J Physiol 1954;123:36–7.
7. Wachtmeister L, Dowling JE. The oscillatory potentials of the mudpuppy retina. Invest Ophthalmol Vis Sci 1978;17:1176–88.
8. Kondo M, Piao CH, Tanikawa A, et al. Amplitude decrease of photopic ERG b-wave at higher stimulus intensities in humans. Jpn J Ophthalmol 2000;44: 20–8.
9. Peachey NS, Alexander KR, Fishman GA, et al. Properties of the human cone system electroretinogram during light adaptation. Appl Optics 1989;28: 1145–50.
10. Yonemura D, Aoki T, Tsuzuki K. Electroretinogram in diabetic retinopathy. Arch Ophthalmol 1962;68:19–24.
11. Miyake Y. Electrodiagnosis of retinal diseases. Tokyo: Springer; 2006.
12. Karpe G, Uchermann A. The clinical electroretinogram. VII. The electroretinogram in circulatory disturbances of the retina. Acta Ophthalmol 1955;33: 493–516.
13. Sabates R, Hirose T, McMeel JW. Electroretinography in the prognosis and classification of central retinal vein occlusion. Arch Ophthalmol 1983;101: 232–5.
14. Hiraiwa T, Horio N, Terasaki H, et al. Preoperative electroretinogram and postoperative visual outcome in patients with diabetic vitreous hemorrhage. Jpn J Ophthalmol 2003;47:307–11.
15. Horio N, Terasaki H, Yamamoto E, et al. Electroretinogram in the diagnosis of endophthalmitis after intraocular lens implantation. Am J Ophthalmol 2001; 132:258–9.
16. Miyake Y, Yagasaki K, Horiguchi M, et al. Congenital stationary night blindness with negative electroretinogram: a new classification. Arch Ophthalmol 1986;104:1013–20.
17. Horiguchi M, Miyake Y. Batten disease: deteriorating course of ocular findings. Jpn J Ophthalmol 1992;36:91–6.
18. Berson EL, Lessell S. Paraneoplastic night blindness with malignant melanoma. Am J Ophthalmol 1988;106:307–11.
19. Heckenlively JR, Aptsiauri N, Holder GE. Autoimmune retinopathy, CAR and MAR syndromes. In: Heckenlively JR, Arden GB, editors. Principles and practice of clinical electrophysiology of vision. 2nd edn. Cambridge, MA: MIT Press; 2006. p. 691–8.
20. Hirose T, Katsumi O, Pruett RC, et al. Retinal function in birdshot retinochoroidopathy. Acta Ophthalmol 1991;69:327–37.
21. Viswanathan S, Frishiman LJ, Robson JG, et al. The photopic negative response of the macaque electroretinogram: reduction by experimental glaucoma. Invest Ophthalmol Vis Sci 1999;40:1124–36.
22. Kohl S, Baumann B, Broghammer M, et al. Mutatons in the *CNGB3* gene encoding the beta-subunit of the cone photoreceptor cGMP-gated channel are responsible for achromatopsia (ACHM3) linked to chromosome 8q21. Hum Mol Genet 2000;9:2107–16.
23. Oguchi C. Über die eigenartige Hemeralopie mit diffuser weissgr ä ulicher Verfärbung des Augenhintergrundes. Graefes Arch Ophthalmol 1912;81: 109–17.
24. Mizuo A. On a new discovery in the dark adaptation in Oguchi's disease. Acta Soc Ophthalmol Jpn 1913;17:1854–9.
25. Miyake Y, Horiguchi M, Suzuki S, et al. Electrophysiological findings in patients with Oguchi's disease. Jpn J Ophthalmol 1996;40:511–9.
26. Fucks S, Nakazawa M, Maw M, et al. A homozygous 1-base pair deletion in the arrestin gene is a frequent cause of Oguchi disease in Japanese. Nat Genet 1995;10:360–2.
27. Yamamoto S, Sipple KC, Berson EL, et al. Defects in the rhodopsin kinase gene in the Oguchi form of stationary night blindness. Nat Genet 1997;15: 175–8.
28. Carr RE, Gouras P. Oguchi's disease. Arch Ophthalmol 1965;73:646–56.
29. Carr RE. Congenital stationary night blindness. Trans Am Ophthalmol Soc 1974;72:448–87.
30. Carr RE, Ripps H, Siegel IM, et al. Rhodopsin and the electrical activity of the retina in congenital night blindness. Invest Ophthalmol 1966;5:497–507.
31. Yamamoto H, Simon A, Eriksson U, et al. Mutations in the gene encoding 11-*cis* retinol dehydrogenase cause delayed dark adaptation and fundus albipunctatus. Nat Genet 1999;22:188–91.
32. Miyake Y, Watanabe I, Asano T, et al. Further studies on EOG in retinitis punctata albescens: effects of change of dark adaptation time on EOG. Folia Ophthalmol Jpn 1974;25:518–27.
33. Miyake Y, Shiroyama N, Sugita S, et al. Fundus albipunctatus associated with cone dystrophy. Br J Ophthalmol 1992;76:375–9.
34. Nakamura M, Hotta Y, Tanikawa A, et al. A high association with cone dystrophy in fundus albipunctatus caused by mutations of the RDH5 gene. Invest Ophthalmol Vis Sci 2000;41:3925–32.
35. Sieving PA. Photopic ON- and OFF-pathway abnormalities in retinal dytrophies. Trans Am Ophthalmol Soc 1993;91:701–73.
36. Miyake Y, Yagasaki K, Horiguchi M, et al. Congenital stationary night blindness with negative electroretinogram. A new classification. Arch Ophthalmol 1986;104:1013–20.
37. Miyake Y, Yagasaki K, Horiguchi M, et al. On- and off-responses in photopic electroretinogram in complete and incomplete types of congenital stationary night blindness. Jpn J Ophthalmol 1987;31:81–7.
38. Bech-Hansen NT, Naylor MJ, Maybaum TA, et al. Mutation in *NYX*, encoding the leucine-rich proteoglycan nyctalopin, cause X-linked complete congenital stationary night blindness. Nat Genet 2000;26:319–23.
39. Dryja TP, McGee TL, Berson EL, et al. Night blindness and abnormal cone electroretinogram ON responses in patients with mutations in the *GRM6* gene encoding mGluR6. Proc Natl Acad Sci USA 2005;102:4884–9.
40. Audo I, Kohl S, Leroy BP, et al. *TRPM1* is mutated in patients with autosomal-recessive complete congenital stationary night blindness. Am J Hum Genet 2009;85:720–9.
41. Strom TM, Nyakatura G, Apfelstedt-Sylla E, et al. An L-type calcium-channel gene mutated in incomplete X-linked congenital stationary night blindness. Nat Genet 1998;19:260–3.
42. Kato K, Miyake Y, Kachi S, et al. Axial length and refractive error in X-linked retinoschisis. Am J Ophthalmol 2001;131:812–4.
43. Sauer CG, Gehrig A, Warneke-Wittstock R, et al. Positional cloning of the gene associated with X-linked juvenile retinoschisis. Nat Genet 1997;17: 164–70.

44. Sieving PA. Juvenile X-linked retinoschisis. In: Heckenlively JR, Arden GB, editors. Principles and practice of clinical electrophysiology of vision, 2nd edn. Cambridge, MA: MIT Press; 2006. p. 823–7.
45. Miyake Y, Shiroyama N, Ota I, et al: Oscillatory potentials in electroretinograms of the human macular region. Invest Ophthalmol Vis Sci 1988;29:1631–5.
46. Sutter EE, Tan D. The field topography of ERG components in man-I. The photopic luminance response. Vision Res 1992;32:433–46.
47. Miyake Y, Shiroyama N, Horiguchi M, et al. Asymmetry of focal ERG in human macular region. Invest Ophthalmol Vis Sci 1989;30:1743–9.
48. Hood DC, Bach M, Brigell M, et al. For the International Society for Clinical Electrophysiology of Vision. ISCEV guidelines for clinical multifocal electroretinography (2007 edition). Doc Ophthalmol 2008;116:1–11.
49. Miyake Y, Miyake K, Shiroyama N. Classification of aphakic cystoid macular edema with focal macular electroretinograms. Am J Ophthalmol 1993;116:576–83.
50. Tanikawa A, Horiguchi M, Kondo M, et al. Abnormal focal macular electroretinograms in eyes with idiopathic epimacular membrane. Am J Ophthalmol 1999;127:559–64.
51. Miyake Y, Shiroyama N, Ota I, et al. Local macular electroretinographic responses in idiopathic central serous chorioretinopathy. Am J Ophthalmol 1988;106:546–50.
52. Miyake Y, Ichikawa K, Shiose Y, et al. Hereditary macular dystrophy without visible fundus abnormality. Am J Ophthalmol 1989;292–9.
53. Miyake Y, Horiguchi M, Tomita N, et al. Occult macular dystrophy. Am J Ophthalmol 1996;122:644–53.
54. Akahori M, Tsunoda K, Miyake Y, et al. Dominant mutations in *RP1L1* are responsible for occult macular dystrophy. Am J Hum Genet 2010;87:424–9.
55. Gass JD. Acute zonal occult outer retinopathy. J Clin Neurol Ophthalmol 1993;13:79–97.
56. Holder GE, Brigell MG, Hawlina M, et al. For the International Society for Clinical Electrophysiology of Vision. ISCEV standard for clinical pattern electroretinography. (2007 update). Doc Ophthalmol 2007;114:111–6.
57. Maffei L, Fiorentini A. Electroretinographic responses to alternating gratings before and after section of the optic nerve. Science 1981;211:953–5.
58. Holder GE. The pattern electroretinogram. In: Heckenlively JR, Arden GB, editors. Principles and practice of clinical electrophysiology of vision, 2nd edn. Cambridge, MA: MIT Press; 2006. p. 341–51.
59. Ogino K, Tsujikawa A, Nakamura H, et al. Focal macular electroretinogram in macular edema secondary to central retinal vein occlusion. Invest Ophthalmol Vis Sci. 2011;52:3514–20.
60. Nakamura H, Miyamoto K, Yokota S, et al. Focal macular photopic negative response in patients with optic neuritis. Eye (Lond) 2011;25:358–64.
61. Machida S, Gotoh Y, Toba Y, et al. Correlation between photopic negative response and retinal nerve fiber layer thickness and optic disc topography in glaucomatous eyes. Invest Ophthalmol Vis Sci 2008;49:2201–7.
62. Kooijman AC, Damhof A. ERG lens with built-in ganzfeld light source for stimulation and adaptation. Invest Ophthalmol Vis Sci 1980;19:315–8.
63. Kondo M, Piao CH, Tanikawa A, et al. A contact lens electrode with built-in high intensity white light-emitting diodes. A contact lens electrode with built-in white LEDs. Doc Ophthalmol 2001;102:1–9.
64. Miyake Y, Yagasaki K, Horiguchi M, et al. Electroretinographic monitoring of retinal function during eye surgery. Arch Ophthalmol 1991;109:1123–6.
65. Miyake Y, Yagasaki K, Ichikawa H. Differential diagnosis of congenital tritanopia and dominantly inherited juvenile optic atrophy. Arch Ophthalmol 1985:103:1496–501.
66. Horiguchi M, Miyake Y, Kondo M, et al. Blue light-emitting diode built-in contact lens electrode can record human S-cone electroretinogram. Invest Ophthalmol Vis Sci 1995;36:1730–2.
67. Kolb H, Lipets LE. The anatomical basis for color vision in the vertebrate retina. In: Gouras P, editor. The perception of colour. London: Macmillan; 1991. p. 128–45.
68. Du Bois Reymond EH. Chapter 3. Von dem ruhen Nervenstrome. Untersuchungen Über Thierische Electricität. Vol. 2. Berlin: G Reimer; 1849; p. 251–288.
69. Marmor MF, Brigell MG, McCulloch DL, et al. For the International Society for Clinical Electrophysiology of Vision. ISCEV standard for clinical electro-oculography (2010 update). Doc Ophthalmol 2011;122:1–7.
70. Arden GB, Barrada A, Kelsey JH. New clinical test of retinal function based upon the standing potential of the eye. Br J Ophthalmol 1962;46:449–67.
71. Arden GB. Origin and significance of the electro-oculogram. In: Heckenlively JR, Arden GB, editors. Principles and practice of clinical electrophysiology of vision. 2nd edn. Cambridge, MA: MIT Press; 2006. p. 123–138.
72. Odom JV, Bach M, Brigell M, et al. ISCEV standard for clinical visual evoked potentials (2009 update). Doc Ophthalmol. 2010;120:111–9.
73. Miyake Y, Hirose T, Hara A. Electrophysiologic testing of visual functions for vitrectomy candidates. I. Results in eyes with known fundus diseases. Retina 1983;3:86–94.
74. American Clinical Neurophysiology Society. Guideline 5: guidelines for standard electrode position nomenclature. J Clin Neurophysiol 2006;23:107–110. Available at https://www.acns.org/.

Chapter 9

Diagnostic Ophthalmic Ultrasound

Rudolf F. Guthoff, Leanne T. Labriola, Oliver Stachs

INTRODUCTION

Ultrasonography is a pervasive diagnostic tool within medicine. It is used to obtain noninvasive images that can aid in the management of patients in almost all fields of medicine. Ultrasound technology has a unique role in ophthalmology since it can provide quantitative and qualitative assessments of the globe and orbit. Ultrasound images are formed by capturing the reflected acoustic signal from different tissues. These images can provide important details of almost every part of the eye from the anterior cornea and ciliary body to the posterior retina and choroid. This chapter will explain the principles involved in ophthalmic ultrasound as well as provide examples of its use within ophthalmology.

ULTRASOUND – PAST AND PRESENT

In 1880, the Curie brothers first demonstrated that a difference in electric potential could be created by mechanically pressing opposing surfaces of a tourmaline crystal.[1-7] This phenomenon is called the piezoelectric effect. This effect is the basis for ultrasound technology and was first applied in underwater sonar systems during World War II.[8] During that same era, the medical community also adopted the use of ultrasound technology. Scientists realized the diagnostic potential of this technology when they were able to use acoustic wavelengths to study the consistency of a material without damaging the material itself.

In 1949, Ludwig used ultrasound to detect gallstones in patients. The first publication on the use of ophthalmologic ultrasound appeared in the medical literature in 1956.[9] By the mid-1970s, ophthalmologists were using ultrasound to determine axial length in a clinical setting. These measurements facilitated calculations of intraocular lens power which led to a revolution in cataract surgery.[10] Further innovations came when Baum and Greenwood introduced their two-dimensional B-mode image to ophthalmology.[11] Soon afterwards, Bronson et al.[12] developed a hand-held contact transducer for this type of image acquisition which led to the rapid dissemination of ultrasound devices within ophthalmology clinics. The B-mode images could be used to delineate accurately retinal detachments, vitreous membranes, and choroidal tumors. In the early 1990s, new technology made it possible to image the anterior segment of the eye with devices that captured images at higher frequencies of 35–50 MHz. This improved image resolution four- to fivefold and is still the gold standard for analysis of certain anterior-segment diseases such as ciliary body effusions, infiltrates, and tumors.

EXAMINATION TECHNIQUES

The ultrasound examination is performed with the patient in a reclined position. The frequency of the ultrasound cannot pass through air; therefore, a coupling medium is needed to transmit the sound waves from the transducer to the ocular tissues. A common coupling agent is methylcellulose (Fig. 9.1). The coupling agent is applied to the tip of the transducer probe, which is then placed on the patient's anesthetized cornea.

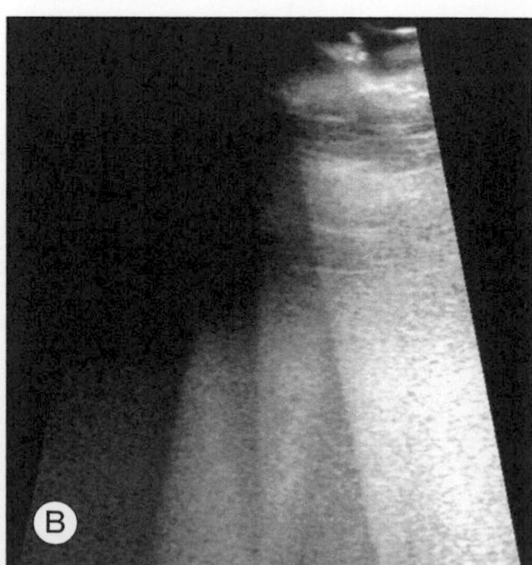

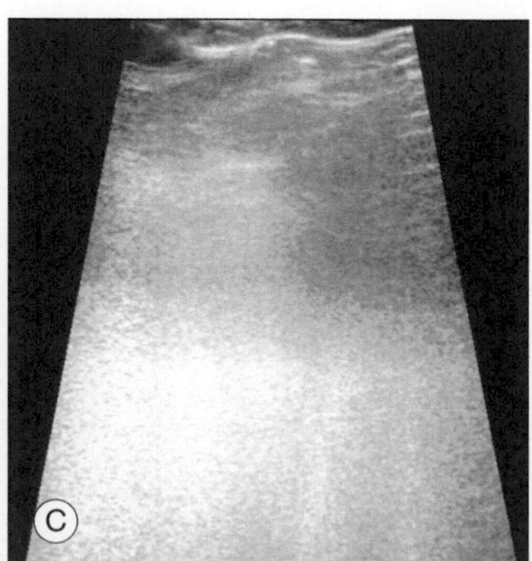

Fig. 9.1 Ultrasound images simulating the effect of transducer (A) without tissue-coupling agent, (B) with partial tissue-coupling agent, and (C) with a complete coupling agent, such as a gel-like contact substance.

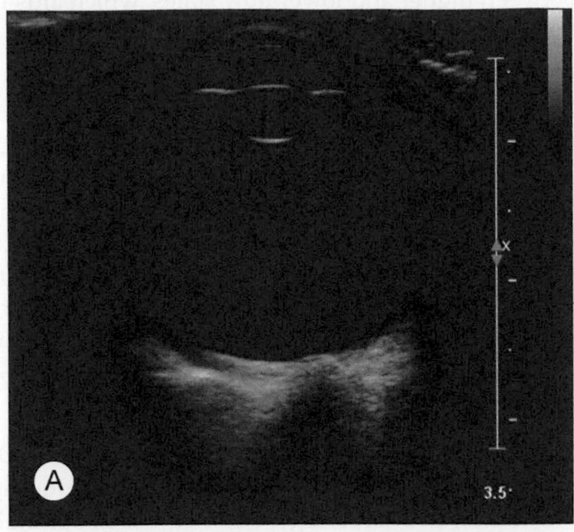

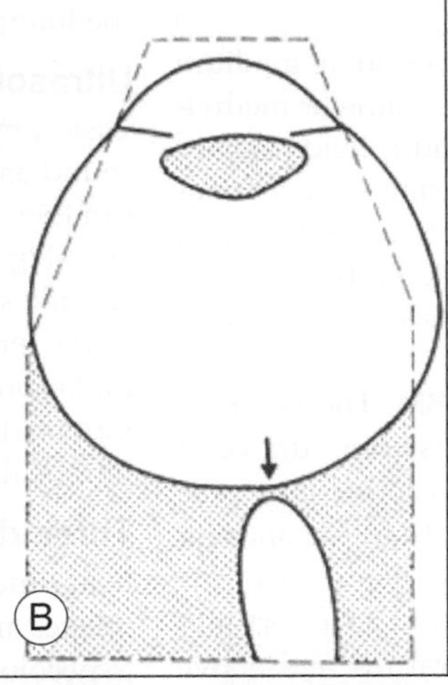

Fig. 9.2 (A) Cross-sectional echogram through a normal globe. (B) Schematic drawing of the eye: the arrow marks the entrance of the optic nerve.

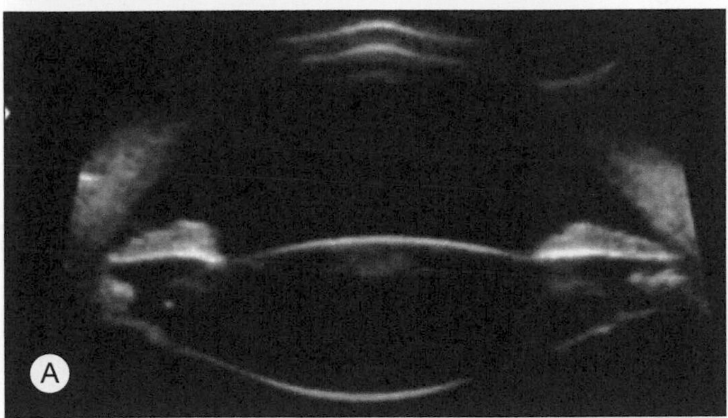

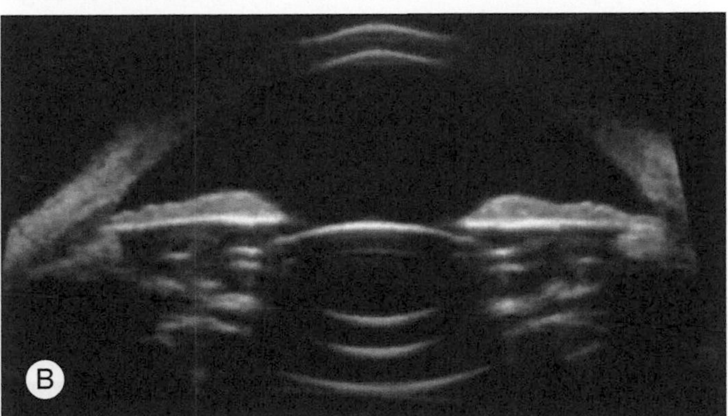

Fig. 9.3 The ultrasound biomicroscopy images of the anterior segment in (A) a phakic and (B) a pseudophakic eye with multiple echo of implant surface.

A-mode technique

The A-scan is a linear representation of echo amplitude that is acquired along a single line of sight. Measurements of the ocular tissue can be achieved using the time interval between emission of the acoustic pulse and echo return to calculate the distance of the tissue being imaged. A-scan images should only be obtained through open lids since the eyelid tissue can attenuate the sound waves and decrease the resolution. The pressure applied by the examiner to the transducer tip is especially important when obtaining A-scan measurements. Excessive pressure can deform the cornea, and lead to inaccurate measurements.

B-mode technique

The B-scan is a two-dimensional cross-section image formed by mechanically sweeping the transducer over an angle of 50–60° with the probe oriented in a specific axis. A systematic approach should be used to acquire all images. One method is first to obtain axial scans of the globe by placing the probe in the center of the cornea with the transducer tip oriented toward 12 o'clock in order to image the posterior pole and optic nerve. Next, the transducer can be turned temporally 90° to obtain images through the macula. Finally, radial and transverse images of the globe can be obtained by placing the probe at each clock-hour around the limbus. Radial scans are acquired when the probe is placed perpendicular to the limbus and the transducer tip is oriented toward the cornea. Transverse scans are obtained by turning the probe 90°, orienting the transducer tip parallel to the limbus. The images obtained are the acoustic reflections from the opposing inner surface of the globe.

The reflected sound waves are recorded by the device and can be viewed as a two-dimensional image on the screen (Fig. 9.2). The ocular structures can be examined individually. The cornea is characterized ultrasonographically by two separate acoustic interfaces. The anterior chamber appears planoconvex in cross-section. The iris diaphragm cannot be satisfactorily imaged because of the limited lateral resolution power of the normal B-mode. A clear lens is acoustically empty and appears as an ellipsoid structure in axial sections. Similarly, normal vitreous does not give an acoustic signal; however, the presence of a detached posterior vitreous membrane presents an interface that can be imaged by increasing the amplification of the echo signal. The sclera is the most strongly reflecting structure on ocular ultrasonography.

High-frequency ultrasound technique

High-frequency echograms can be used for ultrasound biomicroscopy (UBM). The shorter wavelengths provide better resolution of the anterior structures of the eye, including the cornea, lens, aqueous (Fig. 9.3), and ciliary body (Fig. 9.4).[13] High-frequency probes range from 50 to 100 MHz.[14–16] The 50-MHz probe provides the best balance between depth and resolution for UBM technique. One limitation of this technique is that the shorter wavelengths, from the higher frequency, have poor depth of penetration. UBM cannot visualize structures deeper than 4 mm from the surface.

UBM requires immersion of the transducer in a medium to transmit the higher-frequency wavelengths. Saline or methylcellulose can be used as the coupling agent and is held in place over the eye with the use of a custom cup during the examination. UBM is performed through open eyelids in order to obtain a good reflection signal. Images produced by UBM have a resolution of 30–40 µm, which is similar to that seen with a low-power microscope.[17]

The cornea is the first structure seen on UBM. The anterior-chamber depth can be measured from the posterior surface of the cornea to the anterior lens pole. The posterior lens pole cannot be imaged by UBM due to its distance from the anterior surface. The iris is seen as a flat uniform echogenic area. The iris and ciliary body converge in the iris recess and insert into the scleral spur. The area under the peripheral iris and above the ciliary processes is defined as the ciliary sulcus. The angle of the eye can be studied in cross-section by orienting the probe in a radial fashion at the limbus. The scleral spur is the most important landmark in the angle on UBM.

Doppler ultrasound

Doppler images are obtained by using frequency shifts from acoustic reflections to measure movements within a tissue and flow conditions within vessels. These frequency shifts can be observed in tissue volumes of less than 10 mm. False color can be added to the images based on ultrasound frequency to distinguish between higher and lower flow states, which aids in the interpretation of the final result (Fig. 9.5).

Ultrasound biometry

Basic physics formulae can be used to calculate the speed of sound as it passes through various ocular tissues. This number can then be used to calculate distance measurements within the eye (Fig. 9.6). In order to obtain accurate measurements, the specific speed of sound of the different intraocular media, such as the lens, aqueous, and vitreous, must be known.[18] These formulae provide precise measurements that can be used to measure intraocular tumors or to deduce the axial length of the globe for intraocular lens power calculations.

Three-dimensional reconstructions

Real-time three-dimensional (3D) and four-dimensional (4D) images are currently used in some medical specialties, including gynecology, obstetrics, and cardiology, but their use in ophthalmology is limited. 3D ultrasonic images can be produced from a series of scan planes.[19–22] Silverman et al.[23] characterized the ciliary bodies in rabbits and human subjects using 3D high-resolution ultrasound. In the authors' laboratory a simple extension of the Ultrasound Biomicroscope Model 840 (Humphrey Instruments, Carl Zeiss Group) and VuMax UBM 35/50

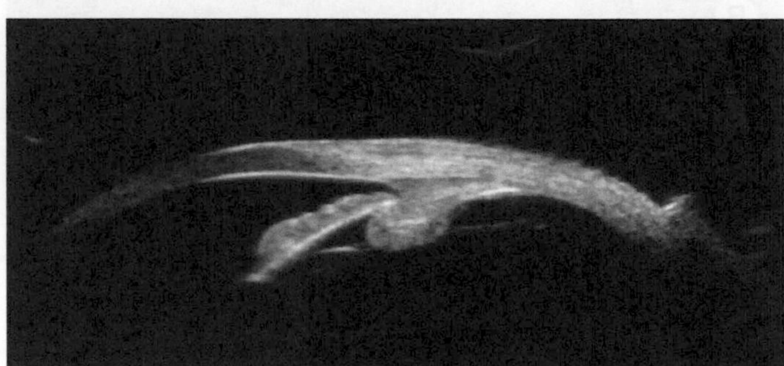

Fig. 9.4 Ultrasound biomicroscopy of the ciliary body.The shorter wavelengths are able to obtain high-resolution images of the anterior structures.

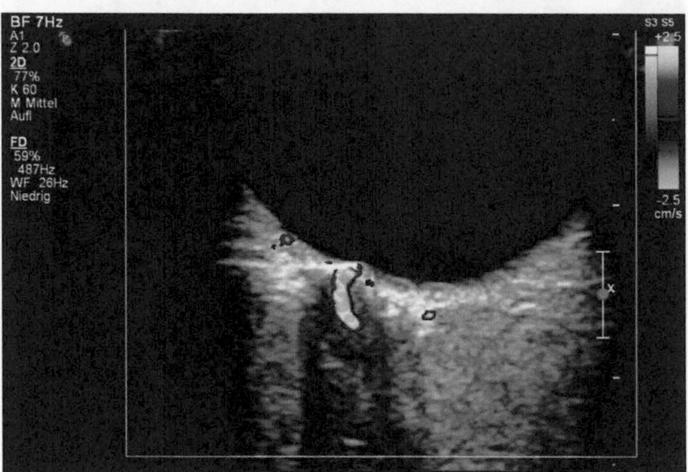

Fig. 9.5 Cross-sectional ultrasonogram through the posterior pole of the eye: color-coded signals from the central retinal artery (red) and the central retinal vein (blue) are displayed inside the optic nerve.

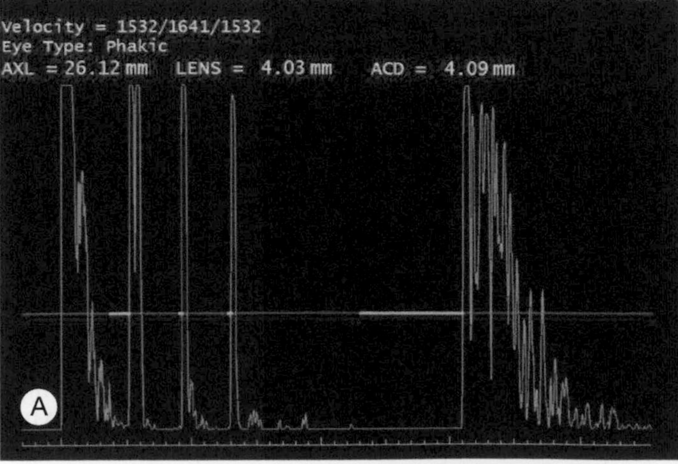

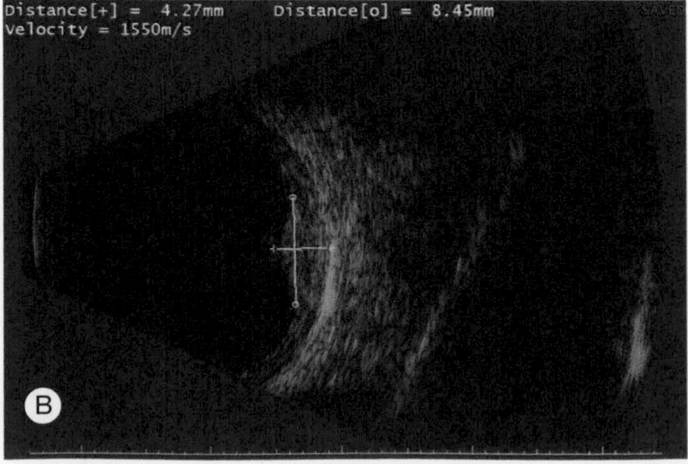

Fig. 9.6 (A) Immersion A-scan biometry showing peak amplitudes of the signal reflection. (B) B-scan image with distance measurement captured on a frozen scan. Measurements are obtained by placing the cursor marks on the image and reading the distance between points.

(Sonomed) into a user-friendly 3D ultrasonic imaging system was developed (Figs 9.7 and 9.8).[24–28]

ULTRASOUND IN INTRAOCULAR PATHOLOGY

Changes in the shape of the globe

Staphyloma

A staphyloma is an abnormal ectasia of the globe that involves uveal tissue. The ectasia typically has a smaller radius of curvature then the normal sclera of the globe. It can be identified on ultrasound by taking axial cross-sectional scans with the transducer probe (Fig. 9.9).

Scleral buckle

A scleral buckle can create a posterior scleral deformity that looks similar to a staphyloma. It can be distinguished from a true staphyloma by a careful history or identification of the encircling band around the anterior sclera. Also, if silicone oil was used for repair, the higher index of refraction within the silicone oil can alter the reflectance of the ultrasound wavelengths, which might provide a false impression of globe deformation (Fig. 9.10).

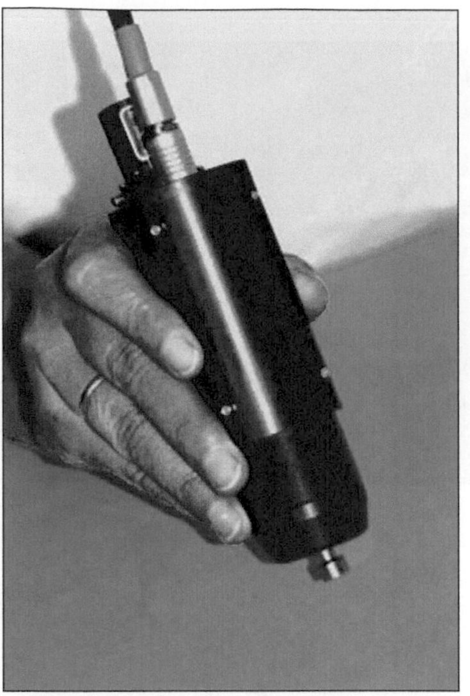

Fig. 9.7 Prototype of a handpiece for three-dimensional high-frequency scanning using the VuMax UBM 35/50 (Sonomed).

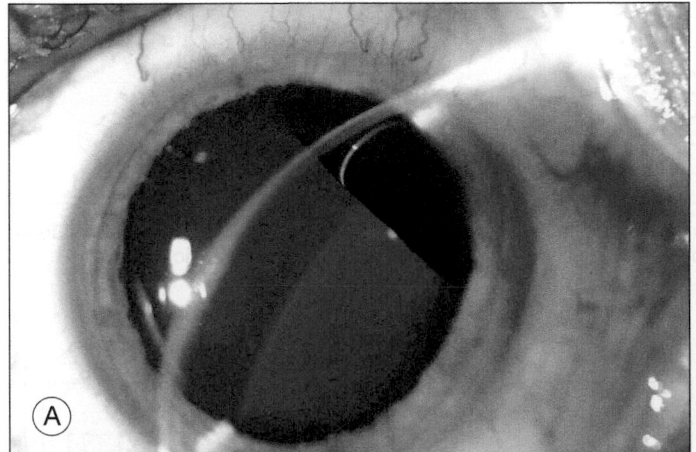

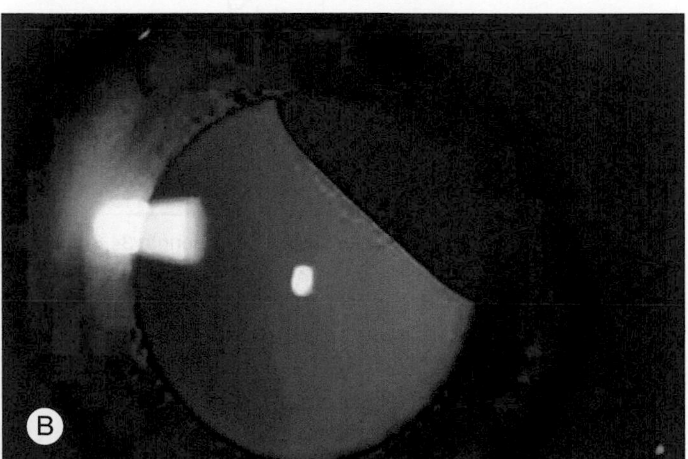

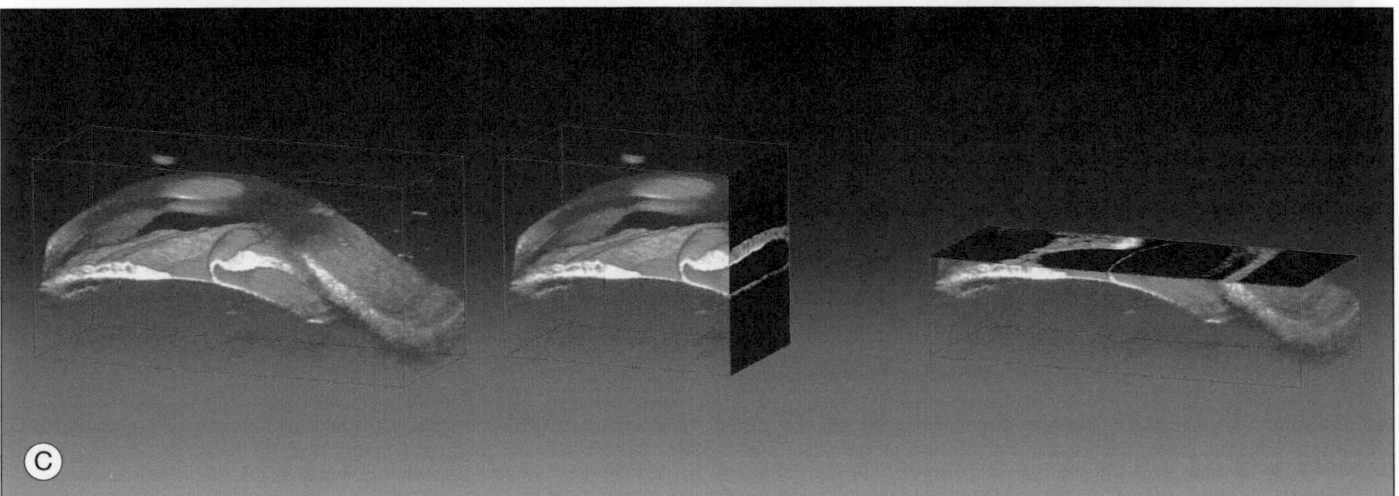

Fig. 9.8 Clinical pictures of the ciliary body with a pigment cyst (A) through a dilated pupil and (B) with retroillumination. (C) The same eye shown with three-dimensional reconstructed volume with oblique sections.

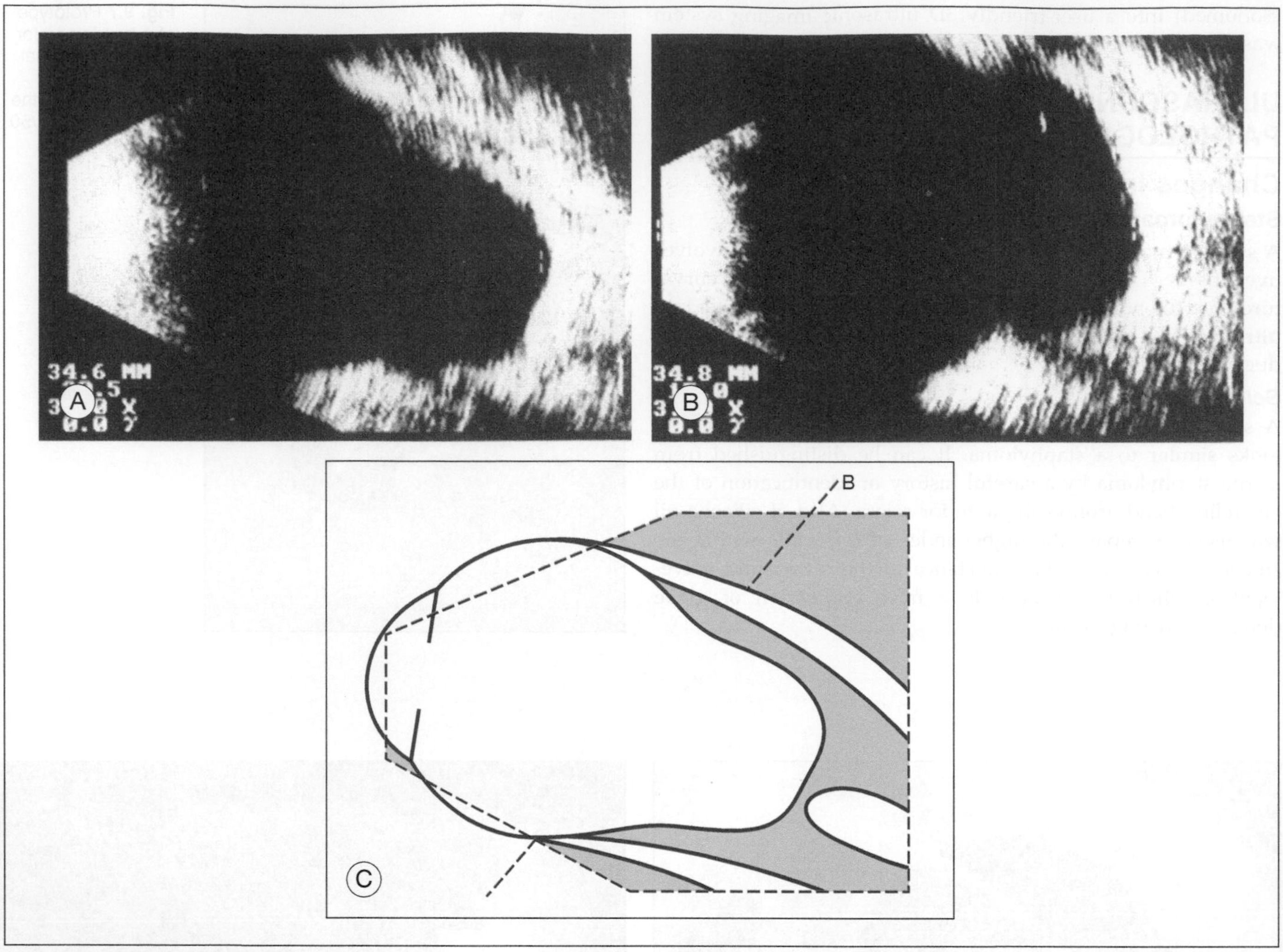

Fig. 9.9 Staphyloma in a highly myopic eye (axial length 34.8 mm). (A) An axial section of the eccentric entrance of the optic nerve can be seen. (B) The misshapen globe is especially well demonstrated on a sectional plane which lies outside the optical axis. (C) Schematic drawing.

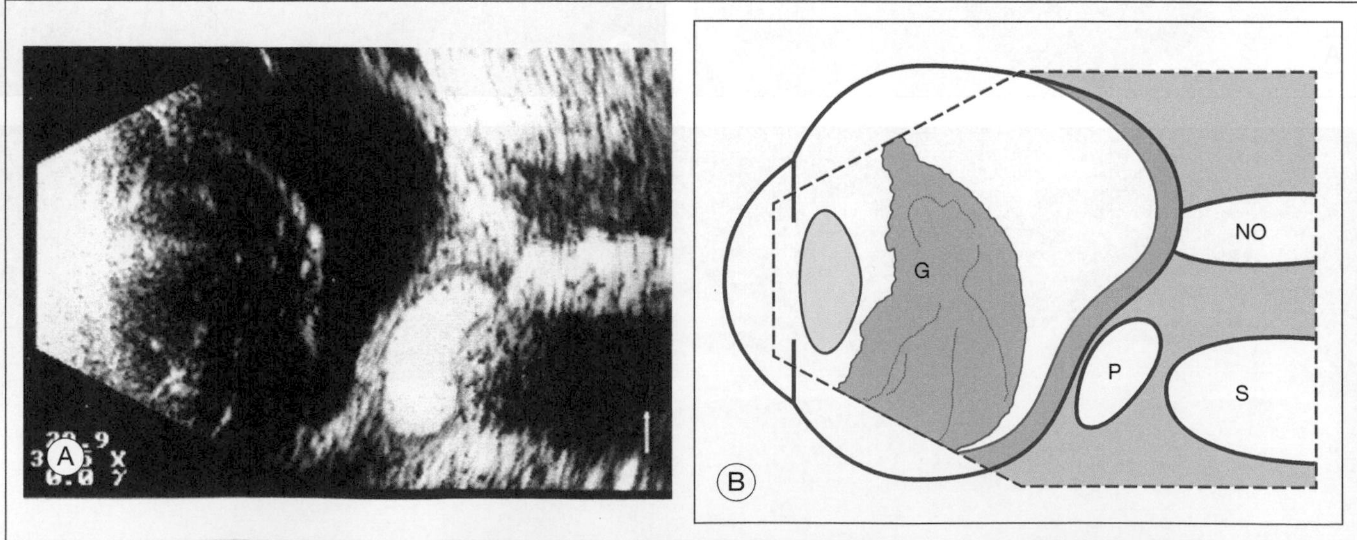

Fig. 9.10 (A) Scleral buckle produced by a silicone sponge explant. After placement of a scleral buckle, the deformity of the globe can be seen in an acoustic cross-section. Silicone explants almost completely reflect the ultrasound. They also cast an acoustic shadow. (B) Schematic drawing. NO, optic nerve; P, explant; S, sound shadow; G, syneretic, densified vitreous.

Microphthalmos

Congenital microphthalmos is an abnormally small eye that can be associated with other ocular abnormalities. The main finding in microphthalmos is axial shortening. This can be identified with A-scan measurements. The B-scan mode can be used to obtain radial and transverse scans to identify abnormalities in the vitreous and posterior segment of the eye, which can also be associated features of microphthalmos. These features include the presence of a coloboma of the retina or optic nerve head, orbital cysts (Fig. 9.11), or persistent hyperplastic vitreous.

Phthisis

Phthisis is defined as severe atrophy of the globe associated with hypotony. Phthisis is characterized ultrasonographically by a thickened outer scleral wall. Occasionally, calcification or ossification may be observed (Fig. 9.12). This may be due to degenerative processes and from metaplasia of the retinal pigment epithelium (RPE). In advanced cases of phthisis, the sclera and choroid can represent up to 70% of the total volume of the globe. The degree of thickening of the globe in chronic hypotony can be an indication of impending phthisis, but the precise thickness threshold for phthisis formation is unknown.

Vitreous

Echographic examination can provide information on vitreous structure which is particularly useful when visualization of the posterior pole is poor due to anterior media opacities. Ultrasonographic findings allow the examiner to differentiate dot-, strand-, and membrane-like reflections (Fig. 9.13). Table 9.1 summarizes the most frequent conditions associated with pathologic changes in the vitreous.

Vitreous degeneration

Vitreous syneresis can appear as dot-like reflections which can be more pronounced in myopia or senile vitreous. During a symptomatic posterior vitreous detachment, the B-mode echo may demonstrate various stages of vitreous syneresis and may reveal the remaining adhesions of the hyaloid membrane to the retinal surface (Fig. 9.14).

Asteroid hyalosis

The calcium-containing lipids of asteroid hyalosis are suspended in the vitreous framework and act as distinctive sound reflectors (Fig. 9.15). They can demonstrate the dynamics of vitreous movements.

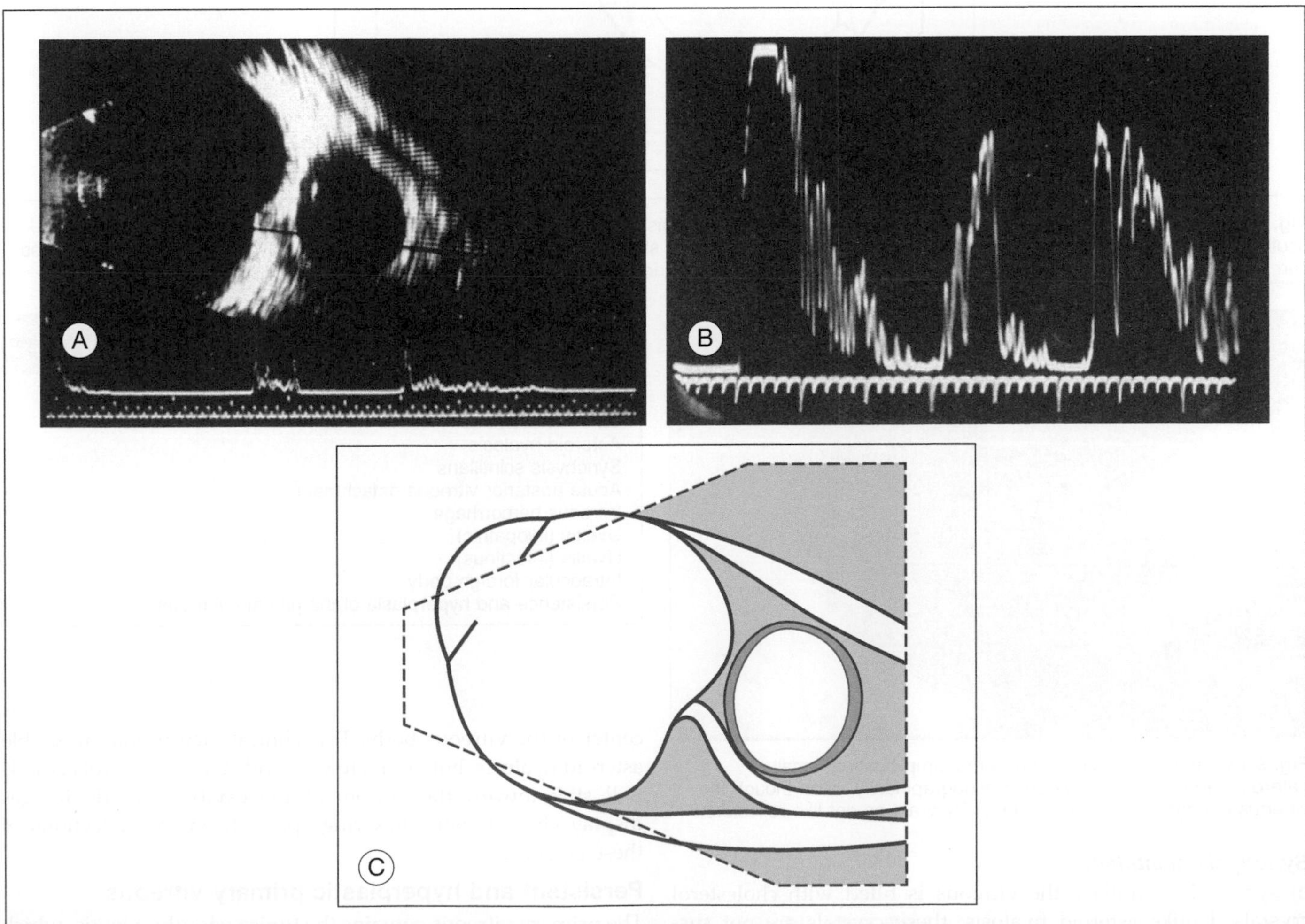

Fig. 9.11 Microphthalmos with orbital cyst. (A) Cystoid space is seen on the B-scan within the muscle cone, which is interpreted as a "completely separated coloboma." (B) A-scan image. (C) Schematic drawing.

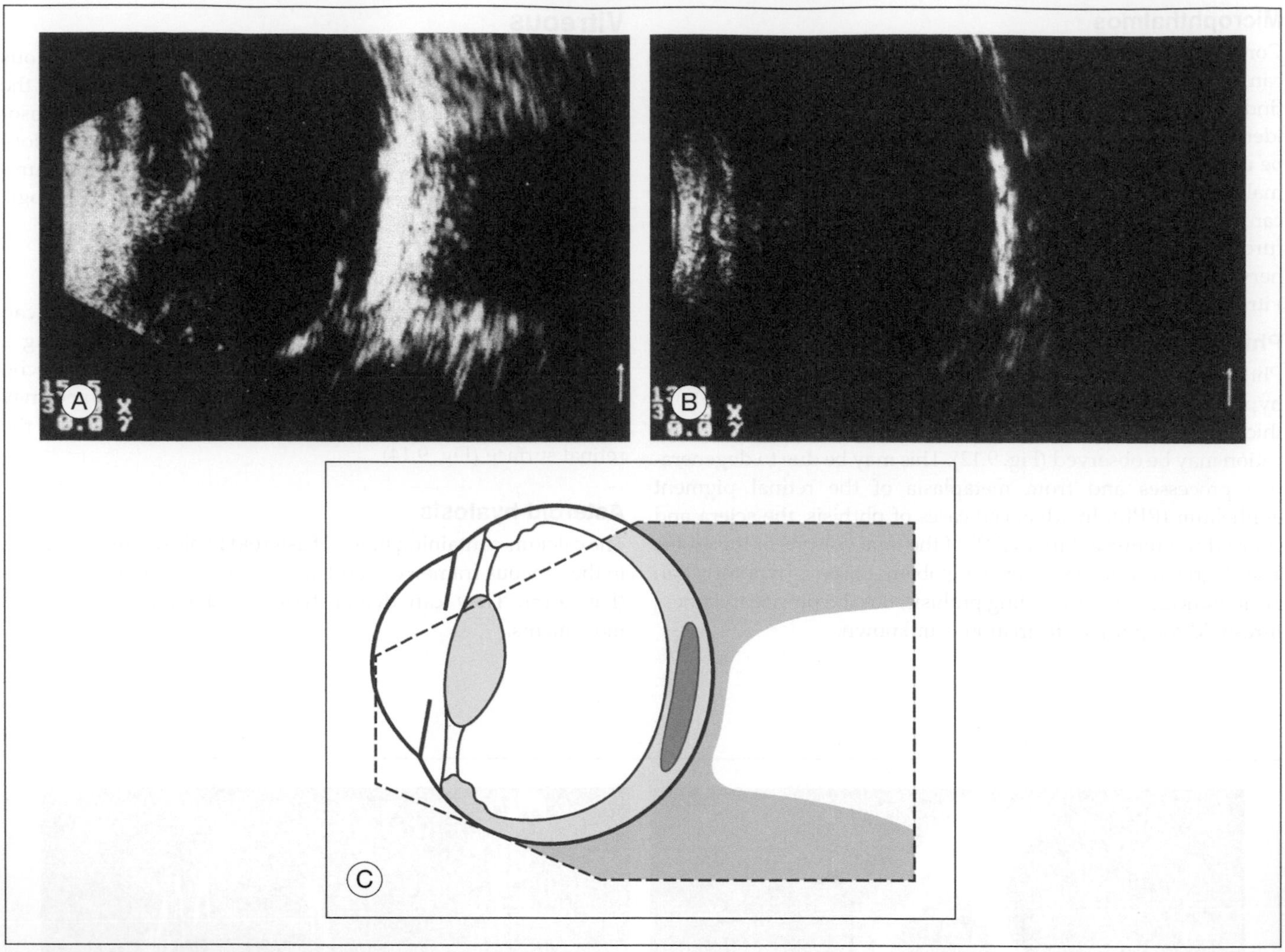

Fig. 9.12 Circumscribed calcification in the ocular wall in advanced phthisis bulbi. (A) Echographically we find highly reflective changes in the ocular wall from calcification or ossification of the choroid which casts a shadow on the soft tissue located posteriorly. (B) These strong echoes can be selectively imaged by reducing the amplification. (C) Schematic drawing.

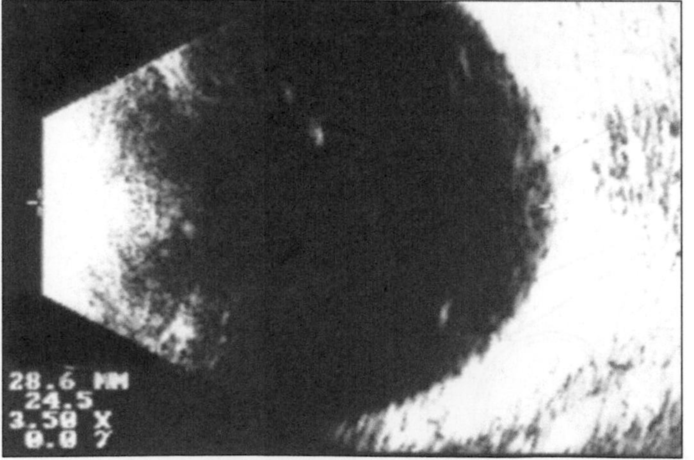

Fig. 9.13 Vitreous opacities. In maximal amplification, small heterogeneous spots can be seen echographically, even though the vitreous appears optically clear (left). They act as dot-like reflectors.

Table 9.1 Clinical conditions with ultrasonographically demonstrable vitreous changes
Changes in the shape of the globe
Vitreous opacities
Asteroid hyalosis
Synchysis scintillans
Acute posterior vitreous detachment
Vitreous hemorrhage
Uveitis (idiopathic)
Uveitis (infectious)
Intraocular foreign body
Persistence and hyperplasia of the primary vitreous

Synchysis scintillans

In synchysis scintillans the vitreous is filled with cholesterol crystals. Unlike asteroid hyalosis, these crystals are not suspended within the vitreous but instead float freely in the vitreous space. When the globe moves, the crystals appear in the center of the vitreous body. This clinical picture may resemble asteroid hyalosis, but after a few seconds the cholesterol crystals will sink toward the bottom of the cavity. A-mode images display characteristic flickering spikes from the reflections of these crystals.

Persistent and hyperplastic primary vitreous

The primary vitreous contains the tunica vasculosa lentis, which is part of the fetal vasculature system. During development, the tunica vasculosa lentis emanates from the optic nerve head

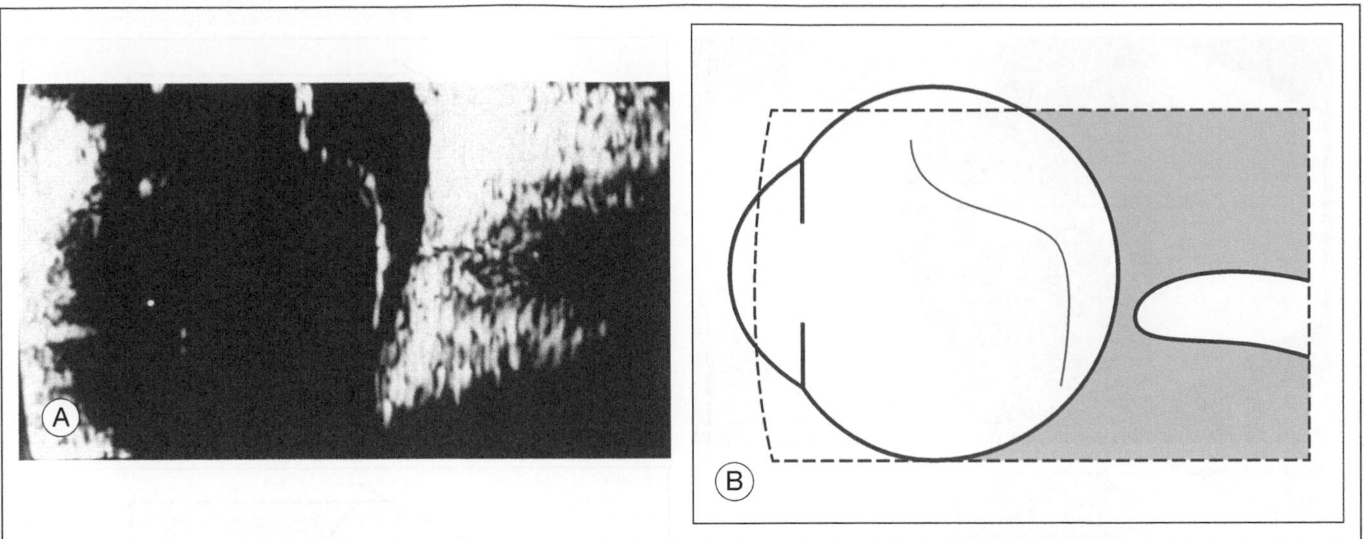

Fig. 9.14 (A) Detached posterior hyaloid membrane imaged as a floating structure of low reflectivity. (B) Schematic drawing.

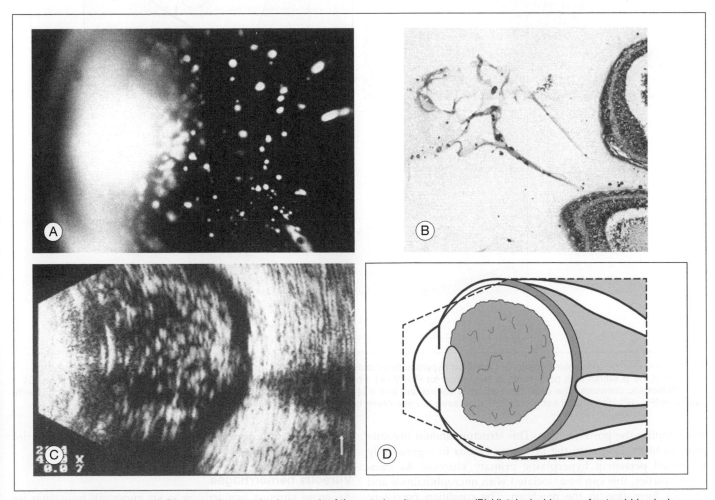

Fig. 9.15 Asteroid hyalosis. (A) Slit-lamp microscopic photograph of the anterior vitreous space. (B) Histological image of asteroid hyalosis shows the calcium crystals adherent to the vitreous scaffold. (C) B-scan cross-section of the crystals, which represent good reflectors for the ultrasound. There is always an echo-free retrovitreal space seen near the ocular walls. (D) Schematic drawing.

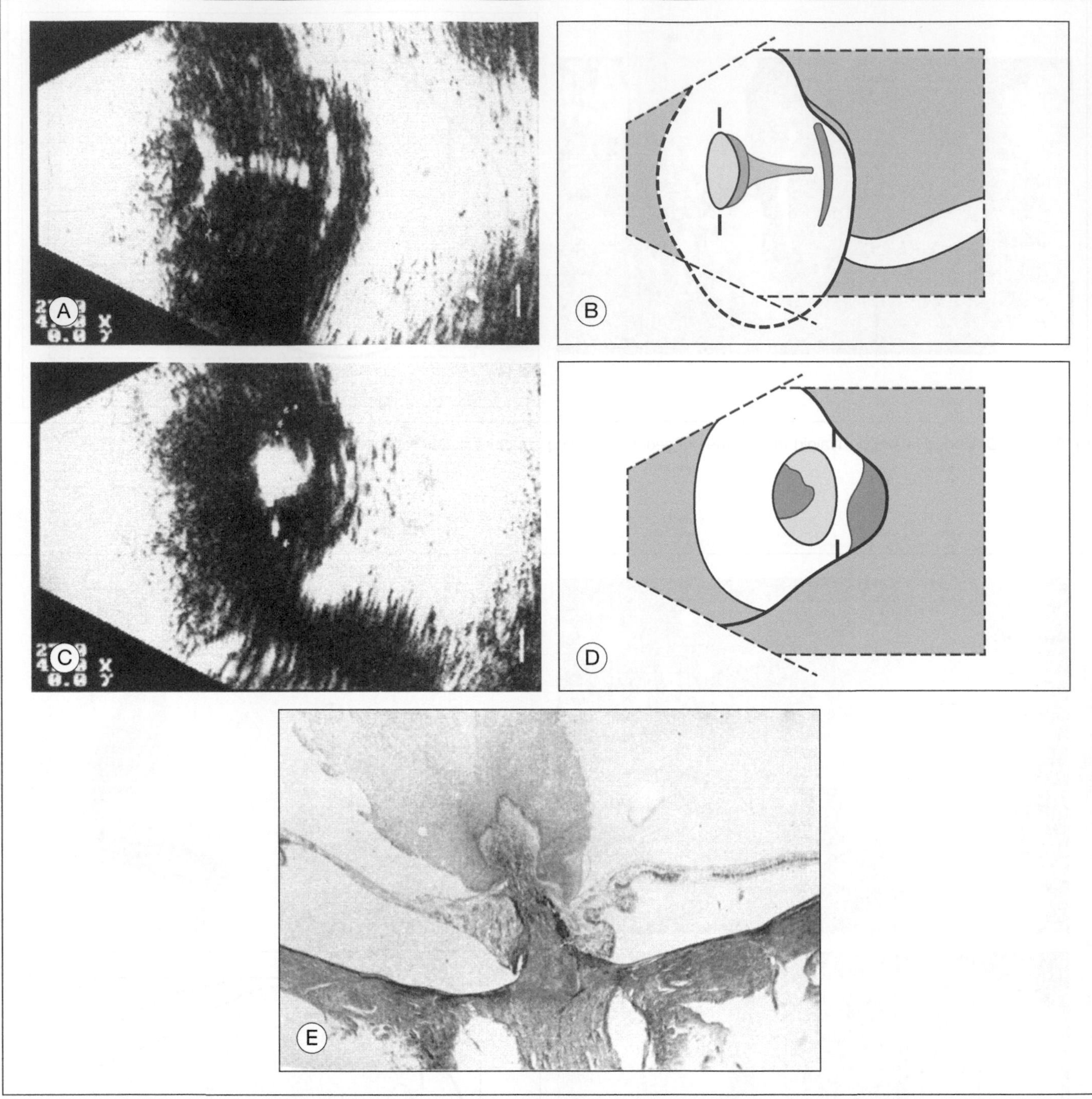

Fig. 9.16 (A–D) Posterior polar cataract in persistent hyperplastic primary vitreous (PHPV). An ultrasonographically demonstrable strand attached to the posterior lens pole points is suspicious for PHPV (A). Frontal plane taken temporally with maximal adduction of the globe (C). (B,D) Schematic drawings. The dark, hatched parts correspond to the opaque area of the posterior cortex and posterior capsule in a child with severe PHPV. (E) Histological section of PHPV as seen at optic nerve head with loupe magnification.

and supplies the posterior lens. This structure should involute prior to birth. Failure of the primary vitreous to regress fully is termed persistent hyperplastic primary vitreous. As mentioned earlier, this can be associated with microphthalmos and cataract formation in the newborn. The condition persistent hyperplastic primary vitreous can be ultrasonographically characterized by two features. The first is a strand of membrane that extends between the posterior surface of the lens and the area of the optic nerve head. The second is the reduced axial length of the globe from microphthalmos on ultrasound biometry (Fig. 9.16). If the anomaly is only mild, the lens may be clear at birth but may become cataractous when the posterior lens capsule ruptures.

Vitreous hemorrhages

An acute vitreous hemorrhage is an important indication for ultrasonography. Acute hemorrhages can fill the vitreous cavity with small opacities from the particles of the red blood cells. These opacities usually accumulate after a few hours in the lower circumference of the vitreous base (Fig. 9.17).

If a detachment of the posterior hyaloid membrane precedes a vitreous hemorrhage, the erythrocytes frequently

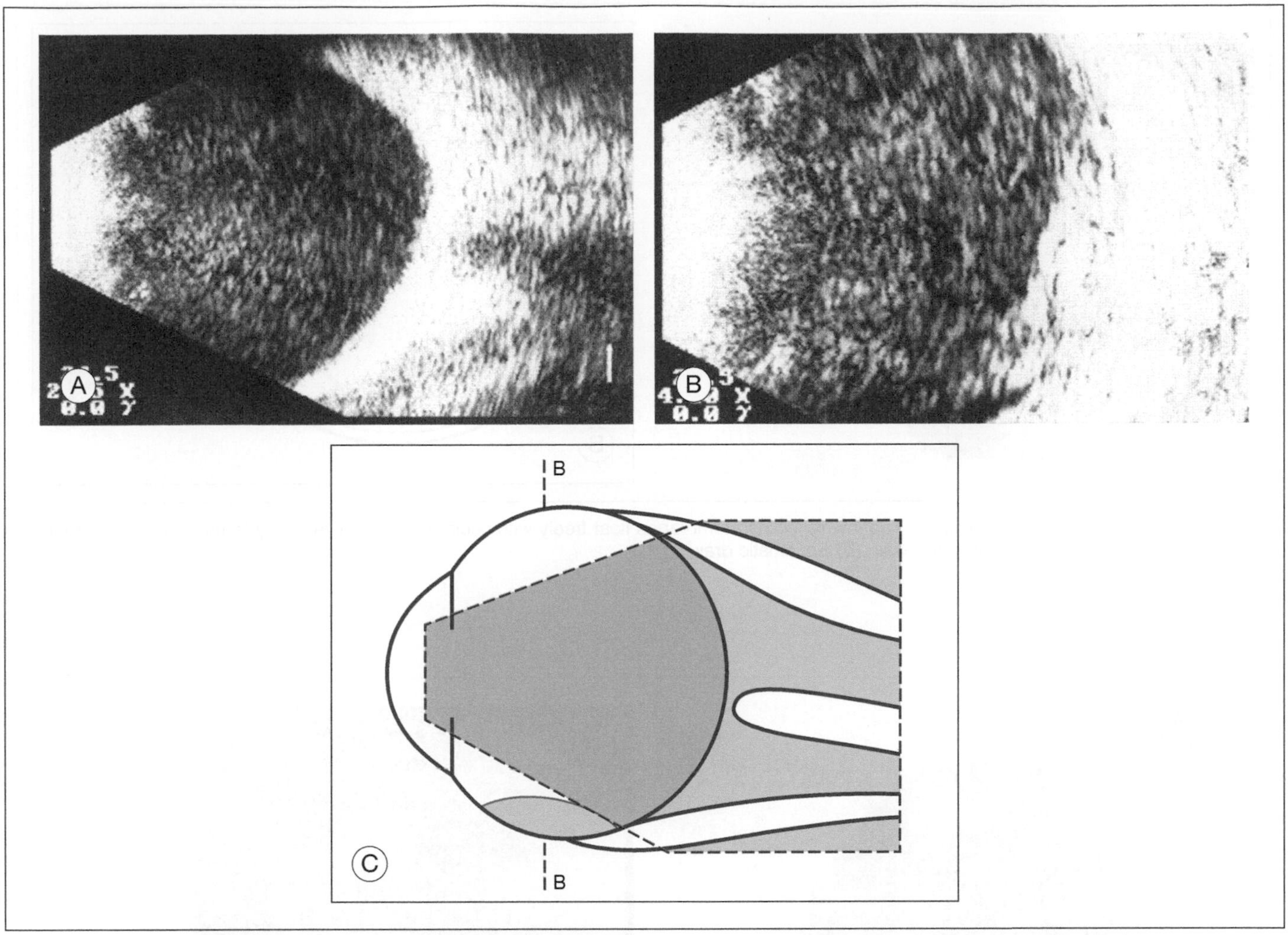

Fig. 9.17 (A) Conspicuous bleeding into syneretic vitreous; erythrocytes within the vitreous create reflective opacities. A static picture may give the impression of a solid lesion. (B) After a few hours the opacities usually accumulate in the lower aspect of the vitreous cavity. (C) Schematic drawing.

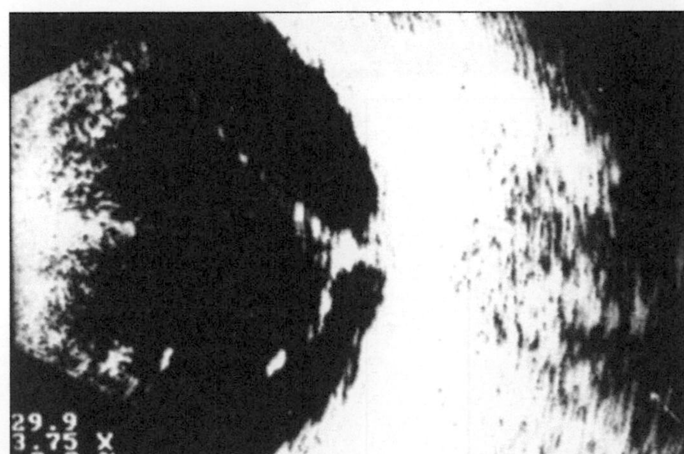

Fig. 9.18 Fresh vitreous hemorrhage. In a cross-sectional echogram the vitreous framework converges towards the ocular wall. Blood precipitates increase the acoustic reflectivity of the vitreous. Traction has to be assumed where the vitreous is in contact with the ocular wall.

precipitate on to a vitreous strand (Fig. 9.18). This strand may be responsible for the development of a retinal tear, and its traction can be demonstrated directly in acoustic sectioning (Fig. 9.19). A circumscribed thickening of the ocular wall in cross-section may indicate the presence of a retinal operculum (Fig. 9.20). This area should be localized echographically and then carefully scrutinized with ophthalmoscopy if possible.

In larger hemorrhages, the blood can also disseminate into multiple pre-existing vitreous compartments. In the early phase of this process, the erythrocytes will collect in the retrovitreal space (Fig. 9.21). The retrovitreal space may completely clear after a few days or weeks due to its high fluid exchange rate; however, blood on the vitreous framework absorbs much more slowly (Fig. 9.22).

Vitreous hemorrhage from neovascularization

Hemorrhages that develop from proliferative changes in patients with diabetic retinopathy and retinal neovascularization will always be accompanied by pathologic changes in the vitreous. Vitreous membranes tent rectilinearly between the adhesions to the retina. The normal aftermovements that should occur in the vitreous after eye movements are extinguished in the presence of peripheral neovascular tufts. The vitreous tufts create adhesions that encircle the posterior pole. This is an ominous sign, which is indicative of early retinal tractional detachment from these circular adhesions (Fig. 9.23). Choroidal neovascularization from age-related macular degeneration will have hemorrhage in multiple layers of the eye (Fig. 9.24).

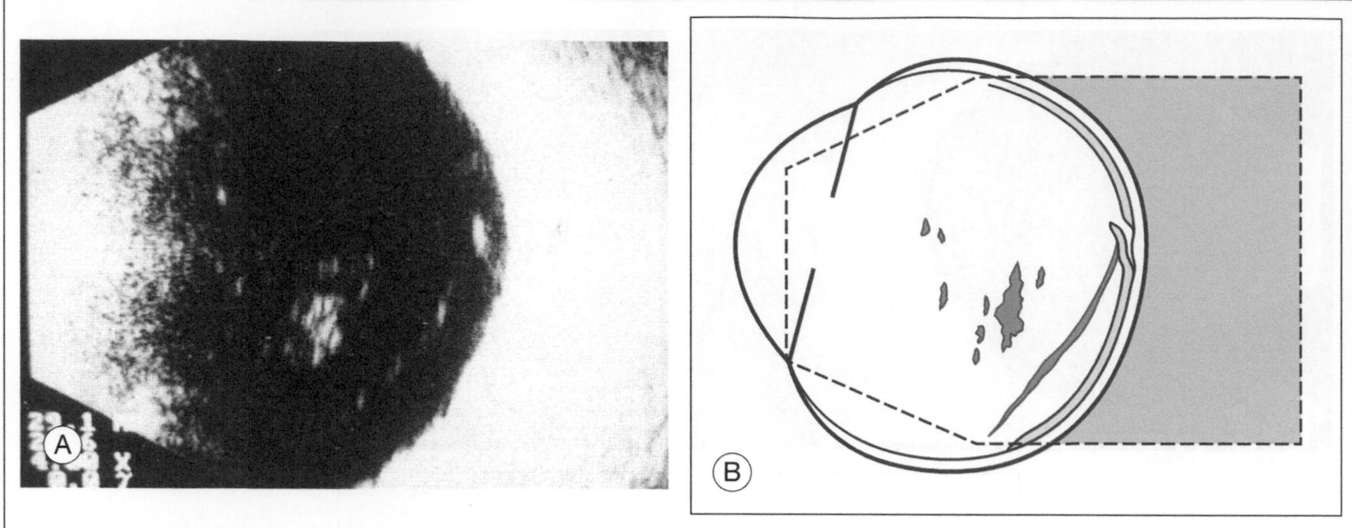

Fig. 9.19 (A) Recent vitreous hemorrhage. The low reflecting membranes float freely with ocular movement. A newly formed horseshoe tear may be present at their connection point to the wall. (B) Schematic drawing.

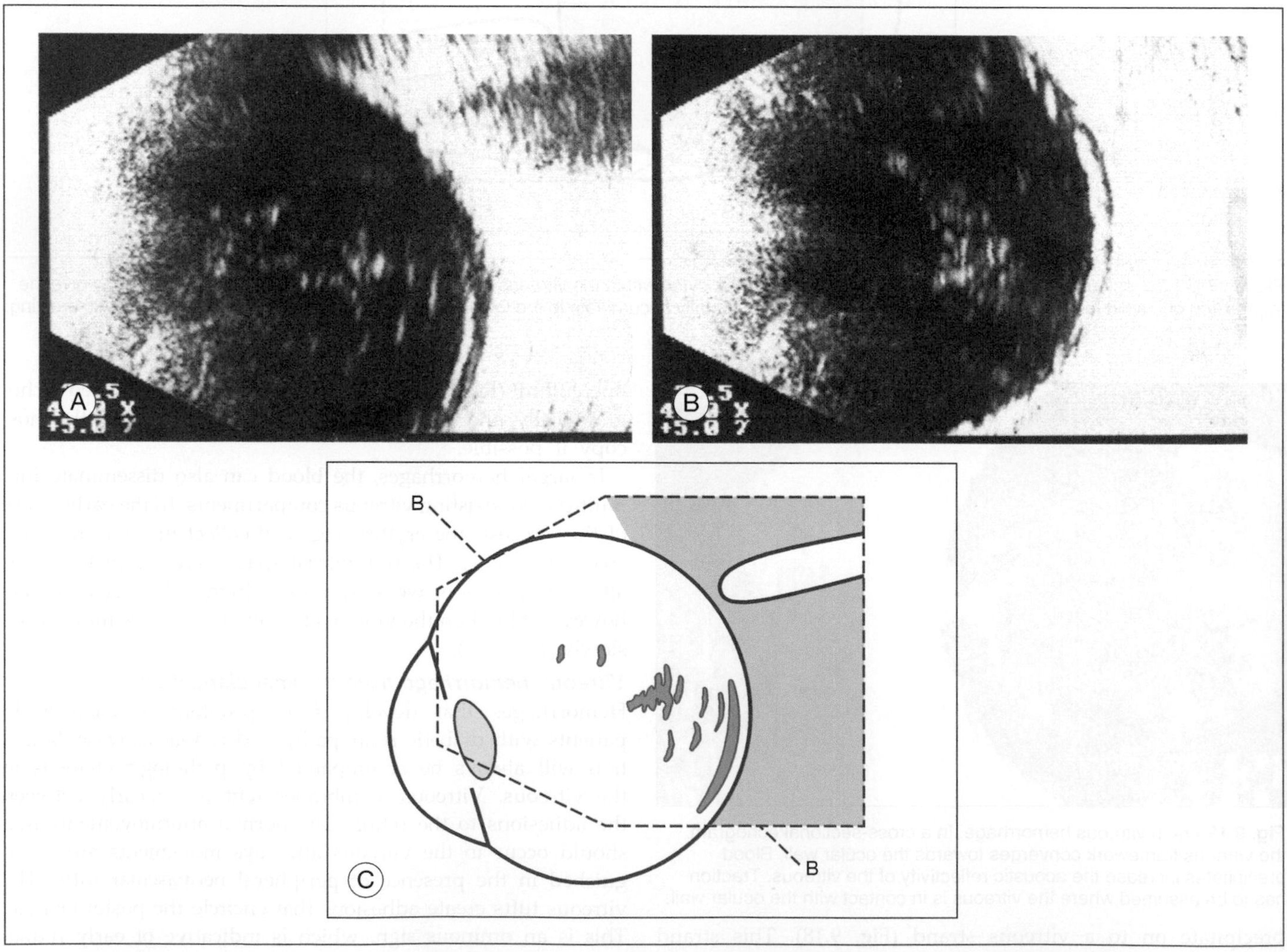

Fig. 9.20 (A,B) Recent vitreous hemorrhage. Erythrocytes have precipitated on to the partly detached posterior hyaloid membrane, increasing its acoustic reflectivity. (C) Schematic drawing.

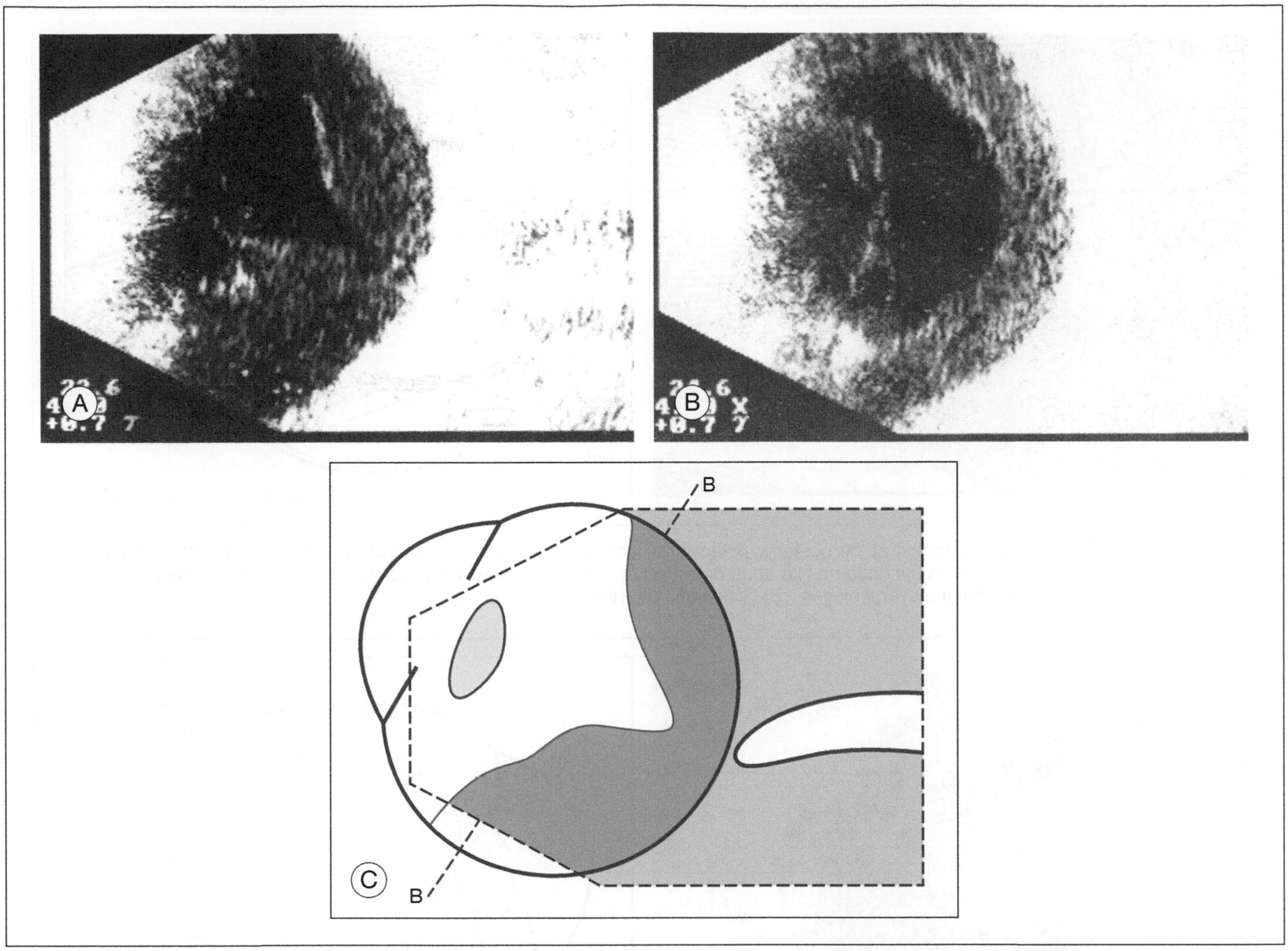

Fig. 9.21 (A) Vitreous hemorrhage with posterior vitreous detachment emphasizing the retrovitreal space. (B) In the early stage after the hemorrhage, erythrocytes accumulate in the retrovitreal space. They may ensheath the part of the vitreous that was free of blood and had a normal structure. (C) Schematic drawing.

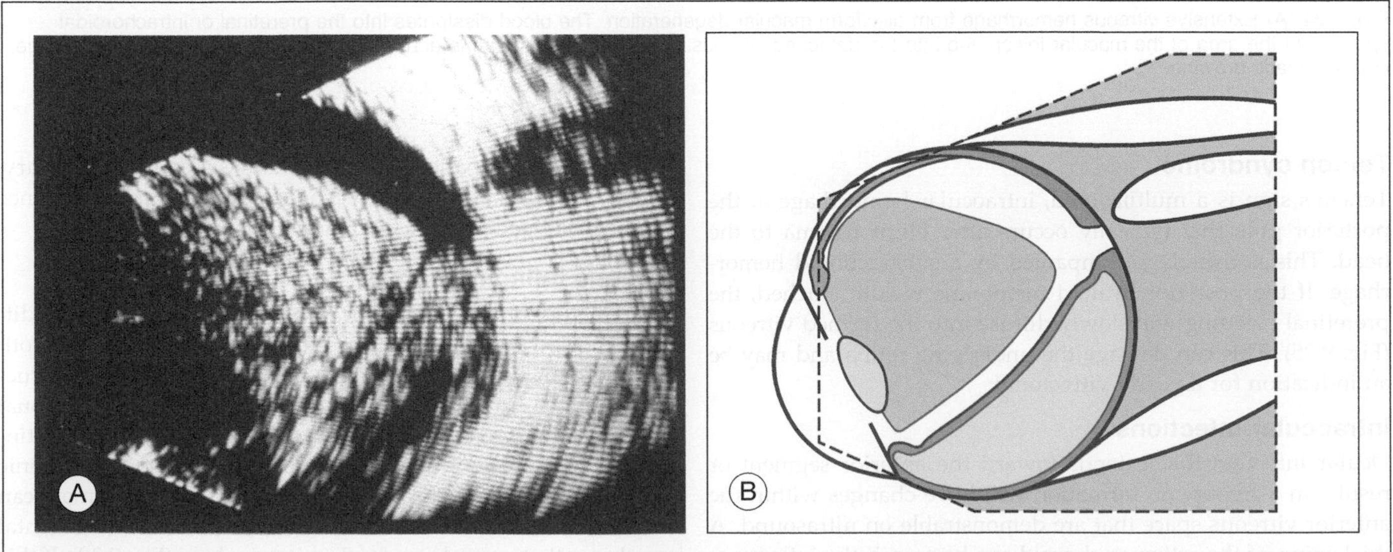

Fig. 9.22 The retrovitreal space may completely clear after a few days or weeks due to its high fluid exchange rate; however, blood on the vitreous framework or located subretinally absorbs much more slowly (A). (B) Schematic drawing.

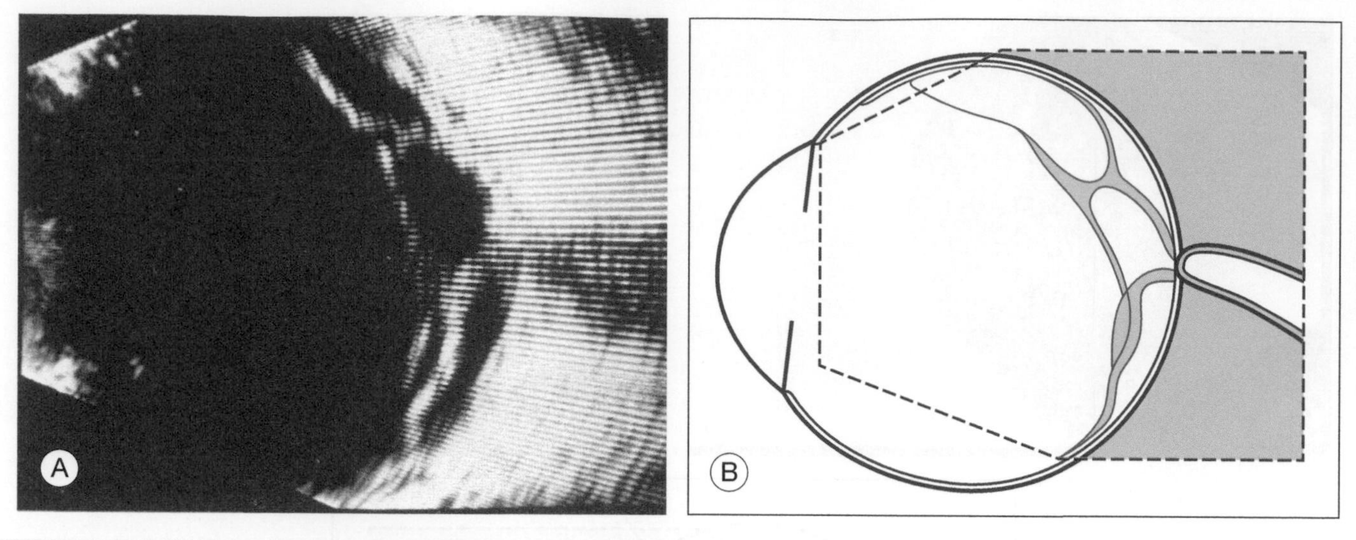

Fig. 9.23 (A) Beginning traction detachment at the posterior pole with vitreous contraction and proliferative diabetic retinopathy, which is hidden behind a diffuse vitreous hemorrhage. A springboard-like, taut, detached hyaloid membrane is still adherent to the retina at the posterior pole and has led to a traction detachment in several places. (B) Schematic drawing.

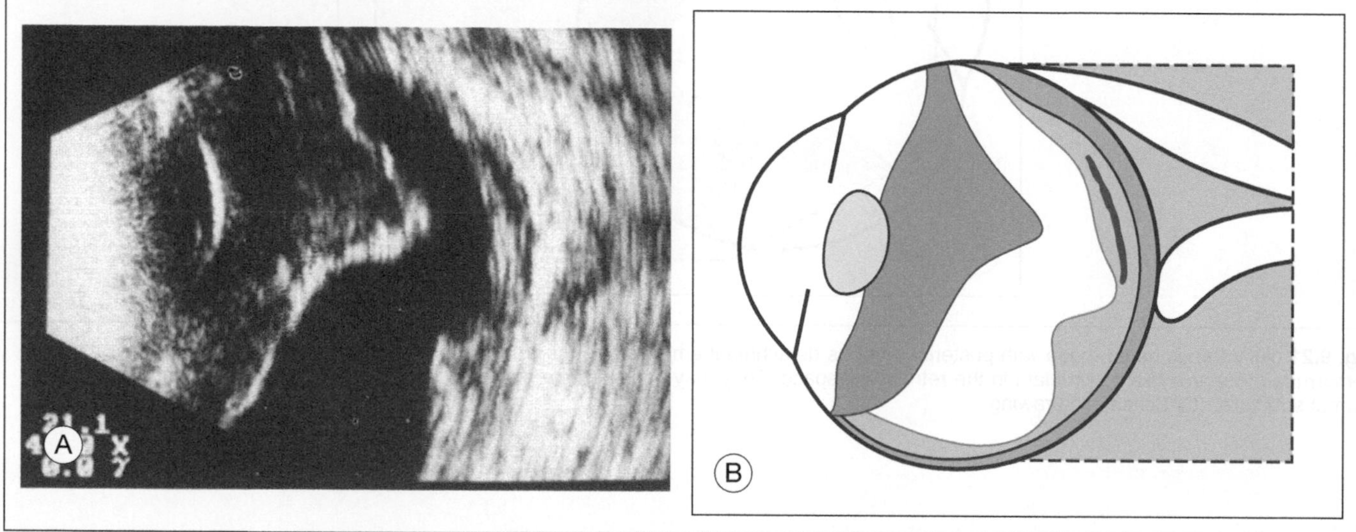

Fig. 9.24 (A) Extensive vitreous hemorrhage from disciform macular degeneration. The blood dissipates into the preretinal or intrachoroidal space, into the area of the macular lesion and into the detached vitreous. The retrovitreal space is echo-free because of its high fluid exchange. (B) Schematic drawing.

Terson syndrome

Terson's sign is a multilayered, intraocular hemorrhage at the posterior pole that typically occurs after blunt trauma to the head. This is usually accompanied by a subarachnoid hemorrhage. If the posterior hyaloid membrane is still attached, the preretinal bleeding will slowly diffuse into the formed vitreous (Fig. 9.25). This can damage the underlying retina and may be an indication for an early vitrectomy.

Intraocular infections

Ocular infection that extends toward the anterior segment or results in a hypopyon formation will have changes within the anterior vitreous space that are demonstrable on ultrasound. A thickening of the retina or choroid can be seen if the inflammation penetrates to the outer layers of the globe (Fig. 9.26). After only a few hours, these changes may involve the entire vitreous body (Fig. 9.27). If panophthalmitis follows a perforating injury, ultrasound evaluation can detect a local reaction at the entrance point of the infection (Figs 9.28 and 9.29).

Vitreous inflammation

Inflammatory and hemorrhagic vitreous changes cannot be differentiated on the basis of ultrasonographic findings alone. Both conditions may cause densification of pre-existing vitreous structures with subsequent shrinkage of the vitreous; tractional detachment of the retina can occur, especially if there are postinflammatory adhesions between the vitreous and retina. In chronic uveitis, an early and complete posterior vitreous detachment can occur and cause the formed vitreous to shrink and form a frontal membrane that extends across the vitreous base (Fig. 9.30). If this membrane adheres to the ciliary body, it may detach the ciliary body and produce subsequent ocular hypotony.[29]

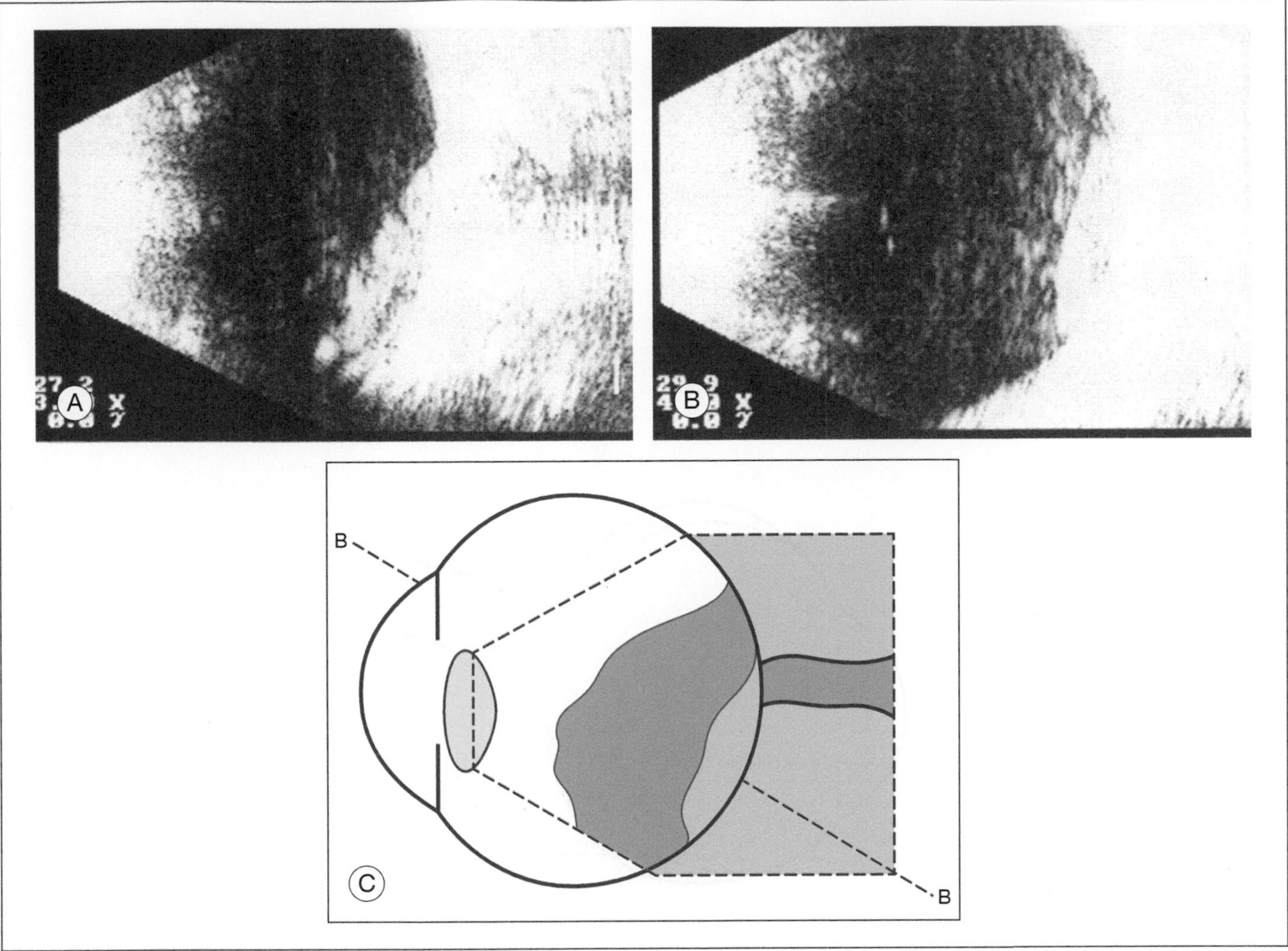

Fig. 9.25 (A,B) Retrovitreal bleeding associated with a subarachnoid hemorrhage (Terson syndrome). The bleeding originates from the area of the optic nerve head. (C) Schematic drawing.

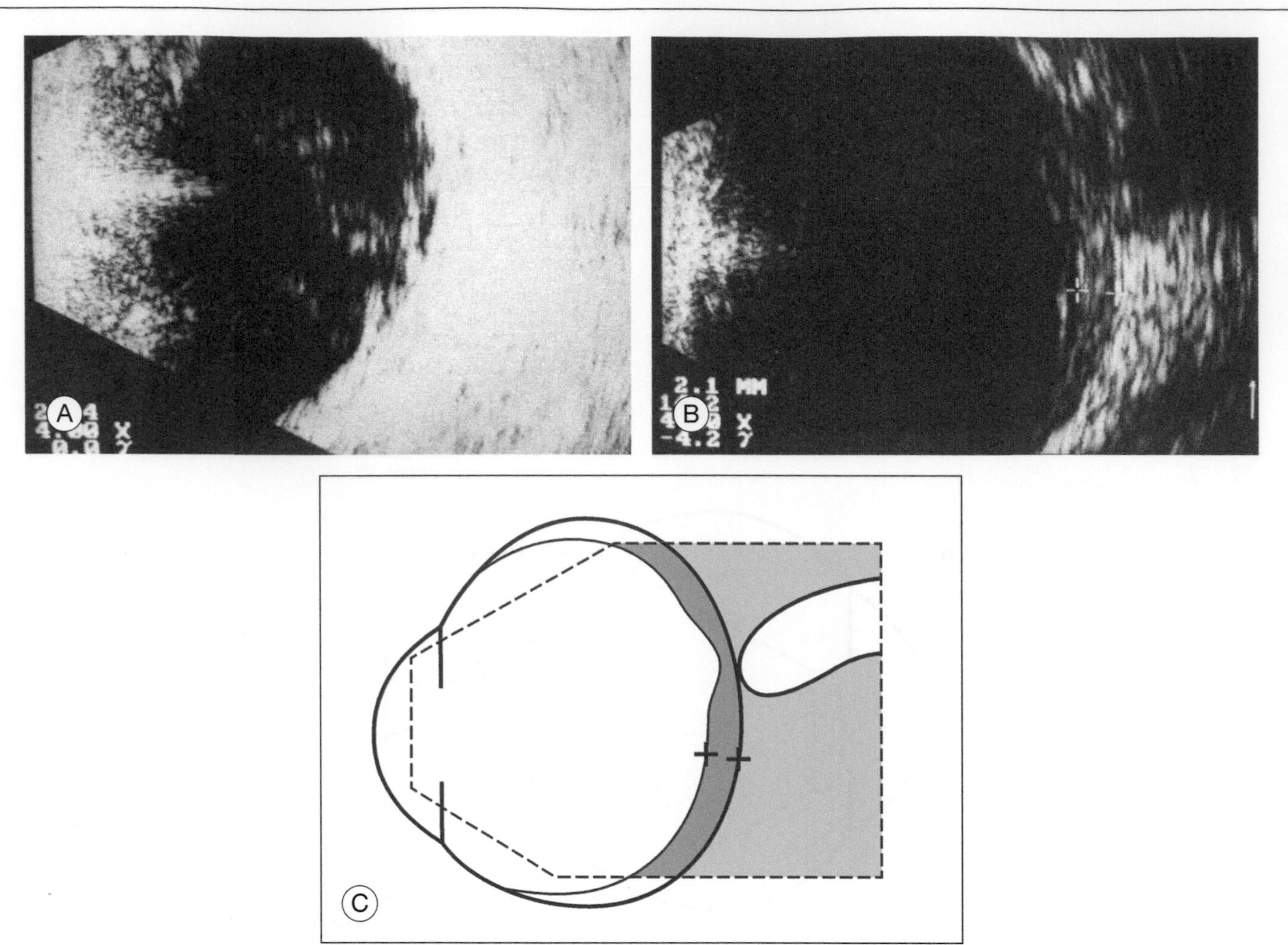

Fig. 9.26 (A,B) Panophthalmitis after an intraocular operation. Widening of the ocular wall to about 2.1 mm indicates inflammatory choroidal infiltrates. (C) Schematic drawing.

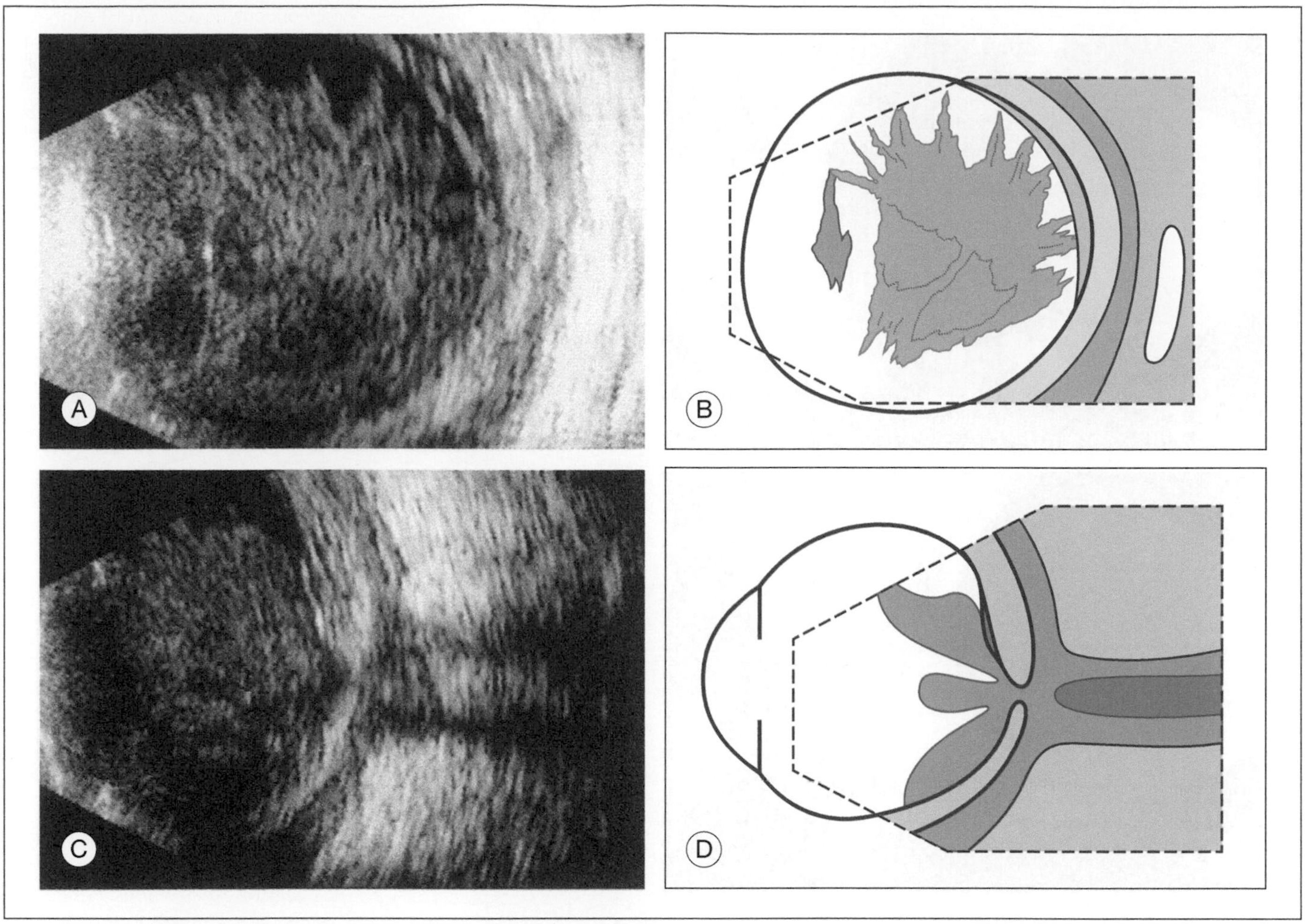

Fig. 9.27 Vitreous abscess that caused a bacterial orbital inflammation. (A) B-scan ultrasonography demonstrates a highly reflective vitreous body which is partly detached from the retina. (B) Schematic drawing of this image. (C) Posterior pole shows infiltration of Tenon's space and widening of the optic nerve sheath. (D) Schematic drawing.

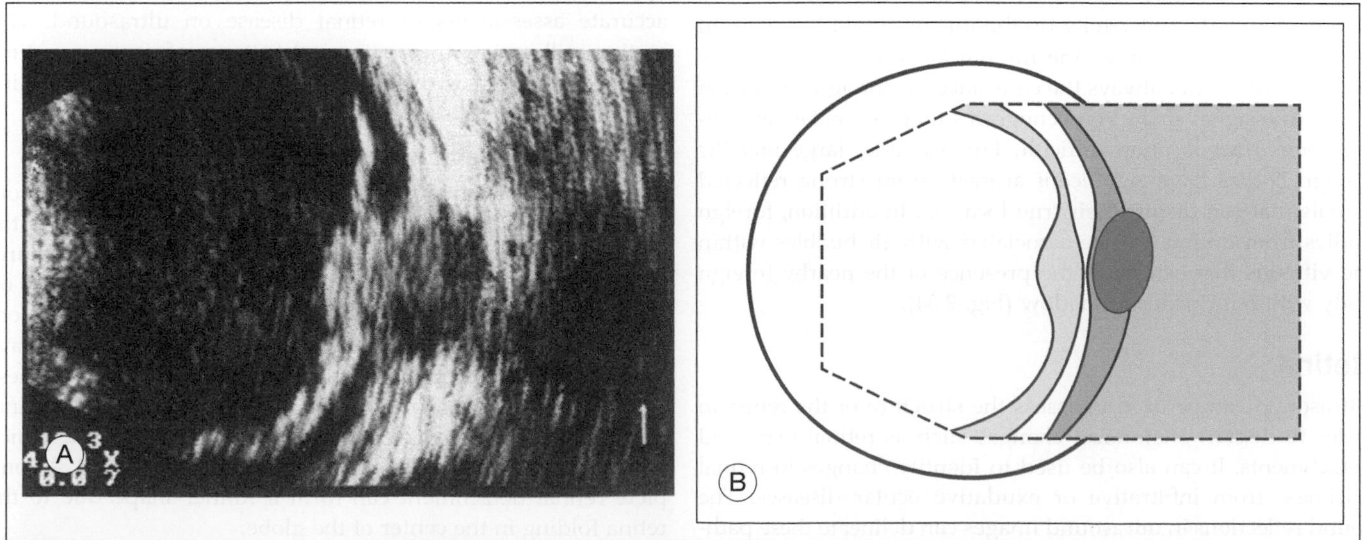

Fig. 9.28 Posttraumatic intraocular infection starting from the side of perforation. (A) B-scan ultrasonography demonstrates localized thickening of the ocular wall indicating the side of the perforation. The vitreous is filled with inflammatory cells, the posterior hyaloid is thickened, and there is a localized retinal detachment. (B) Schematic drawing.

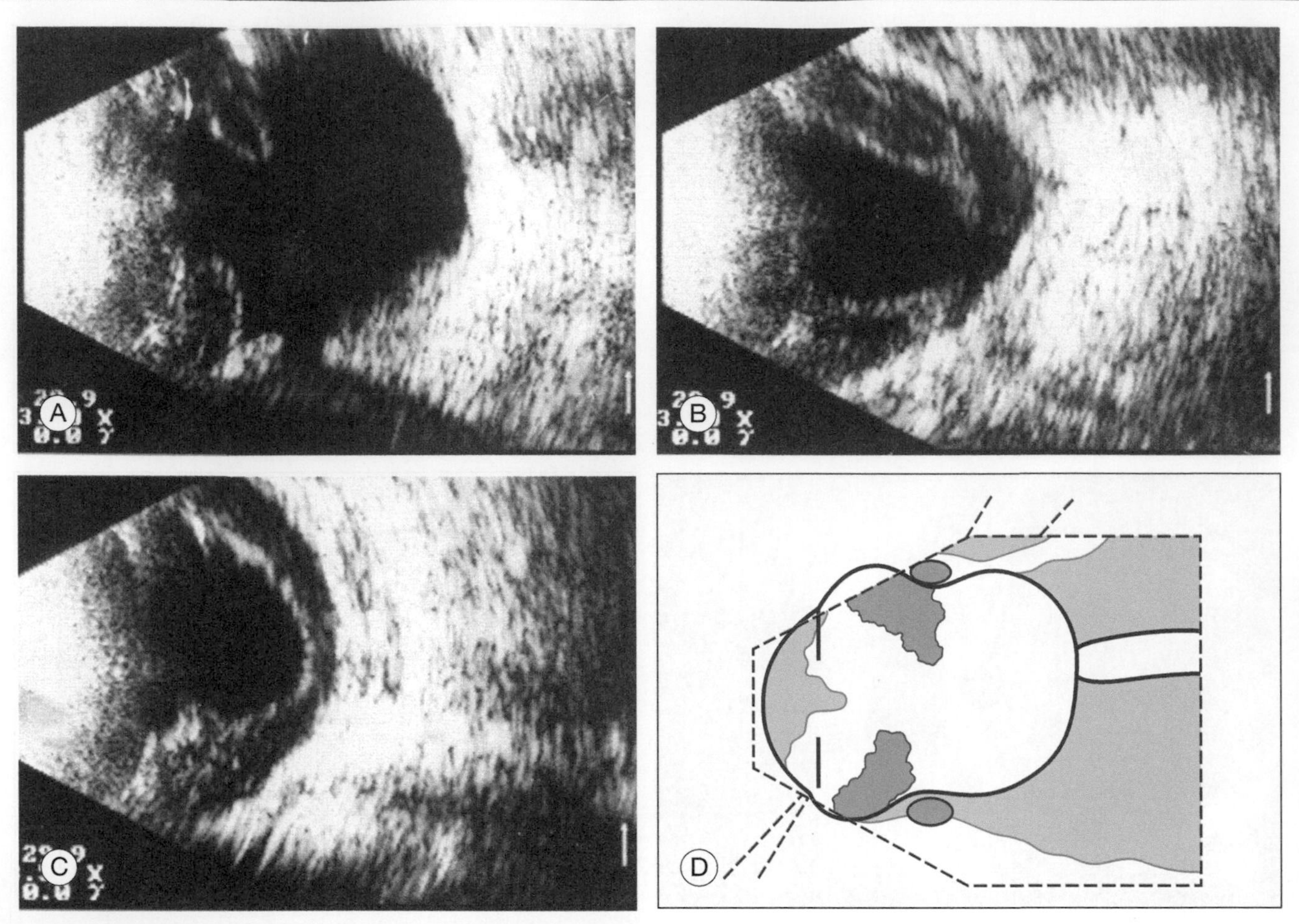

Fig. 9.29 Chronic inflammation with massive vitreous infiltration after pars plana vitrectomy and scleral buckle. (A) Remnants of the infiltrated vitreous can be seen at the vitreous base anterior to the scleral buckle. (B,C) Cross-sections through the vitreous base. (D) Schematic drawing.

Intraocular foreign bodies

Intraocular foreign bodies induce a change in echo reflectivity which is based on the composition of the material (Figs 9.31–9.33). The change in the reflectivity on the image should be a helpful clue in the localization of the foreign body within the globe; however, this is not always the case since the foreign bodies can also create signal artifact on echograms that can make identifying their exact location difficult. For example, large metallic foreign bodies have significant artifacts from strong reflected signals that can distort their true location. In addition, foreign bodies from trauma can be associated with air bubbles within the vitreous that can mask the presence of the nearby foreign body within the acoustic shadow (Fig. 9.34).

Retina

Ultrasound can be used to assess the structure of the retina in order to discern anatomical changes such as retinal tears and detachments. It can also be used to identify changes in retinal thickness from infiltrative or exudative ocular diseases. The sound reflections in ultrasound images can delineate these pathological retinal changes even in eyes with opaque anterior media. This is a particularly useful tool since many diseases that affect the retina can also lead to vitreous changes that limit direct visualization. It is important to have a strong fundamental knowledge of ocular anatomy as well as a good technical approach for acquiring ultrasound images in order to make accurate assessments of retinal disease on ultrasound. This section will review the anatomical features of common retinal conditions as well as the special techniques needed to examine the retina with ultrasound.

Acute retinal detachment

In a retinal detachment, the neurosensory retina separates from the RPE layer. This development allows fluid to collect in the potential space between these two layers. The detached neurosensory retina appears as a membrane in the vitreous space on ultrasound. Partial retinal detachments may still maintain connections to the optic nerve or ora serrata since these areas have the strongest connections to the retina. Identification of these connections on ultrasound can distinguish a partial retinal detachment from a vitreous or choroidal detachment, which would have different anatomical connections (Fig. 9.35). A complete retinal detachment can form a funnel shape due to the retina folding in the center of the globe.

Complicated retinal detachments with severe pathology can make it difficult to identify all the structures on ultrasound (Fig. 9.36). For example, in severe trauma cases that are associated

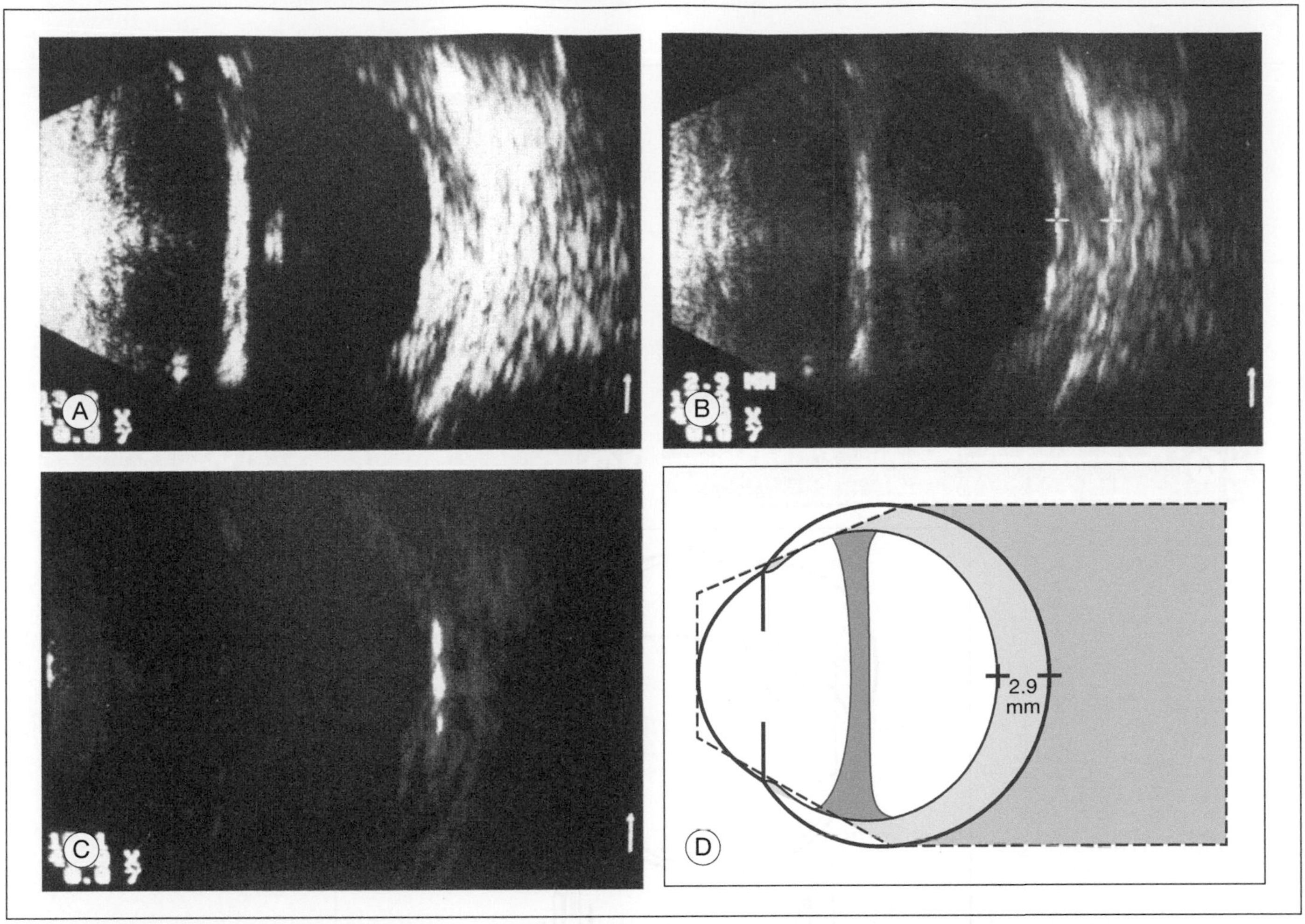

Fig. 9.30 Phthisis oculi in chronic panuveitis. (A) The vitreous has shrunk to form a frontal membrane of high acoustic reflectivity. The ocular wall is widened to 2.9 mm. (B) Using linear amplification, the various layers of the ocular wall have become clearly outlined. (C) Isolated areas of the ocular wall show high acoustic reflectivity, which indicates calcification of the choroid or in the sclera. (D) Schematic drawing highlighting wall thickness.

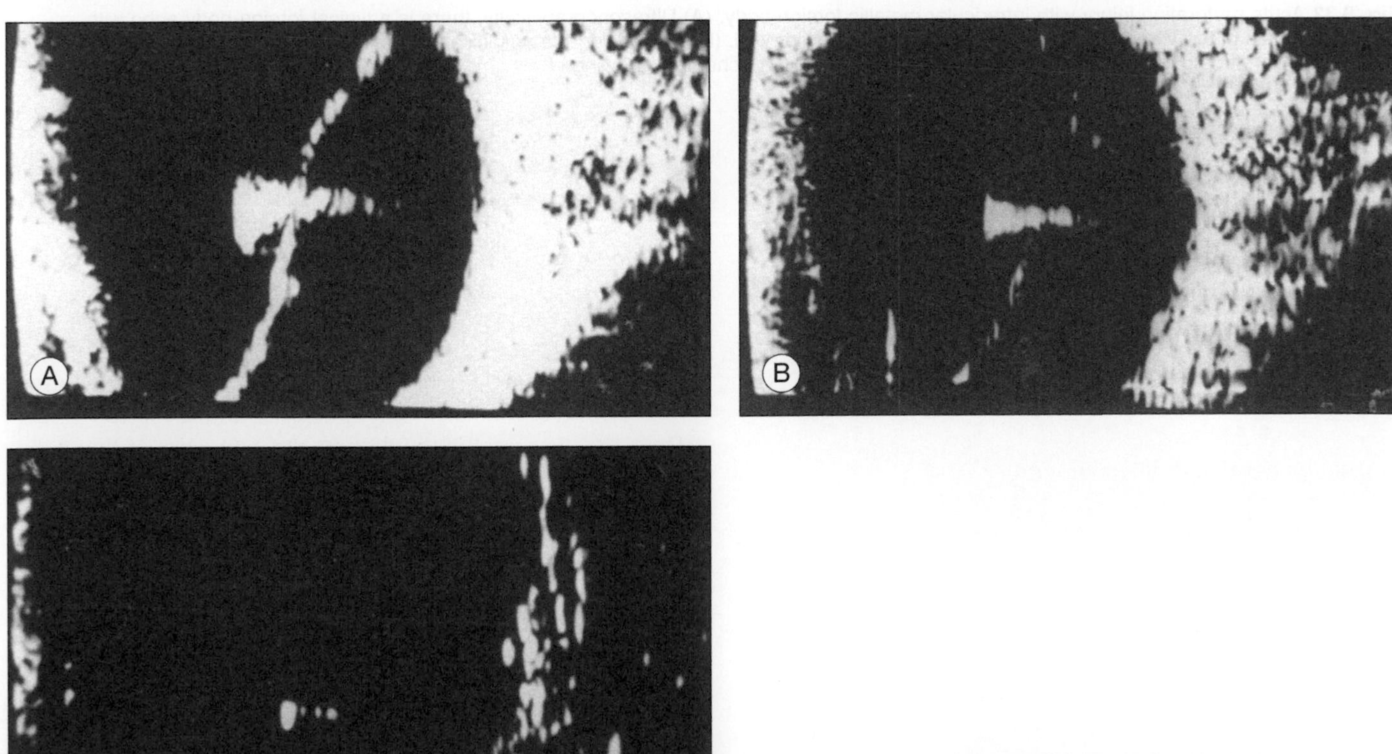

Fig. 9.31 (A) Metallic foreign body in the vitreous with total retinal detachment. (B) The foreign-body spike is characterized by its high amplitude and repetitive echoes. (C) With reduced sensitivity the foreign body can almost be imaged as an isolated echo.

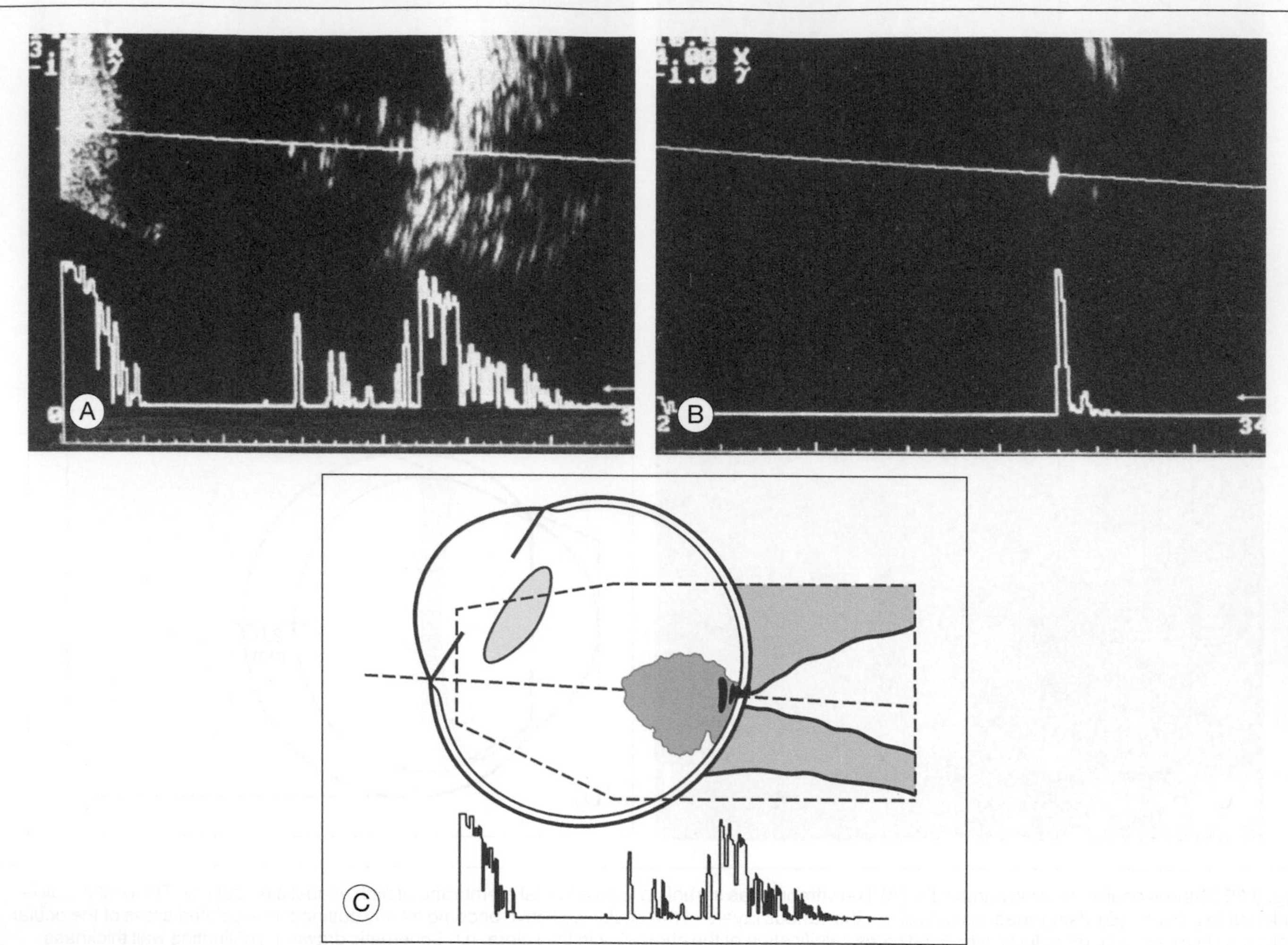

Fig. 9.32 Acute perforating injury with intraocular metallic foreign body. (A) Ultrasonographically, there is a typical foreign-body echo with repetitive spikes in the vitreous about 2 mm in front of the ocular wall. (B) Decreasing the amplification displays the foreign-body echo as the only intraocular structure remaining visible on ultrasonography. (C) Schematic drawing.

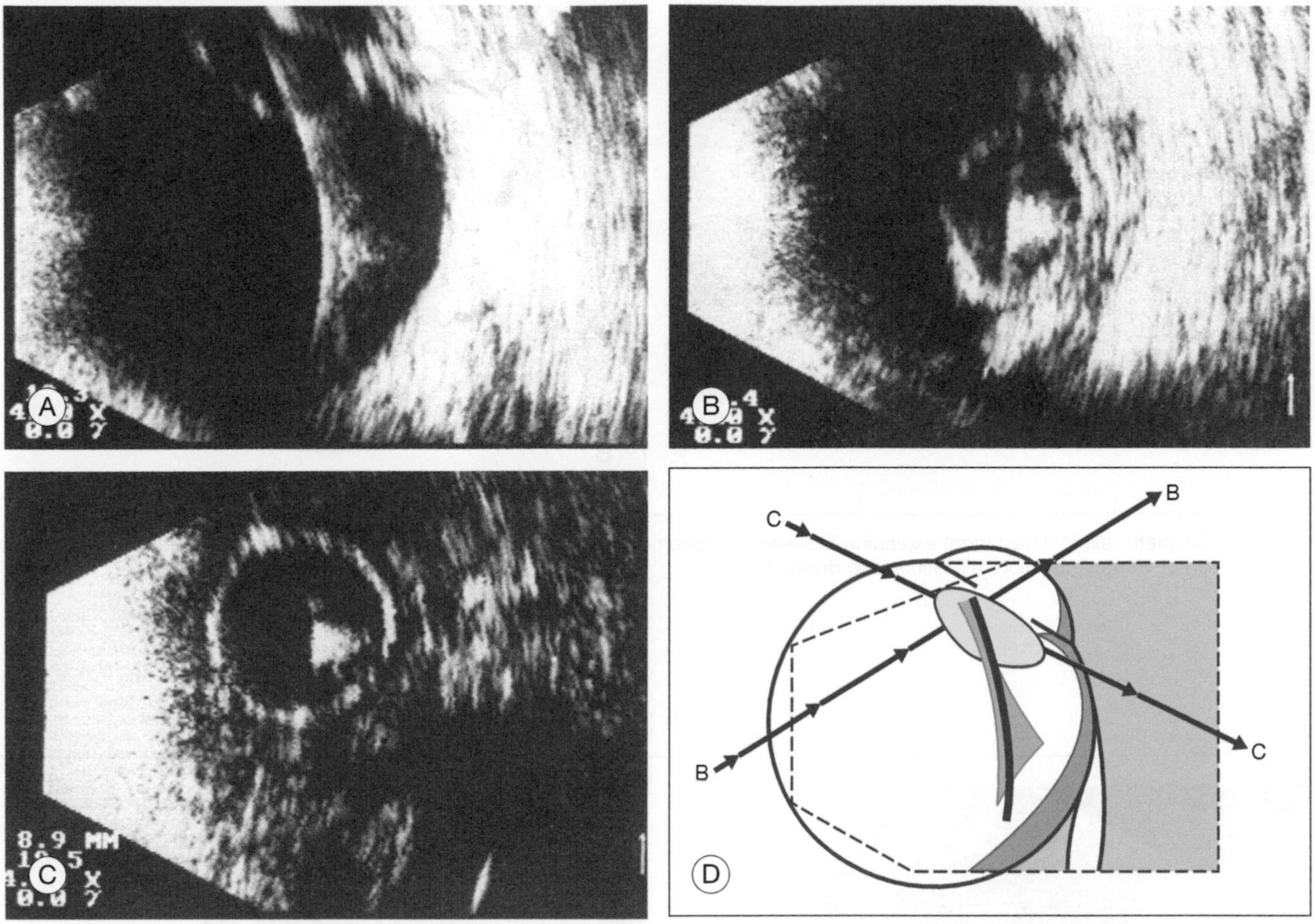

Fig. 9.33 (A) Intraocular foreign body of a piece of wire. (B) The anterior end of the wire remained visible in the lens. Cross-sectional image taken temporally with maximal adduction of the globe. (C) Frontal section through iris and lens. (D) Schematic drawing.

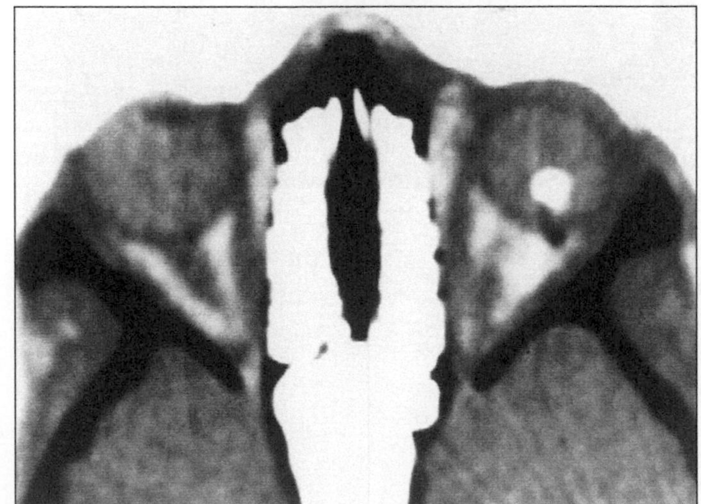

Fig. 9.34 Computed tomography image of a metallic foreign body wedged into the ocular wall with an air bubble adjacent to it.

with proliferative vitreoretinopathy or in advanced diabetic disease associated with proliferative retinopathy, the membranes formed within the vitreous can appear similar to a true retinal detachment. The following questions can guide the ultrasound examination of the retina in order to differentiate these common causes of vitreous membranes:

- What is the spatial extent of the membrane? At which point is there contact with the ocular wall?
- What is the shape of a cross-section of the membrane, especially in the optic nerve head area?
- Which aftermovements occur?
- How great is the difference of the spike from the membrane in question to the scleral standard or to the echo from a standard reflector?

These questions should be clarified in the following way:

1. What is the spatial extent of the membrane? At which point is there contact with the ocular wall? A recent rhegmatogenous retinal detachment can be characterized in cross-section by a membranous structure of high reflectivity that converges in an acute angle toward the ocular wall. If the imaged acoustic section is centered on the optic nerve head, then the border of the detached retina will be captured as it connects to the nerve head (Fig. 9.37). If the membrane passes over the optic nerve head instead of connecting to the optic nerve in the echo image, it is not a retinal detachment (Fig. 9.38). This feature can help identify retinal membranes form vitreous membranes.
2. What is the shape of a cross-section of the membrane, especially at the optic nerve head? In order to appreciate the shape of a retinal detachment, the performance of

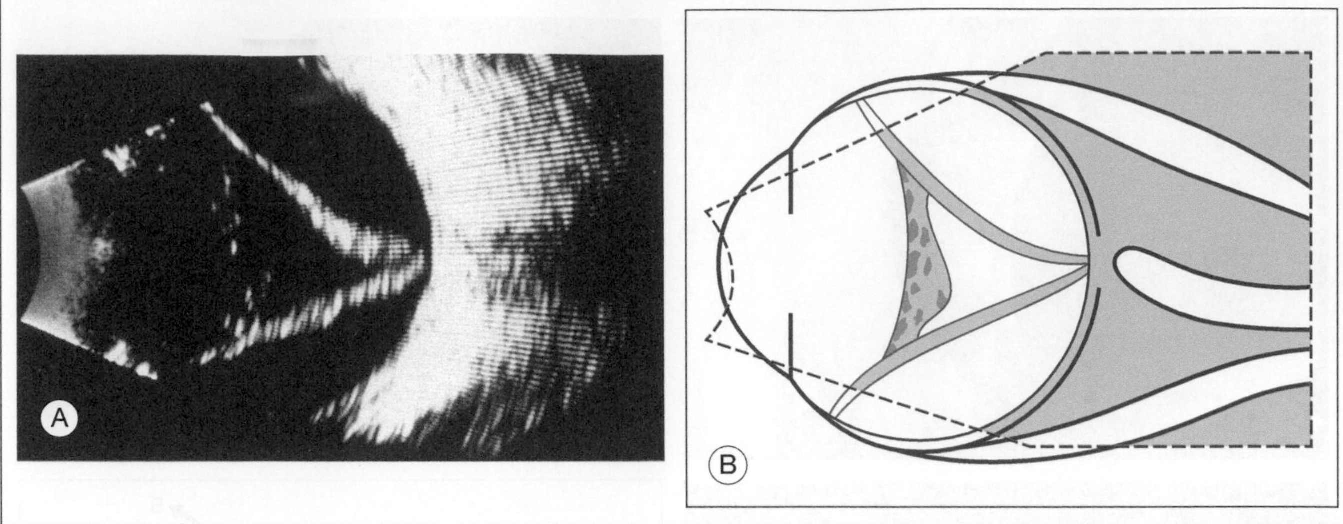

Fig. 9.35 (A) Complete retinal detachment extending between the optic nerve head and the ora serrata. Heterogeneous material in the anterior vitreous is a sign of vitreous reaction. (B) Schematic drawing.

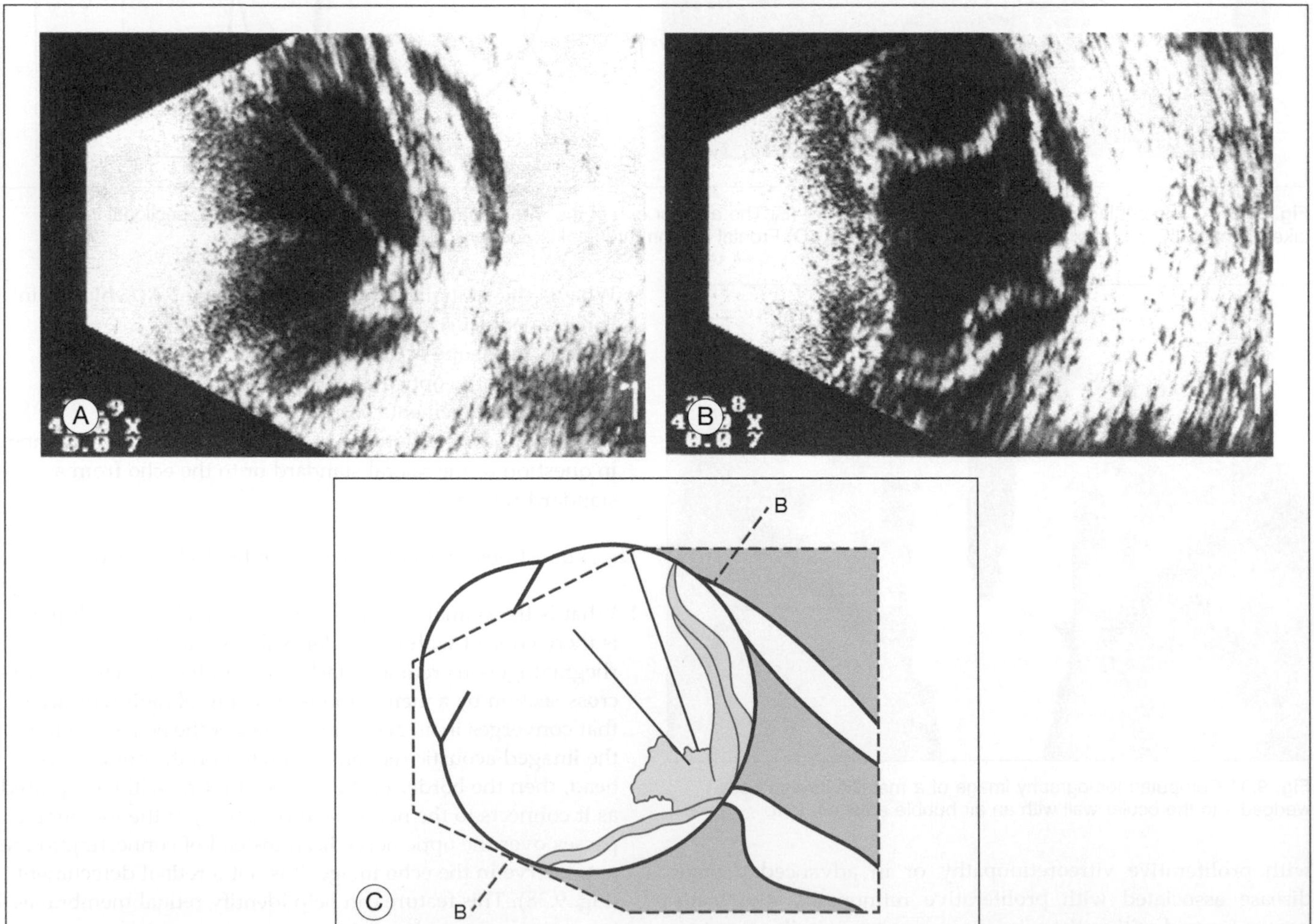

Fig. 9.36 Development of a traction detachment with massive vitreous retraction. (A) Flat subtotal retinal detachment with folds; rigid vitreous strands. (B) In a frontal section, multiple contacts of the retina to the ocular wall can be demonstrated. (C) Schematic drawing.

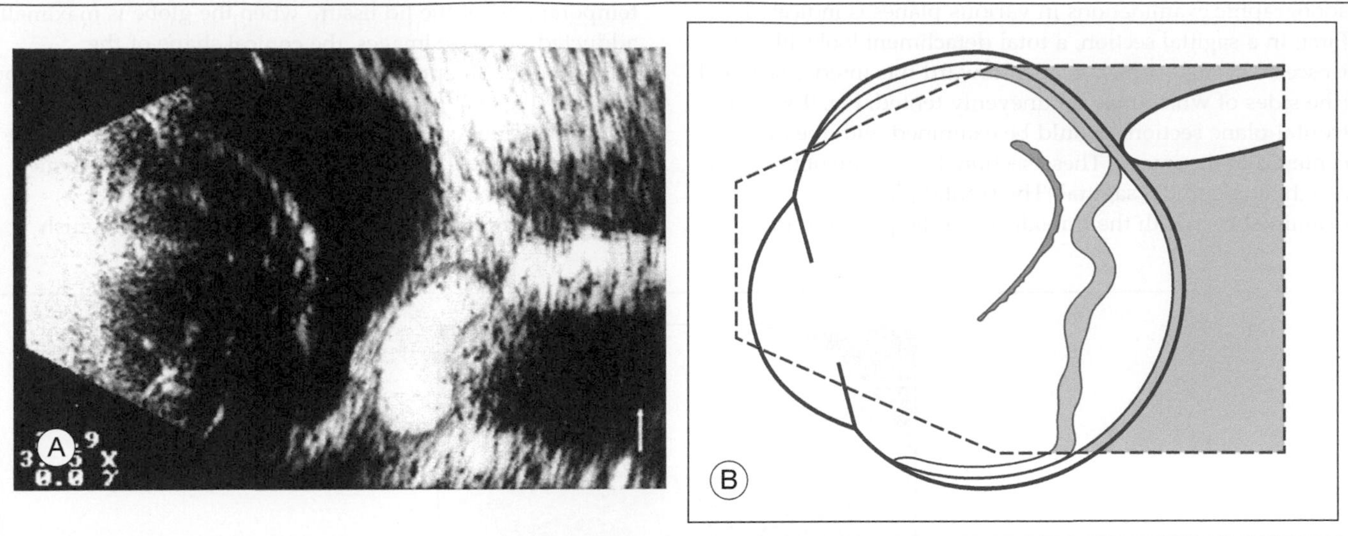

Fig. 9.37 (A) Sectoral retinal detachment. In acute retinal detachment, short aftermovements appear when the globe moves. These aftermovements extend like a whiplash from the area of the contact to the ocular wall. (B) Schematic drawing.

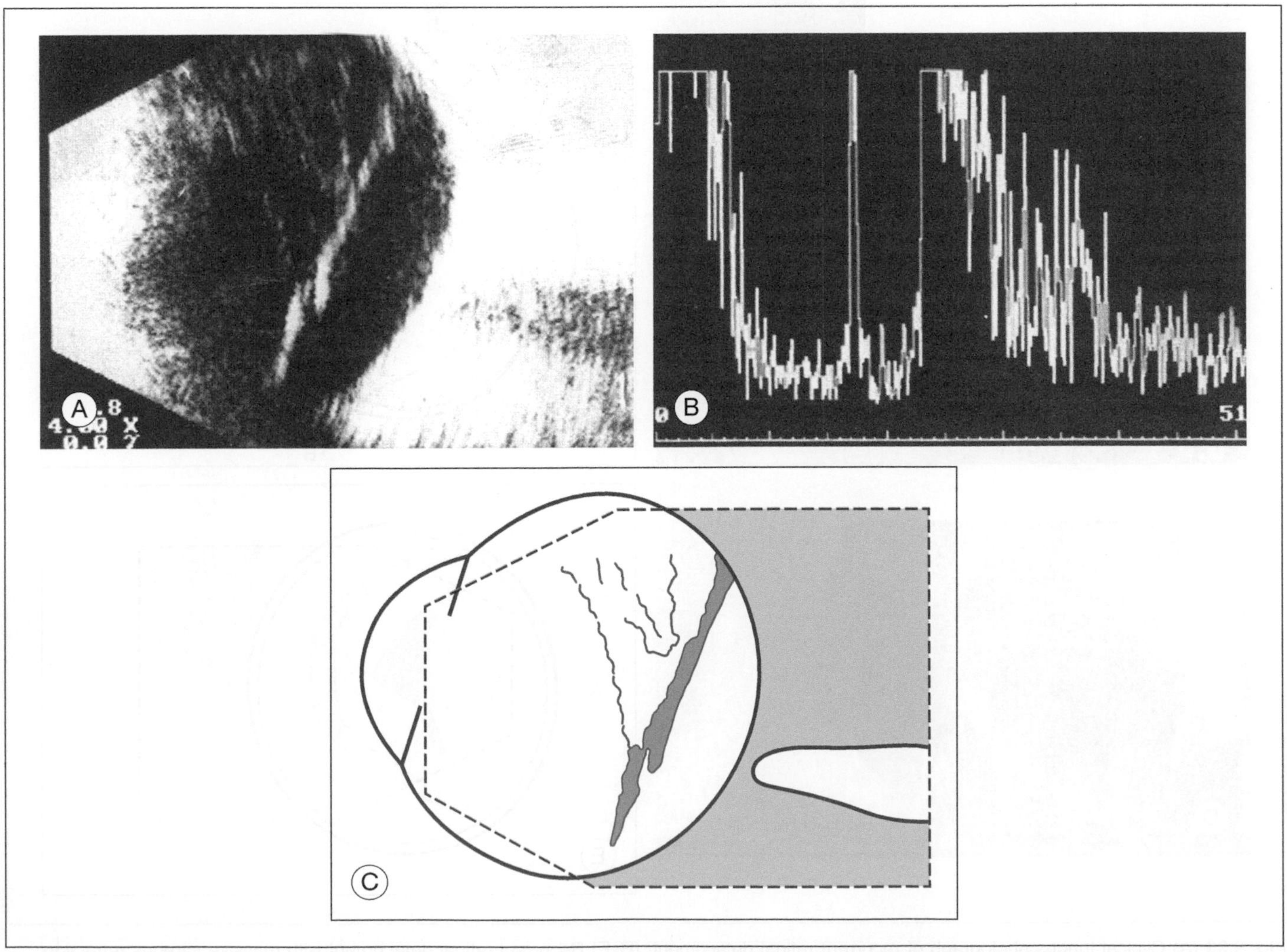

Fig. 9.38 (A,B) Detached posterior hyaloid membrane. Vitreous membranes may reach an acoustic reflectivity similar to that of the retina seen on A-scan. A retinal detachment can be excluded if the membrane tents over the posterior pole without reaching the optic nerve head. (C) Schematic drawing.

sonographic examinations in various planes is indicated. First, in a sagittal section, a total detachment looks like an isosceles triangle which is open toward the anterior segment (the sides of which may be unevenly tented: Fig. 9.35). Next, frontal-plane sections should be examined with the disc centered in the image. These sectional plans are obtained at a right angle to the sagittal. The frontal planes can be examined best with the transducer probe placed in the temporal part of the lid fissure when the globe is maximally adducted. In these images, the conical shape of the detachment will appear oval to nearly circular in the various sections (Fig. 9.39).

3. Which aftermovements occur? Dynamic ultrasound can be obtained with patient participation. The quality of tissue movement at the end of the ocular saccade, or the aftermovement of the tissue, can be used to distinguish

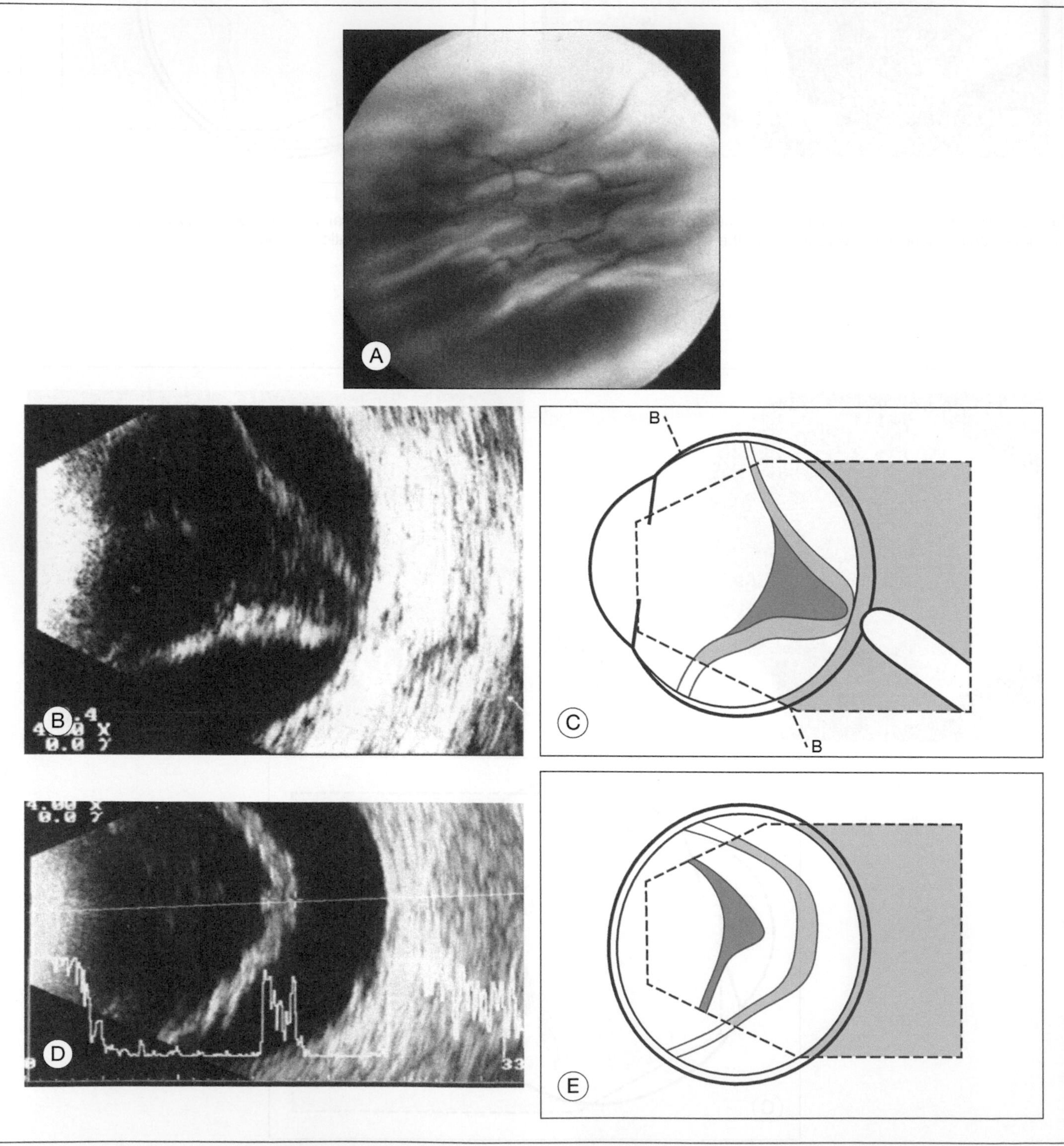

Fig. 9.39 (A) Clinical fundus photograph of recurrent retinal detachment. (B–E) Recurrent retinal detachment with massive vitreous retraction. (B) Axial cross-sectional echogram. The amplitudes of the aftermovements decrease. High-frequency flicker of the taut membrane appears after the eye changes position. (D) Frontal section toward 6 o'clock. An epiretinal membrane of the retinal surface appears echographically as an apparent widening of the retina. (C,E) Schematic drawings.

vitreous tissue from retina tissue. An acute rhegmatogenous retinal detachment shows aftermovements of short duration that extend with a whiplash effect from the area where the retina is still attached, which is usually the optic nerve head. The amplitudes of these aftermovements are smaller and less extensive than those seen in the sinusoidal movements of a vitreous hemorrhage or in asteroid hyalosis.[30]

4. How great is the difference of the spike from the membrane in question to the scleral standard or to the echo from a standard reflector? Quantitative ultrasonography can detect a difference in the echo of the retina compared to that of the sclera, extending from 8 to 15 db.[31] Unfortunately, these measurements provide only guidelines. Well-developed connective tissue membranes may show reflection properties quite similar to those of a detached retina. In complicated cases it may be difficult to correlate an isolated A-spike to the multiple membrane structures as they appear on B-mode.

Chronic retinal detachment

The duration of a retinal detachment can affect the thickness and mobility of the retina, the shape and mechanical properties of the vitreous base, and the contents of the subretinal space. Identifying and understanding these changes can help with the management of these conditions.

A few weeks after a retinal detachment develops, changes in the proliferation of Müller cells and astrocytes will lead to alterations in the mechanical properties of the detached retina. The massive periretinal proliferation of these cells creates a decrease in the aftermovement amplitude of the retina (Fig. 9.40). The large excursions are replaced by a high-frequency flicker and the retina may appear thickened. After a long-standing retinal detachment, cyst-like cavities within the detached retina can be seen on ultrasound (Fig. 9.41). A long-standing detachment can also result in a funnel-shaped retinal detachment. The first step in this process is the proliferation of the epiretinal connective tissue that causes the vitreous to contract. This stage can be identified on ultrasound by the presence of new acoustic interfaces, which are seen as increased vitreous signals that surround the detached retina (Fig. 9.42). The vitreous shrinks, which creates a narrowing of the retinal cavity, which typically begins to narrow anterior to the optic nerve head and continues to the posterior lens. Frontal "cyclitic membranes" can often be seen early, extending from the vitreous base (Fig. 9.43). Next, the peripheral retina is pulled closer to this membrane until the retinal detachment does not show any recognizable cavity of the original funnel. In frontal sections the shrunken retina appears as a strand, only a few millimeters in diameter (Fig. 9.44). Occasionally, a few retinal folds can be observed.

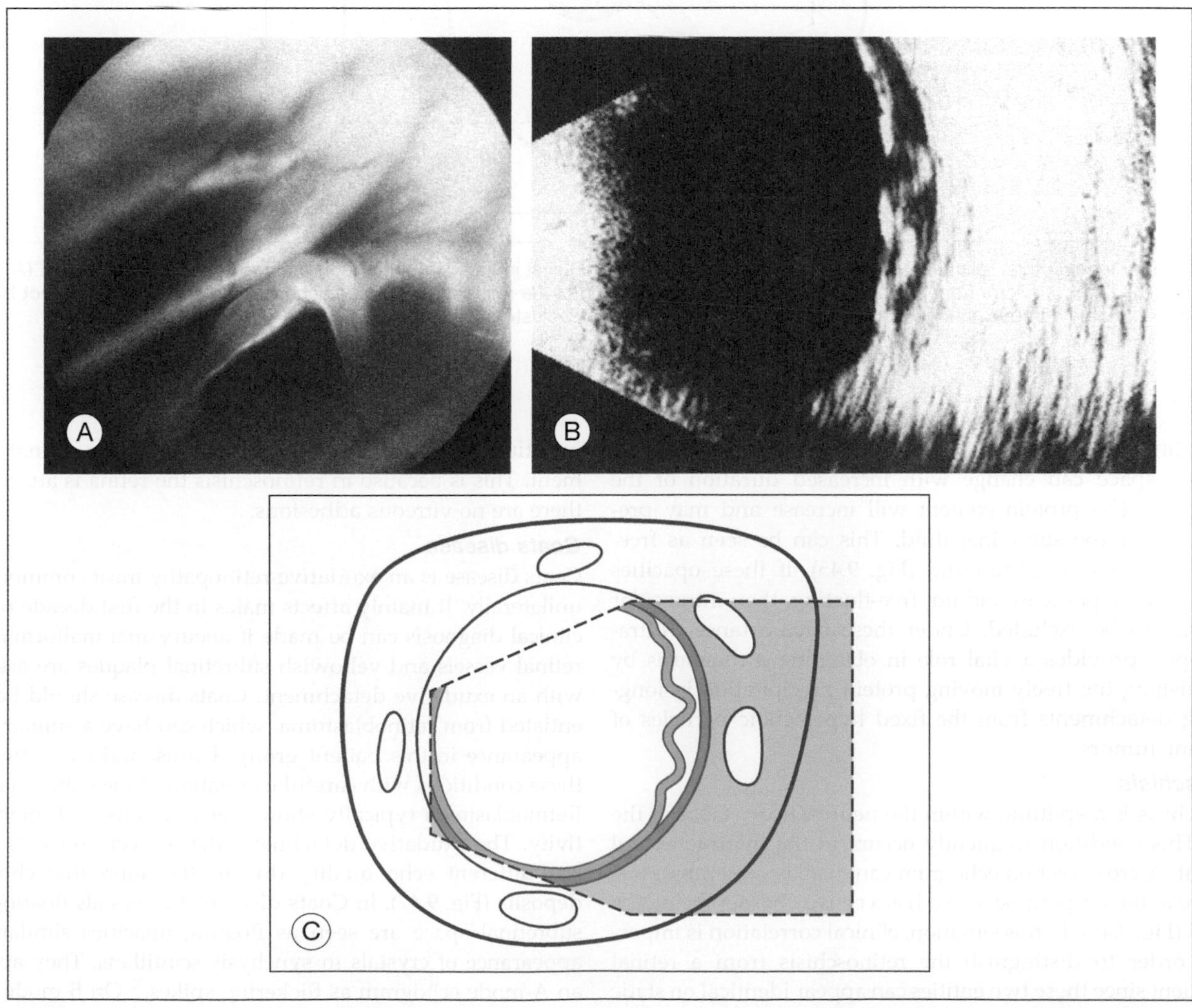

Fig. 9.40 Massive periretinal proliferation with large retinal folds. (A) Ophthalmoscopic picture of large horseshoe tear. (B) The rigid, fixed retinal folds are echographically demonstrable. (C) Schematic drawing.

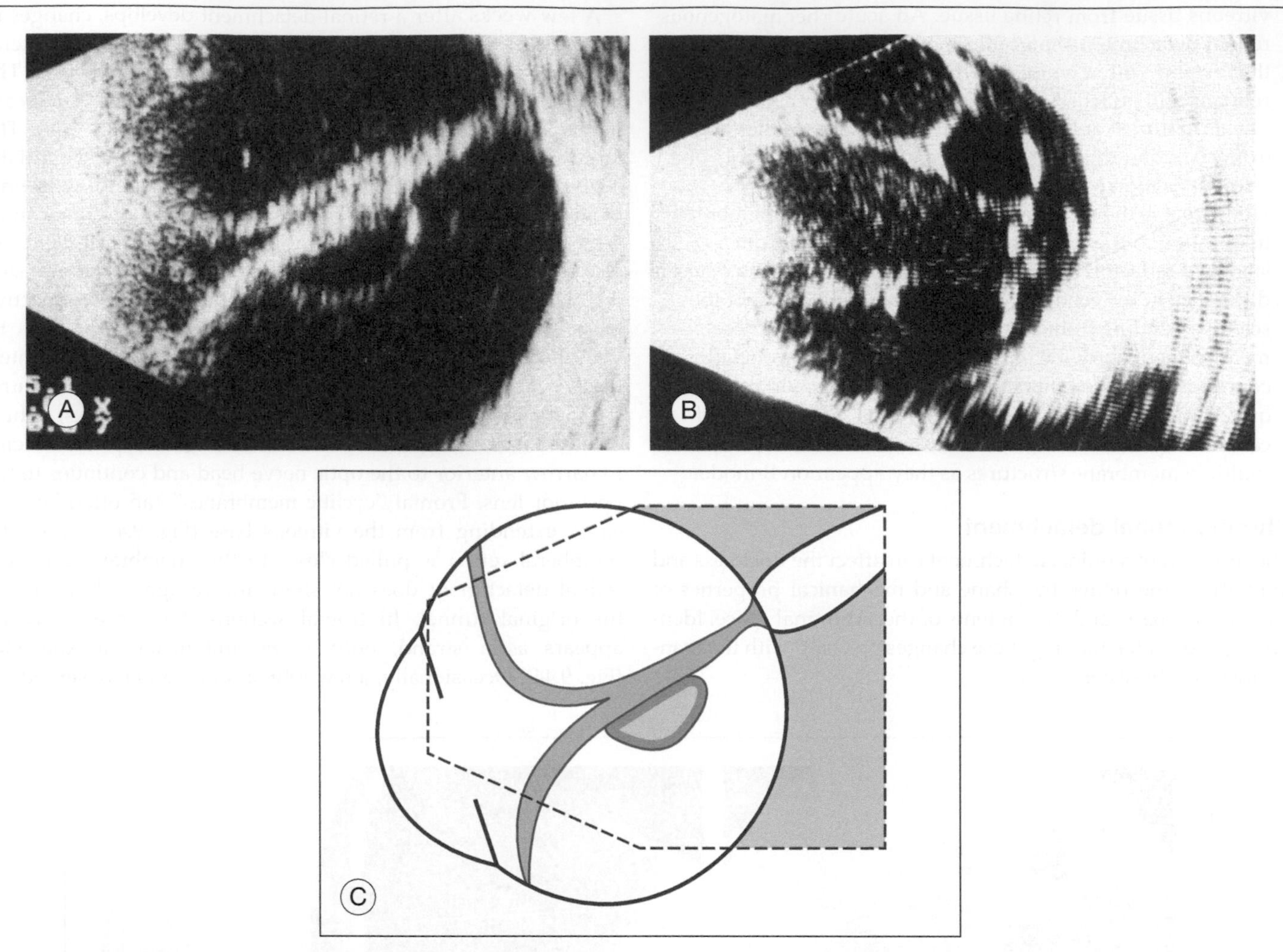

Fig. 9.41 Long-standing total retinal detachment with macrocyst. Intraretinal cyst in the axial area seen on cross-sectional ultrasound (A) and frontal plan (B). The cysts form from coalescing microcystoid degeneration of the retina in chronic detachments. These cavities will not be involved in secondary vitreous changes, such as vitreous hemorrhages or cholesterol deposits. (C) Schematic drawing.

In addition to the above findings, the consistency of the subretinal space can change with increased duration of the detachment. The protein content will increase and may precipitate out of the subretinal fluid. This can be seen as free-floating opacities on ultrasound (Fig. 9.45). If these opacities appear as static particles and not free-floating, then intraocular tumor has to be excluded. Under these circumstances, ultrasonography provides a vital role in obtaining a diagnosis by distinguishing the freely moving protein precipitation in long-standing detachments from the fixed hyperechoic particles of malignant tumors.

Retinoschisis

Retinoschisis is a splitting within the neurosensory layer of the retina. This condition frequently occurs in the inferotemporal quadrant. A cross-section echogram can display a membranous structure in the far periphery that has a convex border facing the vitreous (Fig. 9.46). In this situation, clinical correlation is important in order to distinguish the retinoschisis from a retinal detachment since these two entities can appear identical on static ultrasound. However, use of dynamic ultrasound and evaluation of the aftermovements can show that the aftermovements in retinoschisis are less conspicuous than in a retinal detachment. This is because in retinoschisis the retina is attached and there are no vitreous adhesions.

Coats disease

Coats disease is an exudative retinopathy most commonly seen unilaterally. It mainly affects males in the first decade of life. A clinical diagnosis can be made if aneurysmal malformations of retinal vessels and yellowish subretinal plaques are associated with an exudative detachment. Coats disease should be differentiated from retinoblastoma, which can have a similar clinical appearance in this patient group. Ultrasound can differentiate these conditions with careful evaluation of the subretinal space. Retinoblastoma typically shows calcifications with high reflectivity. The exudative detachment that is seen in Coats disease has different echo quality due to the subretinal cholesterol deposits (Fig. 9.47). In Coats disease, the crystals floating in the subretinal space are seen as floating opacities similar to the appearance of crystals in synchysis scintillans. They appear in an A-mode echogram as flickering spikes.[32] On B-mode images these high-frequency motions of the echo spikes produce a blurred pattern in the subretinal space.

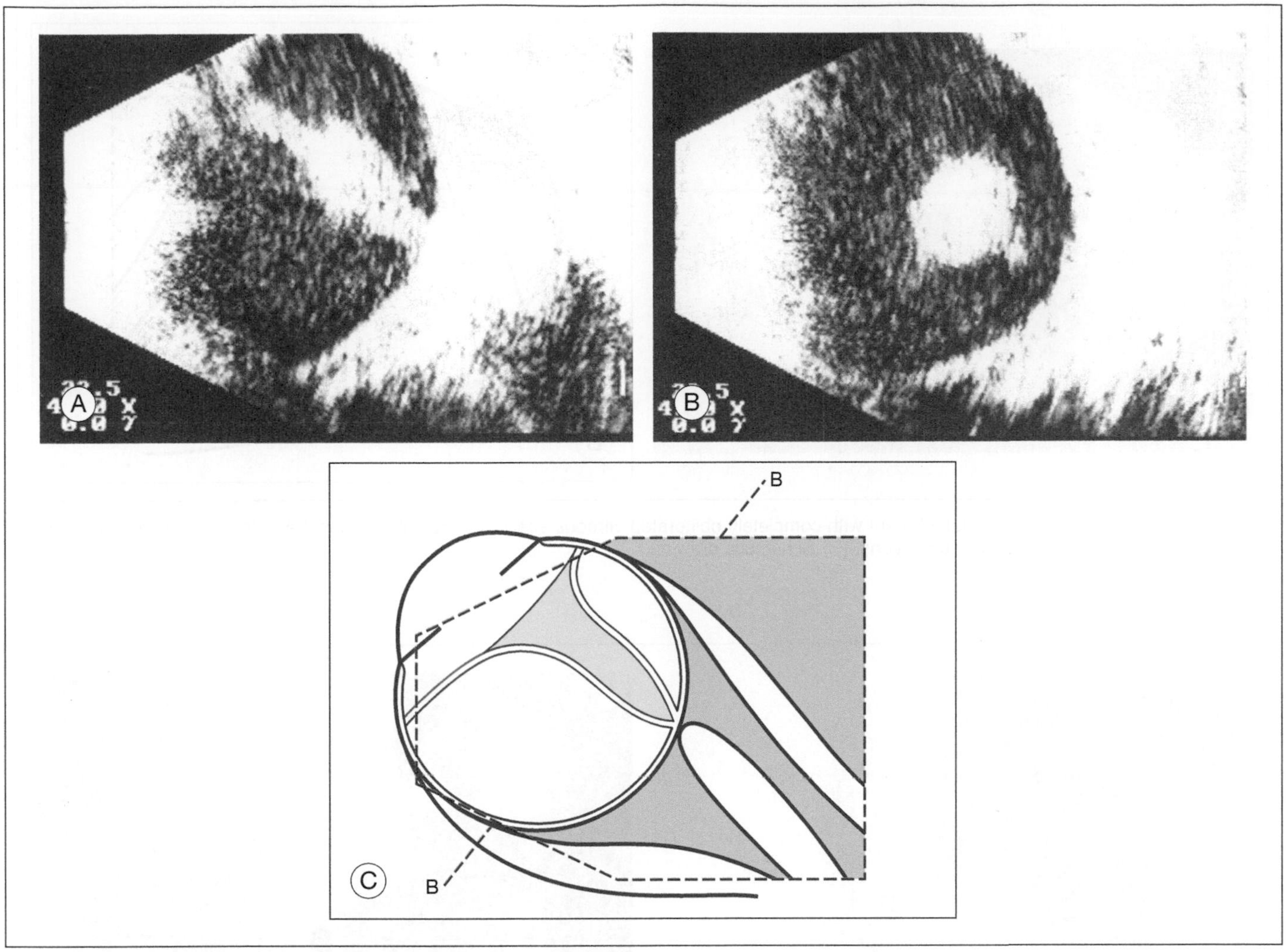

Fig. 9.42 (A,B) Long-standing retinal detachment with increased connective tissue in the vitreous tunnel. Free-floating opacities accumulate in the subretinal space (possibly representing hemorrhage or cholesterol crystals). (C) Schematic drawing.

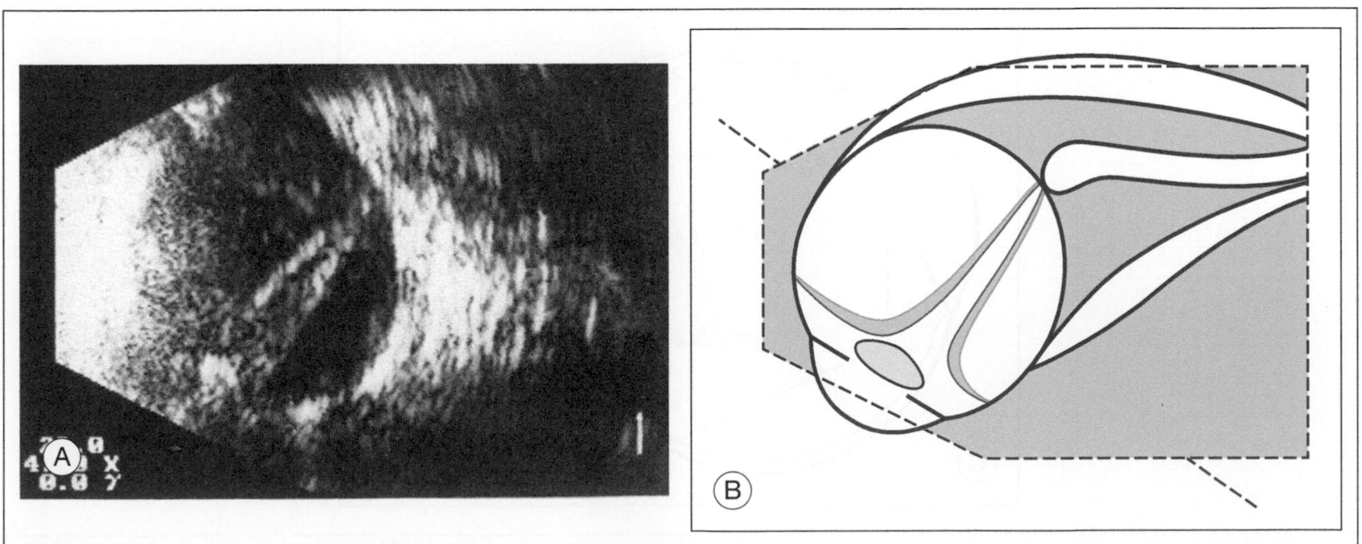

Fig. 9.43 (A) Long-standing total retinal detachment. A tube-like remnant of the vitreous within the shrunken retinal tunnel can be seen. (B) Schematic drawing.

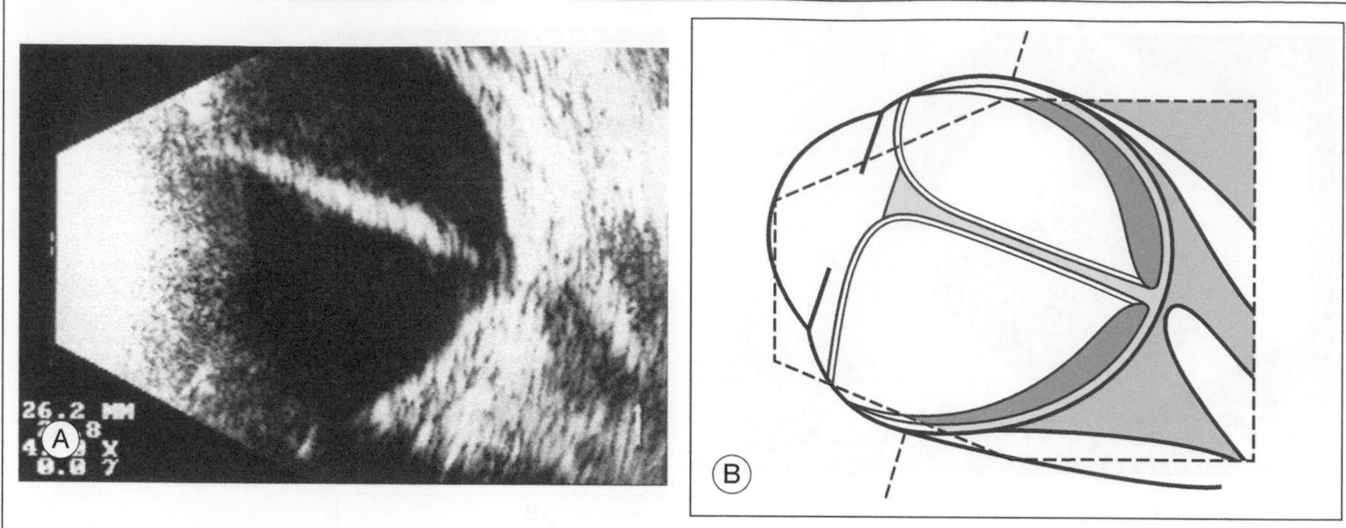

Fig. 9.44 (A) Long-standing retinal detachment with completely obliterated vitreous space. In sagittal sections the extensive adhesions of the retinal leaves produce various acoustic sections. (B) Schematic drawing.

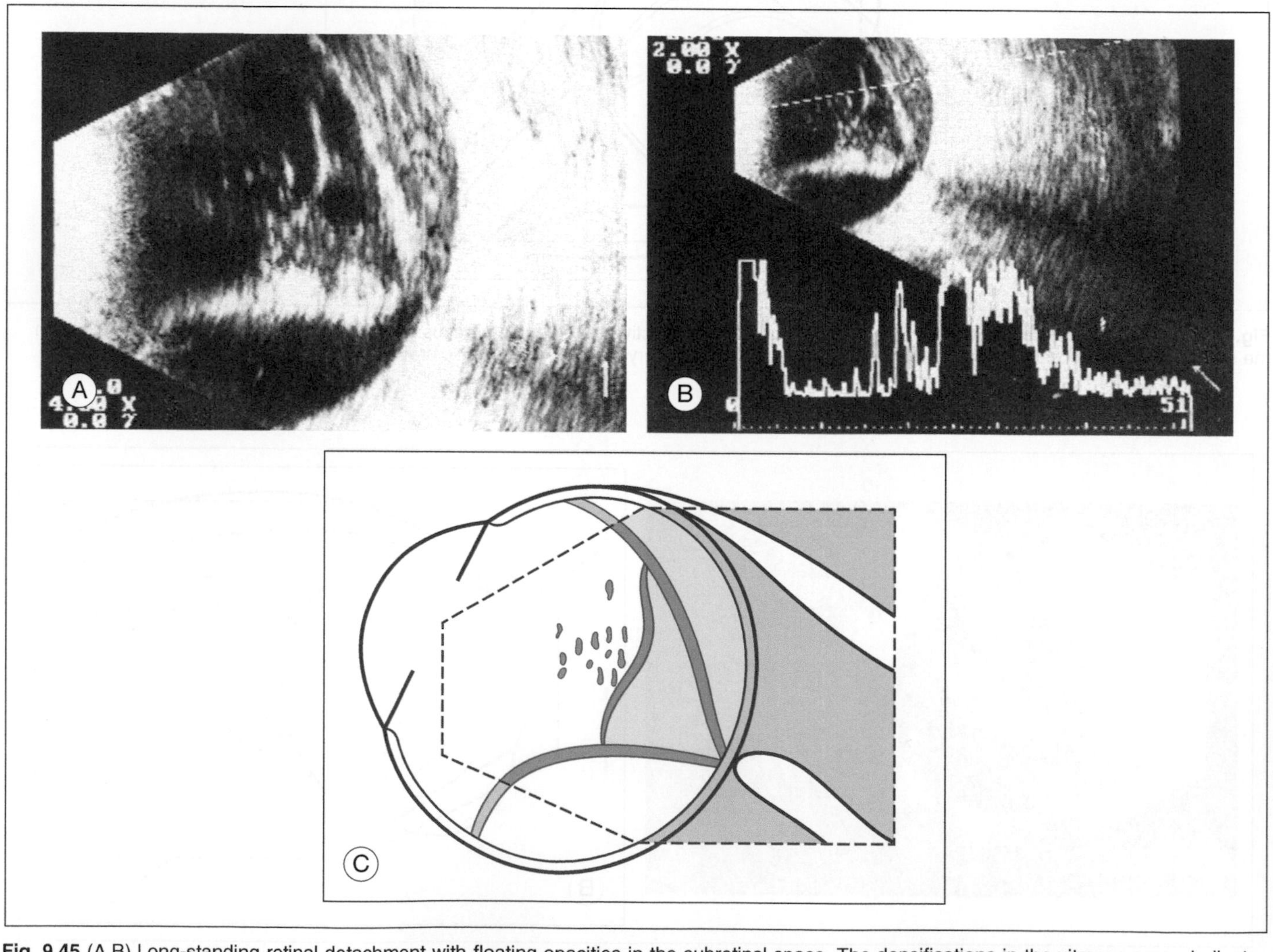

Fig. 9.45 (A,B) Long-standing retinal detachment with floating opacities in the subretinal space. The densifications in the vitreous space indicate a tendency for shrinkage. (C) Schematic drawing.

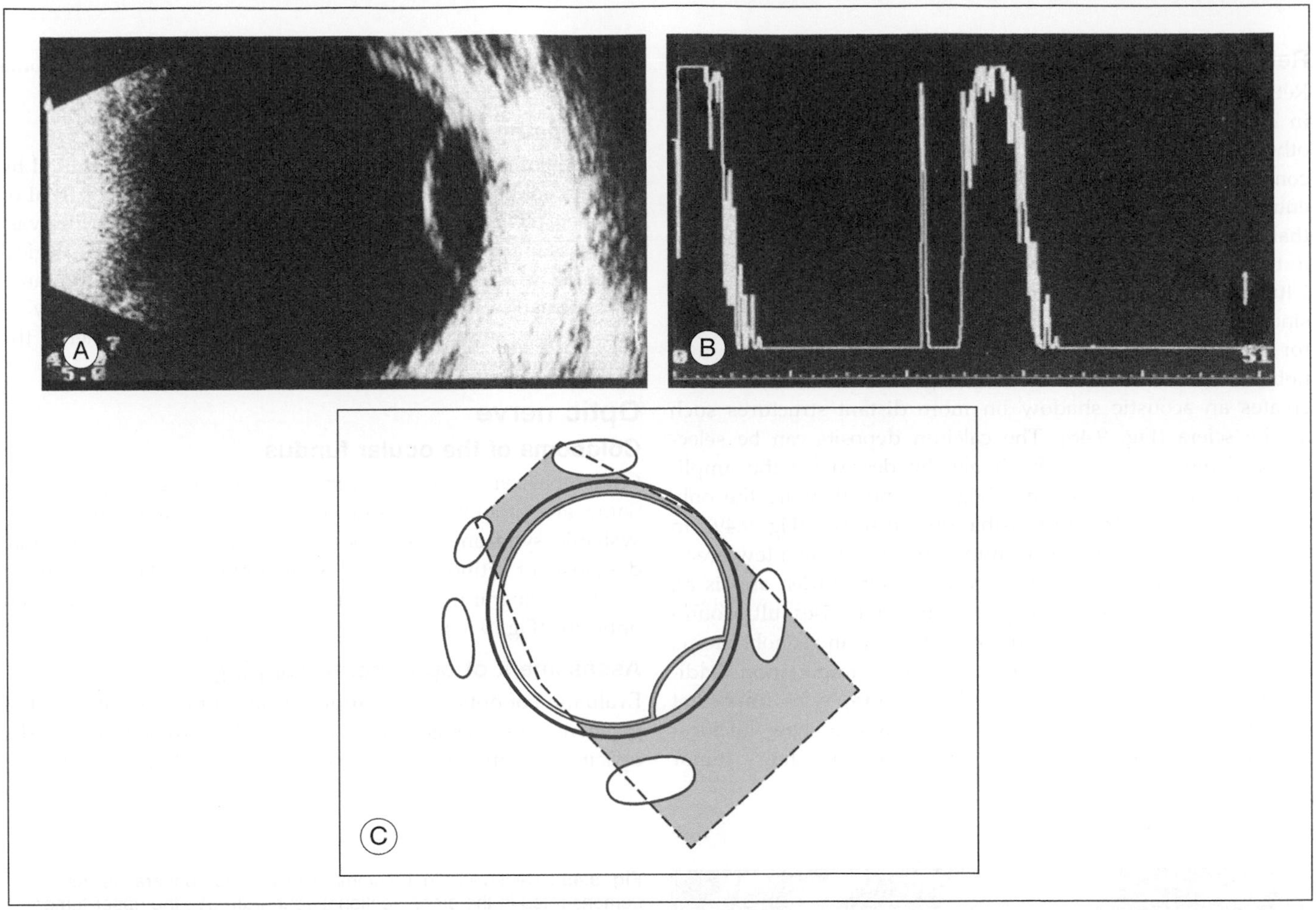

Fig. 9.46 (A) Senile retinoschisis in the inferotemporal quadrant. The typical biconvex cross-sectional image in association with slight aftermovements supports a tentative diagnosis of retinoschisis. (B) The acoustic reflectivity corresponds to that of a detached retina. (C) Schematic drawing.

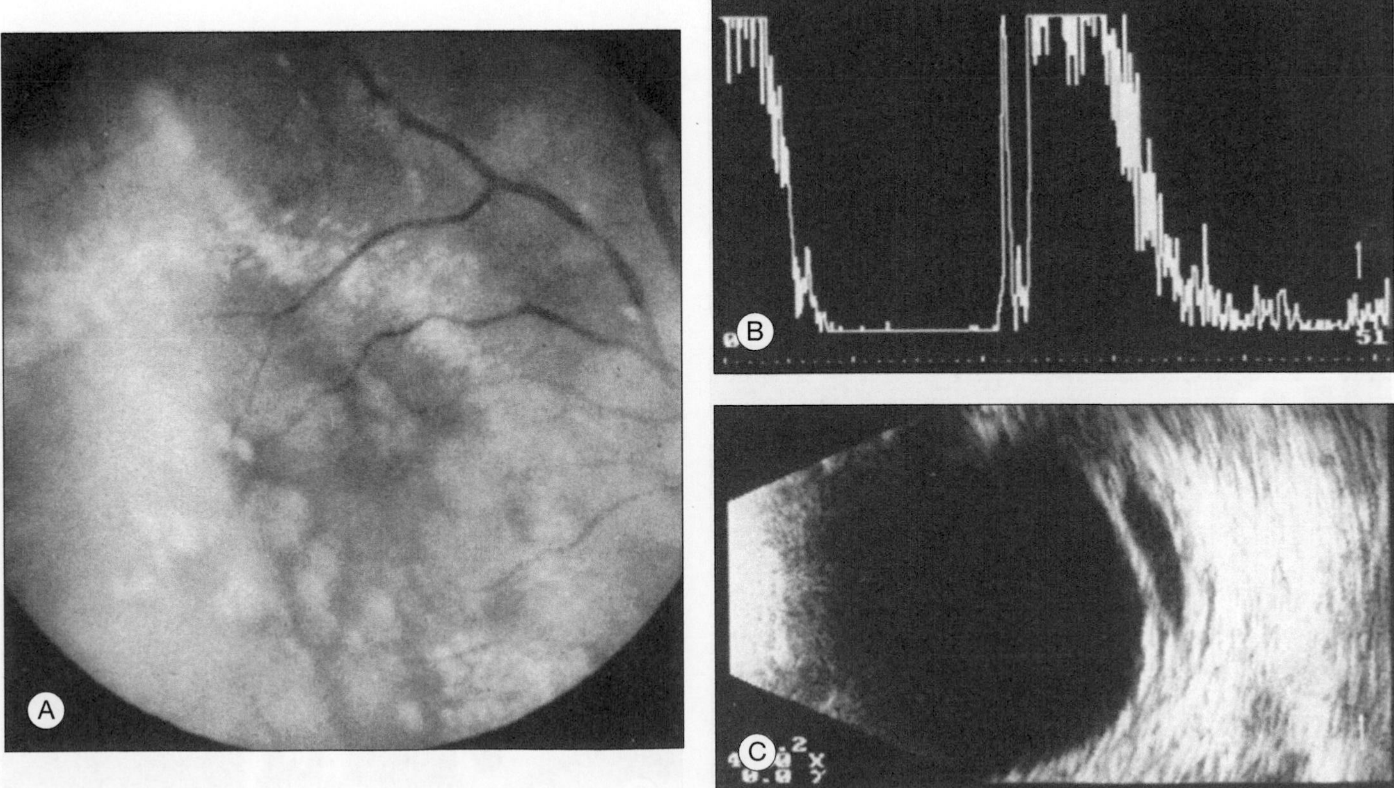

Fig. 9.47 (A) Fundoscopic clinical photo of Coats disease. Circumscribed, strongly reflecting retinal detachment in Coats disease. (B) The A-scan shows the high-intensity signal from the strongly reflecting membrane of the retinal detachment depicted in the image. (C) The B-scan shows the retinal detachment in association with floating opacities in the subretinal space that corroborate the diagnosis of Coats disease.

Retinoblastoma

Retinoblastoma is a life-threatening tumor that can present in children as isolated leukocoria or with a constellation of other ocular findings. Some findings can mimic benign ocular conditions. Since treatment of retinoblastoma can include ocular enucleation, making the appropriate diagnosis is critical. Ophthalmoscopy should be performed but sometimes is limited if there is cataract, hypopyon, vitreous seeding, or opacity. Ultrasound plays a critical role in these patients, especially since certain features on echography can be pathognomonic for retinoblastoma. The presence of calcium deposits in retinoblastoma lesions produces a high sound reflection that creates an acoustic shadow on more distant structures such as the sclera (Fig. 9.48). The calcium deposits can be selectively demonstrated on the image by decreasing the amplification in the cross-section echogram until they are the only remaining tissue structure visible on the screen (Fig. 9.49). In some retinoblastomas the calcium appears only in a few areas, but any calcification is indicative of tumor burden and is an important feature for the diagnosis. In some cases, ultrasound can also define extraocular tumor extension in retinoblastoma and is of great prognostic and therapeutic importance. Additional imaging to supplement ultrasonography is important in retinoblastoma. Computed tomography can show calcification and magnetic resonance imaging can show tumor extension outside the orbit, optic nerve invasion, or pinealoma (Fig. 9.50).

Retinopathy of prematurity

Early stages of retinopathy of prematurity can be diagnosed by indirect ophthalmoscopy. However, later stages with partial or complete tractional retinal detachments from extensive fibrovascular tissue require ultrasonography for diagnosis and surgical planning. Machemer and Aalberg[33] emphasized the importance of information obtained by cross-section ultrasonography in these stages, such as the diameter of the retinal funnel in the retrolental space (Fig. 9.51).

Optic nerve

Coloboma of the ocular fundus

Colobomas can occur in the iris, lens, retina, and optic nerve. Some are spontaneous and some occur in association with systemic syndromes. Colobomas are also in the differential diagnosis of retinoblastoma.[34] Colobomas can be seen clearly by ultrasonography even if the fundus cannot be visualized optically (Fig. 9.52).

Assessment of optic nerve cupping

Evaluation of optic nerve cupping is important for treatment of glaucomatous changes. This is difficult with anterior media opacity. Recently, with improvement of the lateral resolution of

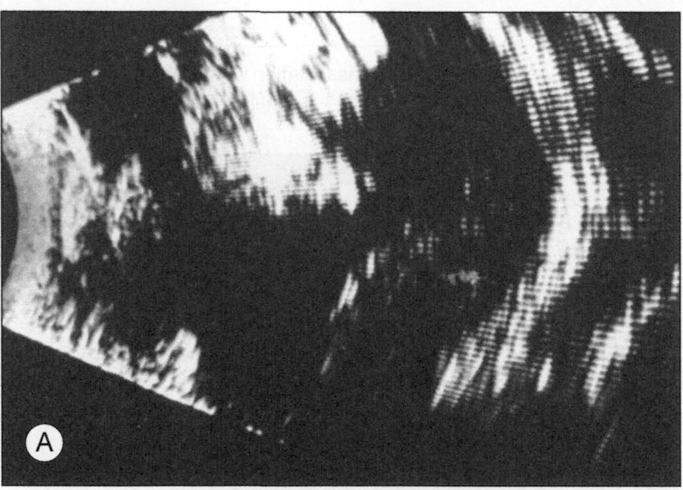

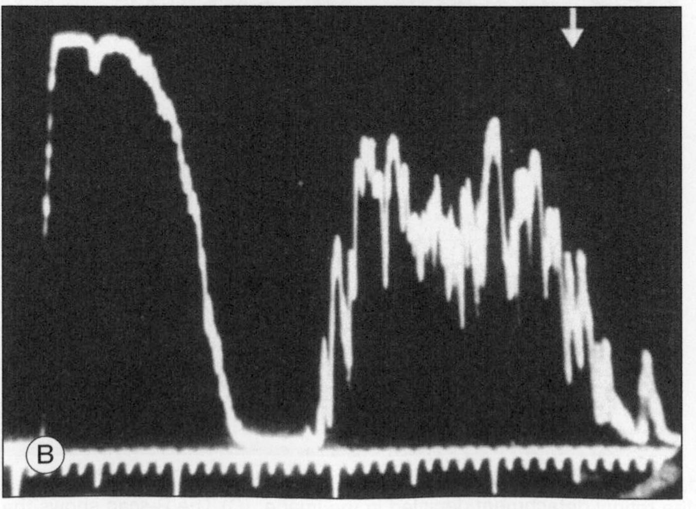

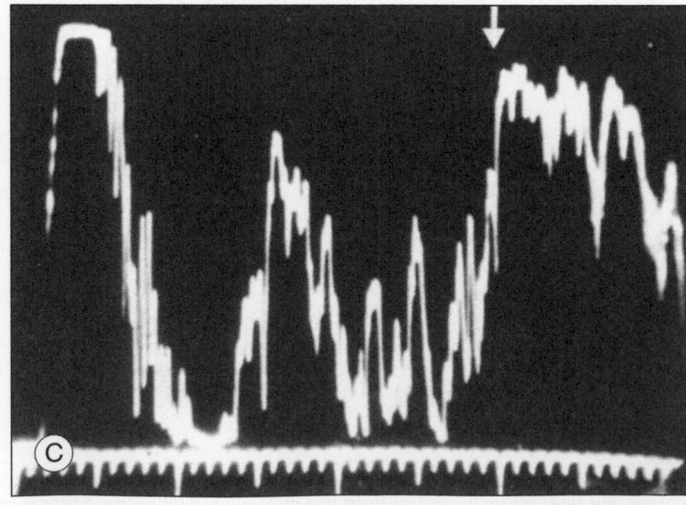

Fig. 9.48 Extensive retinoblastoma with varying appearance. As demonstrated in the cross-sectional echogram (A), the upper tumor portions show high acoustic reflectivity due to massive calcifications. The lower part of the tumor has less acoustic reflectivity than the adjacent sclera. A-scans of the eye (the scleral spikes in the acoustic scans (B,C) are marked by arrows).

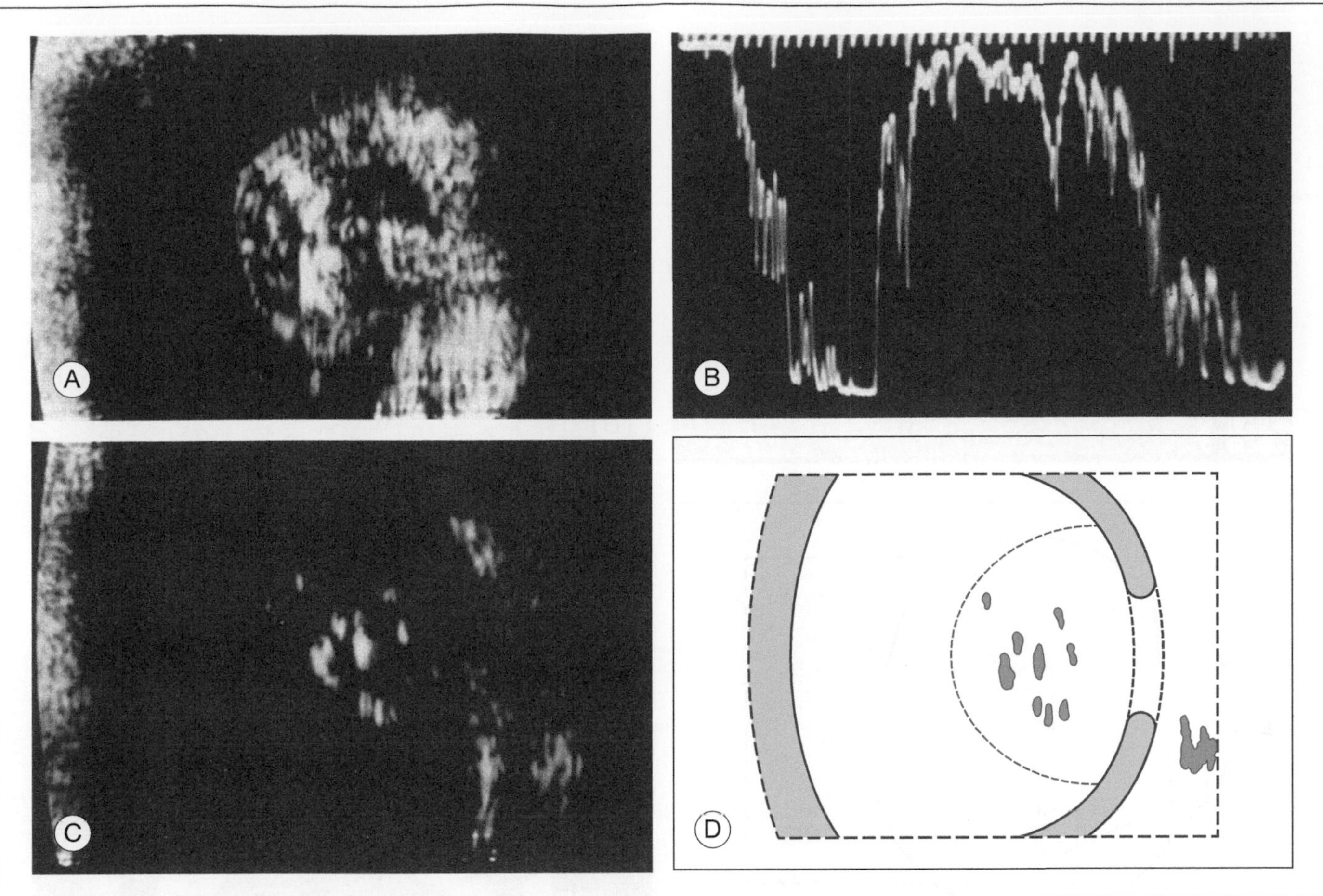

Fig. 9.49 Large retinoblastoma with calcifications and acoustic shadow cast on the adjacent sclera and orbit. (A) The calcifications light up in cross-sectional echograms. (B) In A-mode echograms, they can be quantified as the strongest reflecting structures in the examined area. (C) With reduced amplification, the calcified areas are the only visible signals. (D) Schematic drawing.

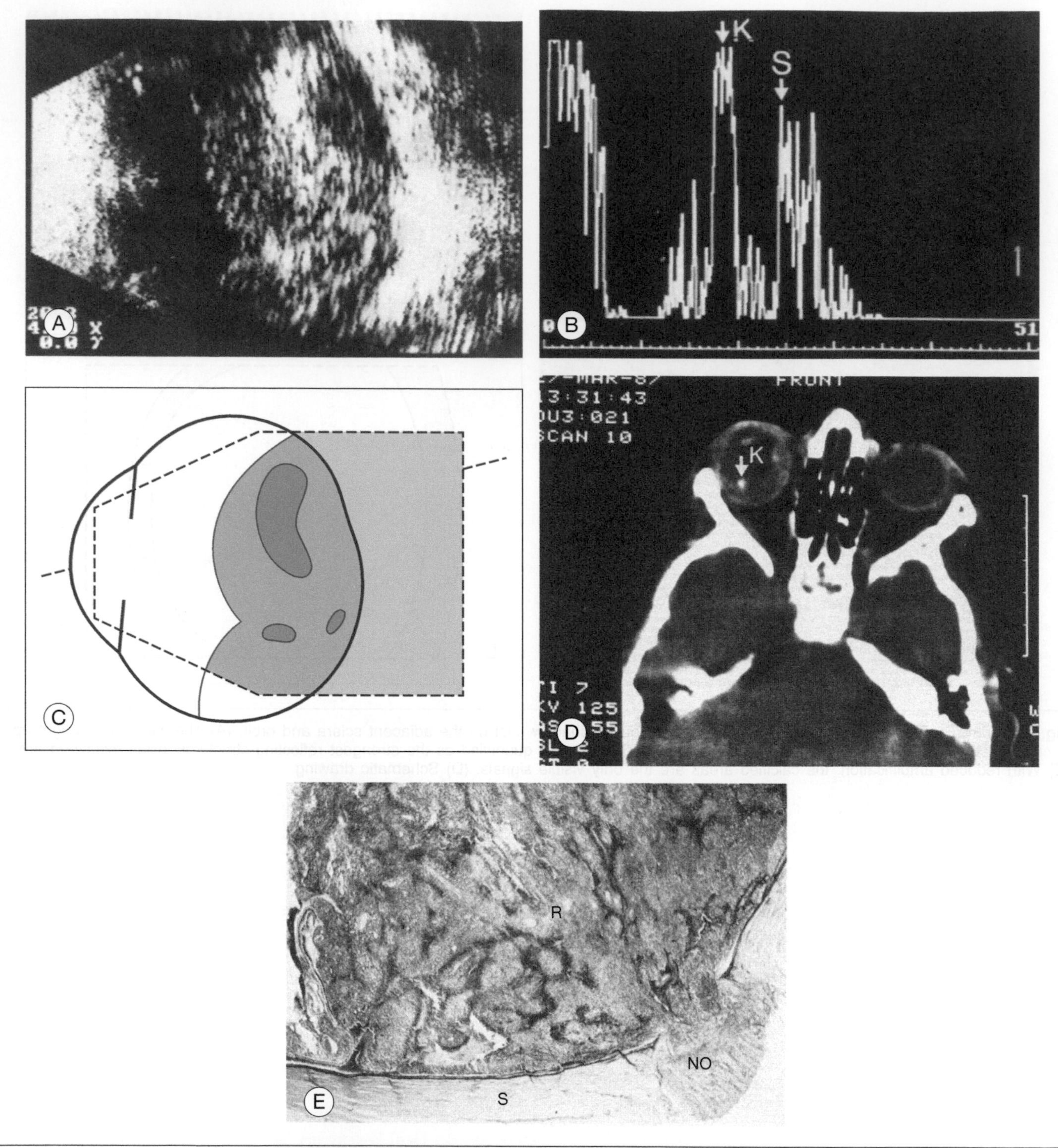

Fig. 9.50 Extensive retinoblastoma. (A) A cross-sectional echographic image. The tumor is characterized by areas of high acoustic reflectivity alternating with areas of low reflectivity. (B) The differences in reflection can be quantified on A-mode echography: calcified parts of the tumor have markedly higher amplitudes as seen at point K as compared to the sclera reflection as seen at point S. (C) Schematic drawing of the ultrasonographical image in (A). (D) Computed tomography scan displays the calcified parts of the retinoblastoma that can be identified with greater certainty than in a plain X-ray picture. (E) A histological sample of the infiltration into the optic nerve. NO, optic nerve; R, retinoblastoma. The calcium deposits explain the nearly pathognomonic echogram.

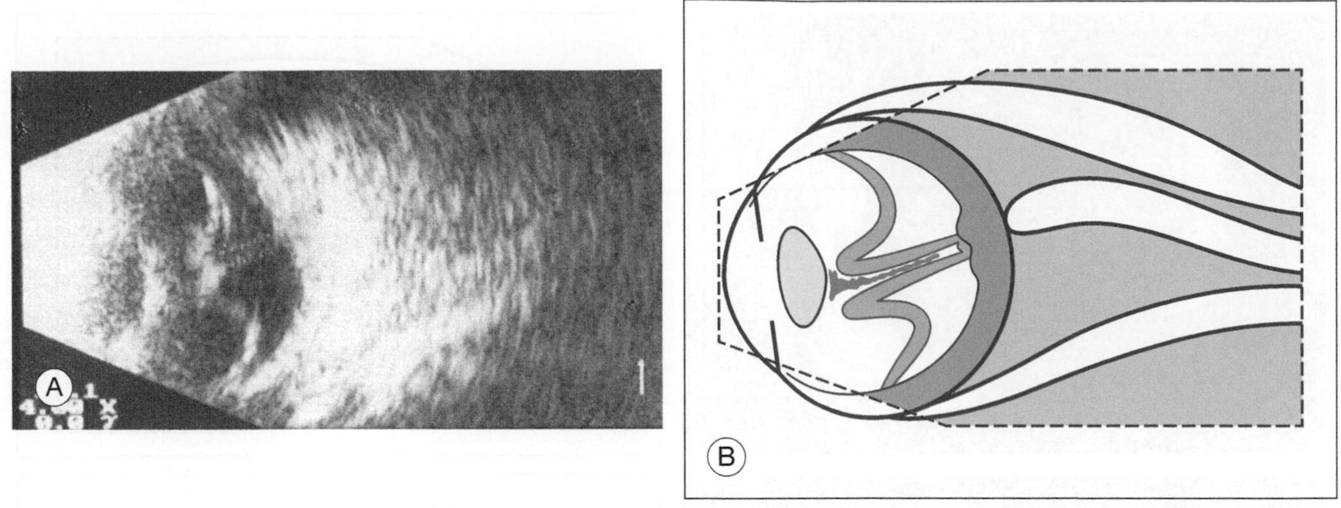

Fig. 9.51 Stage V of retinopathy of prematurity. (A) In cross-sectional images we see a complete retinal detachment with a widening of the avascular peripheral retina toward the subretinal space. (B) Schematic drawing.

B-scan images, optic nerve head cupping can be reliably measured and reproduced on ultrasound images.[35]

Choroid

Changes in the ocular layers due to hypotony

In acute hypotony, exudation into the suprachoroidal space creates an increase in the choroidal vascular pressure. This can lead to a choroidal detachment which will then exacerbate the globe hypotony (Fig. 9.53). This situation is ultrasonographically characterized by a convex border on a cross-sectional image that denotes the location of the choroidal detachment. This convex shape is formed between the pars plana and location of the vortex veins, both of which have strong choroidal attachments. Knowledge of the choroidal anatomic structure and its attachments can aid in ultrasound diagnosis. In addition to the pars plana and vortex veins, the choroid is firmly attached to the optic nerve. The choroid inserts at the optic nerve at a blunt angle, as compared to the retina, which has a steeper insertion. This feature can be used to help differentiate choroidal and retinal detachments of the posterior pole on ultrasound images. In addition, a choroidal detachment would begin at the ciliary body and not the ora serrate, as in a retinal detachment (Fig. 9.54). Occasionally, the detached ciliary body can compress the lens. In severe cases, choroidal detachments may meet in the center of the globe. This feature has been termed "kissing choroidals" and needs to be surgically corrected (Fig. 9.55). In typical cases of serous choroidal detachments the subchoroidal space is acoustically silent. In contrast, an expulsive choroidal hemorrhage can be identified by the hyperechoic signal on ultrasound that the blood clots create within the detachment (Fig. 9.56).

In chronic hypotony with long-standing choroidal detachments, the outer layer of the globe can appear concentrically widened on ultrasound. In advanced stages, the appearance on ultrasound changes, the outer walls appear thickened, and the vitreous cavity becomes substantially reduced. In these eyes, metaplasia of the pigment epithelium can result in calcification and ossification of ocular tissue that is easily identified on ultrasound because of the total reflection of all sound waves noted on the acoustic image.

Choroidal neovascularization

Choroidal neovascularization is a complication seen in many eye diseases, most commonly in macular degeneration. The histological findings include a vascularized collection of connective tissue that extends from the choriocapillaris through defects in Bruch's membrane and then into the subretinal pigment epithelial or subretinal space. This heterogeneous structure produces mixed ultrasound features, including the strong acoustic reflections from the fibrovascular membranes and dense connective tissue septa and the acoustically silent areas of exudate and subretinal fluid (Figs 9.24 and 9.57). Peripheral choroidal neovascularization membranes can appear similar to choroidal melanomas; therefore, familiarity with the ultrasonographic features of these lesions is important, especially if vitreous hemorrhage prevents direct visualization.

Choroidal melanoma

Evaluation of choroidal melanomas includes a comprehensive examination with ophthalmoscopy combined with ultrasound imaging. In choroidal melanomas, the signals produced within the tumor are complicated by overlapping and dampening echo processes. Connective tissue septa and vessels vary in their prominence and interfere with the signals from the tumor tissue. Furthermore, the resolution of the image is limited because the densely packed tumor cells are separated by a considerably shorter distance than the ultrasound wavelength. A thorough understanding of the principles of ultrasonography and a strong knowledge base of the tissue complexity in metastatic processes combined with an extensive case reference aids in the image interpretation of choroidal melanomas. The interpretation of echograms in A- and B-mode is based on reports on this topic which were published by Oksala,[36] Baum,[37] Buschmann and Trier,[38] Till and Ossoinig,[32] Trier,[39] Coleman et al.,[40] and

Text continued on p. e264

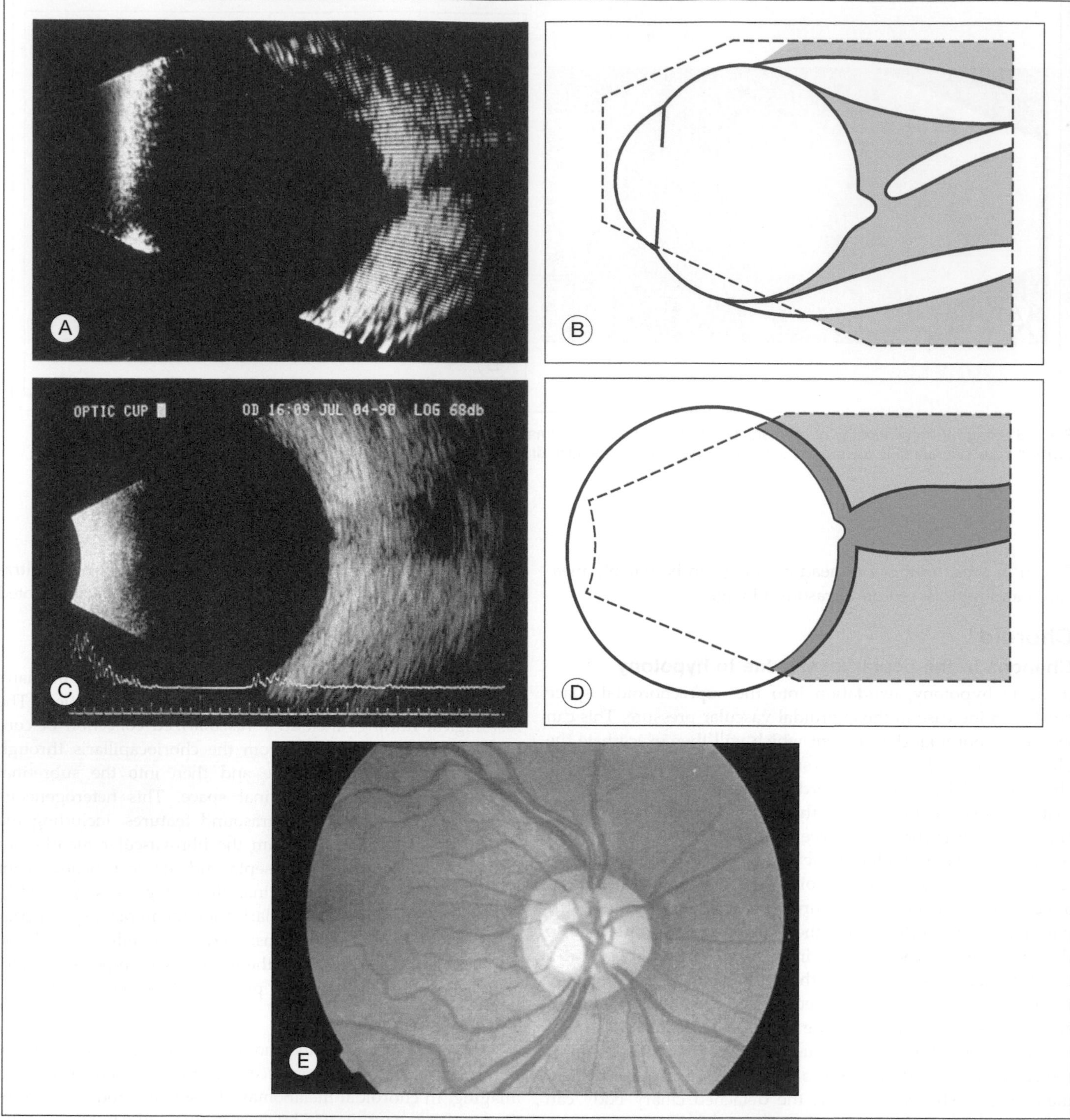

Fig. 9.52 (A) Echogram of the small optic nerve coloboma depicted in (E). In comparision, B-scan section showing normal physiological cupping of an optic nerve head (C). To obtain this vertical section a probe is placed temporal to the limbus, thereby avoiding any artifacts, caused by the lens. (B,D) Schematic drawings. (E) Small coloboma of the optic nerve with a diameter of about 2.5 mm. Fundus photograph showing excavation within the nerve.

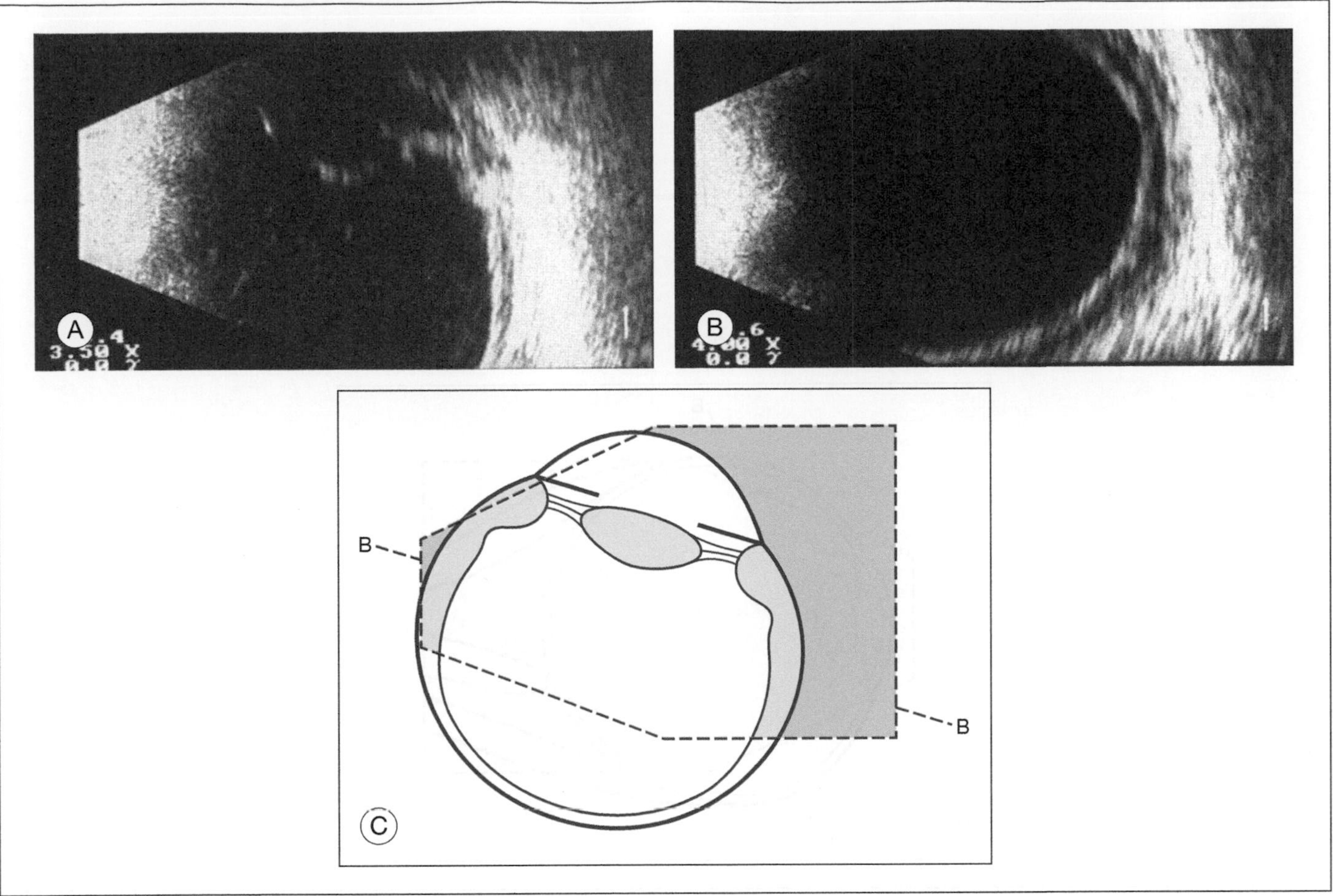

Fig. 9.53 (A) Detachment of the ciliary body and the peripheral choroid due to hypotony. (B) The thickening of the ocular walls begins in the area of the ciliary body and extends to the equator, as seen on the B-scan. (C) Schematic drawing.

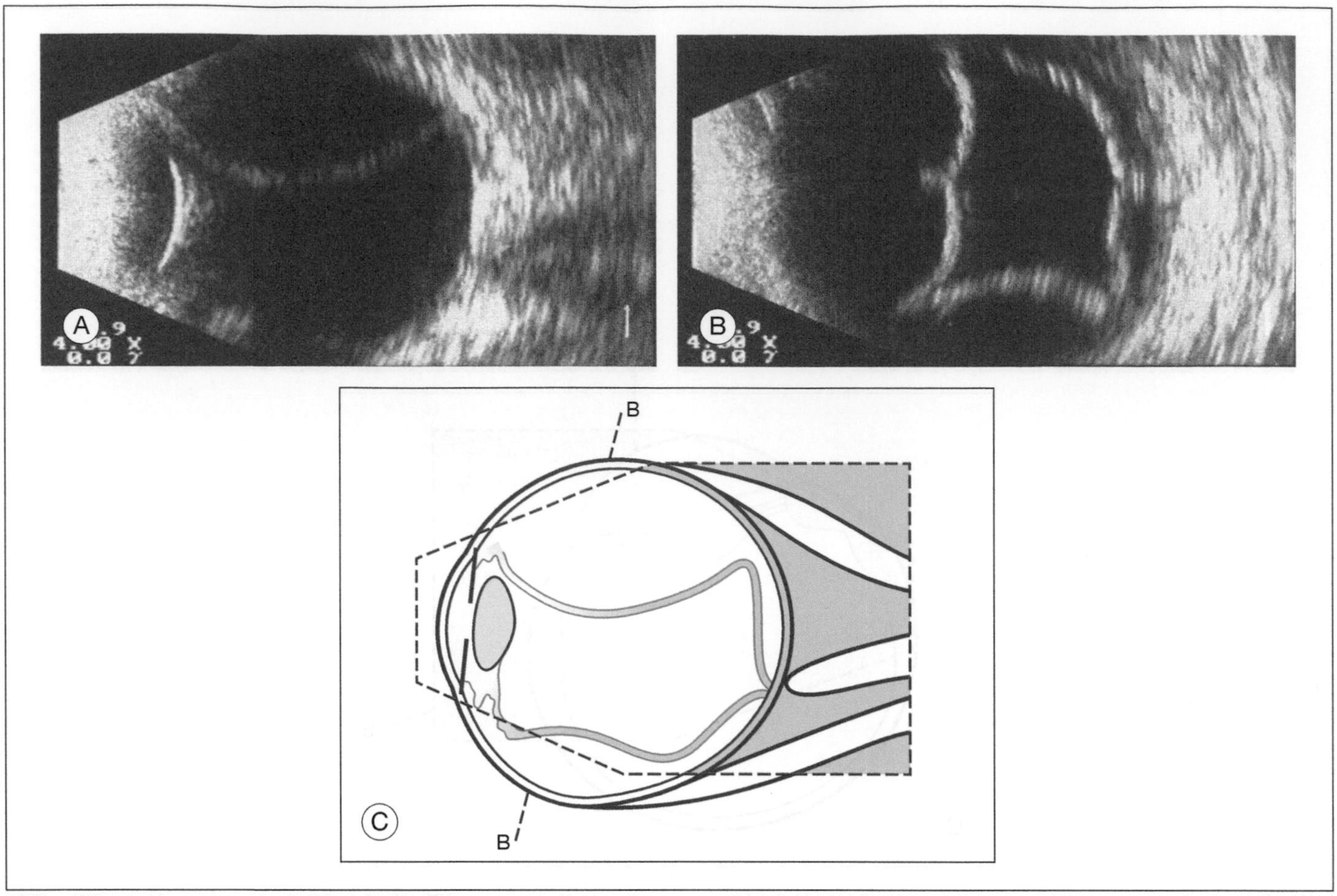

Fig. 9.54 Subtotal exudative choroidal detachment. (A) In contrast to a retinal detachment, the choroidal detachment extends beyond the ora serrata; the detachment extends from the iris diaphragm to the posterior pole without reaching the optic nerve head. (B) The frontal sections depict indentations which are caused by large vessels. (C) Schematic drawing.

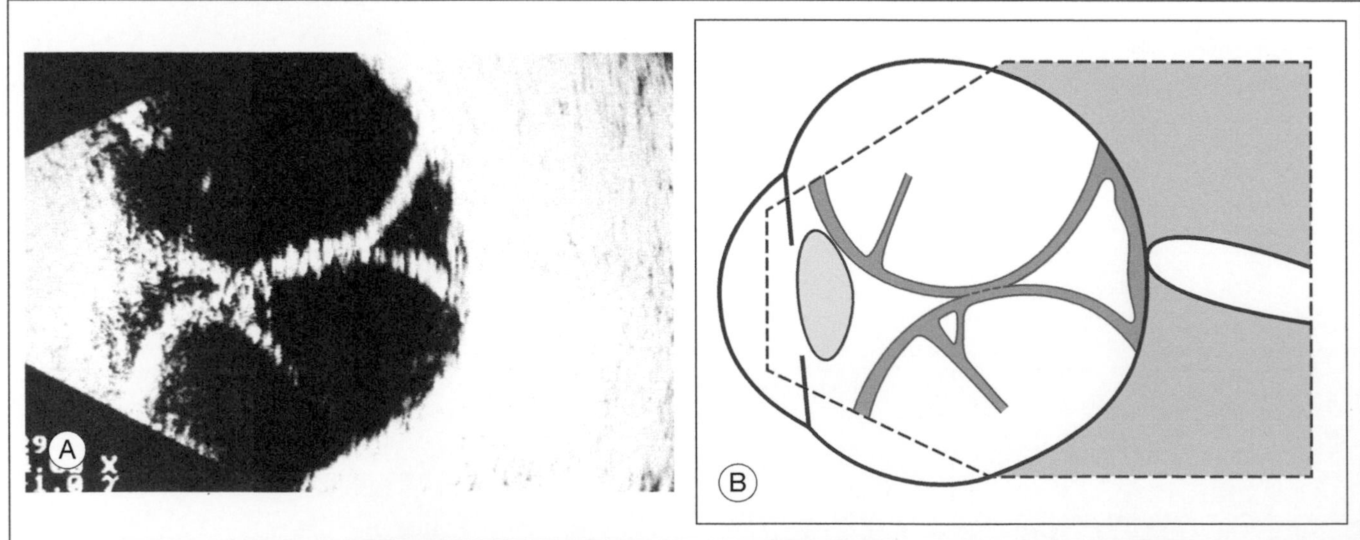

Fig. 9.55 Total exudative choroidal detachment in persistent hypotony after penetrating glaucoma surgery with external fistulation. (A) The apices of the choroidal detachment touch each other in the vitreous and are seen on the echogram. This finding is commonly termed "kissing choroidals." Strand-like structures (possibly taut vortex veins) course through the intrachoroidal space. (B) Schematic drawing.

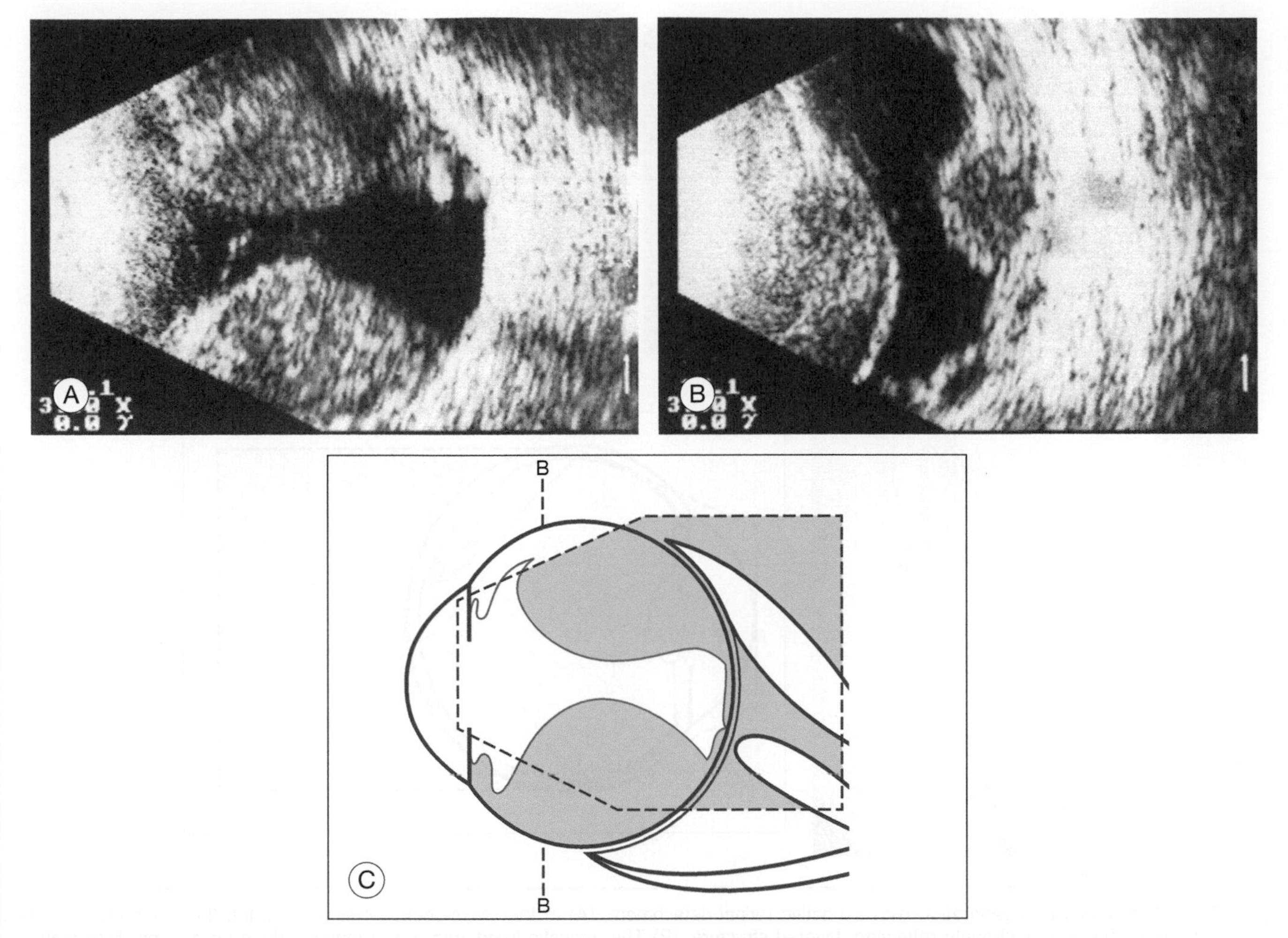

Fig. 9.56 Extensive choroidal detachment in an eye with expulsive hemorrhage. (A) The intrachoroidal space has acquired acoustic reflectivity due to the accumulation of blood. There may be anatomical healing after the absorption of the blood, but we cannot expect visual function to improve. (B) Frontal image of the hemorrhagic choroidal detachments. (C) Schematic drawing.

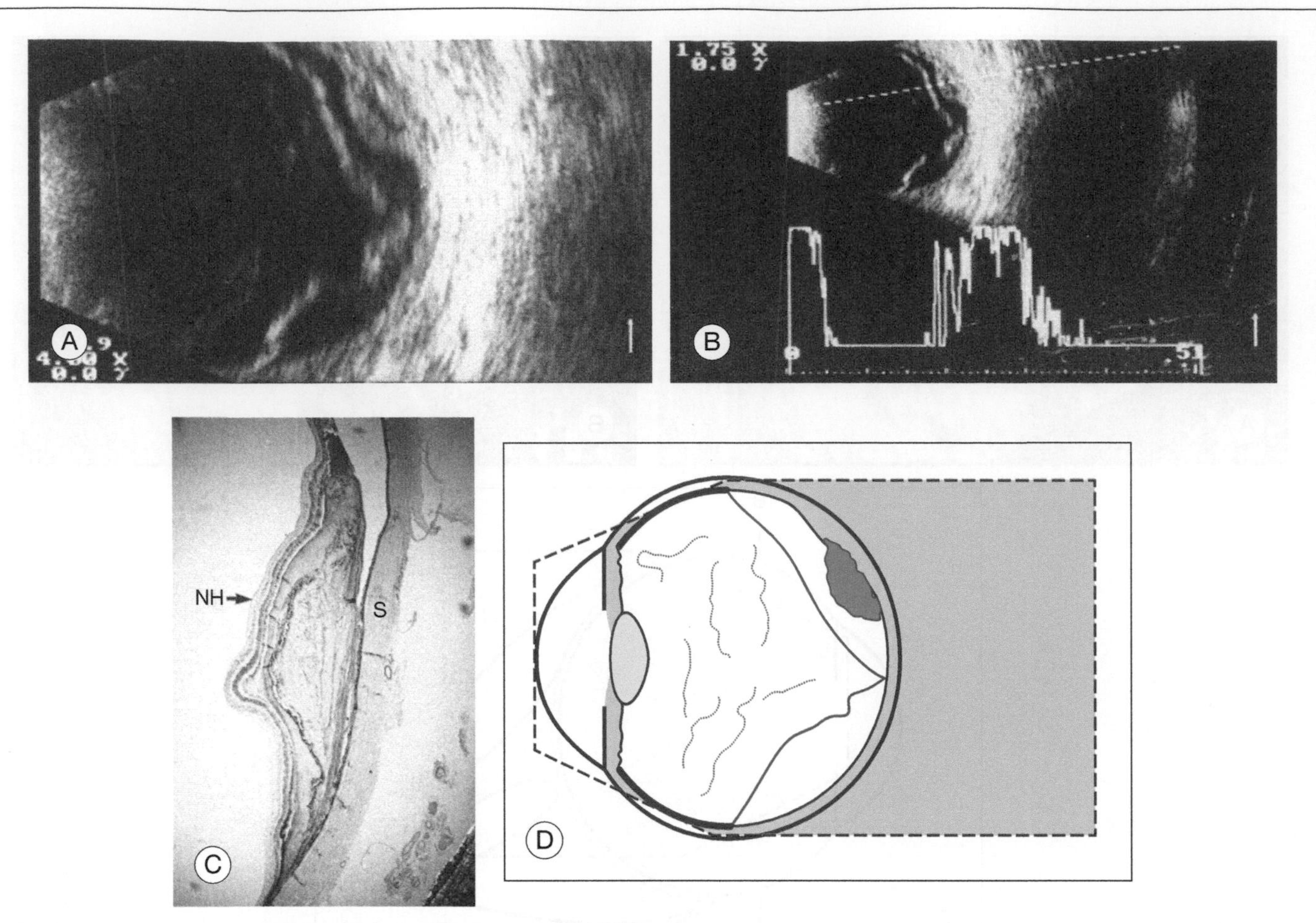

Fig. 9.57 Disciform macular degeneration with exudative retinal detachment. (A) In the cross-sectional echogram, the thickened ocular walls in the macular area appear as a strongly reflecting, layered structure. (B) The acoustic interfaces of the macular degeneration produce high signals. (C) Histologic section of an eye with disciform macular degeneration under loupe magnification. Vascularized connective tissue scars with exudation without acoustic interfaces produce the substrate for the heterogeneous nature of the echogram. NH, retina; S, sclera. (D) Schematic drawing.

Silverman et al.,[41] which include data from the original scans of ocular tissues. The next section will review the principles used to image choroidal tumors and the features of a choroidal melanoma on B-mode and A-mode imaging.

The characteristics of a choroidal melanoma on B-mode echography

In B-mode echograms, a melanoma appears as a biconvex lesion. The internal structure is relatively homogeneous so produces markedly fewer signals than the tumor surface or the sclera (Fig. 9.58). If the tumor has broken through Bruch's membrane, then a mushroom-shaped lesion, or a collar button, can be demonstrated in cross-section and serves as a pathognomonic sign (Fig. 9.59). If present, this perforation does not necessarily occur at the peak of the tumor; careful ultrasound examination of the entire lesion is needed (Fig. 9.60). In some sections, the collar button of a tumor may even simulate a tumor mass lying free in the vitreous (Fig. 9.59). In addition, the collar button portion of the lesion has unique ultrasound features due to the presence of the mass above Bruch's membrane in some places and below Bruch's membrane in other places. Previously this feature was attributed to sound attenuation, which is the continuous decay of spike altitudes in the A-mode and was called the angle kappa. However, the change in signal is most likely due to more than just an attenuation phenomenon. The features of the collar button can be explained on the basis of echographic–histopathologic correlations (Fig. 9.61). Usually, a tumor lying immediately beneath the sensory retina reflects ultrasound more than the portion of the tumor beneath Bruch's membrane. In a collar button, the part of the tumor growing in front of Bruch's membrane will be drained less well, leading to a dilatation of the vessels in this part of the tumor.[31,42] This creates new acoustic interfaces with higher signal intensity, resulting in brighter dots in B-mode and higher spikes in A-mode. In the area of the tumor base, a "choroidal excavation" can be seen (Figs 9.62 and 9.63). This excavation in the acoustic section develops at the edge of the tumor where melanoma tissue intersects the adjacent strongly reflecting intact choroid.[37,43]

The characteristics of a choroidal melanoma on A-mode ultrasonography

The ultrasonographic internal structure of a tumor is quantitatively best described in the A-mode echogram. An unfocused A-mode transducer can obtain a summation signal from the large tissue area,[31] which typically demonstrates spikes of relatively uniform amplitudes within the large biconvex tumor if the lesion has not extensively broken through Bruch's membrane

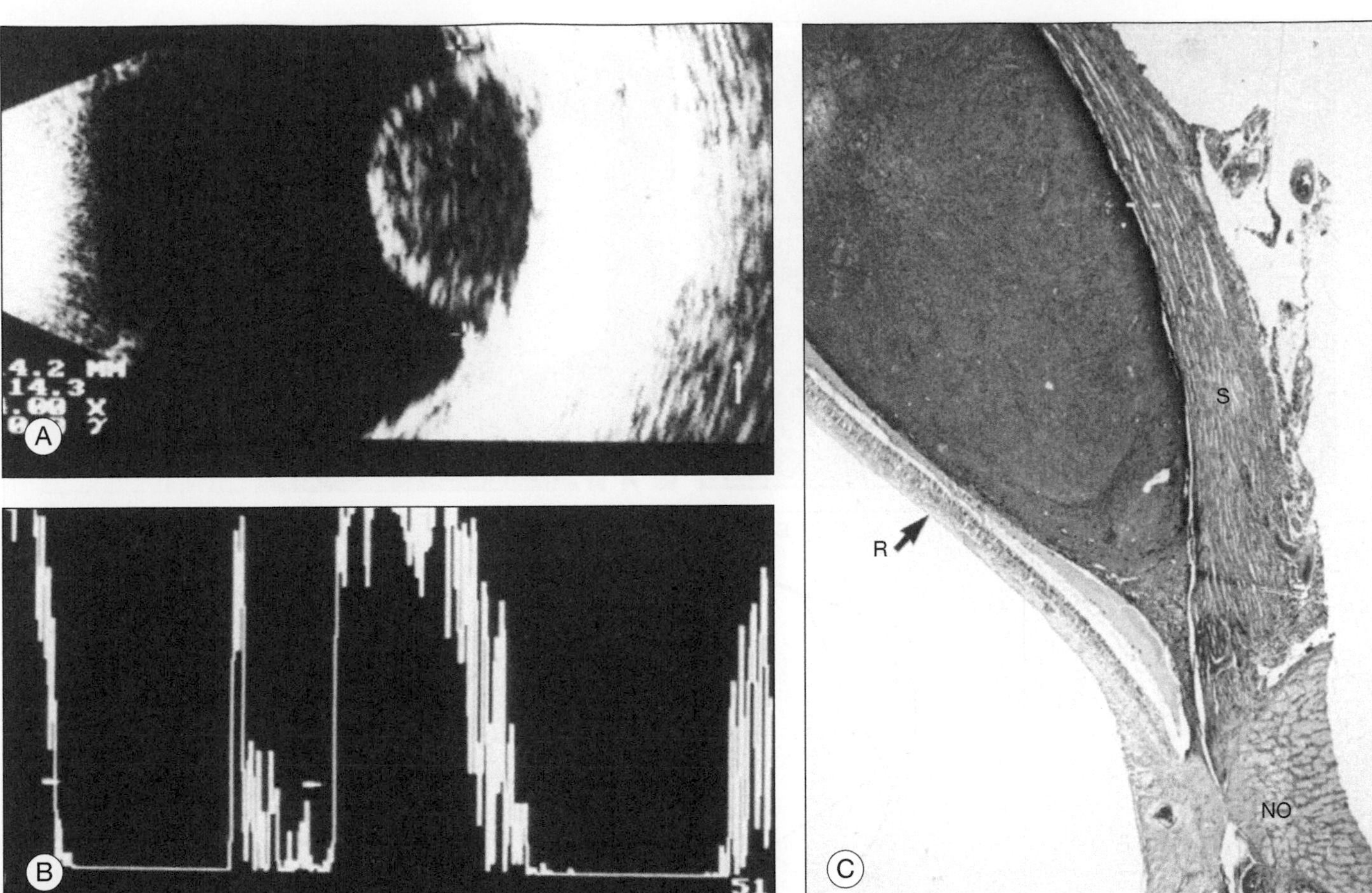

Fig. 9.58 Typical findings of a choroidal melanoma. (A) In cross-section the tumor is biconvex. The diameter of the base is 14 × 14 mm; elevation, 8.5 mm; calculated tumor volume, 750 mm^3. (B) With standardized A-mode, the spike amplitude within the tumor amounts to about 20% of the scleral spike. (C) Histological section visualized under loupe magnification of a peripapillary choroidal melanoma. The reason for the low homogeneous acoustic reflectivity of a choroidal melanoma is the densely packed tumor cells, the margins of which are separated by a distance much smaller than the wavelength of ultrasound. R, retina; S, sclera; NO, optic nerve.

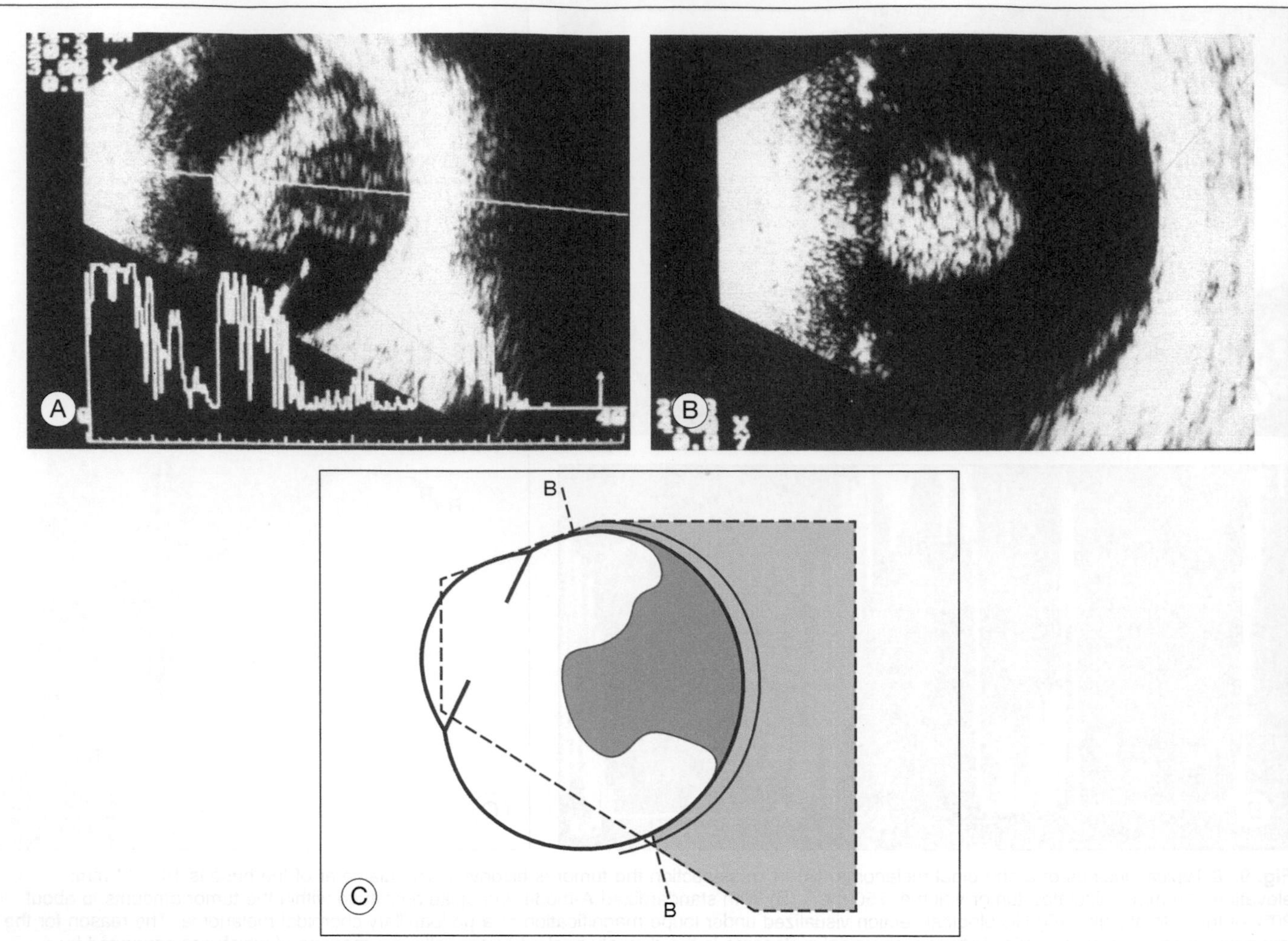

Fig. 9.59 Large choroidal melanoma, mushroom-shaped after perforating Bruch's membrane. (A) Sagittal section. (B) In the frontal plane, one part of the tumor does not seem to have contact with the ocular outer walls, which demonstrates the principle of the necessity to image tumors in multiple planes to define the full extent of invasion. (C) Schematic drawing.

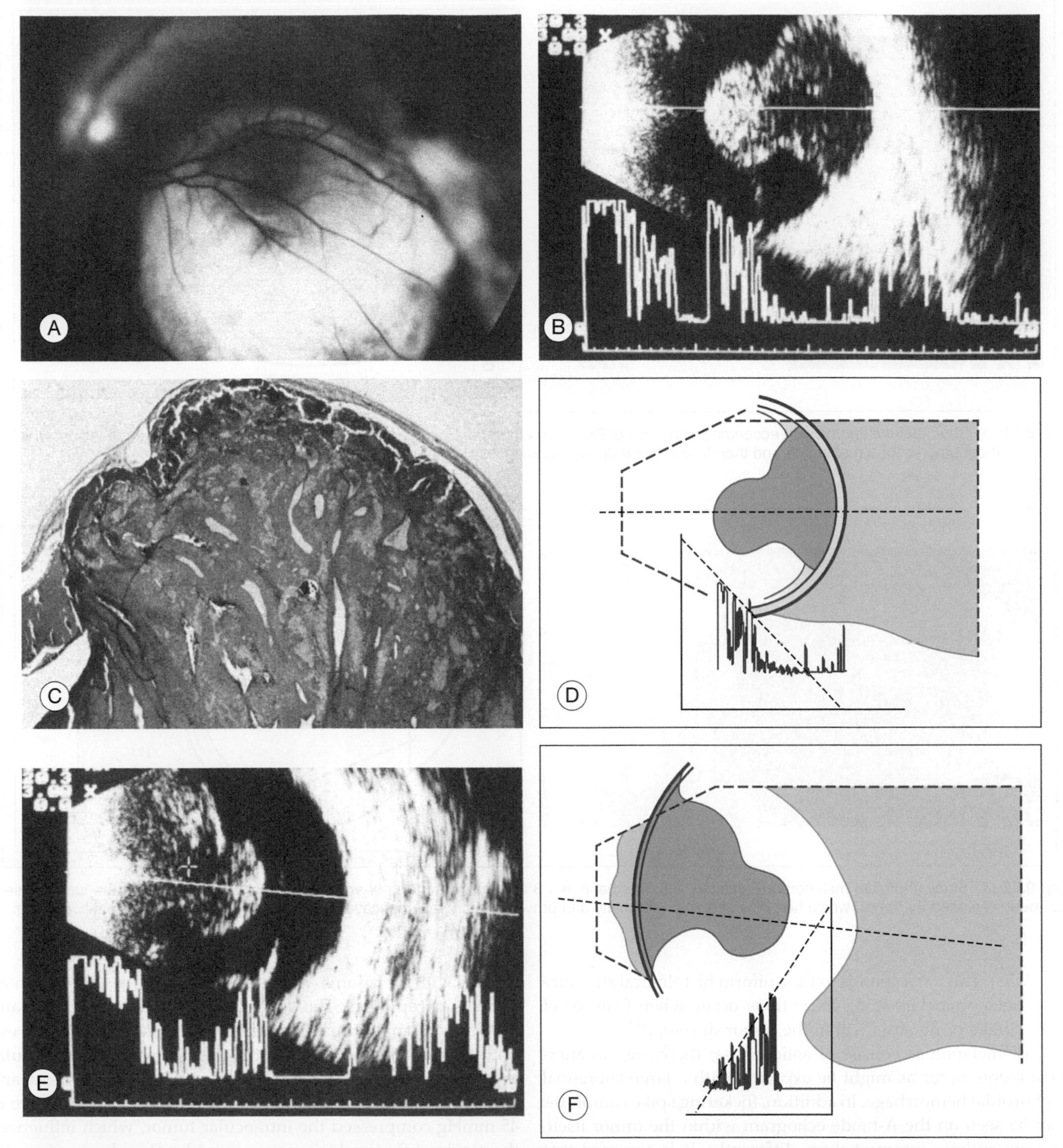

Fig. 9.60 (A) Large mushroom-shaped choroidal melanoma with collar button seen on fundus photography. (B) Sagittal echogram cross-section with A-mode echogram. There is markedly increased reflection in the area of the tumor peak. The part of the tumor in front of Bruch's membrane often shows dilated vessels, which act as interfaces to increase the acoustic reflectivity. (C) Histological section through the tumor. (D) Schematic drawing. (E) Echogram from the tumor base. This image was obtained with maximal adduction of the globe, and made possible because of the far temporal location of the tumor base. Also in this direction of examination, the part of the tumor anterior to Bruch's membrane demonstrates high reflectivity. (F) Schematic drawing.

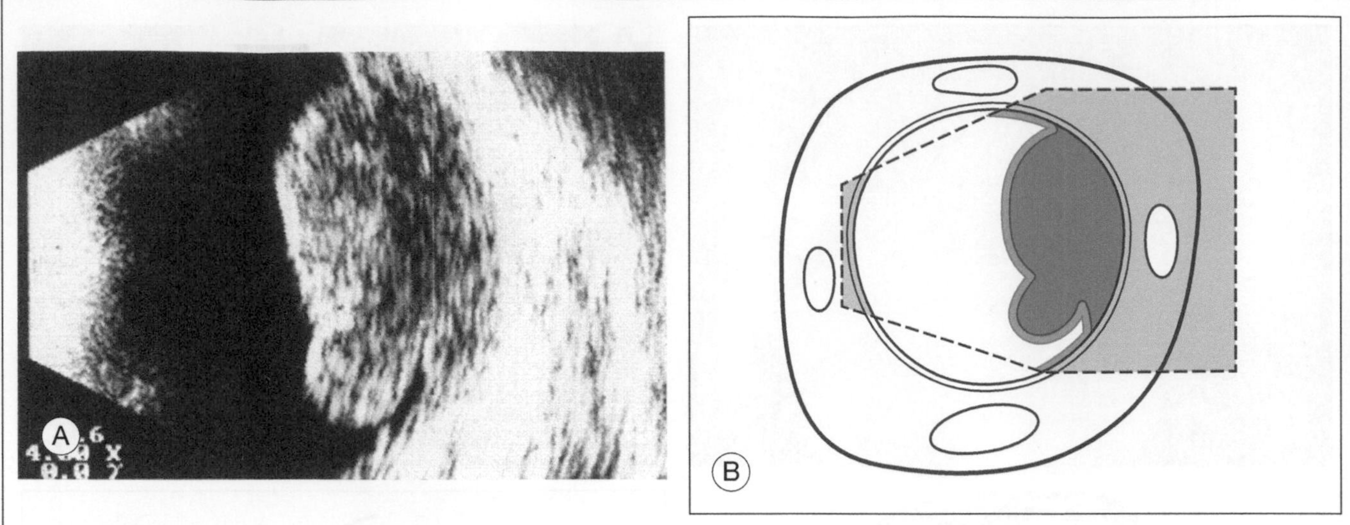

Fig. 9.61 (A) Choroidal melanoma with eccentric perforation of Bruch's membrane. Echogram shows a mushroom-like shape of the lesion, which is nearly pathognomonic for a melanoma and therefore of great differential diagnostic value. (B) Schematic drawing.

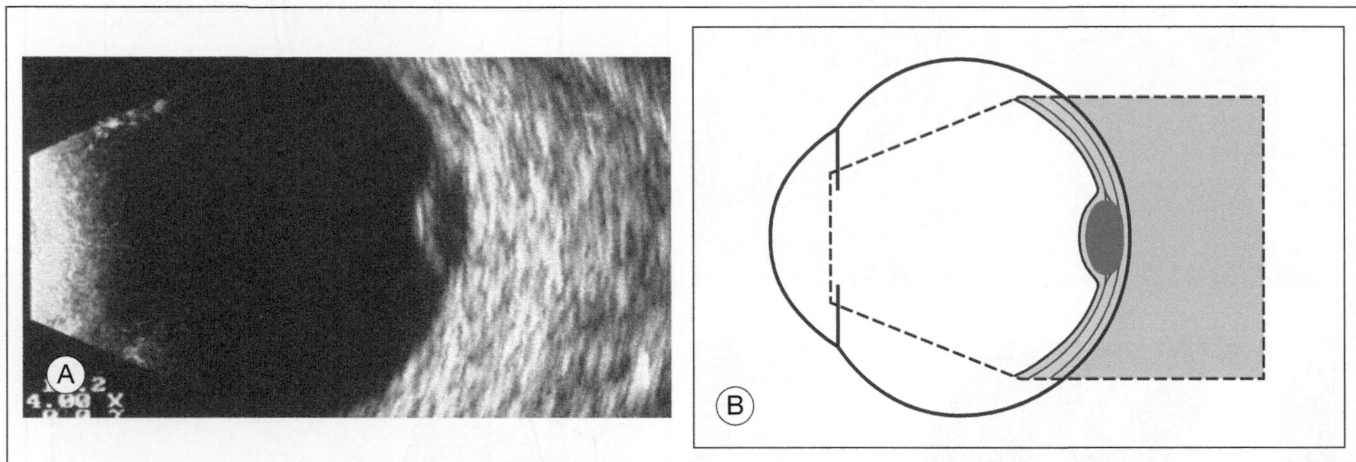

Fig. 9.62 (A) Small choroidal melanoma. Elevation, 2.5 mm; base, 8 × 8 mm; calculated tumor volume: 66 mm^3. The choroid at the tumor base has been replaced by tumor, which has less acoustic reflectivity and provokes a choroidal excavation echographically. (B) Schematic drawing.

(Fig. 9.58). This corresponds to the uniform histological structure of a melanoma (Fig. 9.58). Exceptions occur when features of hemorrhage or necrosis within the tumor develop.[44,45]

Most melanomas consist of solid tissue; therefore, no after-movements occur as might be expected with a large subretinal or choroidal hemorrhage. In addition, flickering spike complexes may be seen on the A-mode echogram within the tumor itself. Various authors interpret them differently. It is assumed that they are due to blood circulating in large tumor vessels. Although the features of the ultrasound combined with a thorough clinical examination can establish the diagnosis of choroidal melanoma with enough certainty to recommend treatment, a preoperative correlation between the sonographic pattern and the histopathological findings is currently still in debate.[40,41]

B-mode Doppler devices can obtain signals from the interior of the tumor by using a high-resolution power and a frequency between 7 and 20 MHz. This method is more sensitive than the visual evaluation of a time amplitude echogram[46] (Fig. 9.64). In some patients it was possible to determine the blood flow within the tumor using Doppler color-coding technology. In a series of 50 eyes with melanoma, Doppler shifts could be detected in all patients except one. The tumor size varied between 80 and 1500 mm^3. Doppler imaging has also been used to study an eye with secondary glaucoma and significantly increased intraocular pressure. In this patient the tumor perforated the sclera and invaded the muscle cone (Fig. 9.65). An intraocular pressure of 45 mmHg compressed the intraocular tumor, which influenced the maximal flow velocities measured by Doppler sonography (Fig. 9.65).

The use of Doppler ultrasonography in studying ocular blood flow in disease states is increasing; however, at the present time this method does not allow exact measurements of maximal flow velocities.

Determining the volume of a choroidal melanoma by ultrasonography

Ultrasonography produces spikes in the recorded signal when interfaces with different media are encountered. In a normal eye, the first acoustic interface after the signal passes through the vitreous is the retina. In the case of a choroidal tumor the apex is adjacent to the retina spike and the base is anterior to the

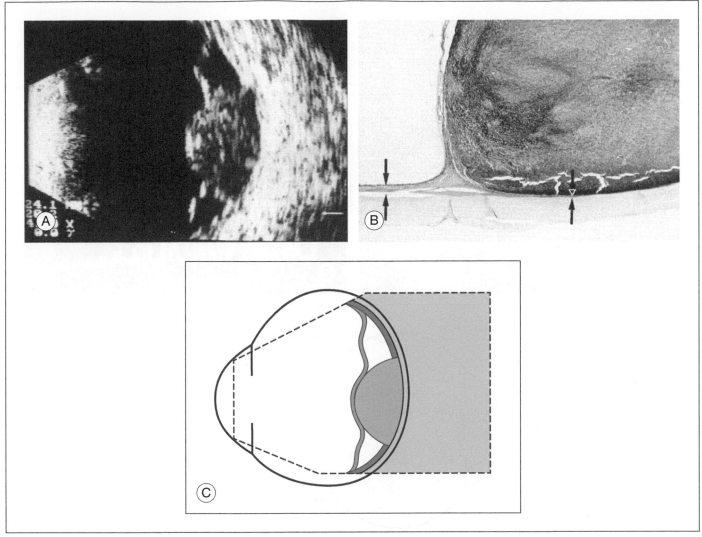

Fig. 9.63 Choroidal melanoma. (A) Elevation, 6 mm; diameter at the base, 11 × 12 mm; calculated tumor volume, 330 mm^3. The highly reflecting choroid has been replaced by the poorly reflecting melanoma, producing a choroidal excavation in the cross-section. (B) Histologic section through the margin of a choroidal melanoma. At the base, normal choroid is replaced by tumor. (C) Schematic drawing.

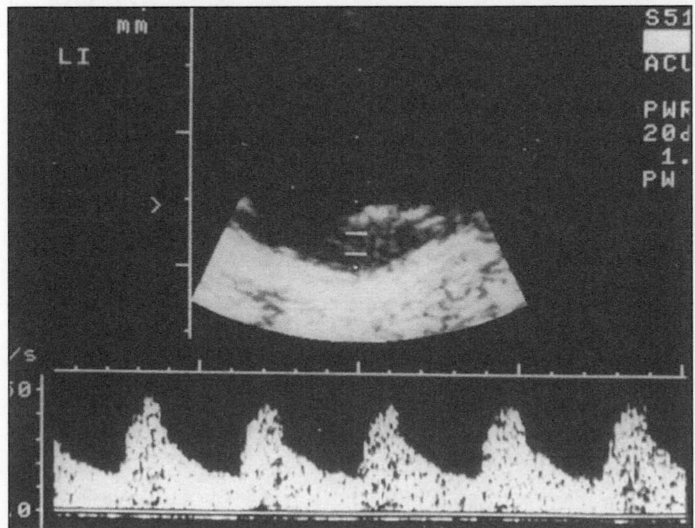

Fig. 9.64 B-mode Doppler sonography (duplex technique) of a choroidal melanoma of average size. In A-mode the occasionally observed flickering amplitudes are produced by the blood flow. They can be quantified when using a B-mode Doppler instrument of high resolution.

scleral spike. Identifying these positions, however, can be challenging in some settings. For example, if the retina is attached to the tumor surface, no separate discrimination of the two interfaces is possible (Fig. 9.58). On the other hand, if the accompanying retinal detachment is also present over the peak of the tumor, then the retina will be imaged as a separate membranous structure lying in front of the lesion (Fig. 9.66). Then the transition between tumor and scleral must be identified. In most cases, the scleral spike is still the strongest signal even in the presence of a choroidal tumor. If the tumor breaks through the scleral barrier, the continuity of this strong signal is interrupted at the site of perforation. An exact measurement of the volume of the tumor is important when measuring the lesion height, planning a treatment, or analyzing the effect of therapy.

Ultrasonography is capable of providing precise measurements of tumor size. Ultrasound devices have measurement tools that can be applied in the window of the image. The examiner can use this feature to measure the height of the largest and smallest diameter of the tumor. In biconvex tumors, volume data and tumor can be calculated from these linear measurements or it can be evaluated using special equipment designed for 3D evaluation (Fig. 9.67).

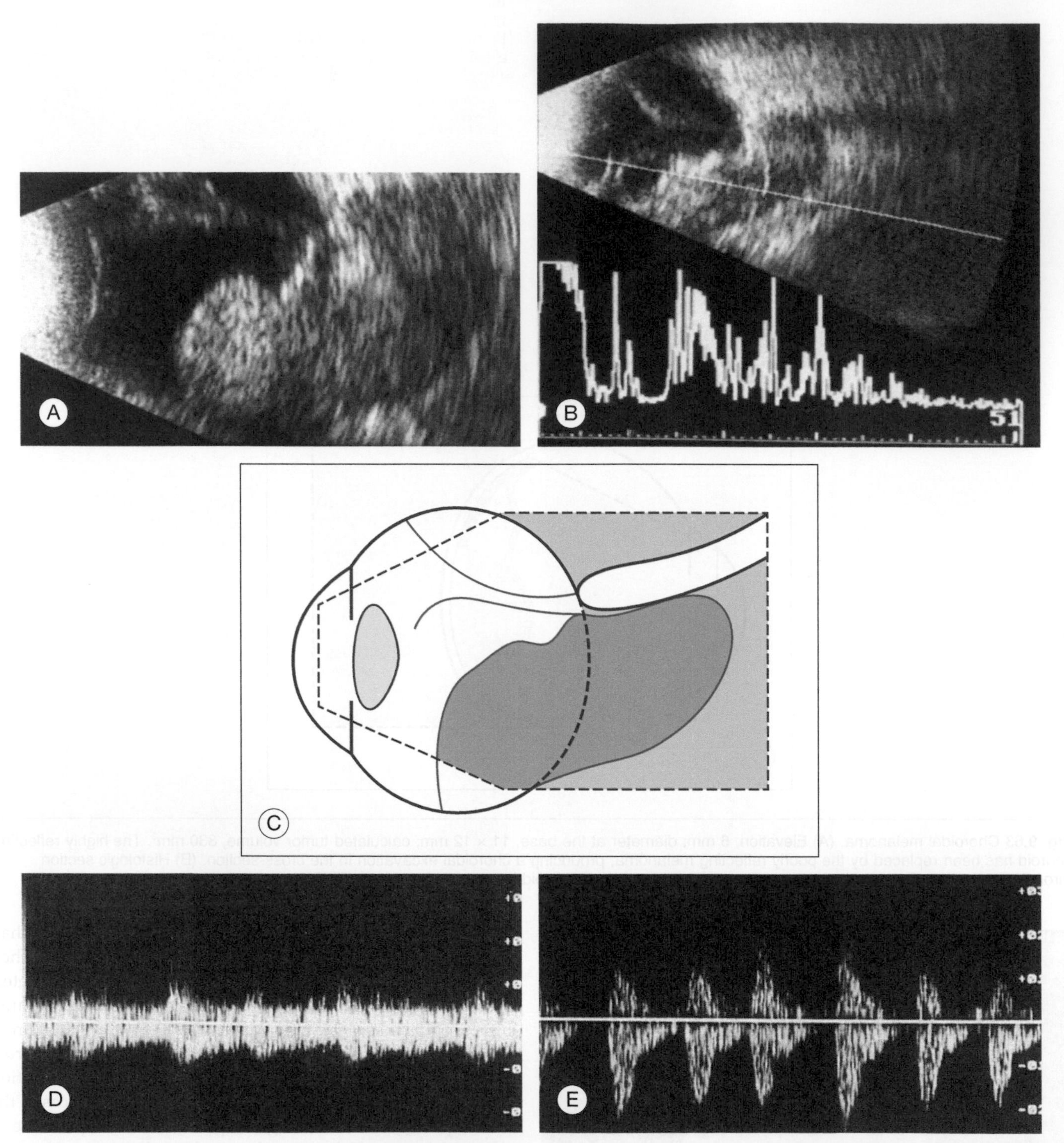

Fig. 9.65 Choroidal melanoma with orbital invasion in a 65-year-old woman. Referral diagnosis was orbital cellulitis. Echographic findings include a large intraocular tumor with wide invasion of the orbital tissues (A). Remnants of the sclera can be demonstrated within the tumor in both A- and B-mode echograms because of their strong acoustic reflectivity (B). Additional findings include a total retinal detachment as seen in both images. (C) Schematic drawing of the echogram. (D,E) Doppler signal of the choroidal tumor. (D) Frequency shift from the intraocular tumor, maximum velocity: 10 cm/s. (E) Frequency shift from the extraocular tumor, maximum velocity: 2 cm/s. With Doppler technique the intraocular part of the tumor shows reduced blood flow compared to the extraocular part.

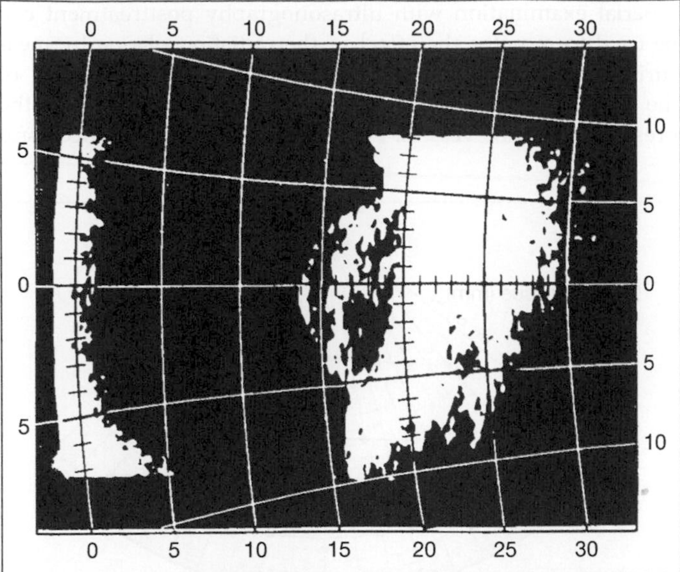

Fig. 9.66 Choroidal melanoma with associated retinal detachment over the peak of the tumor. Tumor size: base, 9 × 9 mm; elevation, 3.5 mm. The detached retina lies about 2 mm in front of the tumor. The calculated tumor volume is about 150 mm^3. If the retinal detachment were erroneously included, the volume would be about 230 mm^3.

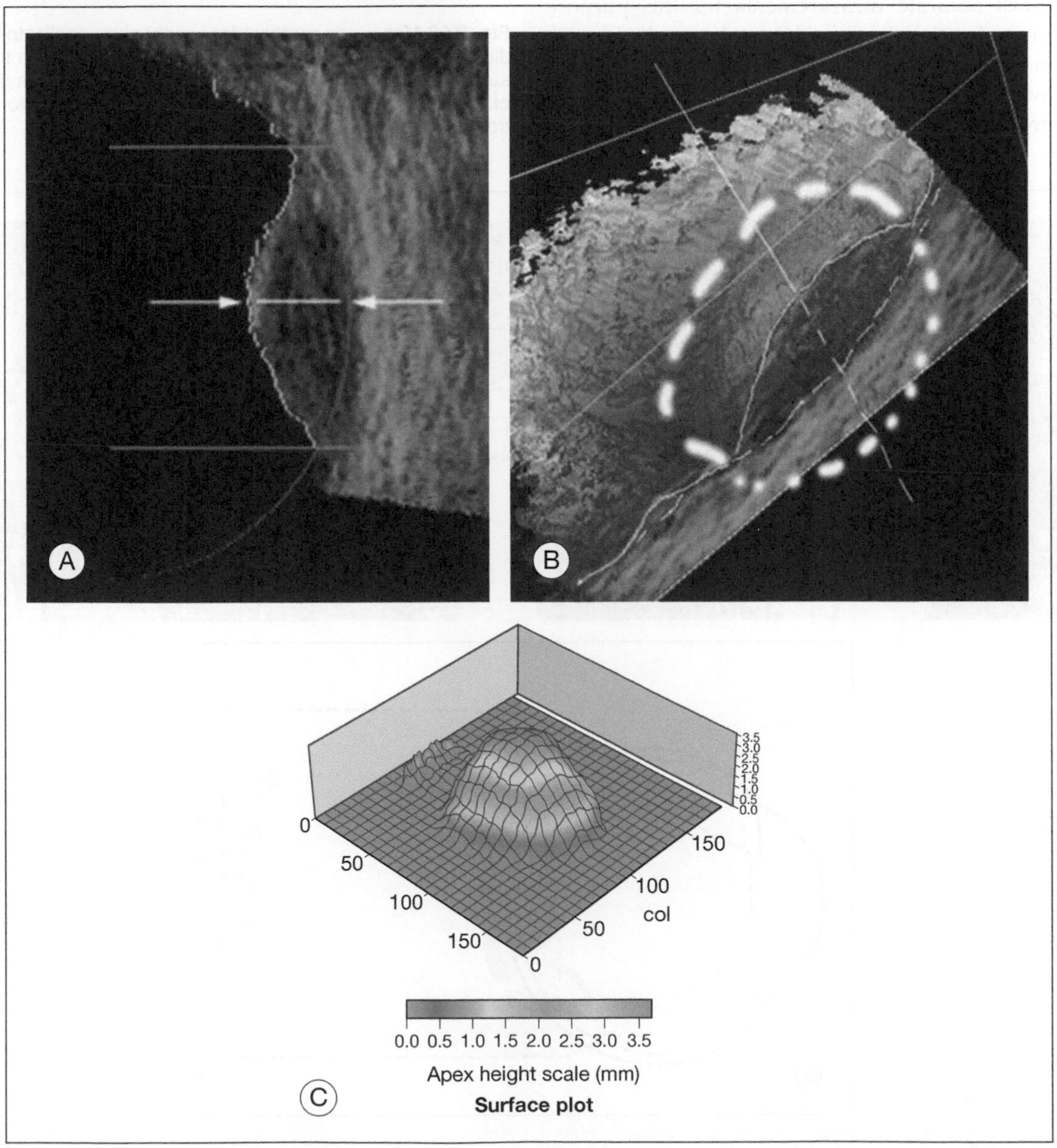

Fig. 9.67 Example of three-dimensional rendering of the posterior segment tumor. (A) Area of interest marked. (B) Contour-finding procedure with outlining of the space-occupying lesion. (C) Surface plot for volume determination.

The role of ultrasonography for planning the treatment of choroidal melanomas

After a choroidal melanoma is diagnosed by careful clinical examination and ultrasound interpretation, the next step for the physician is to formulate a treatment plan. Radiation therapy is successfully used for the treatment of medium or small ocular melanomas. Scleral contact radiotherapy using ruthenium-106, cobalt-90, or iodine-125 applicators shows a relatively steep decay of radiation dosage. At a distance of 8 mm from the radiation surface, only 10% of the energy is still available. In order to achieve complete tumor necrosis in this area, an application of 10 times the duration of radiation is needed. Figure 9.68 shows the isodose curves for ruthenium-106 applicators. The aim of any radiation therapy is to destroy the tumor tissue and to spare the adjacent normal ocular tissues as much as possible. The radiation pellets are placed on custom scleral plaques that are designed to cover the full extent of the tumor. It is therefore important to have an exact measurement of the size of the tumor and have precise placement of the scleral plaque over the tumor (Figs 9.69 and 9.70). Ultrasonography provides the most accurate measurements for this purpose. Dynamic imaging using the ultrasound B-mode can also provide information on adjacent pathology such as overlying retinal detachments, which may overestimate the total height of the tumor if not properly identified.

Serial examination with ultrasonography posttreatment can be used to monitor the effect of the radiation plaque by measuring the tumor elevation, tumor base, and reflectivity of the internal tumor structure as well as by identifying the presence of tumor vessels. Figure 9.71 illustrates the successful

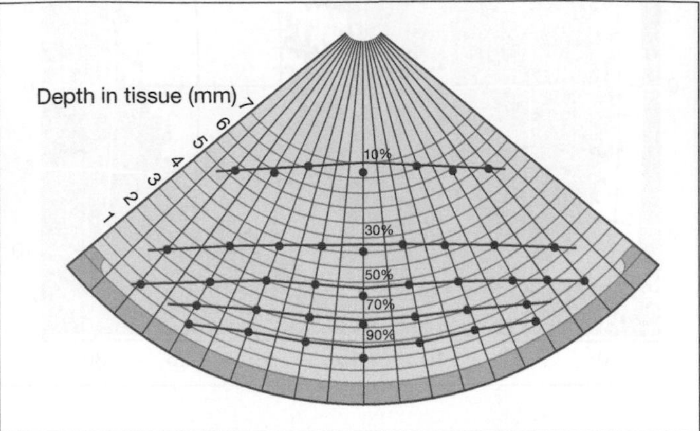

Fig. 9.68 Measuring protocol for a ruthenium applicator type CCC; diameter of the emitting plane, 21 mm. At 5 mm from the applicator surface, only 25% of the scleral contact dose is still available. Because of this steep decay of effective radiation, it is critical to plan the treatment exactly.

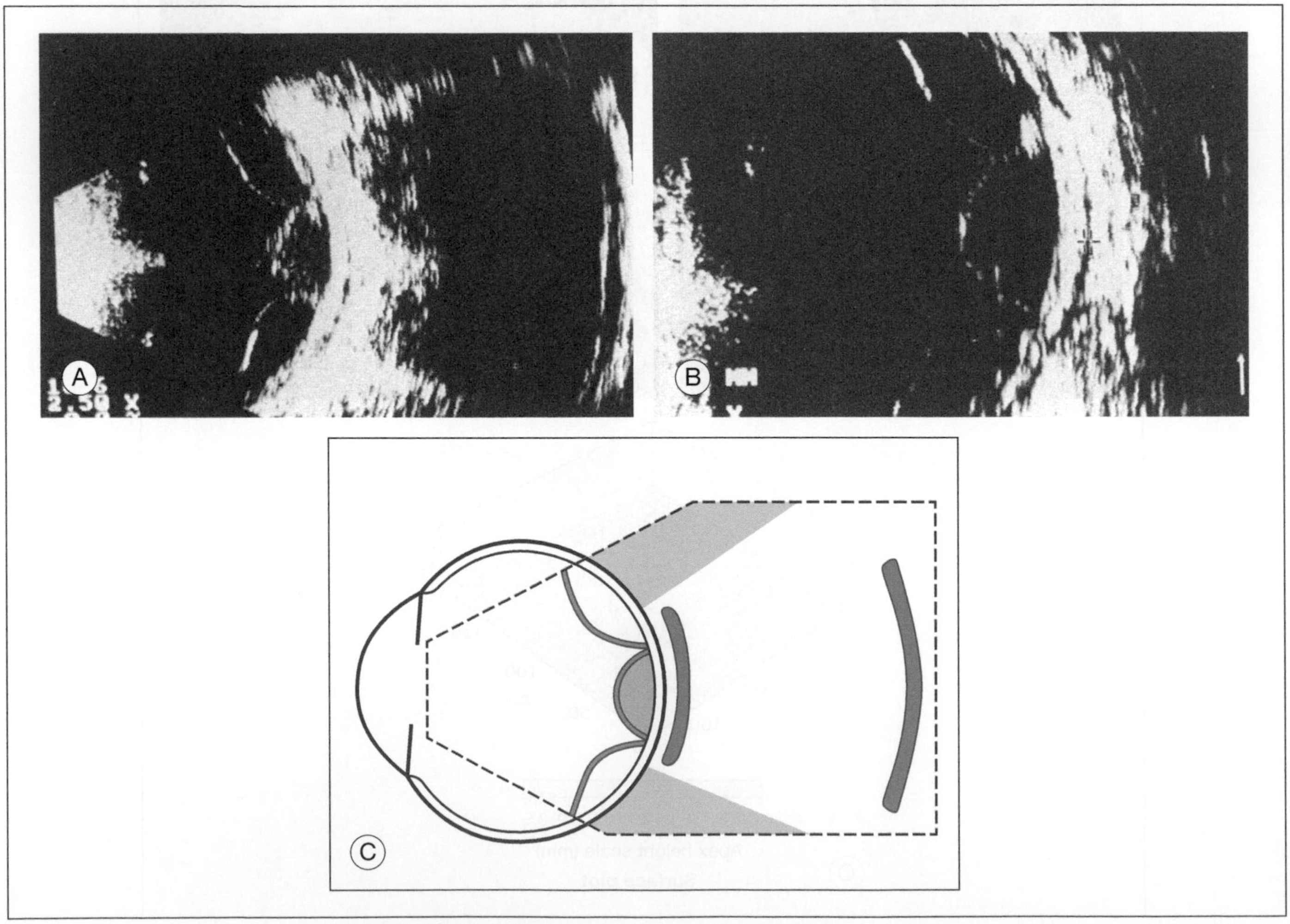

Fig. 9.69 (A,B) Echogram of an eye with the ruthenium-beta applicator in place. The slit between the posterior scleral surface and the applicator is filled with fluid and is less than 0.5 mm wide. The lateral extent of the applicator is marked by the sound shadow. (C) Schematic drawing.

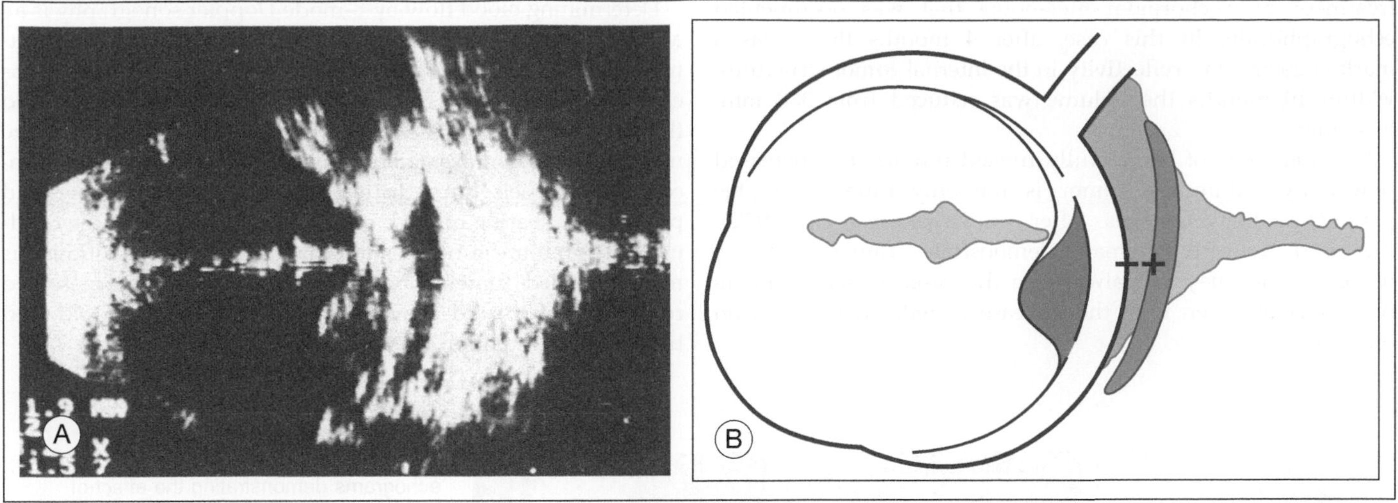

Fig. 9.70 (A) Ruthenium-beta applicator in place with a wide slit between the sclera and the applicator surface. On the basis of this echographic finding, the position of the applicator should be changed or the duration of the treatment has to be prolonged. Distance of the measuring marks: 1.9 mm. (B) Schematic drawing.

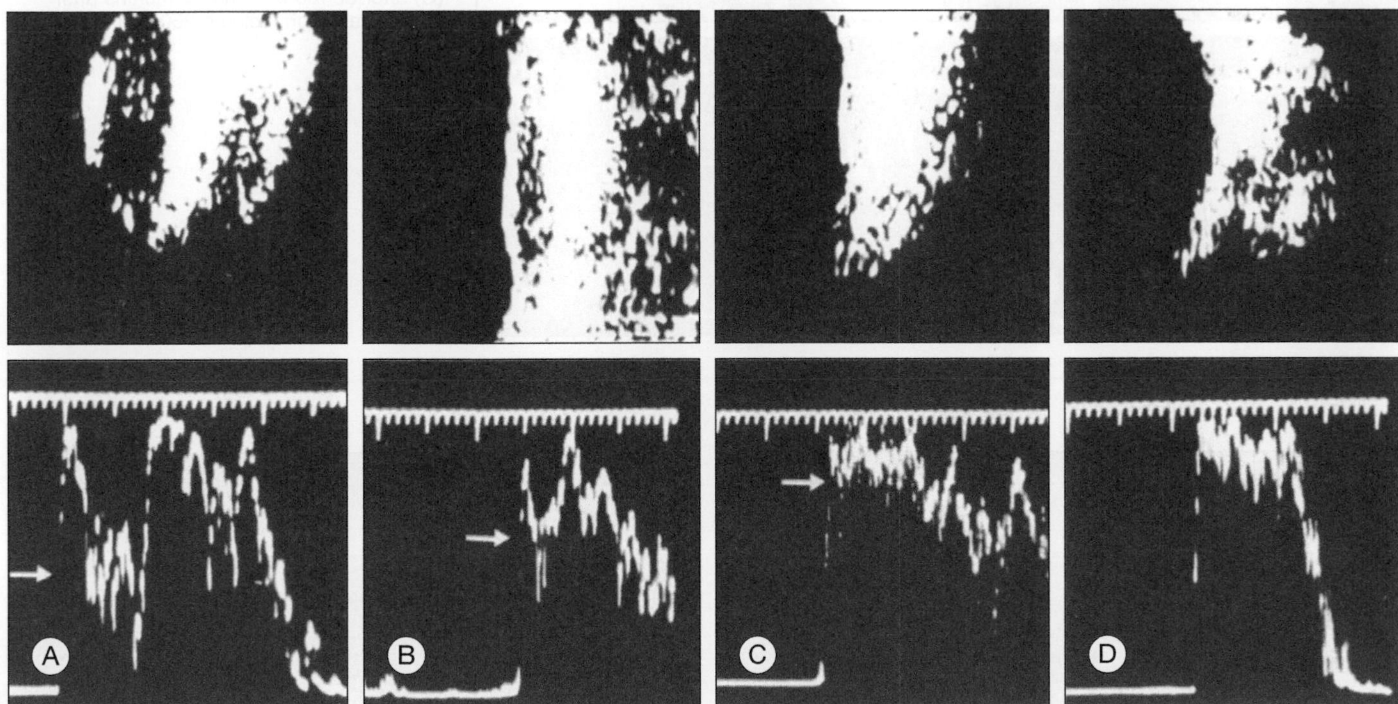

Fig. 9.71 A-mode (bottom) and B-mode (top) echograms during follow-up assessments of a successfully treated choroidal melanoma. The tumor volume was reduced from 380 to 0 mm^3 within 10 months. After 8 months the spikes within the tumor increased from about 40% of the scleral spike to about 90% (white arrows). (A) Before radiation, 380 mm^3, reflection 40%; (B) after 4 months, 230 mm^3, reflection 80%; (C) after 8 months, 100 mm^3, reflection 90%; (D) after 10 months, 0 mm^3, no reflection.

treatment of a choroidal melanoma that was documented echographically. In this case, after 4 months there was a marked increase in reflectivity in the internal tumor structures. Within 10 months the volume was reduced from 380 mm^3 to 0 mm^3.

In some cases of successfully treated tumors, the increased reflectivity within the tumor is the only ultrasonographic parameter that changes after radiotherapy (Fig. 9.72). Increased reflectivity may demonstrate tumor necrosis; however, this may not always be the case, as some tumors remain viable even with the increase in reflectivity noted on ultrasound.

Determining blood flow by B-mode Doppler sonography is an additional parameter that could be used to monitor the treatment response in highly vascularized choroidal tumors, such as choroidal melanomas. Doppler can detect a decrease in blood flow in the necrotic mass that is left after radiation therapy. The necrotic tissue from treated tumors can be absorbed by the adjacent blood vessels, but radiation may damage these vessels and prevent the clearing of these products, which explains the residual mass on ultrasound seen after treatment with radiation: this mass is called tumefaction. This may explain the increased reflectivity of treated tumors. Figure 9.73 shows an elevated tumor before radiation.

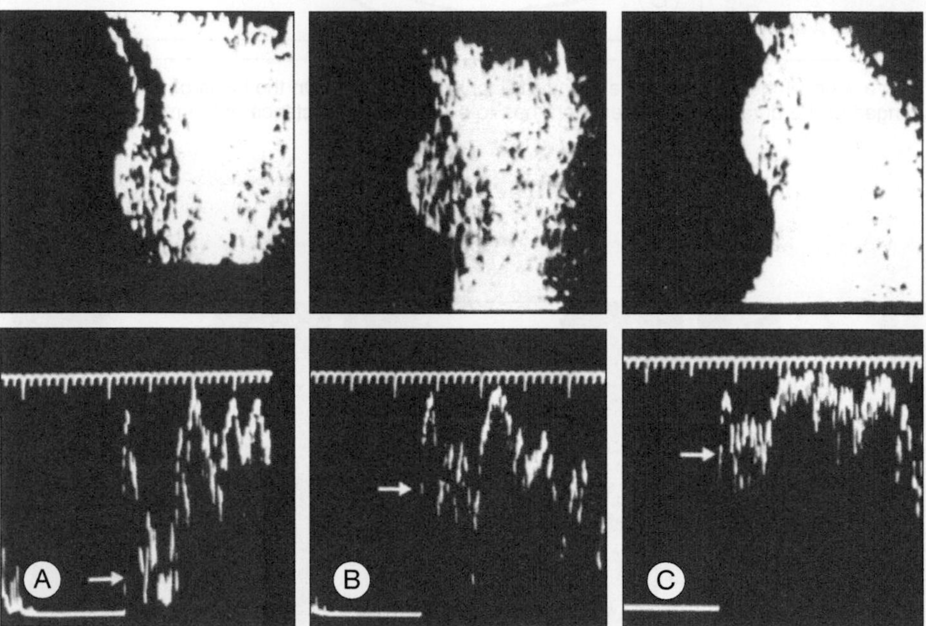

Fig. 9.72 A-mode (bottom) and B-mode (top) echograms demonstrating the effect of brachyradiotherapy on a choroidal melanoma. The external shape of the tumor also remains unchanged after a second series of radiation; the reflectivity of the tumor increases from about 20% of the scleral spike before radiation to about 80% after radiation (white arrows). (A) Before radiation, volume 250 mm^3, reflection 20%; (B) after 8 months, 250 mm^3, reflection 70%; (C) after 36 months and 22 months after second radiation, volume 250 mm^3, reflection 80%.

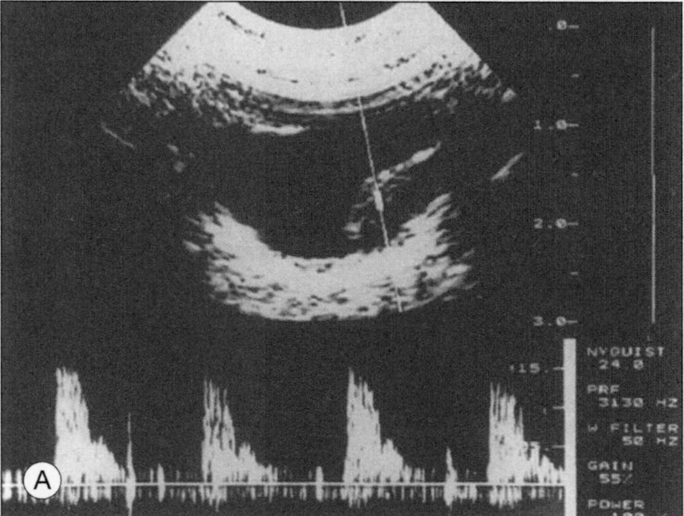

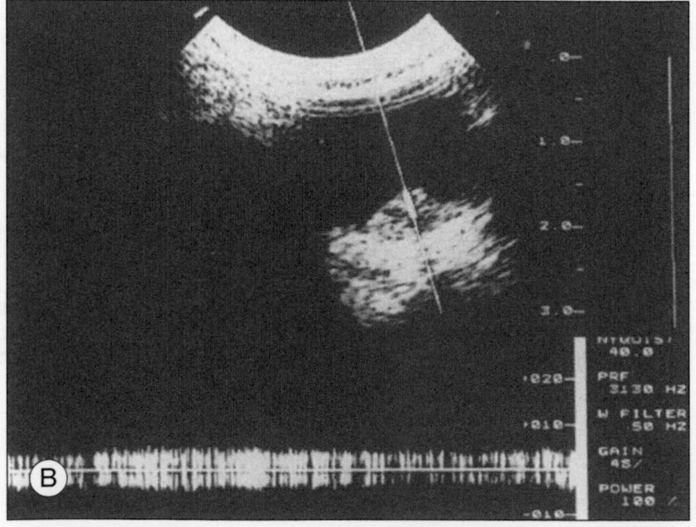

Fig. 9.73 (A) Choroidal melanoma with an elevation of 5 mm. Cross-sectional echogram obtained with the duplex instrument ATL mark 8. The sample volume is identified by the marks on the aiming beam. In this area Doppler spectra are obtained, indicating a high blood flow velocity (represented in the lower part of the illustration). (B) Same patient as in panel A, 4 months after radiation treatment of the choroidal melanoma with ruthenium. There is still a considerable volume of tumor remaining (maximal elevation, about 3.5 mm). No frequency shift can be obtained from the interior of the tumor when using duplex examination. The tissue lying in the guiding beam produces only a biphasic noise (illustrated in the lower part of the image).

Metastatic choroidal tumors

Choroidal metastasis is a known complication of several cancers, including all types of carcinomas and sarcomas. The most frequent primary tumors are breast (40%) and lungs (29%). One study examined 230 eyes from deceased patients with known systemic carcinoma and showed that 12% of the eyes had choroidal metastasis on pathological specimens.[47] Many of these tumors remained undetected at the time of death. The detection of such lesions can be a poor prognostic factor. The average survival time after treatment for choroidal metastasis is 7.4 months.[48] Therefore, many of these patients are not followed for extended periods of time by their ophthalmologist.

Typically carcinoma metastasis presents as a large, highly reflective thickening of the ocular outer layers. The internal acoustic properties can resemble a disciform macular degeneration or a choroidal hemangioma. A metastatic adenocarcinoma typically presents with high reflectivity from the strong acoustic interfaces from its adenoid-like histological structure (Fig. 9.74).

In contrast, there are several atypical presentations of choroidal metastasis that have also been reported.[49,50] Pathological examination of an eye that was enucleated because of suspicion for choroidal melanoma from ultrasound examination revealed a choroidal metastasis from small-cell bronchial carcinoma (Fig. 9.75).[49]

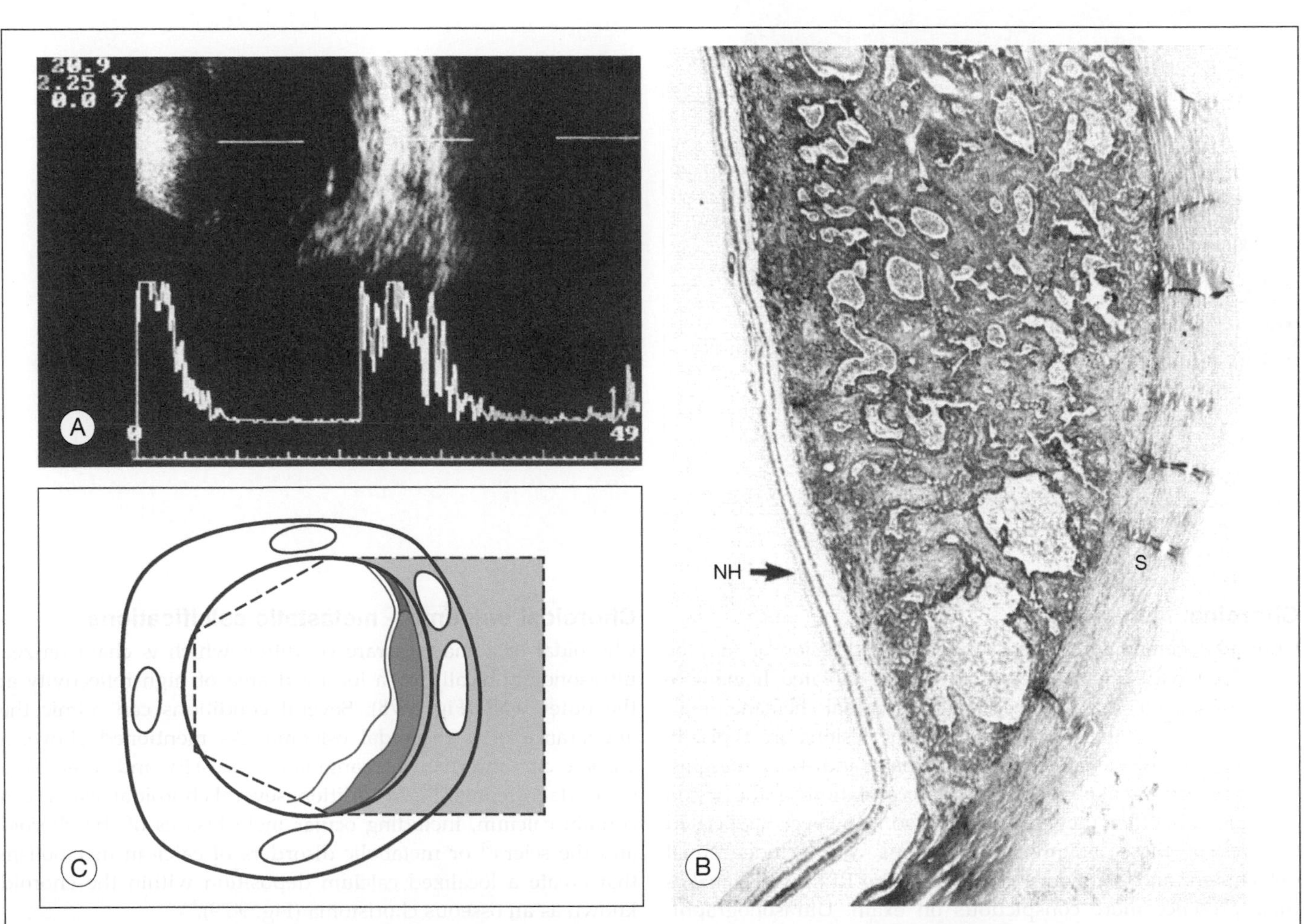

Fig. 9.74 Extensive choroidal metastatic tumor in the lower nasal quadrant. (A) On the echogram the choroid is widened to about 2.5 mm; the retina is partly detached by an exudate. The tissue inside the metastatic tumor shows high acoustic reflectivity. (B) Histologic section of a metastatic adenocarcinoma in the choroid. The gland-like structure provides good acoustic interfaces. NH, retina; S, sclera. (C) Schematic drawing.

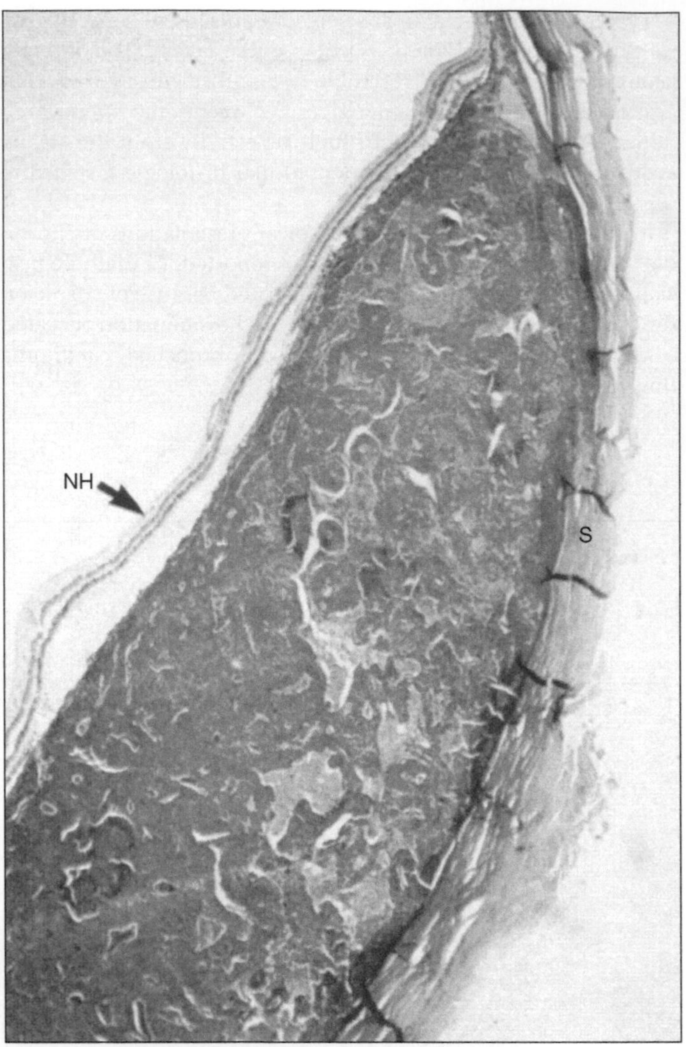

Fig. 9.75 Histological metastatic tumor from a small-cell bronchial carcinoma. The echogram (not shown) resembled that of a typical choroidal melanoma. Similar findings have been seen in choroidal metastases from cutaneous melanoma. NH, retina; S, sclera.

Choroidal hemangioma

Choroidal hemangioma may be an isolated lesion or may be associated with Sturge–Weber syndrome. Isolated hemangiomas, described as circumscribed choroidal hemangiomas, usually occur at the posterior pole. The lesions are typically diffuse, slightly elevated, and may have indistinct margins. These features make ophthalmic interpretation of the lesion difficult and often they can be missed. However, associated features of these circumscribed lesions can include retinal detachment and secondary changes of the RPE, which makes their presence more conspicuous on exam. Ultrasonographically, choroidal hemangiomas appear as a strongly reflecting, nearly concentric widening of the outer layers of the eye (Fig. 9.76). In spite of the abundant vascularization, ultrasound images of choroidal hemangiomas do not show the circulating blood as in choroidal melanomas. Instead, the echogram of a choroidal hemangioma is similar to that of metastatic adenocarcinoma or disciform macular degeneration, which may be indicative of a slower circulation more consistent with laminar flow in the cavities of dilated blood vessels shown by Doppler ultrasonography (Fig. 9.77). In long-standing cases the epichoroidal layer may ossify and produce sound shadows. In this stage, a hemangioma may appear identical to an osteoma or a metastatic calcification of the choroid.[51,52]

Choroidal osteoma – metastatic calcifications

Choroidal osteoma is a rare condition which is characterized ultrasonographically by a localized area of high reflectivity at the outer wall (Fig. 9.78). Several conditions can mimic the appearance of a choroidal osteoma. As mentioned above, a chronic circumscribed hemangioma can ossify and resemble a choroidal osteoma.[53–55] In addition, several choroidal lesions can contain calcium, including ocular metastasases of the choroid and the sclera[51] or metabolic disorders of calcium metabolism that create a localized calcium deposition within the choroid known as an osseous choristoma (Fig. 9.79).[54]

Choroidal tuberculoma

Choroidal tuberculomas are another extremely rare choroidal lesion (Fig. 9.80).[56] Tuberculomas can also appear similar to choroid melanoma (Figs 9.81). Images that are suggestive of choroidal tuberculomas exemplify the importance of placing the ultrasound image in context with the rest of the patient examination in order to make the proper diagnosis. Tuberculomas are found in patients with disseminated tuberculosis and a complete examination can identify other tuberculomas to confirm the diagnosis. Laboratory confirmation of mycobacterium by blood or sputum sampling is also helpful. In addition, these lesions should respond to antituberculous treatment.

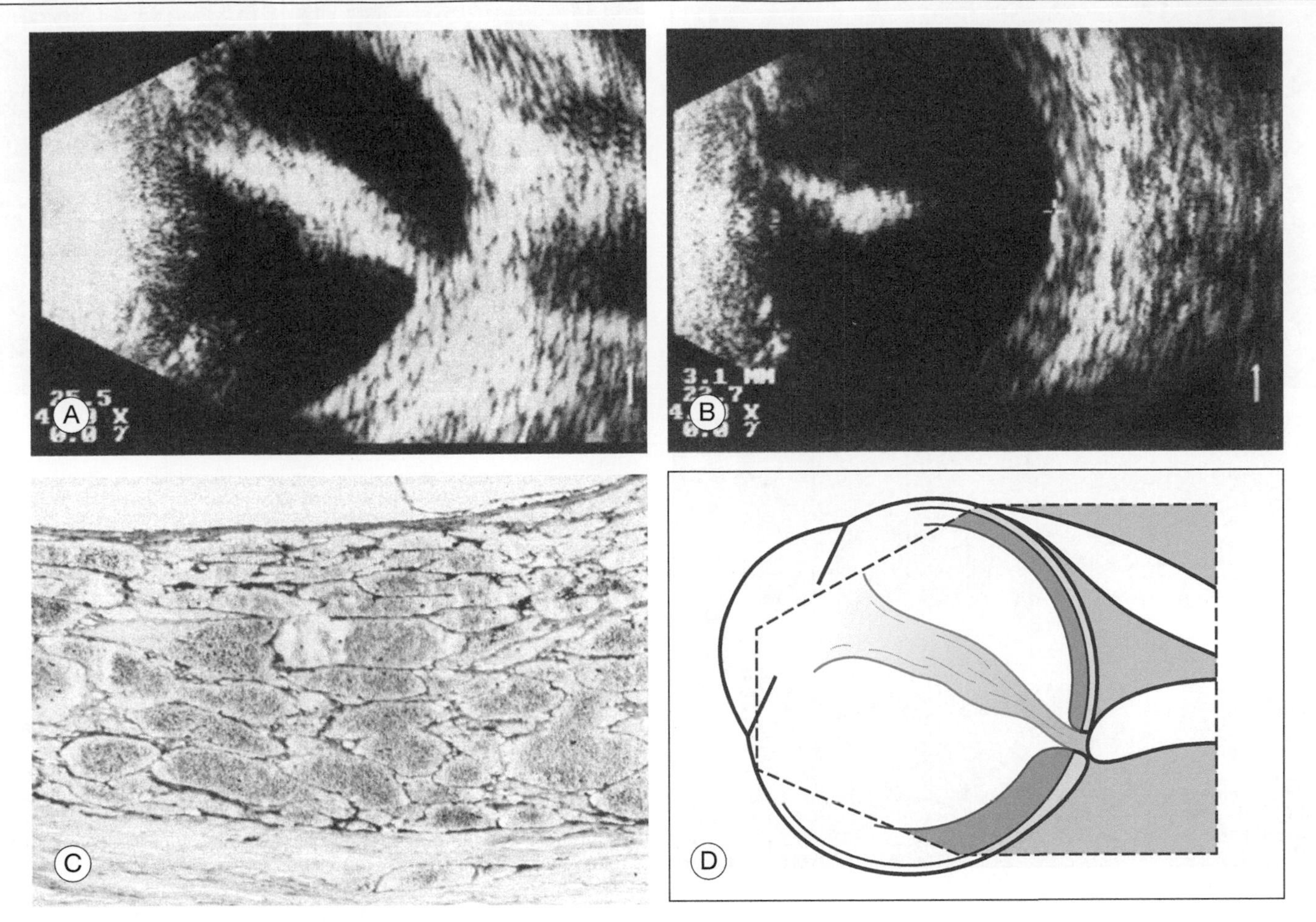

Fig. 9.76 Extensive choroidal hemangioma in Sturge–Weber syndrome (additional finding: total retinal detachment). (A) Cross-sectional echogram through the area of the optic nerve head. In the lower quadrant, the ocular walls are markedly thickened. (In spite of the associated retinal detachment, the intraocular pressure was 50 mmHg by applanation.) (B) With reduced sensitivity, the scleral surface can be delineated in spite of the high acoustic reflectivity within the tumor (distance of the measuring marks, 3.1 mm). (C) Histologic section through the tumor illustrated in (A) and (B): the septa of the cavities are thin and lined with endothelium. They produce strong reflectivity within the lesion. (D) Schematic drawing.

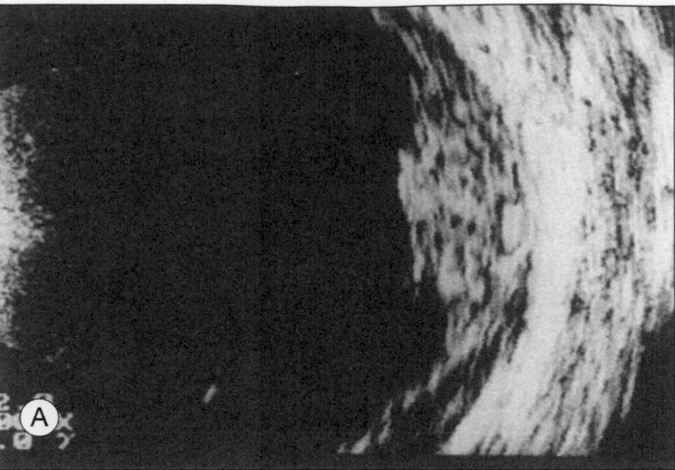

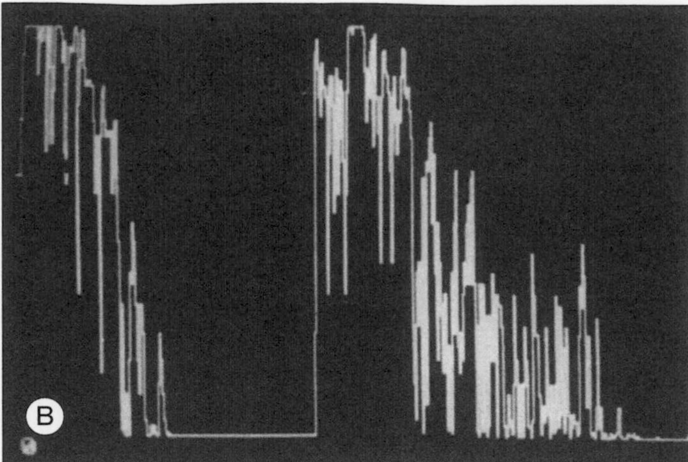

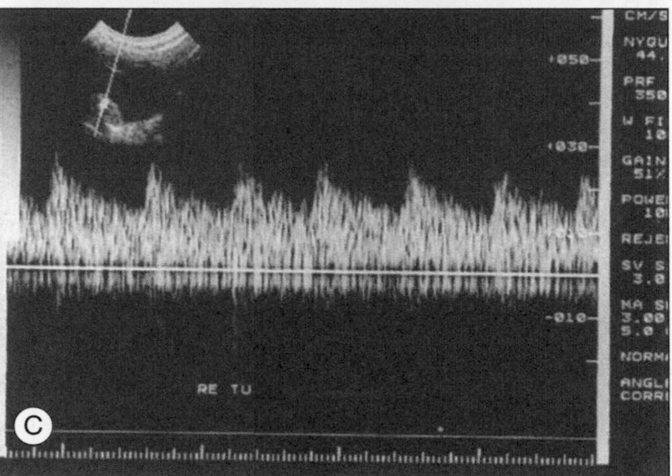

Fig. 9.77 (A) Cross-sectional echogram of a circumscribed choroidal hemangioma in a 12-year-old boy. The tumor has an elevation of 4 mm. (B) In an A-mode echogram with S-shaped amplification the cross-sectional picture corroborates the high reflectivity of the tumor. (C) On Doppler sonography, we see blood circulating within the tumor, synchronous with the pulse. The illustrated velocity profile speaks for a relatively low resistance by the blood vessels.

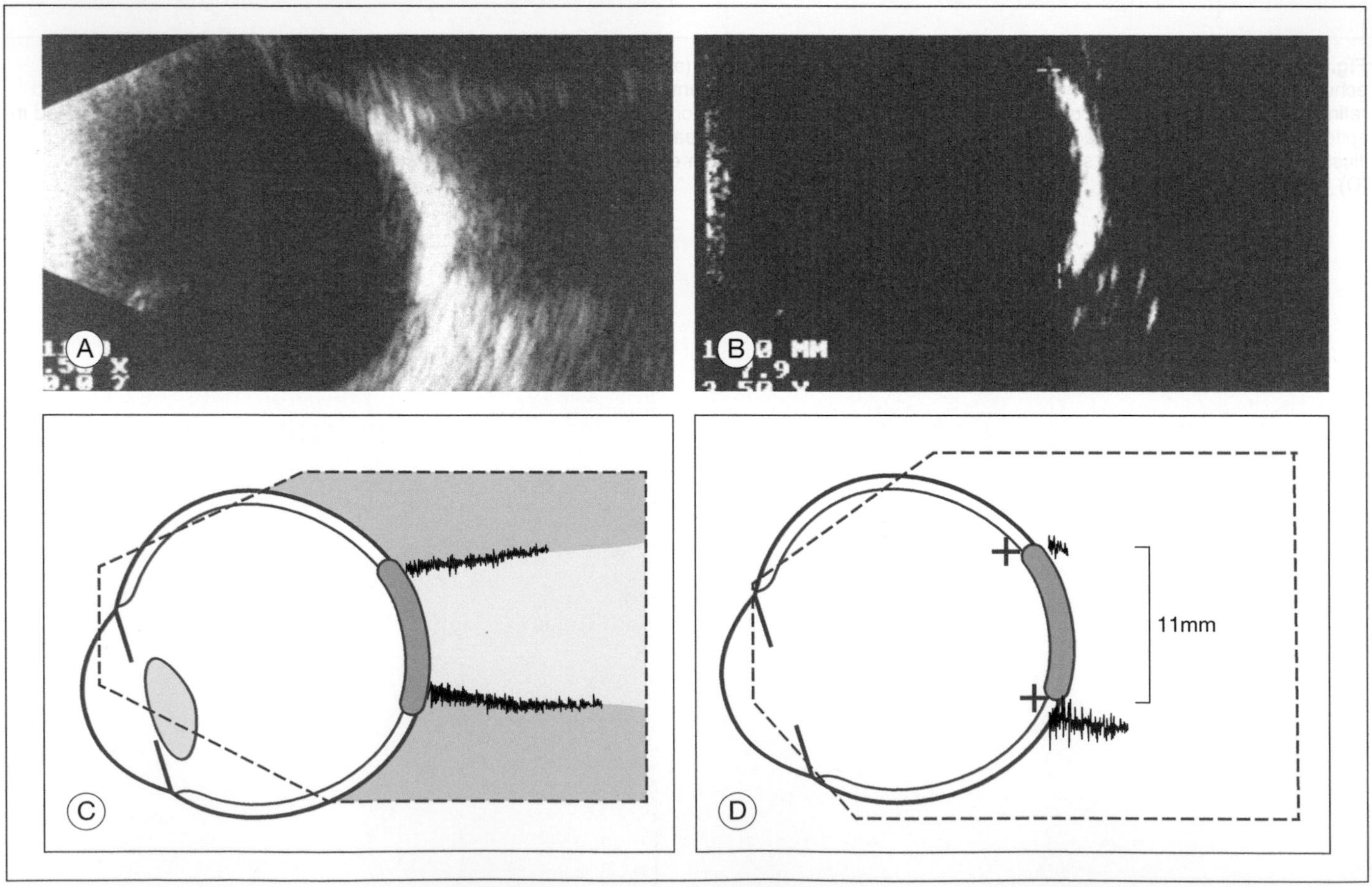

Fig. 9.78 Cross-sectional echogram of the choroidal osteoma. (A) The echogram of the lesion is characterized by total reflection of the ultrasound, and shadow formation. An elevation cannot be unequivocally documented. (B) With reduced amplification it is possible to image the ossification as an isolated signal. The horizontal diameter is 11.0 mm. (C,D) Schematic drawings.

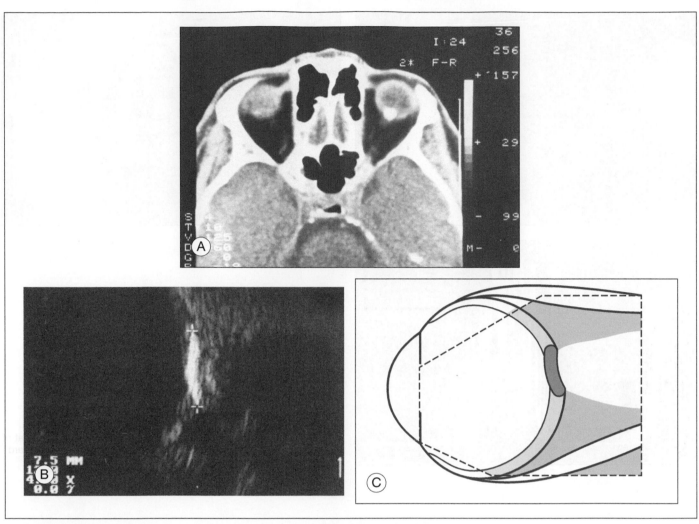

Fig. 9.79 Metastatic calcification of the ocular walls of unknown etiology. Differential diagnosis includes choroidal osteoma. (A) A computed tomography scan was obtained because of nonophthalmological problems. A circumscribed calcified structure within the ocular walls was found incidentally. (B) In cross-sectional echograms, a lesion of the ocular walls above the optic nerve head showed total reflection of the ultrasound signal. The lateral extension was about 7.5 mm. There was no corresponding lesion seen on fundus examination that would be typical of an osteoma. The etiology of this lesion is unknown. (C) Schematic drawing.

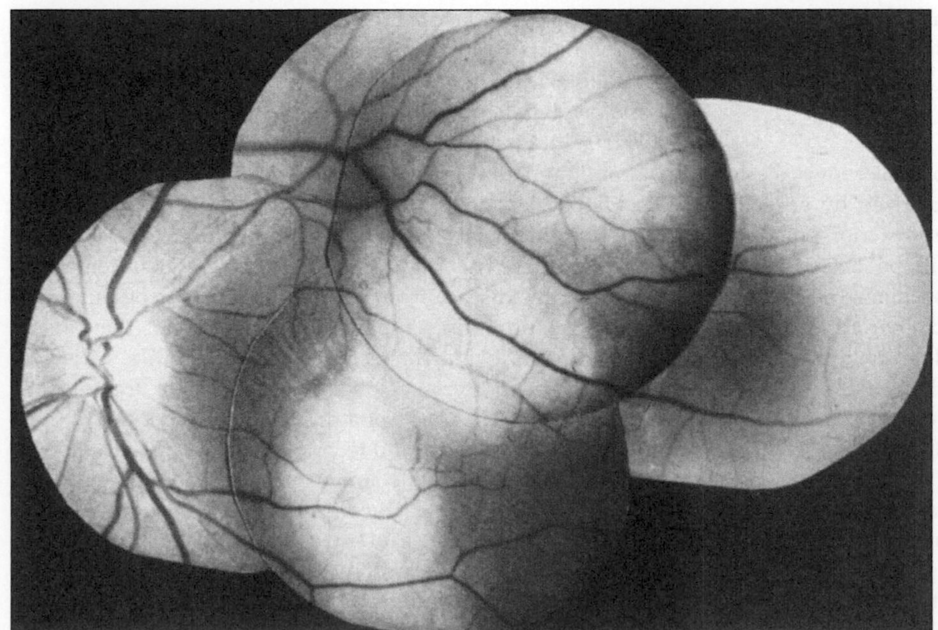

Fig. 9.80 Fundus picture of a 52-year-old woman with active pulmonary tuberculosis. This lesion resolved with antituberculosis treatment.

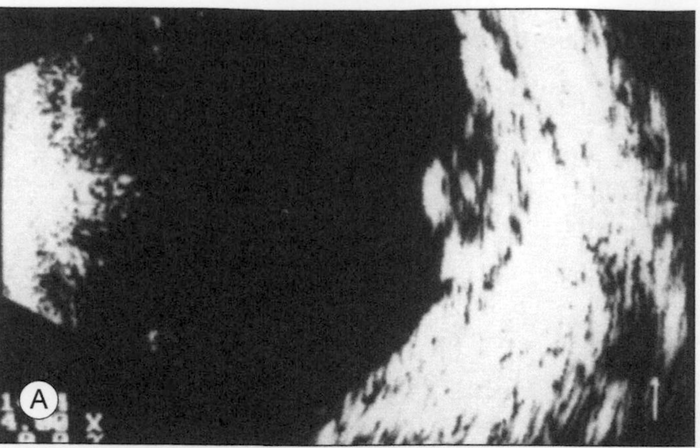

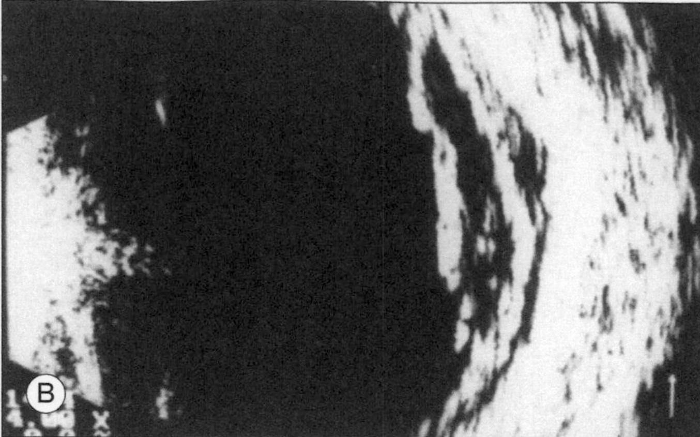

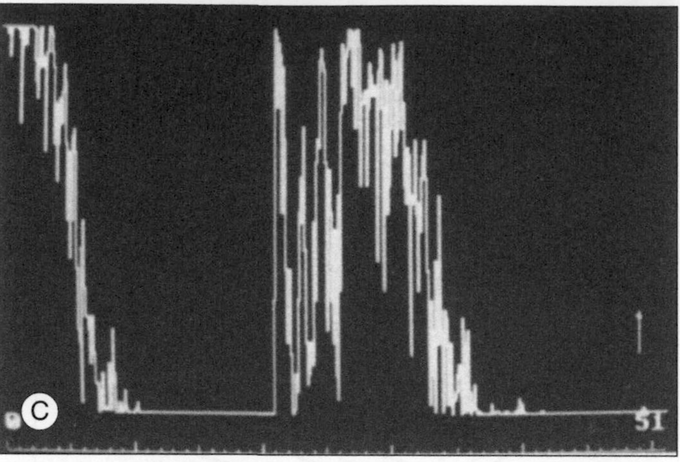

Fig. 9.81 (A,B) Echogram of the fundus lesion shown in Fig. 9.80. (C) The lesion is characterized by low acoustic reflectivity. Tenon's space can be well demonstrated. The reflectivity corresponds to that of a choroidal melanoma. The infiltration of Tenon's space points toward inflammatory etiology.

The uveal effusion syndrome

Patients with uveal effusion syndrome can have partial or circular choroidal detachment combined with an exudative retinal detachment (Fig. 9.82). Ultrasonography is very important in this condition. It can reveal fluid in the suprachoroidal space or differentiate choroidal hemorrhage or tumor from the serous fluid seen on imaging from choroidal effusion syndrome.[49,57]

Sclera

Posterior scleritis

Ultrasonography is the diagnostic method of choice for posterior scleritis.[52,58,59] The clinical picture is characterized by an acute loss of vision associated with folds at the posterior pole. The normal high reflectivity of the sclera will be decreased by changes in the tissue from inflammatory swelling. The result is a low reflective signal from a thickened choroid, which is suggestive of posterior scleritis. Choroid and vitreous may appear normal. Occasionally, there is a slight exudation into the subretinal space with accompanying disc edema. In 50% of the patients, fluid accumulates in the Tenon's space.[60] This signal can be similar to a diffuse choroidal melanoma. There is one case report of an eye that was enucleated because of suspicion of an ocular melanoma based on the finding of brawny scleral thickening (Figs 9.83 and 9.84). This case highlights the importance of proper ultrasound interpretation in the clinical context of each patient.[61]

ULTRASOUND IMAGING USED TO DIFFERENTIATE OCULAR DISEASE

Ultrasonography is invaluable in the diagnosis of certain ocular and orbital conditions. Proper imaging with ultrasound can narrow the differential diagnosis in certain conditions and guide further workup and management. These conditions include choroidal folds (Tables 9.2–9.4 and see Fig. 9.85), leukocoria (Table 9.5 and see Fig. 9.86), and vitreous hemorrhage (Table 9.6 and see Fig. 9.87). First, choroidal folds can be from orbital masses, ocular inflammation, disc edema in an atypical presentation, or from idiopathic causes.[49] Next, leukocoria is a condition of a white pupil that blocks ophthalmic examination, typically diagnosed in infancy. This finding can be from retinoblastoma. Differentiating this disease from other benign causes of leukocoria is critical for providing appropriate treatment of the patient. Finally, vitreous hemorrhage may manifest from a variety of changes in the posterior globe; the urgency of treatment is dependent on the diagnosis of a retinal detachment. All of these conditions require ultrasound technology to establish the proper diagnosis. The tables listed above provide information on the differential diagnosis of each condition and ultrasound features that will help guide image interpretation.

Furthermore, ultrasonography can aid in the preoperative planning and patient counselling for surgery. Table 9.7 lists some of the possible ultrasonographic information and

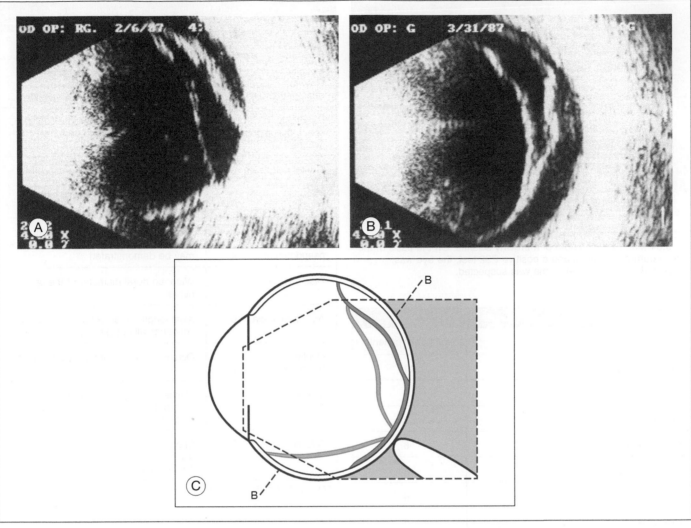

Fig. 9.82 Uveal effusion syndrome in a 55-year-old woman. (A) In the axial cross-section, the retina is attached to the optic nerve head. There is an associated, strongly reflecting choroidal detachment. (B) Cross-section of image in (A). (C) Schematic drawing.

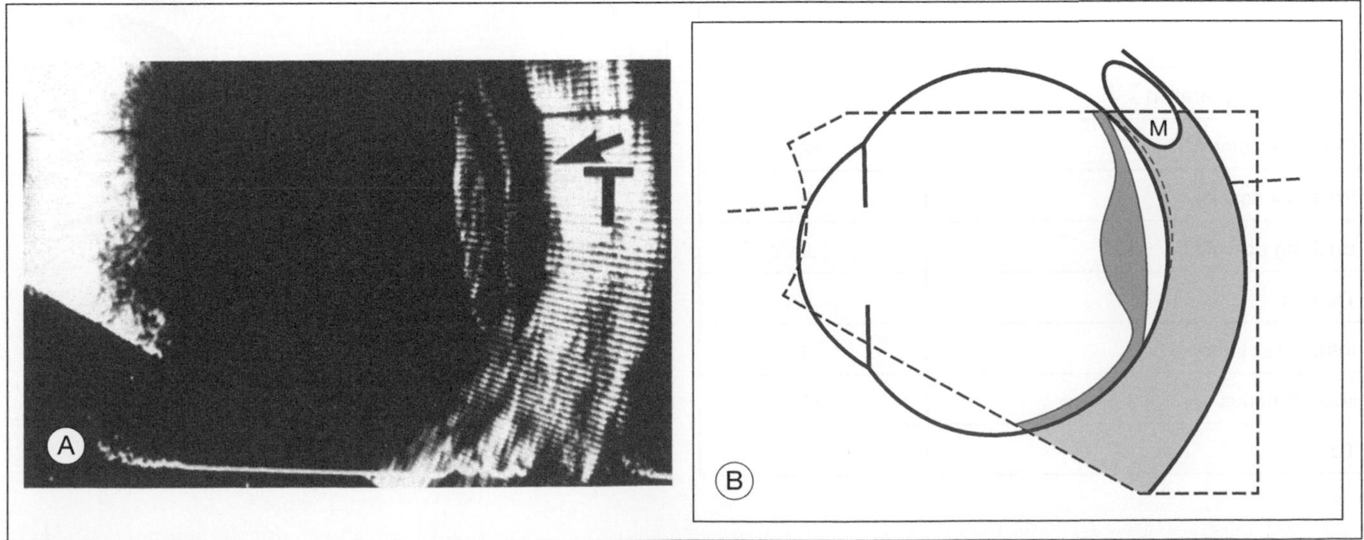

Fig. 9.83 (A) Brawny scleritis with inflammatory infiltration of Tenon's space. This disease entity can be clinically and ultrasonographically identical to a choroidal melanoma. T, Tenon's space. (B) Schematic drawing. M, muscle.

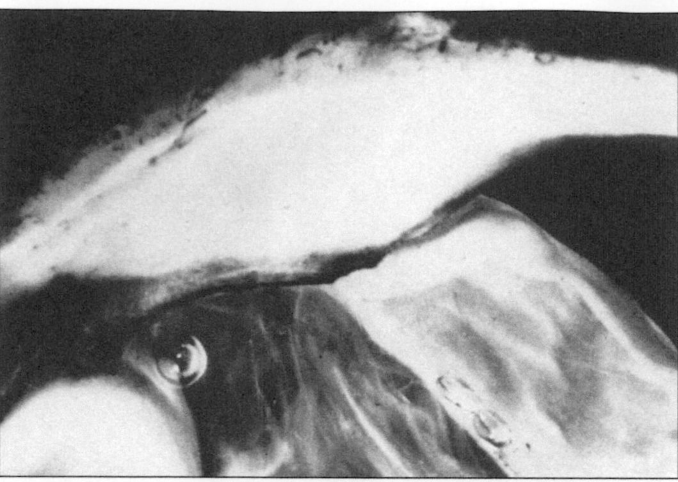

Fig. 9.84 Macroscopic photo of a brawny scleritis. On the basis of the ultrasonographic findings and a positive P32 test, the eye was enucleated because a melanoma was suspected.

Table 9.2 Orbital causes of orbital folds[49]

Diagnosis	Number of patients
Graves orbitopathy	11
Sinusitis	5
Mucocele	2
Hemangioma	6
Orbital pseudotumor	5
Various orbital tumors	8
Unexplained	6
Total	43

Table 9.3 Ocular causes of choroidal folds

Diagnosis	Number of patients
Hyperopic eye	17
Macular degeneration	12
Ocular hypotony	12
Posterior scleritis	9
Buckling operation	9
Trauma	6
Intraocular tumor	3
Miscellaneous	10
Total	78

Table 9.4 Choroidal folds: ultrasonographic findings helpful for differential diagnosis

Diagnosis		Ultrasonographic findings
Myositis Graves orbitopathy	1	Thickened extraocular muscles
Periorbital space-occupying lesions	2	Change in the relief of the orbital wall, sound propagation into perinasal sinuses
Orbital neoplasm	3	Directly evident (it may be difficult to demonstrate a small cavernous hemangioma because of its high acoustic reflectivity)
Inflammatory orbital pseudotumor	4	Widening of normal orbital structures, low acoustic reflectivity, Tenon's space may be demonstrated
Disc edema	5	Widened dural diameter of the optic nerve
Axial hyperopia	6	Axial length below 22 mm, ocular walls concentrically thickened
Ocular hypotony	7	Ocular walls concentrically thickened
Macular degeneration		Thickening of the ocular walls in the area of the macula, high acoustic reflectivity
Scleritis	8	Circumscribed widening of the ocular walls Tenon's space apparent

For companion schematic drawing, see Fig. 9.85.

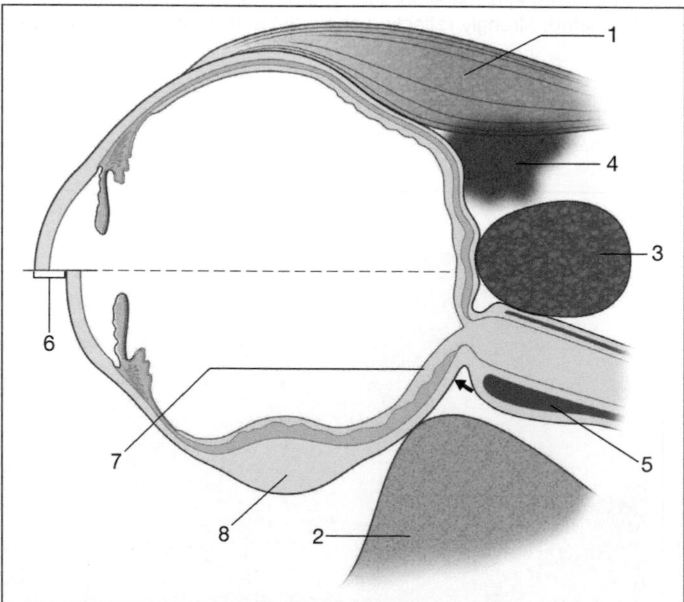

Fig. 9.85 Choroidal folds: ultrasonographic contribution to the differential diagnosis (for detail, see Table 9.4).

Table 9.5 Leukocoria: ultrasonographic findings helpful for differential diagnosis

Diagnosis		Ultrasonographic findings
Normal axial length for the patient's age		
Retinoblastoma	1	Widening of the ocular walls, extremely high acoustic reflectivity, shadowing effect, atypical findings possible
Congenital cataract	2	Increased reflectivity from the posterior lens surface, vitreous space empty, ocular walls normal
Shortened axial length		
Retinopathy of prematurity	3	In stages IV and V, beginning or complete traction detachment (normal findings in stages I–III)
Persistent hyperplastic primary vitreous (PHPV)	4	Dense strand of tissue between optic nerve head and posterior lens pole; formes frustes may occur (posterior or anterior PHPV)
Retinal anomalies		Membranes in the vitreous, atypical detachment, which in part appears solid (no typical echogram)
Fundus coloboma	5	Directly demonstrable protrusion of ocular wall, sometimes with orbital cyst (microphthalmos with cyst)
Coats disease	6	Floating crystals in the vitreous and subretinal space (fast-flickering spikes on A-mode)

For companion schematic drawing, see Fig. 9.86.

Table 9.6 Vitreous hemorrhage: ultrasonographic findings helpful for establishing the etiology

Diagnosis		Ultrasonographic findings
Symptomatic posterior vitreous detachment	1	Thickened detached posterior hyaloid membrane, occasionally early retinal detachment
Recently formed retinal break with torn vessel	2	Blood-covered vitreous strands converge toward the retinal break; occasionally a high-floating operculum may be detected
Proliferative retinopathy	3	Strands or membranes extending from the optic nerve head or the posterior pole, high acoustic reflectivity
Terson syndrome (vitreous hemorrhage after subchoroidal bleeding)	4	Vitreous opacities in front of the optic nerve head or behind the detached vitreous
Disciform macular degeneration	5	Widening of the ocular walls in the macular area, high acoustic reflectivity, vitreous strands extending from the macula
Choroidal melanoma	6	Biconvex thickening of the ocular wall, low acoustic reflectivity, sometimes mushroom-shaped; accompanying retinal detachment distant from the tumor

For companion schematic drawing, see Fig. 9.87.

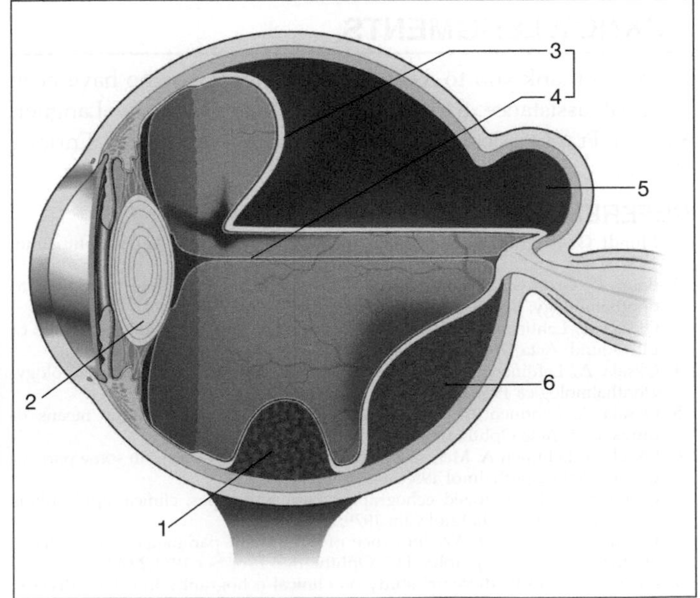

Fig. 9.86 Leukocoria: echographic contribution to the differential diagnosis (for detail, see Table 9.5).

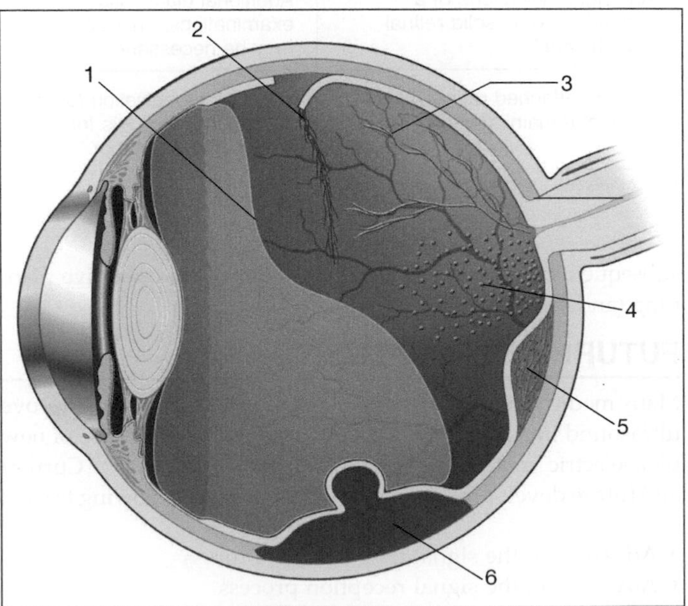

Fig. 9.87 Vitreous hemorrhage: echographic contribution to determine the pathogenesis (for detail, see Table 9.6).

Table 9.7 Examination before a vitrectomy: ultrasonographic findings helpful for planning the operation

Questions on the ultrasonographic examination		Consequences for planning the operation
Is the choroidal detachment including the pars plana?	1	Avoiding this area when inserting the ports
Is the posttraumatic vitreous hemorrhage associated with a detached retina?		If retina is detached, strong indication for vitrectomy
Is an intraocular foreign body demonstrable? If so, where is it in regard to ocular outer wall?	2	Choice of surgical approach, magnet extraction possible?
		Estimating the prognosis
Is there a choroidal detachment caused by blood?	3	Extremely poor prognosis that may not benefit from surgical intervention
Is there a free-floating retinal detachment?	4	Reattachment probable, can be achieved without tamponade from the inside
Is there a rigid retinal detachment? Is there a thickened retina?	5	Removal of preretinal membranes necessary
Are there vitreous strands with traction effect demonstrable?	6	Consider intraoperatively cutting the strands
Is there retinal detachment that is displaced anteriorly to be near the lens?	7	Special care indicated when entering the vitreous space
Are there thickened ocular walls in the macula that may indicate a disciform lesion from macular degeneration?	8	Poor prognosis for central vision
Are there indications of a secondary, e.g., solid retinal detachment?	9	Additional diagnostic examinations; enucleation may be necessary
Is there attached retina with minimal remaining vision?		Reconsider indication for operation, prognosis for vision extremely poor

For companion schematic drawing, see Fig. 9.88.

subsequent conclusions that can be obtained for operative planning (and see Fig. 9.88).

FUTURE DEVELOPMENTS

Many medical fields are using advances in technology to improve ultrasound images. These improvements involve the use of new piezoelectric materials and broadband transducers.[62] Current and future developments can be focused on the following trends:

- Advances in the signal transmission process
- Advances in the signal reception process
- Compounding, equalization, and extended-field acquisitions
- 3D and 4D imaging
- Elastographic imaging
- Miniaturization of units and probes, transfer, and archiving ultrasonic data.

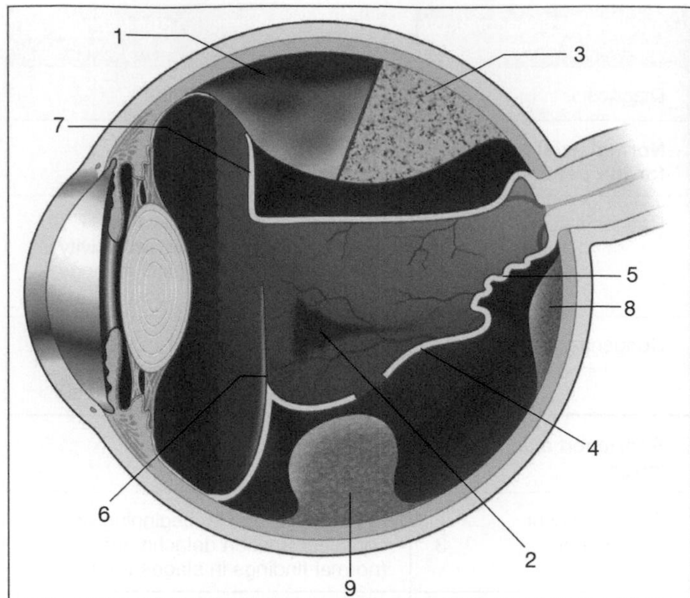

Fig. 9.88 Examination before a vitrectomy: echographic contribution to the planning of the operation (for detail, see Table 9.7).

In the field of ophthalmology new Doppler modes for analyzing retinal blood flow are currently being utilized in research initiatives. A new technique is elastographic imaging. Recently, this technique has been used to image ocular and periocular tissues. Patterns of elastic imaging in the vitreous cavity could be attributed to posterior vitreous detachment, whereas that of medial and lateral rectus muscles may be related to the level of muscle fiber strain. With improved resolution, higher frequencies, and spatial images on ultrasound, new frontiers in ophthalmic imaging are being reached and further research is still under way. These advancements, as well as the safety in image acquisition, maintain the utility of ultrasound imaging within all fields of medicine.

ACKNOWLEDGMENTS

A special thank you to a number of colleagues who have been of great assistance in creating this chapter: Sönke Langner, Kirsten Franke, Beate Stroteich, Angrit Stachs, and Enrique Pfeiffer.

REFERENCES

1. Mundt G, Hughes W. Ultrasonics in ocular diagnosis. Am J Ophthalmol 1956;41:488.
2. Baum G, Greenwood J. The application of ultrasonic locating techniques to ophthalmology, part 1. Am J Ophthalmol 1958;46:319.
3. Oksala A, Lehtinen A. Diagnostic of detachment of the retina by means of ultrasound. Acta Ophthalmol 1957;35:461–7.
4. Oksala A, Lehtinen A. Diagnostic value of ultrasonics in ophthalmology. Ophthalmologica 1957;134:387–95.
5. Oksala A, Lehtinen A. Diagnostic of rupture of the sclera by means of ultrasound. Acta Ophthalmol 1958;36:37–42.
6. Oksala A, Lehtinen A. Measurement of the velocity of sound in some parts of the eye. Acta Ophthalmol 1958;36:633–9.
7. Ossoinig K. Standardized echography: basic principles, clinical applications and results. Int Ophthalmol Clin 1979;19:127.
8. Buschmann W, Haigis W. Influence of equipment parameters on results in ophthalmic ultrasonography. Doc Ophthalmol Proc Ser 1981;29:487.
9. Ossoinig K, Till P. 10 years' study on clinical echography in orbital disease. Bibl Ophthalmol 1975;83:200.
10. Gernet H. Ultrasonic biometry of the eye. Klin Monatsbl Augenheilkd 1967; 151:853–71.
11. Baum G, Greenwood J. Ultrasound in ophthalmology. Am J Ophthalmol 1960; 49:249–61.
12. Bronson N, Fisher Y, Pickering N, et al. Ophthalmic contact B-scan ultrasonography. Westport, CT: Intercontinental; 1976.

13. Pavlin C, Foster F. Ultrasound biomicroscopy of the eye. New York: Springer; 1995.
14. Sherar M, Starkowski B, Taylor W, et al. A 100 Mhz B-scan ultrasound backscatter microscope. Ultrasound Imaging 1989;11:95–105.
15. Pavlin C, Harasiwicz K, Sherar M, et al. Clinical use of ultrasound biomicroscopy. Ophthalmology 1991;98:287–95.
16. Sherar M, Foster F. The design and fabrication of high frequency transducer. Ultrasound Imaging 1989;11:75–94.
17. Pavlin C, Harasiwicz K, Foster F. Ultrasound biomicroscopy of anterior segment structures in normal and glaucomatous eyes. Am J Ophthalmol 1992;113:381–9.
18. Atta HR. New applications in ultrasound technology. Br J Ophthalmol 1999; 83:1246–9.
19. Iezzi R, Rosen R, Tello C, et al. Personal computer-based 3-dimensional ultrasound biomicroscopy of the anterior segment. Arch Ophthalmol 1996;114: 520–4.
20. Cusumano A, Coleman D, Silverman R, et al. Three dimensional ultrasound imaging - clinical applications. Ophthalmology 1998;105:300–6.
21. Coleman D, Silverman R, Daly S. Advances in ophthalmic ultrasound. Radiol Clin North Am 1998;36:1073–82.
22. Reinstein D, Raevsky T, Coleman D. Improved system for ultrasonic imaging and biometry. J Ultrasound Med 1997;16:117–24.
23. Silverman R, Lizzi F, Ursea B, et al. High-resolution ultrasonic imaging and characterization of the ciliary body. Invest Ophthalmol Vis Sci 2001;42: 885–94.
24. Stachs O, Martin H, Behrend D, et al. Three-dimensional ultrasound biomicroscopy, environmental and conventional scanning electron microscopy investigations of the human zonula ciliaris for numerical modelling of accommodation. Graefes Arch Clin Exp Ophthalmol 2006;244:836–44.
25. Stachs O, Martin H, Kirchhoff A, et al. Monitoring accommodative ciliary muscle function using three-dimensional ultrasound. Graefes Arch Clin Exp Ophthalmol 2002;240:906–12.
26. Kirchhoff A, Stachs O, Guthoff R. Three-dimensional ultrasound findings of the posterior iris region. Graefes Arch Clin Exp Ophthalmol 2001;239: 968–71.
27. Stachs O, Schneider H, Stave J, et al. Potentially accommodating intraocular lenses - an in vitro and in vivo study using three-dimensional high-frequency ultrasound. J Refract Surg 2005;21:37–45.
28. Schneider H, Stachs O, Göbel K, et al. Changes of the accommodative amplitude and the anterior chamber depth after implantation of an accommodative intraocular lens. Graefes Arch Clin Exp Ophthalmol 2006;244:322–9.
29. Jaffe NS. Complications of acute posterior vitreous detachment. Arch Ophthalmol 1968;79:568–71.
30. McLeod D. (chair) Round table discussion on vitreous pathology. Doc Ophthalmol Proc 1981;Ser. 547.
31. Ossoinig KC. Advances in diagnostic ultrasound. Acta 14th Int Congr Ophthalmol 1983:89.
32. Till P, Ossoinig KC. 10 years' study on clinical echography in intraocular disease. Bibl Ophthalmol 1975;83:49.
33. Machemer R, Aalberg TM, editors. Glaskörperchirurgie, Vitrektomie. Indikationen und Technik. Berne: Huber Verlag; 1981.
34. Shapiro DR, Stone RD. Ultrasonic characteristics of retinopathy of prematurity presenting with leucokoria. Arch Ophthalmol 1885;103:1690.
35. Darnley-Fisch DD, Frazier-Byrne S, Hughes JR, et al. Contact B-scan echography in the assessment of optic nerve cupping. Am J Ophthalmol 1990; 109:55.
36. Oksala A. Echogram in melanoma of the choroid. Br J Ophthalmol 1959; 43:408.
37. Baum G. Use of ultrasonography in the differential diagnosis of ocular tumors. In: Boniuk M, editor. Ocular and adnexal tumors. St Louis: Mosby; 1964. p. 308.
38. Buschmann W, Trier H. Ophthalmologische Ultraschalldiagnostik, mit Atlas, Standardisierung und Einordnung in den ophthalmologischen Untersuchungsbefund. Berlin: Springer; 1989.
39. Trier H. Gewebsdifferenzierung mit Ultraschall. Bibl Ophthalmol 1977;86:92.
40. Coleman DJ, Silverman R, Rondeau MJ, et al. Explaining the current role of high frequency ultrasound in ophthalmic diagnosis (ophthalmic ultrasound). Expert Rev Ophthalmol 2006;1:63–76.
41. Silverman R, Kong F, Chen Y, et al. High-resolution photoacoustic imaging of ocular tissues. Ultrasound Med Biol 2010;36:733–42.
42. Guthoff R. Ultraschall in der ophthalmologischen Diagnostik. In: Naumann GOH, Hollwich F, Gloor B, editors. Ein Leitfaden für die Praxis. Stuttgart: Enke-Verlag; 1988.
43. Wolter J. Parallel horizontal choroidal folds secondary to an orbital tumor. Am J Ophthalmol 1974;77:669.
44. Coleman D, Lizzi S, Jack R. Ultrasonography of the eye and orbit. Philadelphia: Lea and Febiger; 1977.
45. Bujara K, von Domarus D, Guthoff R. Necrotic malignant melanoma of the choroid with unusual clinical, echographical and histological case study. Ophthalmologica 1980;180:222–7.
46. Guthoff R, Berger R, Helmke K, et al. Doppersonographische Befunde bei intraokulären Tumoren Forstschr Ophthalmol 1989;86:239.
47. Bloch RS, Gartner S. The incidence of ocular metastatic carcinoma. Arch Ophthalmol 1971;85:673.
48. Ferry AP, Font RI. Carcinoma metastatic to the eye and the orbit: a clinical pathological study of 227 cases. Arch Ophthalmol 1974;92:276.
49. Verbeek A. Echographic findings in 36 patients with choroidal folds. Doc Ophthalmol Proc Ser 1981;29.
50. Manschot WA. The relation between histopathological and ultrasonographyin intraocular tumors. Doc Ophthalmol Proc Ser 1981;29:71.
51. Shields CL, Shields JA, Augsburger JJ, editors. Update on choroidal osteomas. Proceedings of the 2nd international meeting on the diagnosis and treatment of intraocular tumors; Lyons; 1987.
52. Wende S, Aulich A, Nover A, et al. Computer tomography of orbital lesions: a cooperative study of 210 cases. Neuroradiology 1978;13:123.
53. Gass JDM, Guerry RK, Jack RI, et al. Choroidal osteoma. Arch Ophthalmol 1978;96:428.
54. Gass JDM. New observations concerning choroidal osteomas. Int Ophthalmol 1979;71.
55. Wing GI, Schepenz CL, Trempe CL, et al. Serous choroidal detachment and the thickened choroidal sign detected by ultrasonography. Am J Ophthalmol 1982;94:499.
56. Blodi FC. Ein Tuberkulom der Aderhaut, ein melanom vortäuschend. Klin Monatsbl Augenheilkd 1977;170:845.
57. Wirold J, Orlowski-Szczypinski J. Ultrasonography of the subretinal space in rhegmatogeneous retinal detachment. Z Mod Probl Ophthalmol 1976;18:40.
58. Cappaert W, Purnell E, Frank K. Use of B-scan ultrasound in the diagnosis of benign choroidal folds. Am J Ophthalmol 1977;84:375.
59. Singh G, Guthoff RF, Foster S. Observations on long-term follow-up of posterior scleritis. Am J Ophthalmol 1986;101:570.
60. Guthoff RF. Die differentialdiagnostische Bedeutung des Tenon'schen Raumes. Fortschr Ophthalmol 1974;81:388.
61. Feldon S, Sigelman J, Albert D, et al. Clinical manifestations of brawny scleritis. Am J Ophthalmol 1978;85:781.
62. Claudon M, Tranquart F, Evans DH, et al. Advances in ultrasound. Eur Radiol 2002;12:7–18.

Section 2 Retinal Diagnostics

Chapter 10

Color Vision and Night Vision

Dingcai Cao

OVERVIEW

Day vision and night vision are two separate modes of visual perception and the visual system shifts from one mode to the other based on ambient light levels. Each mode is primarily mediated by one of two photoreceptor classes in the retina, i.e., cones and rods. In day vision, visual perception is primarily cone-mediated and perceptions are chromatic. In other words, color vision is present in the light levels of daytime. In night vision, visual perception is rod-mediated and perceptions are principally achromatic. Under dim illuminations, there is no obvious color vision and visual perceptions are graded variations of light and dark. Historically, color vision has been studied as the salient feature of day vision and there has been emphasis on analysis of cone activities in color vision. Night vision has historically been studied in terms of rod activity and considerations of the shift from day vision to night vision.

This chapter will review basic aspects of rods and cones and neural pathways that process rod and cone information. Measurement of sensitivity during dark adaptation is discussed as the established measure of the shift between day vision (cone vision) and night vision (rod vision). Clinical assessment of rod and cone sensitivities using dark adaptation function as a means of assessing retinal disease is also discussed. Color vision is discussed in terms of experimental paradigms and theoretical considerations and variations in human color vision are described. Evaluation of color vision can be helpful in understanding the underlying mechanisms of some retinal diseases and suggestions for clinical evaluation of color vision are offered. In the last section of this chapter, new developments in color vision research are discussed.

ROD AND CONE FUNCTIONS

Differences in the anatomy and physiology (see Chapters 4, Autofluorescence imaging, and 9, Diagnostic ophthalmic ultrasound) of the rod and cone systems underlie different visual functions and modes of visual perception. The rod photoreceptors are responsible for our exquisite sensitivity to light, operating over a 10^8 (100 millionfold) range of illumination from near total darkness to daylight. Cones operate over a 10^{11} range of illumination, from moonlit night light levels to light levels that are so high they bleach virtually all photopigments in the cones. Together the rods and cones function over a 10^{14} range of illumination. Depending on the relative activity of rods and cones, a light level can be characterized as photopic (cones alone mediate vision), mesopic (both rods and cones are active), or scotopic (rods alone mediate vision).[1] In the literature, the terms photopic vision and scotopic vision are used to reflect cone and rod vision, respectively. Table 10.1 shows this overlapping range of activity.

The distribution of rods and cones in the retina (see Chapter 4, Autofluorescence imaging) is also reflected in visual function. The greatest sensitivity to light occurs in the midperiphery of the visual field, which has a predominance of rods, while high-acuity and good color vision are mediated by the fovea, which has a predominance of cones. Nonetheless, the entire retina, with the exception of a very small area within the fovea, is capable of mediating night vision, and color vision is present throughout the visual field with daylight stimulation of the entire retina. The following will introduce rod and cone differences in light adaptation, spectral sensitivity, and spatial/temporal sensitivity.

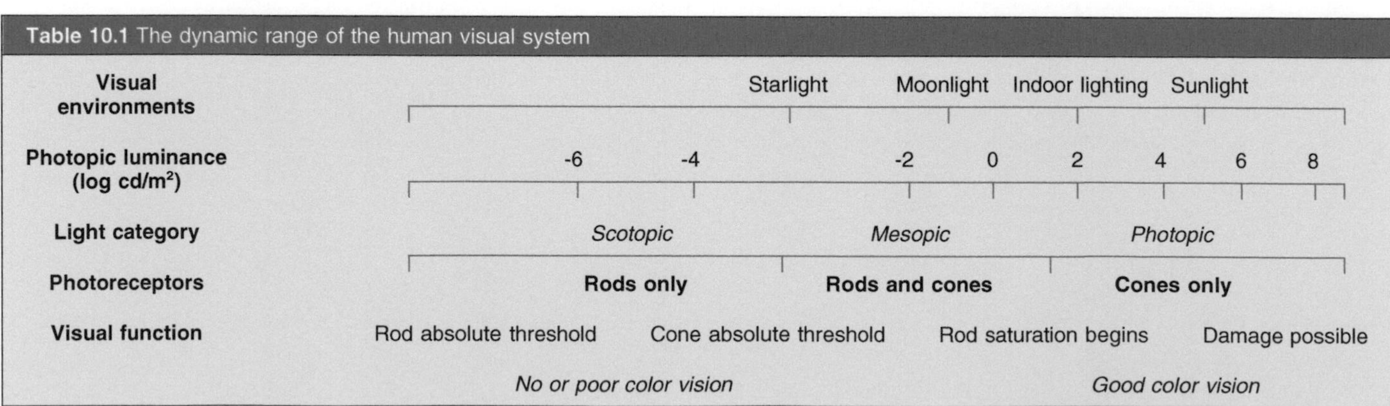

Table 10.1 The dynamic range of the human visual system

Visual environments			Starlight	Moonlight		Indoor lighting	Sunlight	
Photopic luminance (log cd/m²)	-6	-4	-2	0	2	4	6	8
Light category	Scotopic			Mesopic		Photopic		
Photoreceptors	Rods only			Rods and cones		Cones only		
Visual function	Rod absolute threshold		Cone absolute threshold		Rod saturation begins		Damage possible	
	No or poor color vision					Good color vision		

Modified from Hood DC, Finkelstein MA. Sensitivity to light. In: Boff KR, Kaufman L, Thomas JP, editors. The handbook of perception and human performance, vol. 1. Sensory processes and perception. New York: John Wiley; 1986.

Light adaptation

Photoreceptors, whether they are rods or cones, respond well to only a small range of variations in illumination within a steady adapting background.[2] However, adaptation mechanisms adjust photoreceptor sensitivity so that this small range of responses is always centered near the current adaptation level, even though adaptation levels can vary over a wide range. This behavior forms the basis for the large operating range of the visual system.

It is possible to measure a threshold for the perception of an increment in light on a large, steady background field. As the background light level is increased, the increment threshold starts to increase. Rods and cones behave somewhat differently in this regard. For the rod system, as shown in Fig. 10.1A, the increment threshold increases steadily over almost a thousand-fold range. With further increases in background adaptation levels, an increment is not detected, no matter how much additional test light is presented as an increment, due to rod saturation. In comparison, the cone system, as shown in Fig. 10.1B, shows a continuous steady increase in the increment threshold with increases in background illumination, even at levels that bleach almost the entire amount of available photopigment. The portion of the curve that rises linearly with illumination levels is called the Weber region (Fig. 10.1). In the Weber region, an incremental light can be detected when it is a constant proportion (i.e., the Weber fraction) of the background light level. Different photoreceptor systems have a characteristic Weber fraction. Cones have lower Weber fractions than rods and the M and L cones have lower Weber fractions than S cones. Under optimal conditions, the cone system can detect a light level difference of 1%, while rods need a light change of 20%.

In addition to photoreceptor adaptational properties, other factors, including pupil size, the temporal and spatial summation characteristics, and photopigment depletion, can also contribute to extend the operating range of the visual system over a large luminance range. While some adaptation operates within the photoreceptors themselves, other properties of adaptation may reflect the effects of the complex neural circuitry of the retina.[2]

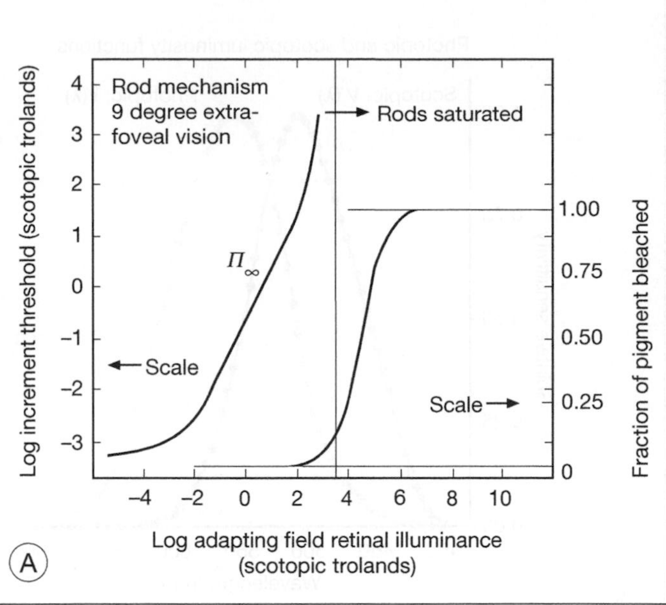

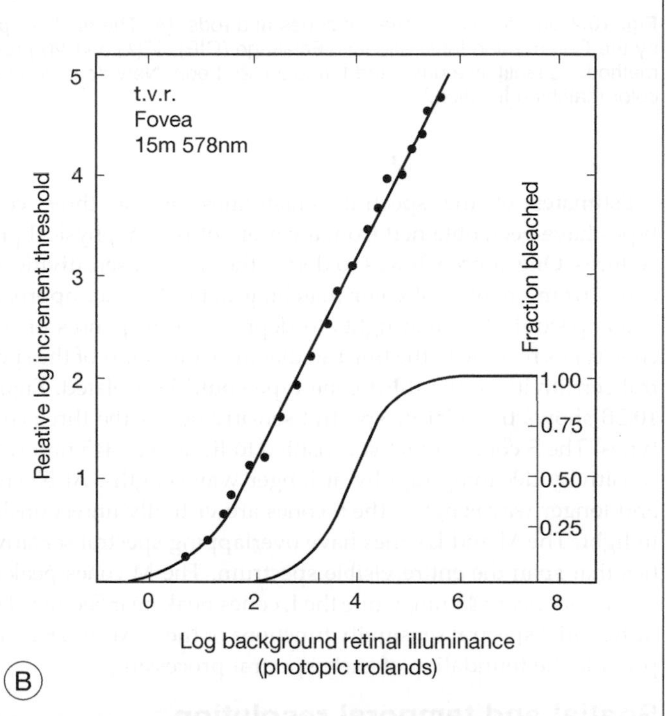

Fig. 10.1 The increment threshold functions for scotopic (rod) and photopic (cone) vision as a function of background illuminance. (A) Rod increment thresholds measured at 9° in the parafovea. The dashed line has a slope of 1. The portion where the curve has unit slope (in parallel to the dashed line) is the Weber region, followed at higher levels by the region of rod saturation. To the right is shown the fraction of rod photopigment bleached. The rods are saturated before there is substantial photopigment bleaching. (B) Cone increment thresholds measured at the fovea. To the right is shown the fraction of photopigment bleached. The Weber region extends to luminances (6 million tds) that bleach virtually all the cone photopigment. (Reproduced with permission from Enoch JM. The two-color threshold technique of Stiles and derived component color mechanisms. In: Jameson D, Hurvich L, editors. Visual psychophysics: handbook of sensory physiology, vol. VII/4. Berlin: Springer-Verlag; 1972.)

Spectral sensitivity

Day vision is primarily mediated by three types of cone photoreceptors with different but overlapping spectral sensitivities. Each is identified by the relative position of the peak in spectral sensitivity. The three cone types are called the long-, middle-, and short-wavelength-sensitive (L, M, and S) cones. When overall sensitivity to light is measured at the light-adapted fovea, a broad sensitivity spectrum peaking near 555 nm is found. This sensitivity spectrum represents the combined activity of the L and M cones and is called the $V(\lambda)$ function. When sensitivity to light is measured in the dark-adapted peripheral retina, where rods dominate, a broad-sensitivity spectrum is found with a peak sensitivity at 507 nm. This rod spectral sensitivity function is called $V'(\lambda)$ (Fig. 10.2A). Both $V(\lambda)$ and $V'(\lambda)$ functions have practical significance and have been accepted by the International Commission of Illumination as representative of human vision relative luminous efficiency at photopic and scotopic levels. They are also used to relate luminous (perceived energy of light) to radiant (emitted light) energy.

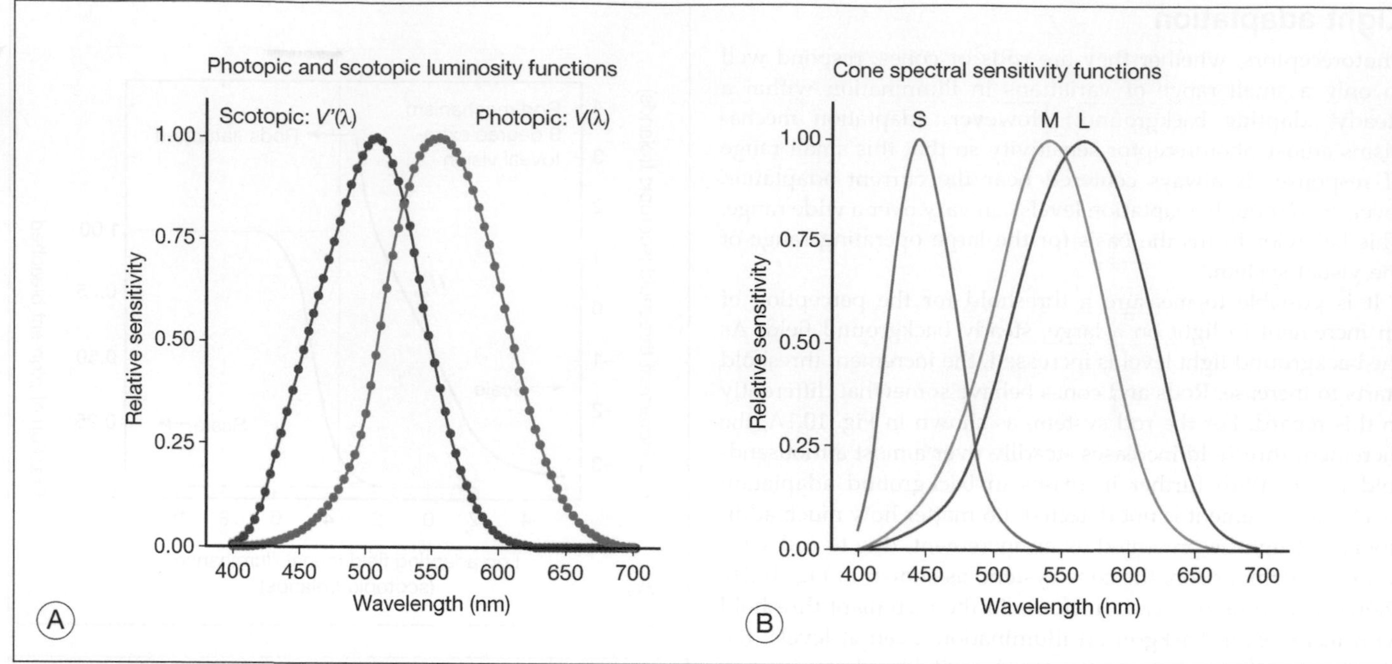

Fig. 10.2 Spectral sensitivities of cones and rods. (A) The relative spectral luminous efficiency functions for scotopic and photopic vision adopted by the Commission International d'Eclairage (CIE), $V'(\lambda)$ and $V(\lambda)$ respectively. (Data from Wyszecki G, Stiles WS. Color science – concepts and methods, quantitative data, and formulae, 2nd edn. New York: John Wiley; 1982). (B) Spectral sensitivities of the S, M, and L cones derived from color-matching function.[14]

Estimates of the spectral sensitivities of the three cone types have been obtained from a variety of psychophysical procedures. One approach was to derive the spectral sensitivities of cones from analysis of color-matching data. Another approach used spectral bleaching lights to depress the responses of two cone types relative to the third so that measurements of the spectral sensitivity of the third cone type could be isolated. Figure 10.2B shows the relative spectral sensitivities of the three cone types. The S cones are most sensitive to light near 445 nm, with sensitivity declining rapidly at longer wavelengths. At 555 nm and longer wavelengths, the S cones are virtually unresponsive to light. The M and L cones have overlapping spectral sensitivities that span the entire visible spectrum. The M cones peak in sensitivity near 543 nm, while the L cones peak near 566 nm. The differential spectral sensitivity functions of the L, M, and S cones provide the foundation of early spectral processing.

Spatial and temporal resolution

Compared with the cone system, the rod system has poorer spatial resolution (acuity). For an observer with 20/20 photopic acuity, scotopic acuity would be about 20/200 (10 times worse than photopic acuity). The rod system also has poorer temporal resolution, which refers to the ability to perceive a physically alternating light as steady or flickering in time. The transitional temporal frequency at which the light appears from flickering to steady is called the critical fusion frequency (CFF). CFFs increase with light adaptation level, reaching a maximum of 20 Hz for rods and 55–60 Hz for cones. This means that flickering lights can be perceived at higher frequencies in brighter light conditions. Interestingly, dark-adapted rods can suppress cone-mediated flicker detection[3] and this suppression mainly occurs in the magnocellular (MC) pathway (explained below).[4]

VISUAL PATHWAYS FOR ROD AND CONE FUNCTIONS

Retinal pathways

Rod signals are conveyed by two primary neural pathways that are dependent on the illumination level.[5] One pathway is via ON rod bipolars, AII amacrine cells, and ON and OFF cone bipolars, which are all cells in the retina. This is a temporally sluggish pathway that mediates rod vision at low scotopic light levels. The second pathway transmits rod information via rod–cone gap junctions and ON and OFF cone bipolar cells in the retina. This is a fast pathway that mediates vision at higher scotopic and mesopic light levels. A third insensitive rod pathway between rods and OFF cone bipolars has been identified in rodents but, thus far, not in primates. The significant point here is that rods and cones share neural pathways and have joint inputs to retinal ganglion cells.

Retinogeniculate pathways

There are three major neural retinogeniculate pathways in primates that convey retinal information to the visual cortex.[6,7] The pathways are named after the layers of the lateral geniculate nucleus (LGN) that receive input from distinct types of ganglion cells and project to different areas of the primary visual cortex. The MC layer of the LGN receives inputs from parasol ganglion cells. The MC pathway processes the summed output of the L and M cones to signal luminance information. The parvocellular (PC) layer of the LGN receives input from midget ganglion cells. The PC pathway mediates spectral opponency of L and M cones (discussed later) to signal chromatic information. The koniocellular (KC) layer of the LGN, which receives input from small bistratified as well as other ganglion cells, detects changes in

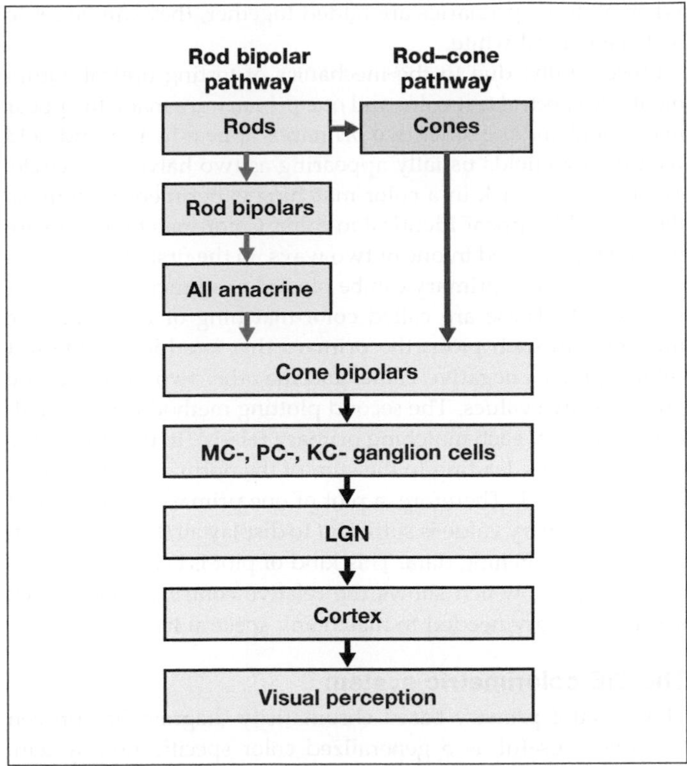

Fig. 10.3 The schematic diagram of visual pathways carrying rod and cone inputs for visual perception. MC, magnocellular; PC, parvocellular; KC, koniocellular; LGN, lateral geniculate nucleus.

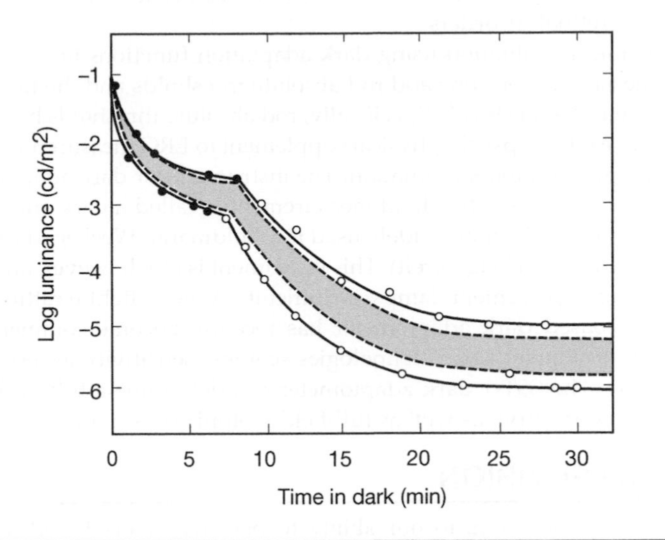

Fig. 10.4 The time course of dark adaptation. The range of threshold sensitivities of 110 normal observers is shown. The circular points represent data of the most and least sensitive individuals. The area enclosed by the dashed lines represents 80% of this population. The cone absolute thresolds are obtained during the cone and rod plateaus, respectively. (Data from Hecht S, Mandlebaum J. The relationship between vitamin A and dark adaptation. JAMA 1939;112:1910–6.)

S-cone signals compared to the sum of the L- and M-cone signals. These three pathways mediate different aspects of vision, with the MC pathway mainly carrying out luminance and motion processing, the PC pathway mainly processing red–green color, acuity, and shape information, and the KC pathway mainly handling blue–yellow color processing.

The sharing of neural pathways between rods and cones implies that rods should have input to the MC, PC, and KC pathways. Indeed, physiological studies have shown that there is strong rod input to the MC pathway, but weak input to the PC pathway.[8] Demonstration of rod input to the KC pathways is less clear. An earlier study[8] did not find rod input to the bistratified ganglion cells in the parafovea, while two recent studies demonstrated strong rod input in the peripheral retina.[9,10] Figure 10.3 shows a schematic diagram of the visual pathways conveying rod and cone inputs to the MC, PC, and KC ganglion cells, which would then produce signals that are projected into the cortex to mediate different aspects of visual perception.

DARK ADAPTATION FUNCTIONS: ASSESSMENT OF THE SHIFT FROM DAY VISION TO NIGHT VISION

Measurements of sensitivity thresholds during adaptation to darkness have produced a characteristic biphasic function with an initial segment that is attributed to cone responses and a subsequent segment attributed to rod responses. Figure 10.4 shows a characteristic dark adaptation function measured in the peripheral retina. Thresholds decrease quickly initially and this rapid recovery is attributed to cones. Thresholds then reach a plateau in about 5 minutes and remain invariant for another 5 minutes (cone plateau, reflecting cone absolute thresholds). Then, there is a second rapid decrease in thresholds due to sensitivity recovery of the rods, referred to as the rod–cone break, to a new plateau that is reached in 40–50 minutes (rod plateau, reflecting rod absolute thresholds).

The shape of the dark adaptation function depends on testing parameters, including retinal location, wavelength, and temporal and spatial characteristics.[1,11] The effects of these parameters on dark adaptation curves can be understood by the differences between rods and cones in terms of their distributions, spectral sensitivity, and spatial/temporal resolution characteristics. For instance, because there are only cones in the fovea, dark adaptation measured at the fovea using a small test light reveals a rapid monophasic branch attributable to the cones. On the other hand, because the rod and cone systems have similar absolute sensitivities at long wavelengths, dark adaptation measured with long-wavelength lights is monophasic, resembling the cone function. As the test wavelength is changed to shorter wavelengths, a biphasic curve emerges because the rods show greater absolute sensitivity than cones at shorter wavelengths.[12]

Clinical evaluation using dark adaptation functions

It is known that certain retinal disorders may selectively affect rods (e.g., retinitis pigmentosa) or cones (e.g., cone dystrophies). Clinically, rod and cone functions can be evaluated electrophysiologically by measuring rod and cone electroretinograms (ERG: see Chapter 7, Electrogenesis of the electroretinogram) or, psychophysically, by measuring dark adaptation functions. Dark adaptation functions quantify the ability of the rod and cone systems to recover sensitivity (i.e., regenerate photopigment) after exposure to light. The recovery is faster for cones, but the absolute level of sensitivity is greatest for rods. Variations in sensitivity and sensitivity recovery times can be used to characterize retinal disorders.

Clinical evaluation using dark adaptation functions involves a measure of the cone and rod absolute thresholds and the time of the rod–cone break. Specifically, rod absolute thresholds have been used as a psychophysical supplement to ERG measurement for night-blindness evaluation. The instrument for dark adaptation rod absolute threshold measurement is called a dark adaptometer and the most widely used is a Goldmann–Weekers dark adaptometer (Haag-Streit). This instrument is old, however, and finding replacement lamps is difficult. A new light-emitting diode-based dark adaptometer has recently become commercially available (LKC Technologies scotopic sensitivity tester-1: SST-1). The SST-1 dark adaptometer can determine a full dark adaptation curve as well as full-field scotopic sensitivities.

COLOR VISION

Color vision refers to our ability to perceive colors based on spectral variations in light absorbed by the photoreceptors. Color vision includes both chromatic discrimination and color appearance appreciation. Color matching and color discrimination experimental tasks are two fundamental psychophysical procedures that have provided theoretical insights into the nature of color vision and have also been developed for clinical diagnosis of color vision. Color matching and color discrimination results, however, do not address questions of color appearance, for example, why an object appears red. Color appearance is far more complex because it depends on not only the chromatic properties of an object but also the spatial, temporal, and spectral characteristics of the neighboring objects.[13] Neural processing beyond the retina is required for color appearance perceptions.

Color matching

Color matching as the foundation for the theory of trichromacy

The psychophysical procedure in which an observer sets a mixture of three primary lights to match the color of a test stimulus is called color matching. It has been known since the 19th century that different colors perceived by humans can be specified by an economical three-variable (trichromatic) system. In the 1800s, Thomas Young and Hermann von Helmholtz proposed that there must be three kinds of physiological entities in the eye accounting for this trichromacy and their theory is called the Young–Helmholtz trichromatic theory of color vision. We now know the basis for trichromacy is the existence of three cone types in the retina. Color matching was the means to uncover the spectral sensitivity functions of the three different cone types (Fig. 10.1B).[14]

Color-matching experimental techniques and data

Theoretically, a color match occurs when the photoreceptor quantal catch for the test stimulus and the quantal catch for the stimulus that is a combination of the three primary lights are the same. Color matches are unperturbed by changes in luminance levels, as long as no significant photopigment bleaching occurs, which means that the basic nature of trichromacy exists under wide variations in light levels. In a classical color-matching experiment, three spectral lights are chosen as the three primaries and the precise setting of the relative percentages of the three primaries to match a test light is the data for that match. When all three primaries are added together, they can be set to match a neutral white.

Procedurally, due to the mechanics of testing optical equipment, the spectral test color and one primary are made to appear in one field and the other two primaries appear in a second field with the two fields usually appearing as two halves of a circle. The observer's task in a color-matching experiment is to make the two fields appear identical in color. Color-matching data are usually represented in one of two ways. In the first, the amounts of energy of each primary can be plotted as a function of the test wavelength. These are called color-matching or color mixture functions. In such plots, the primary that is added to the test color is given a negative value, and the other two primaries are given positive values. The second plotting method is to normalize the value of each matching primary relative to the sum of the three primaries, leading to the sum of the normalized primaries being equal to 1. Therefore, a plot of one primary value against a second primary value is sufficient to display all the information in the color-matching data. This kind of plot is called a chromaticity diagram, which shows the relative contributions of each spectral primary needed to match any spectral light.

The CIE colorimetric system

This spectral primary-based chromaticity diagram has proven to be very useful as a generalized color specification system. However, linear transformation is needed to compare data collected with different choices of primaries. In 1931, the Commission Internationale d'Eclairage (CIE) standardized the spectral-primary-based chromaticity system by adopting three imaginary primaries (*X, Y, Z* primaries) that are out of the spectral locus and therefore do not exist physically. The choices of the imaginary primaries were based on two important considerations: first, to ensure that the chromaticities of all physical lights have positive values and, second, to relate colorimetric functions to the previously adopted luminosity function, $V(\lambda)$. In the system, the color-matching function for the *Y* primary is identical to $V(\lambda)$ of the photometric system as designed.

Figure 10.5A shows the 1931 CIE chromaticity chart, in which the coordinates of the *Y* primary [$y = Y/(X + Y + Z)$] are plotted against those of the *X* primary [$x = X/(X + Y + Z)$]. The spectrum loci (their wavelengths are indicated on the graph) form the horseshoe-shaped curve. Equal-energy-spectrum (EES) light is plotted in the center, with the coordinates of $x = 0.3333$ and $y = 0.3333$. A straight line connects 400 nm to 700 nm for purples, which result from mixtures of short- and long-wavelength light. All possible lights occur within the boundaries of the spectrum locus and the purple line. Highly saturated colors occur near the locus and desaturated (pale) colors occur near the white point.

The 1931 CIE system was based on 2° field color-matching functions that were derived from color matches of many observers. The averaged color-matching function from these observers was treated as the standard. Therefore, an observer with the standard color-matching function is referred to as the standard observer. Since the color-matching data are affected by the size of the stimulus field presented to the observer, in 1964, the CIE also adopted a large-field *XYZ* system that was based on the 10° field standard observer color-matching functions. For large stimuli, such as those generated by Ganzfeld for ERG measurements, it is recommended to use the 1964 CIE chromaticities to reflect more accurately the large field color-matching functions.

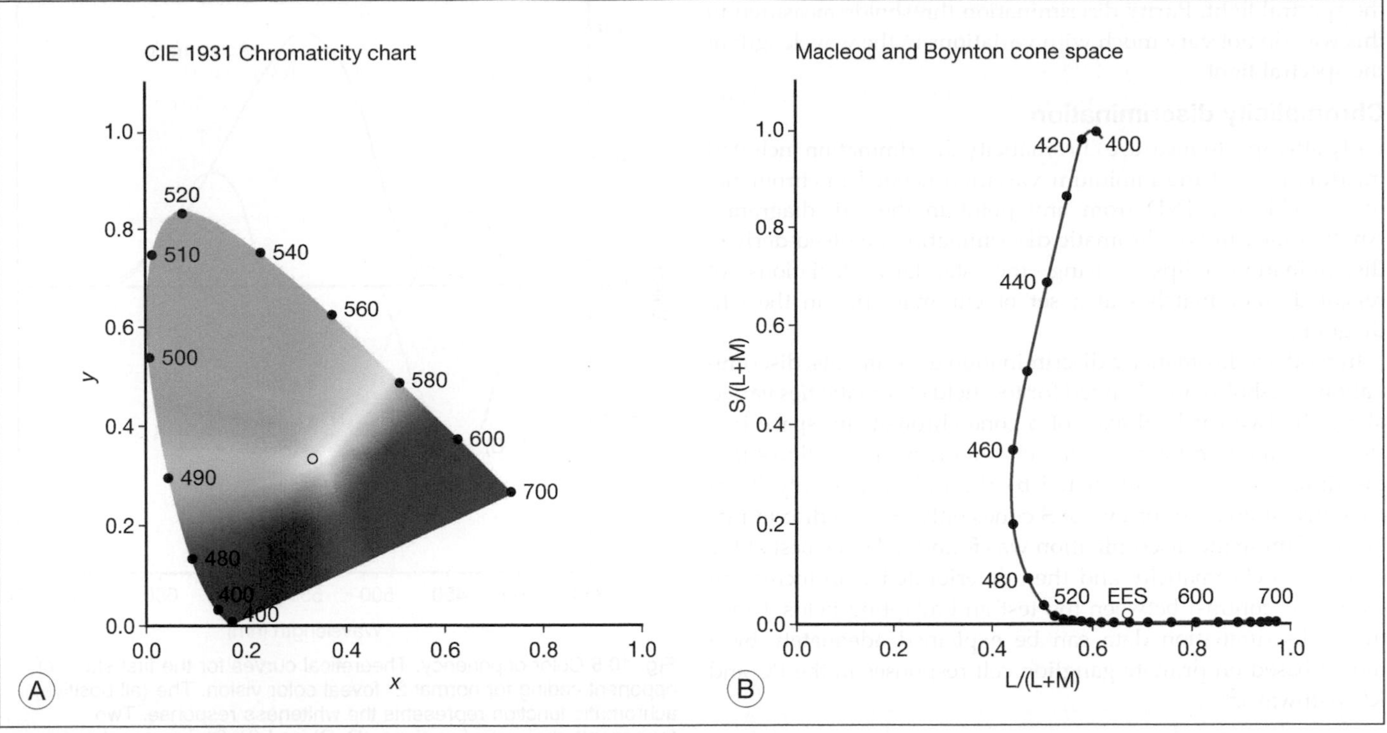

Fig. 10.5 Chromaticity spaces. (A) The Commission International d'Eclairage (CIE) 1931 *x*, *y* chromaticity diagram. An equal-energy-spectrum (EES) light has a coordinate of $x = 0.3333$ and $y = 0.3333$. Spectral wavelengths are represented on the horseshoe-shaped spectrum locus. All lights can be represented in this diagram. (Data from Wyszecki G, Stiles WS. Color science – concepts and methods, quantitative data, and formulae, 2nd edn. New York: John Wiley; 1982.) (B) The MacLeod and Boynton cone space, which plots S-cone excitation versus relative L/M-cone excitations. In this space, the S/(L + M) chromaticity of 400 nm spectral light is normalized to be 1. In such a normalization, an EES light has a chromaticity of L/(L + M) = 0.665 and S/(L + M) = 0.016. In a relative cone troland space, the S/(L + M) for an EES light is normalized to be 1. The chromaticities of the spectral loci form an "L" shape in this space.

Cone chromaticity space

The CIE colorimetric system is valuable for light specifications; however, psychophysical experiments using the CIE system cannot yield results that allow easy interpretation of the underlying physiological mechanisms. When the physiological mechanisms of color vision are of interest, a cone chromaticity space that can represent cone stimulations, as well as the postreceptoral pathways, is preferred.

The concept of cone chromaticity space appeared in the early 20th century. It was not until 1979 that MacLeod and Boynton[15] published a cone chromaticity space based on modern estimates of the cone spectral sensitivities.[14] In the MacLeod and Boynton cone chromaticity space (Fig. 10.5B), the horizontal axis [L/(L + M)] represents the variation of relative L- versus M-cone stimulation at equiluminance, while the vertical axis [S/(L + M)] represents the variation of S-cone stimulation. The space normalizes in that S/(L + M) = 1 for spectral light of 400 nm. Later, a relative cone troland space that normalizes S/(L + M) for EES light to be 1 was proposed to link cone excitations with retinal illuminance, which is measured in trolands.[16] Another spectral opponency space normalizes the cone chromaticity based at the EES-white to reflect both cone contrasts and postreceptoral opponency signals.[17] These cone chromaticity spaces are a major breakthrough for vision research because neurons in the PC and KC pathways show preferred responses to stimuli along the two axes of the cone chromaticity spaces.[17,18] Therefore, psychophysical experiments can be designed to infer the functions of the postreceptoral pathways by generating stimuli along the two theoretical axes.

Chromatic discrimination

Chromatic discrimination refers to the ability of an observer to discriminate two colors. Chromatic discrimination has been investigated using three approaches: wavelength discrimination, purity discrimination, and chromaticity discrimination (reviewed by Pokorny and Smith[19]). Chromatic discrimination is usually measured at a constant luminance level to avoid potential interactions between the luminance pathway (MC pathway) and the chromatic pathway (PC or KC pathway).

Wavelength discrimination

In a typical wavelength discrimination experiment, the stimulus consists of two equiluminant semicircular fields, one filled with a narrow band of spectral light to serve as the standard field and the other as the comparison field. The observer is instructed to change the wavelength of the comparison field to achieve a just noticeable difference (JND) from the standard wavelength. Typical wavelength discrimination thresholds, as a function of standard wavelengths, form a skewed "W" shape with two minima, one at 490 nm and the other at 580 nm.[20]

Purity discrimination

There are two ways to measure purity discrimination. The first method measures the minimum amount of spectral light the observer adds into a white field to achieve a JND from the same white in another juxtaposed field. Discrimination thresholds measured in this way are the largest at 570 nm and the smallest at 400 nm. The second method measures the minimum amount of white light added into a spectral light to achieve a JND from the spectral light. Purity discrimination thresholds measured in this way do not vary much with variations in the wavelength of the spectral light.

Chromaticity discrimination

Early attempts to measure chromaticity discrimination included measurement of the minimum variation needed in chromaticity to achieve a JND from any point in the CIE diagram.[21] Another measure of chromatic discrimination involved derived discrimination ellipses using the standard deviations of repeated color matches at a set of chromaticities in the CIE diagram.[22]

In modern chromaticity discrimination experiments, discrimination thresholds are obtained for test field chromaticities varied along the two cardinal axes of a cone chromaticity space in a steady adaptation field. A cone chromaticity space allows that discrimination can be mediated by the L/M cones only (L/M cone discrimination) or by the S cones only (S-cone discrimination).[23] Chromatic discrimination was found to be the best at the adaptation chromaticity and then deteriorated with increasing chromatic contrast between the test and adapting fields. Chromatic discrimination data can be explained adequately by a model based on primate ganglion cell responses in the PC and KC pathways.[24]

Color appearance

In color-matching and color discrimination experiments, observers determine whether two colors appear the same or different but they do not determine which color is perceived. Color appearance has three perceptual dimensions: hue, saturation, and brightness. Hue is the perceptual dimension that differs from white, such as red, orange, green, blue, yellow, purple, and pink. Saturation indicates how different the hue is from white. For instance, colors on the spectral locus are highly saturated compared with desaturated colors near white (Fig. 10.5A). Brightness is the perceptual dimension related to luminance variance.

An important feature of color appearance is that colors do not simultaneously appear red and green, nor do they simultaneously appear blue and yellow. However, colors do appear as mixtures of red and yellow or red and blue and they also appear as mixtures of green and yellow or green and blue. Further, human observers can separately abstract the qualities of redness–greenness or blueness–yellowness in an arbitrary test color. These facts have led to the concept that color appearance can be represented in a double-opponent system, with red and green placed in opposite directions on one dimension and blue and yellow placed in opposite directions in the other dimension (Fig. 10.6). Red and green are said to be opponent sensations, as are blue and yellow. This observation triggered Ewald Hering, a German physiologist, to propose the "opponent-color" theory in the late 19th century.

The theories of opponency and trichromacy were two competing theories in the history of color vision research; however, the two theories have been reconciled in that chromatic processing starts with three types of cones, supporting trichromacy, and spectral responses from the cones are transmitted in bipolar and ganglion cells that have antagonistic receptive field structures, consistent with opponency. This interpretation of color vision, first proposed by von Kries in 1905,[25] is referred to as the two-stage or two-process model of color vision.

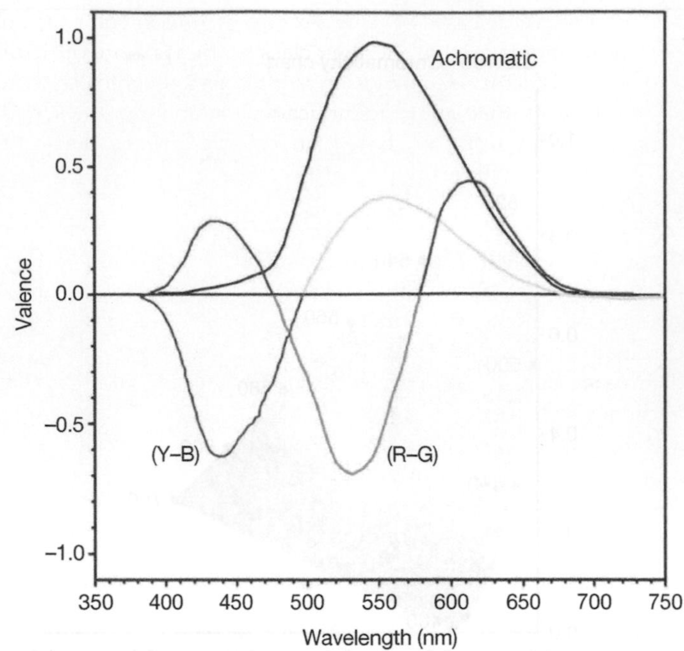

Fig. 10.6 Color opponency. Theoretical curves for the first stage of opponent coding for normal 2° foveal color vision. The (all-positive) achromatic function represents the whiteness response. Two (opponent) chromatic functions, (R–G) and (Y–B), represent redness–greenness and yellowness–blueness, respectively. (Reproduced with permission from Hurvich LM, Jameson D. Some quantitative aspects of an opponent-colors theory. II. Brightness, saturation and hue in normal and dichromatic vision. J Opt Soc Am 1955;45:602–16.)

In a complex visual scene, the perceived color of a light (emitted from a source or reflected from an object) cannot be predicted from its spectral power distribution because the context of other nearby light affects color appearance. For instance, chromatic induction occurs when perception changes because of the presence of other lights nearby in space or time. Chromatic induction includes both chromatic contrast and chromatic assimilation. Chromatic contrast occurs when the color appearance of a test light shifts away (in terms of color opponency) from the color appearance of a nearby light. Chromatic assimilation occurs when the color appearance of a test light shifts toward the color appearance of inducing nearby light. Therefore, the color of a light seen in isolation (surrounded by darkness) is called an unrelated color while the color perceived in the presence of a complex context is called a related color; that is, its percept is related to the surrounding colors. Cortical mechanisms are likely involved in color perception in a complex scene.[26]

VARIATIONS IN HUMAN COLOR VISION

Abnormal color vision that is either inherited or acquired is present in about 4.5% of the population. Congenital color vision defects are stationary over the lifespan and do not result from other visual problems. These color vision defects have been studied extensively and their classification is well established based on psychophysical and genetic works. The most common are the congenital X-chromosome-linked red–green color vision defects, which have been associated with alterations in the gene sequences encoding the opsins on the X chromosome.[27,28] Acquired color vision defects refer to abnormalities that accompany eye diseases or drug toxicity. Acquired color vision defects are more variable and their classification is more difficult and less satisfactory. Color vision is often tested clinically with screening tests that allow identification of abnormalities and most screening tests are based on color discrimination and color-matching abilities.[29]

Color vision classifications

Color vision classifications are based on both the number of functioning cone types and the presence of abnormal cones. An observer with three functioning cone types is called a trichromat, an observer with two functioning cone types is a dichromat, and an observer with one functioning cone type is a monochromat (monochromacy sometimes is also termed achromatopsia in the literature since it is believed that vision based on a single cone type cannot produce color perception, assuming rods are not involved). An observer with normal color vision has three normal cone types, in terms of spectral sensitivity, and is called a normal trichromat. Observers who are said to have defective color vision have at least one abnormal cone type or are missing at least a cone type with conventional color-matching techniques. Observers with rods only (lack of any cones) are called rod monochromat or complete achromatopsia.[30]

X-linked color vision defects have been recognized since the 18th century and were subdivided into two qualitatively different types: protan ("red-blind") and deutan ("green-blind"). The term "protanope" is used for a dichromat who is thought to be missing L cones and the term "deuteranope" is used for a dichromat who is thought to be missing M cones, based on color-matching characteristics using a 2° visual field in the fovea. Anomalous trichromacy is a variation in color vision that is attributed to the presence of a cone type that is shifted in spectral sensitivity. A protanomalous observer has trichromatic color vision but the L cones have spectral sensitivity that is shifted to shorter wavelengths compared to normal L cones. A deuteranomalous observer also has trichromatic color vision but the M cones have spectral sensitivity that is shifted to longer wavelengths compared to normal M cones. A third qualitively different type of color vision is tritan ("blue-blind"). Tritan color vision defects are thought to arise from variations in S cones.

The genes encoding the human photopigments

It has been known for many years that the spectral sensitivities of rods and cones reflect the absorption spectra of the visual photopigments. In a major advance, the genes encoding the opsins of the human visual photopigments were cloned and mapped in the human genome in 1983.[27,31] The gene for rhodopsin was found on chromosome 3 and the human rhodopsin gene showed high homology (93.4%) to that of bovine rhodopsin.[31] A visual photopigment gene for the opsin of S cones (*OPN1SW* gene) was found on chromosome 7. A tandem array of visual photopigment genes for the opsins of the M and L cones (*OPN1MW* and *OPN1LW* genes) was found on the X chromosome. The human opsin genes show about 45% homology between rhodopsin and any of the three cone photopigment genes and between the chromosome 7 and the X-chromosome pigment genes. This similarity among the photopigment genes suggests a common ancestor. The genes on the X chromosome have a high homology to each other (about 96%), suggesting a more recent evolutionary appearance. An unexpected finding was that of multiple genes in a tandem array on the X chromosome, which has been proposed to range from 2 to 6. Nathans et al.[28] postulated that the multiple genes in the tandem array on the X chromosome arose as a result of unequal homologous recombination. Subsequent study has suggested there are polymorphisms among these genes in color-normal and color-defective individuals.[27]

The initial study of the opsin genes on the X chromosome was based on the long-standing conventional ideas about X-linked congenital color vision defects[28]; that is, protanopes are missing L cones and deuteranopes are missing M cones, and that the genetics of these types of defective color vision may be based on missing genes for either L or M cones. Specifically, protanopes were thought to be dichromats who lacked an L-cone gene and deuteranopes were dichromats who lacked an M-cone gene.

The initial work with the X-chromosome opsin genes, in attempting to link color vision defects with these genes, was carried out using restriction fragment length polymorphisms (RFLPs), an early molecular genetic technique that simplified the study of DNA sequences. The initial RFLP analysis of the X-chromosome genes was done on DNA from one observer with normal color vision and a few protanopes and deuteranopes. Comparisons were carried out to determine which of the fragments found in the normal observer's RFLPs were missing in the protanopes and deuteranopes. A fragment found in the normal observer that was missing in the protanope was said to be part of the assumed missing L-cone gene. Similarly, a fragment found in the normal observer that was missing in the deuteranope was said to be part of the assumed missing M-cone gene. In the initial study, observers with dichromatic as well as anomalous trichromatic color vision defects showed the presence of hybrid genes (genes comprising the head of one type of gene and the tail of the other type of gene). The hybrid genes were said to be the basis for the altered spectral sensitivity of anomalous L or M cones associated with X-linked anomalous trichromacy (discussed previously).

Subsequent studies that have been carried out on both normal and X-linked defective color vision have their roots in the initial RFLP analysis based on the conventional idea of missing cone types and missing genes using one normal observer and a few color-defectives. The variations that have been found in subsequent studies on the visual pigment genes have correlated largely, but not absolutely, with phenotypes established by color vision testing. The current view is that the X-chromosome tandem array consists of one or more opsin genes encoding L-cone photopigment, followed by one or more opsin genes encoding the M-cone photopigment. The expression of the genes in the tandem array is believed to be governed by a stochastic process.[27]

There have been advances in molecular genetic technology and in the understanding of the human genome since the initial RFLP studies of the opsin genes. Knowledge derived from the Human Genome Project, which has spurred an understanding of the scarcity of genes in the human genome, and the developing knowledge of epigenetics, such as the editing processes of microRNAs, may contribute to future studies and understanding of the genetics of color vision variations.

CLINICAL EVALUATION OF COLOR VISION

Screening tests

Screening tests are rapid tests (requiring 2–3 minutes) and color-defective observers are identified due to their inability to see the difference between certain colors that are easily discriminated by normal observers. Screening tests can be administered to both children and adults.

Pseudoisochromatic plate tests

The most commonly used screening tests are the pseudoisochromatic plate tests. First introduced by Stilling, a pseudoisochromatic plate presents a figure composed of colored dots in a background of differently colored dots. Usually, the colors are chosen so that an X-linked color-defective observer does not see the figure that is easily seen by normal observers. The cleverest designs use four sets of colors, chosen so that the normal observer sees one figure and the defective observer sees a different figure.

The majority of pseudoisochromatic plate tests (such as the Ishihara) were designed to identify observers with X-linked congenital color defects (i.e., protan or deutan color anomalies). The choice of colors was optimized to take advantage of the particular discrimination losses found in X-linked color vision defects and the tests are successful in detecting 90–95% of color-defective observers. Pseudoisochromatic plate tests cannot be used to identify acquired color vision defects, which are most likely to affect blue/yellow color vision. More recently developed pseudoisochromatic plates (such as the HRR and SPP2 plates) have been designed specifically for acquired color vision deficiencies, including tritan (blue/yellow) anomalies.

Other rapid tests of color vision

Other rapid tests of color vision involve sorting colored pieces. In principle, this approach can be used successfully with acquired color vision abnormalities since it does not involve the choice of a particular pair of colors that has a prediction based on common X-linked color vision defects.

Chromatic discrimination ability tests

Clinical assessment of color discrimination ability involves arrangement tests that require the observer to arrange a set of colored samples according to their similarity in color. If the samples are closely spaced in chromaticity (e.g., the Farnsworth–Munsell 100-hue test: Fig. 10.7), the task becomes one of fine chromatic discrimination. Tests involving fine chromatic discrimination are usually relatively time-consuming. If the samples are widely spaced in chromaticity (e.g., the Farnsworth panel D-15), the test evaluates color confusions that occur with defective color vision that would not be perceived by a normal observer. Tests with widely spaced colors are conducted rapidly and can even be used for screening. An arrangement test may use samples that differ only in chromaticity to test hue discrimination (e.g., the Farnsworth–Munsell 100-hue test, Farnsworth panel D-15, Farnsworth desaturated panel D-15, and Lanthony new color test), may vary in luminance only to test lightness discrimination (Verriest's lightness discrimination test), or may vary only in grayness to test saturation discrimination (Sahlgren's saturation test, Lanthony new color test). Arrangement tests are easy to administer but require the concept of abstract ordering, manual dexterity, and patience. As a result, they are rarely suitable for children under 10 years of age.

The best known of the arrangement tests is the Farnsworth–Munsell 100-hue test. The test includes 85 black plastic caps with inserted papers that vary in hue but have constant lightness and saturation. The caps are divided into four boxes with each box covering one-quarter of the color circle. Observers being tested arrange the caps in a natural color order according to their unique perception. An error occurs if the caps are misplaced from the ideal color order. A numeric score can be calculated and displayed on a polar graph. Age norms have been prepared giving the range of the expected total error scores for an unselected population as well as the expected intereye variability.

Observers with congenital color vision deficiencies make characteristic errors on arrangement tests because their chromatic discrimination ability is weakened or lost on particular axes in chromaticity space. Discrimination loss in acquired color vision defects is more variable. However, following the idea that discrimination of blueness content is, to a first order, independent of discrimination of redness–greenness, it is possible to partition the caps into those where correct ordering depends on normal function of the S-cone system (caps 1 through 12, 34 through 54, and 76 through 84) and those where correct ordering depends on normal function of the M- and L-cone opponent system (caps 13 through 33 and 55 through 75). The partitioned scores can be examined to determine whether an acquired color vision defect causes a particular type of discrimination loss, i.e., the S or L/M systems.[32]

Importance of the test illuminant for plate and discrimination color vision tests

The plate and discrimination tests described above use reflective materials as colored test objects and the perceived color presented to an observer depends on the illuminating light as well as the reflective properties of the test materials. The original pseudoisochromatic plate tests were designed to be viewed under afternoon daylight in the northern hemisphere, and more recent tests have followed this design convention. Standardized illuminants (called illuminant C or illuminant D65) that closely simulate the spectra of afternoon daylight are more preferable to natural daylight, which may vary substantially in both spectrum and radiance with time of day and weather. Light sources that approximate these standard illuminants are commercially available and are suitable for use in illuminating clinical color vision tests. Most fluorescent light sources, however, do not accurately mimic the colors produced in natural light and, therefore, they are not appropriate illuminants for color vision tests.

Color-matching tests

Adjusting three primaries to match a test color is not intuitive for many observers and research experimental methods are therefore not appropriate for clinical purposes. To adapt color-matching procedures for clinical evaluation, simplified methods have been developed by using two-variable matches and rapid, less complicated tasks. The instruments that allow these matches to be carried out are called anomaloscopes and the color-matching paradigms are called equations. The equations are named after the researchers who first proposed or used them.

Anomaloscope color matching test using the Rayleigh equation

In a Rayleigh match, a spectral "yellow" test field (589 nm) is presented in one-half of a circular field with an adjustable brightness. In the half field, a mixture of two "green" and "red" spectral primaries (545 and 670 nm) is presented. The mixture field can appear green (545 nm), green–yellow, yellow, orange, or red (670 nm) as the ratio of the primaries is varied. The task of the observer is to adjust the primary red–green ratio and brightness of the yellow to make the two fields appear identical. Observers with normal color vision accept a narrow range of ratios near the middle of the red–green range, but color-deficient observers will pick ratios shifted away from this range, depending on the specific deficiency. Matching abnormalities accompanying ophthalmic disease or X-linked color vision variations may include a widened matching range or acceptance of an abnormal match.[33]

The Rayleigh equation assesses the normality of M- and L-cone functions, since S cones are not contributing to the match because they are unresponsive to the primary wavelengths.

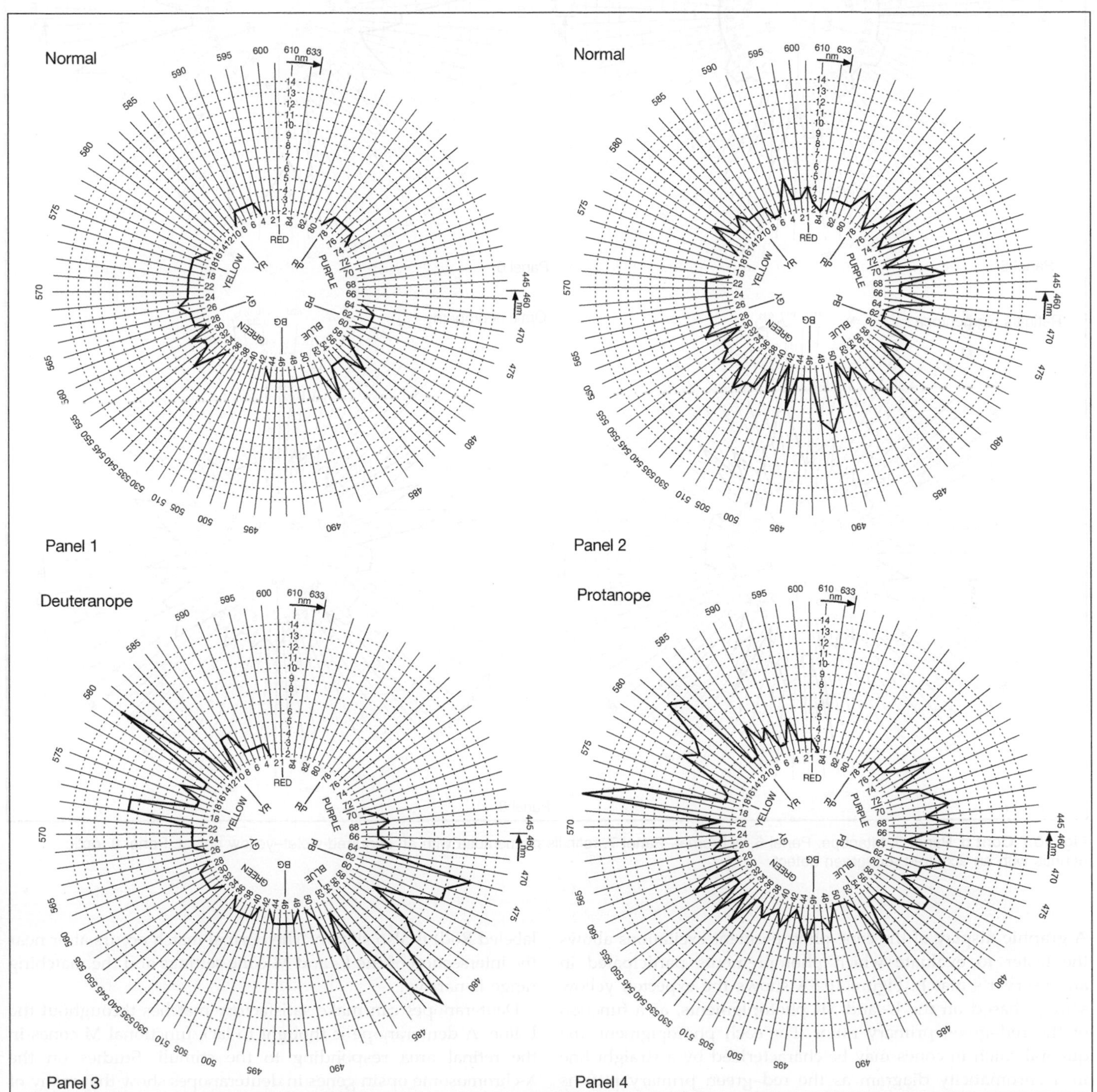

Fig. 10.7 Examples of Farnsworth–Munsell 100-hue test error patterns in normal subjects (panels 1 and 2) and in observers with congenital (panels 3–6) and later onset or acquired (panels 7 and 8) color vision defects. Panel 1, normal with good discrimination. Panel 2, normal with poor discrimination. Panel 3, deuteranope. Panel 4, protanope.

Continued

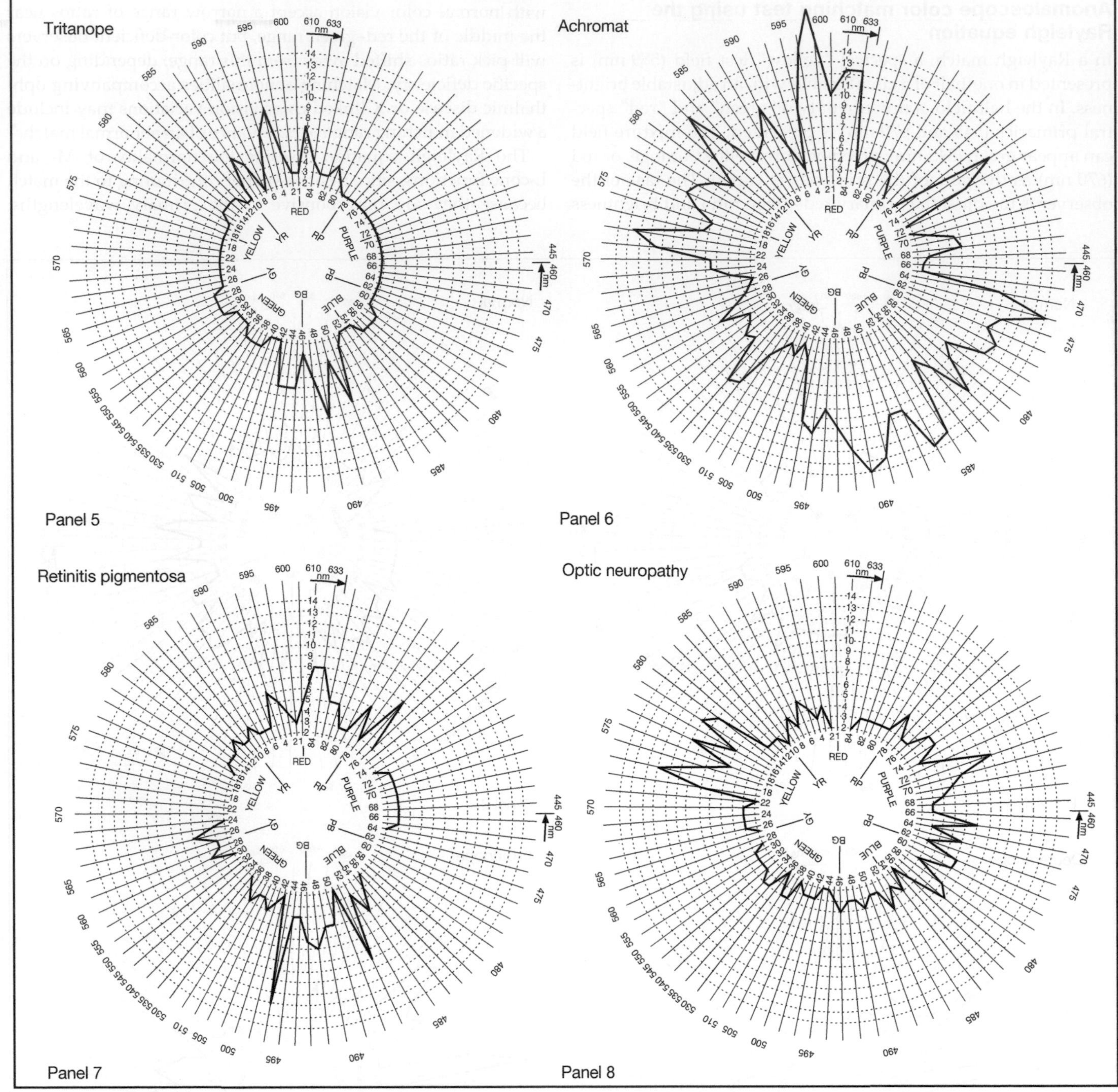

Fig. 10.7 Cont'd Panel 5, tritanope. Panel 6, achromat. Panel 7, retinitis pigmentosa with an acquired violet–yellow defect. Panel 8, optic neuritis with an acquired red–green defect.

A graphic display of the cone photopigment excitations allows the tester to evaluate which photopigments participated in an observer's match. Figure 10.8A shows the expected yellow setting, based on the L- and M- photopigments, as a function of the red–green primary ratios. For each photopigment, the quantal catch in cones may be characterized by a straight line in a chromaticity diagram as the red–green primary ratio is changed. Two lines show the predicted responses of the L cones alone (dashed and labeled L) and the M cones alone (dotted and labeled M). The rod photopigment is responsive at these wavelengths as well and the predicted rod response (solid and labeled Rod) is also shown. The normal match occurs at or near the intersection of the L- and M-cone settings and the matching range is narrow.

Deuteranopes can make satisfactory matches throughout the L line. A deuteranope is thought to lack functional M cones in the retinal area responding to the stimuli. Studies on the X-chromosome opsin genes in deuteranopes show that many of these observers have only a single gene that is thought to encode the L photopigment. Protanopes can make matches throughout the extent of the M line. It has been speculated that the protanope lacks functional L cones in the retinal area responding to the

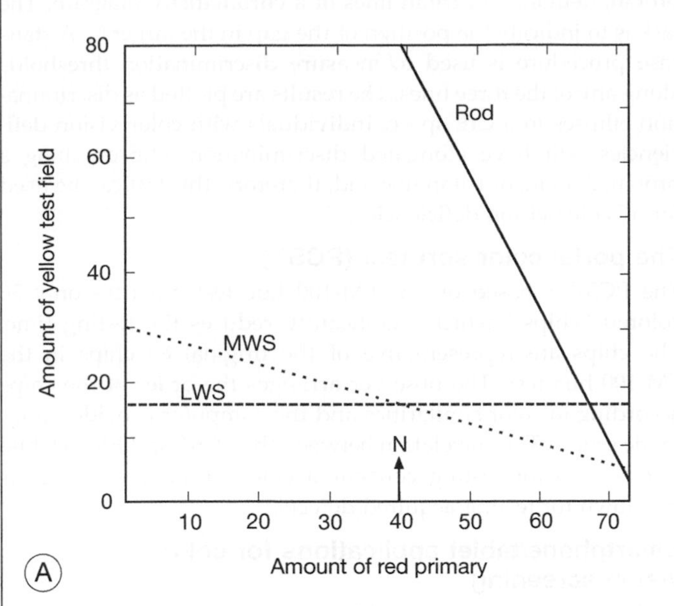

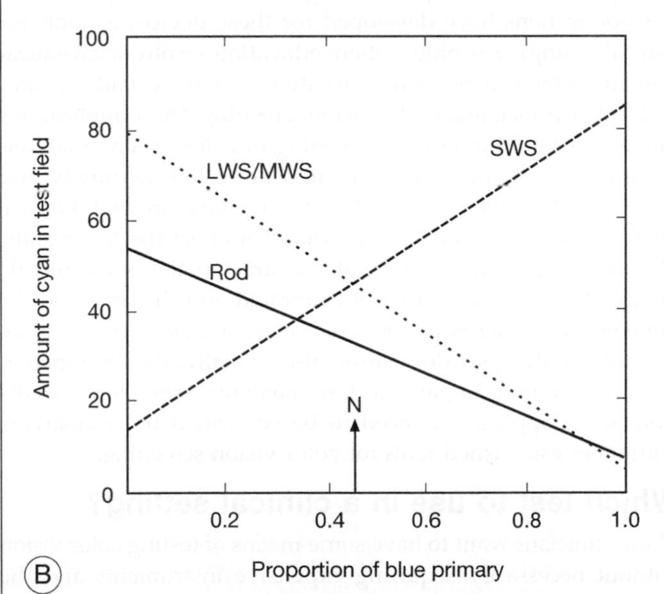

Fig. 10.8 Graphic analysis of the Rayleigh equation and Moreland equation. (A) The Rayleigh equation. The relative light in the "yellow" (589 nm) test is plotted as a function of the proportion of the "red" (670 nm) primary. The lines are calculated from the cone and rod photopigment excitations. The line marked LWS represents the L-cone response of Figure 10.2B and predicts the matching behavior of deuteranopes. The line marked MWS represents the middle-wavelength cone response of Figure 10.2B and predicts the matching behavior of protanopes. The normal match (N) occurs at the intersection of the L and M lines. The line marked Rod represents the rod response of Figure 10.2A and predicts the matching behavior of achromats. (B) The Moreland equation. The relative light in the bicolor (480 nm + 580 nm) test is shown as a function of the proportion of the 440-nm primary. The lines are calculated from the cone and rod photopigment excitations. The line marked LWS/MWS represents the L- and M-cone response and predicts the matching behavior of tritanopes. The line marked SWS represents the short-wavelength cone response. The normal match (N) occurs at the intersection of the L/M line with the S line. The line marked Rod represents the rod response and predicts the matching behavior of achromats.

stimuli; genetic studies have suggested that these observers usually have only a single gene on the X chromosome that has been described as a hybrid gene composed of a piece of the normal L- and a piece of the normal M-opsin genes.

Other X-linked color-defective observers, called anomalous trichromats, have a wider range of acceptable matches that are displaced from the normal match. Such observers are trichromatic but have one cone photopigment with an abnormal spectral sensitivity. Deuteranomalous matches occur along the L line (indicating a normal L-cone photopigment) but are shifted to low red-green primary ratios. The psychophysical interpretation is that the deuteranomalous trichromat has an abnormal M-cone photopigment that is shifted so that its spectral sensitivity closely overlaps that of the normal L-cone photopigment. Protanomalous matches occur along the M line (indicating a normal M-cone photopigment) but are shifted to high red–green primary ratios. The interpretation of these psychophysical studies is that the protanomalous trichromat has an abnormal L-cone photopigment, shifted so that its spectral sensitivity closely overlaps that of the normal M-cone photopigment. Anomaloscope color matching using the Rayleigh equation is recognized as the only clinical method that allows definitive classification of the X-linked color vision defects.

Anomaloscope analysis is important in ophthalmic disease assessment since it can be used to recognize a number of clinical entities, such as rod-dominated vision characteristic of cone degenerations and incomplete and complete achromatopsias. These diseases are characterized by Rayleigh matches extending along the rod line (solid line in Fig. 10.7A). Matching abnormalities that are characteristic of choroidal disorders affecting the fovea lead to Rayleigh matches that extend along or just below the L line but are shifted to higher red primary ratios (pseudoprotanomaly). The discrimination loss characteristic of optic nerve disorders leads to matches that widen around the normal match on the L line.

Anomaloscope color-matching test using the Moreland equation

The Moreland equation[34] is a match of a bicolor test field (480 and 580 nm) to a mixture of two primaries (440 and 500 nm). The test field appears blue–green to a normal observer, while appearance of the mixture field appearance ranges from violet, to blue, to blue–green, to green–blue, to green as the primary ratio is changed from mostly 440 nm to mostly 500 nm. The primary ratio is expressed in terms of the amount of the 440 nm ("violet") primary required for the match. As with the Rayleigh equation, an observer with normal color vision can find a primary ratio and test field luminance at which both fields appear identical.

The Moreland equation assesses the normality of S-cone function. Figure 10.8B shows the predicted function for a single photopigment to the bicolor test field as a function of the violet–green primary ratio. The L and M cones share the same line (dotted and labeled as L/M). The S-cone response crosses this on the diagonal (dashed and labeled as S). The predicted rod (solid line labeled as Rod) line has the same direction as the L- and M-cone lines. The normal match occurs at the intersection of the S-cone line with the L/M line. Both congenital and acquired color vision defects can be recognized using the Moreland equation.[35] The tritanope (an observer lacking S-cone function) has matches extending along the L/M line, as do observers with acquired defects that affect S-cone function. Point mutations in the S-cone opsin gene on chromosome 7 have been reported in affected individuals in tritan pedigrees.[36]

Patients with X-linked achromatopsia (i.e., S-cone monochromacy) have matches that extend along the S-cone line. The majority of X-linked achromat pedigrees show major deletions of the region just preceding the cone opsin tandem gene array on the X chromosome in affected individuals.[37] This region is thought to be a regulatory area controlling expression of the L- and M- cone opsin genes. Additionally, some X-linked achromat pedigrees show only a single abnormal gene instead of the normal tandem array. Patients with complete achromatopsia have matches extending along the rod line.

Considerations in the use of anomaloscopes

Even though the color-matching task on an anomaloscope is simplified compared with usual research color-matching procedures, anomaloscope testing procedures are not easily explained and an observer may require some practice before being able to complete a match. Correct use of an anomaloscope requires extensive operator training and these instruments are therefore usually found only in research centers. However, if properly used, the anomaloscope is a diagnostic instrument of great power.

Computerized color vision tests

Computer-controlled color vision tests have been developed using a similar principle as that used for pseudoisochromatic plate tests or discrimination ability tests (such as the FM-100 hue test). Computerized tests are automated and therefore easy to use. Further, computerized tests can avoid the illuminating light issue that exists for reflective materials. However, the sensitivity and specificity of the computerized tests largely rely on the accurate presentation of color on computer monitors, including cathode ray tubes (CRTs) or liquid crystal displays (LCDs). A CRT is typically preferred over an LCD because CRTs have reliable temporal characteristics. To present color accurately, the displays have to be calibrated, including spectral distribution measurements and linearization. Caution must be taken when using a computerized color vision test that does not incorporate specific display calibration.

Color assessment and diagnosis (CAD) test

The CAD test was developed by Dr Barbur and coworkers at City University, London.[38] The web-based CAD uses a color square that moves against a flickering luminance contrast noise. The color of the square changes along different chromaticity directions. Color-defective observers have difficulty seeing the square moving, whereas normal observers easily see the square move. The web-based CAD test requires a monitor to be balanced at around 9000 K and the ambient illumination must be kept at a minimum. It is reported that this web-based test has good sensitivity and specificity for red–green color deficiencies.[39]

Cambridge color test (CCT)

The CCT is a computer-controlled, easy-to-use color vision test. The CCT was developed by Drs Mollon, Reffin, and Regan at the University of Cambridge, England.[40] The CCT system provides 14-bit color and luminance control on a calibrated CRT display. The stimulus is a Landolt C on an achromatic background. The chromaticity of the target C is varied along the protan, deutan, and tritan lines of a chromaticity diagram. The task is to indicate the position of the gap in the target C. A staircase procedure is used to measure discrimination thresholds along any of the three lines. The results are plotted as discrimination ellipses in a CIE space. Individuals with color vision deficiencies will have elongated discrimination ellipses along a protan, deutan, or tritan line and, therefore, this test can be used for all color vision deficiencies.

The portal color sort test (PCST)

The PCST is based on the FM-100 hue test but uses only 36 colored "chips," which significantly reduces the testing time. The chips are representative of the original 85 chips in the FM-100 hue test. The observer arranges the order of the chips according to color similarities and the computer provides automatic scores. The correlation between the PCST and FM-100 hue test is high for testing congenital color vision defects but is unknown for testing acquired defects.[41]

Smartphone/tablet applications for color vision screening

With the popularity of mobile communication devices (e.g., smartphones or tablets) increasing in medical settings, numerous applications have developed for these devices as tools for clinical testing/screening, patient education, or physician education and reference. Several applications use the pseudoisochromatic plate principle for color vision screening. These applications might be useful for a quick screening of color vision; however, these tools have not been validated and their sensitivity and specificity for color vision defect screening are not known. Further, there are many factors that can affect the test results. The most important is the display characteristics of the mobile device. These displays are not calibrated and they may not be homogeneous; therefore, the tests for color vision screening are not necessarily "pseudoisochromatic." Finally, the illumination in the office may impair the test reliability. Therefore, results from these applications need to be confirmed by comparison with other established tools for color vision screening.

Which test to use in a clinical setting?

Many clinicians want to have some means of testing color vision without necessarily acquiring expensive instruments and the expertise needed for professional evaluation and diagnosis. Tests using colored papers (pigment tests) and the proper illuminant offer office clinicians the possibility of some color vision evaluation.

A screening plate test with the proper illuminant would be minimal equipment for testing color vision. Approximately 8–10% of American males have one of the X-linked color vision defects. Identification of color vision defects in children before they enter grade school allows the clinician to provide counseling to the parents. Many children with color vision defects have memories of being teased or ridiculed in the early grades and early testing allows appropriate counseling. Also, many males with color vision defects may inadvertently choose careers, for example, as pilots or firefighters, from which they will be barred due to their color vision status. It should be noted, however, that the screening plate tests that may be very useful for the common genetic color vision defects are less successful at identifying acquired color vision defects.

A more ambitious plan to test color vision in an office would be to combine a screening plate test with a test of color discrimination. A discrimination test (e.g., the Farnsworth–Munsell 100-hue test) allows the clinician to follow changes in color vision over time, such as might occur with optic neuritis. Occasionally, a clinician will see a patient who has an extremely rare form of color defect and color vision testing may be informative. For example, cerebral achromatopsia is a fascinating case that likely arises from damage to higher-order visual processes. In these cases, a more complete color vision testing (such as spectral sensitivity and saturation discrimination evaluation) should be considered and case reports would be of wide interest in the medical community. Patients should be referred to a psychophysics laboratory for more visual function testing, such as contrast discrimination evaluation.

NEW DEVELOPMENTS IN COLOR VISION RESEARCH

Color vision has been studied considering genetics, evolution, physiology, and psychophysics. A few newer research areas related to color vision are provided here.

Gene therapy for color vision defects

Drs Jay and Maureen Neitz and coworkers have carried out pioneering studies on "curing" red-green color deficiency in dichromatic adult squirrel monkeys that were missing the L-cone opsin gene at birth.[42,43] As gene therapy, the human L-cone opsin gene was delivered into the photoreceptor layers of the retinas of the monkeys. A few months after the introduction of the new opsin gene, these monkeys exhibited trichromatic color vision behavior with spectral sensitivity shifted, chromatic discrimination improved, and color perception enriched. An experiment involving gene therapy in humans would require approval from the National Institutes of Health Office of Recombinant DNA Activities (ORDA)/Recombinant DNA Advisory Committee (RAC) and the Food and Drug Administration and this would not be expected to be granted without a long and thorough approval process. However, the fundamental question of whether it is necessary to "cure" color deficiencies is currently the point of debate since the majority of dichromats live a normal life and most are not significantly affected by having the color vision deficiency.

Adaptive optics (AO) retinal imaging system

AO was initially used in astronomy to remove the effects of atmospheric distortion to improve the performance of telescopes and laser communication systems.[44] An AO system has three components: (1) a wavefront sensor for ocular aberration measurement; (2) a deformable mirror for aberration correction; and (3) a control system that compares the sensor output and adjusts the deforming mirrors to achieve optimal resolution. This technology was first adopted for retinal imaging in the 1990s by Dr David Williams to reduce ocular aberrations in the eyes.[45] After its initial introduction, the AO imaging system was considered to have great scientific and clinical application potential because it had the capability of imaging photoreceptors, the retinal pigment epithelium, retinal blood vessels and, potentially, ganglion cells at a high magnification. For instance, AO made it possible to measure color perception[46] or cell responses in the postreceptoral pathways[47] associated with tiny flashes of light stimulating a single cone in the eye. For color vision screening, in particular, the AO system can provide high resolution of the cone mosaic and it can show whether a particular type of cone (e.g., L cones) is missing in the retina. Combining this information with genetic studies is potentially informative because AO imaging can provide insights about cone distributions that can be related to the cone opsin genes.[48] (See Chapter 5, Advanced imaging technologies, for more details about this topic.)

Rod and cone interactions in color vision

Duplex theory states that rods and cones independently contribute to different aspects of visual perception. However, rods and cones share common neural pathways from the retina to the brain and this provides a neural basis for rod–cone interactions in visual function, including color vision.[49] Conventionally, rod vision has been considered to be achromatic. However, numerous psychophysical studies have indicated that rods contribute to color vision at either mesopic[50] or even scotopic light levels.[51] Psychophysical evidence for rod contributions to color vision comes from measurements of scotopic color contrast,[52] photochromatic intervals during the course of dark adaptation following a light bleach,[53] chromatic discrimination,[54] and color-matching or color appearance methods using unique hue measurement or hue-scaling methods.[55,56]

Recently, rod contributions to color vision were studied using a four-primary Maxwellian-view photostimulator[57] that allowed independent control of rod and cone excitations at the same chromaticity, retinal locus, and light level. This new method has yielded new insights into rod contributions to color vision. Specifically, rods contribute to color percepts in a manner analogous to M-cone signals at all mesopic light levels and analogous to S-cone signals only at low mesopic light levels near cone thresholds.[50] Also, the strength of rod contributions is linearly related to rod contrasts.[58]

ACKNOWLEDGMENTS

The preparation of this chapter is partially supported by a National Institutes of Health grant (R01 EY019651). I express my great appreciation to Drs Vivianne Smith and Joel Pokorny for allowing me access to the materials they prepared for an earlier version of the chapter in a previous edition of *Retina*. I thank Dr Margaret Lutze for her assistance in preparing this chapter.

REFERENCES

1. Hood DC, Finkelstein MA. Sensitivity to light. In: Boff KR, Kaufman L, Thomas JP, editors. Handbook of perception and human performance, vol I: Sensory processes and perception. New York: John Wiley; 1986. p. 5-1–5-66.
2. Smith VC, Pokorny J, Lee BB, et al. Sequential processing in vision: The interaction of sensitivity regulation and temporal dynamics. Vision Res 2008;48:2649–56.
3. Goldberg SH, Frumkes TE, Nygaard RW. Inhibitory influence of unstimulated rods in the human retina: evidence provided by examining cone flicker. Science 1983;221:180–2.
4. Cao D, Zele AJ, Pokorny J. Dark-adapted rod suppression of cone flicker detection: evaluation of receptoral and postreceptoral interactions. Vis Neurosci 2006;23:531–7.
5. Sharpe LT, Stockman A. Rod pathways: the importance of seeing nothing. Trends Neurosci 1999;22:497–504.
6. Dacey DM. Parallel pathways for spectral coding in primate retina. Annu Rev Neurosci 2000;23:743–75.
7. Lee BB. Visual pathways and psychophysical channels in the primate. J Physiol 2011;589.1:41–7.
8. Lee BB, Smith VC, Pokorny J, et al. Rod inputs to macaque ganglion cells. Vision Res 1997;37:2813–28.
9. Crook JD, Davenport CM, Peterson BB, et al. Parallel ON and OFF cone bipolar inputs establish spatially coextensive receptive field structure of blue-yellow ganglion cells in primate retina. J Neurosci 2009;29:8372–87.
10. Field GD, Greschner M, Gauthier JL, et al. High-sensitivity rod photoreceptor input to the blue-yellow color opponent pathway in macaque retina. Nat Neurosci 2009;12:1159–64.

11. Bartlett NR. Dark adaptation and light adaptation. In: Graham CH, editor. Vision and visual perception. New York: John Wiley; 1965. p. 185–207.
12. Graham CH. Vision and visual perception. New York: John Wiley; 1965.
13. Shevell SK, Kingdom FA. Color in complex scenes. Annu Rev Psychol 2008;59:143–66.
14. Smith VC, Pokorny J. Spectral sensitivity of the foveal cone photopigments between 400 and 500 nm. Vision Res 1975;15:161–71.
15. MacLeod DIA, Boynton RM. Chromaticity diagram showing cone excitation by stimuli of equal luminance. J Opt Soc Am 1979;69:1183–5.
16. Boynton RM, Kambe N. Chromatic difference steps of moderate size measured along theoretically critical axes. Color Res Appl 1980;5:13–23.
17. Derrington AM, Krauskopf J, Lennie P. Chromatic mechanisms in lateral geniculate nucleus of macaque. J Physiol (Lond) 1984;357:241–65.
18. Lee BB, Martin PR, Valberg A. Sensitivity of macaque retinal ganglion cells to chromatic and luminance flicker. J Physiol (Lond) 1989;414:223–43.
19. Pokorny J, Smith VC. Chromatic discrimination. In: Chalupa LM, Werner JS, editors. The visual neuroscience. Cambridge, MA: MIT Press; 2004. p. 908–23.
20. Pokorny J, Smith VC. Wavelength discrimination in the presence of added chromatic fields. J Opt Soc Am 1970;69:562–9.
21. Wright WD. The sensitivity of the eye to small colour differences. Proc Phys Soc (Lond) 1941;53:93–112.
22. MacAdam DL. Visual sensitivities to color differences in daylight. J Opt Soc Am 1942;32:247–74.
23. Cao D, Zele AJ, Smith VC, et al. S-cone discrimination for stimuli with spatial and temporal chromatic contrast. Vis Neurosci 2008;25:349–54.
24. Krauskopf J, Gegenfurtner K. Color discrimination and adaptation. Vision Res 1992;32:2165–75.
25. von Kries J. Influence of adaptation on the effects produced by luminous stimuli. In: MacAdam DL, editor. Sources of color science. Cambridge, MA: MIT Press; 1905.
26. Shevell SK, Cao D, editors. Chromatic assimilation: evidence for a neural mechanism. Oxford: Oxford University Press; 2003.
27. Neitz J, Neitz M. The genetics of normal and defective color vision. Vision Res 2011;51:633–51.
28. Nathans J, Piantanida TP, Eddy RL, et al. Molecular genetics of inherited variation in human color vision. Science 1986;232:203–10.
29. Working-Group-41. Procedures for testing color vision, NAS-NRC Committee on Vision. Washington, DC: National Academy Press; 1981.
30. Pokorny J, Smith VC, Pinckers AJLG, et al. Classification of complete and incomplete autosomal recessive achromatopsia. Graefes Arch Clin Exp Ophthalmol 1982;219:121–30.
31. Nathans J, Hogness DS. Isolation and nucleotide sequence of the gene encoding human rhodopsin. Proc Natl Acad Sci USA 1984;81:4851–5.
32. Smith VC, Pokorny J, Pass AS. Color-axis determination on the Farnsworth-Munsell 100-hue Test. Am J Ophthalmol 1985;100:176–82.
33. Pokorny J, Smith VC, Verriest G, et al., editors. Congenital and acquired color vision defects. New York: Grune and Stratton; 1979.
34. Moreland JD, Kerr J. Optimization of stimuli for trit-anomaloscopy. Mod Probl Ophthalmol 1978;19:162–6.
35. Pokorny J, Smith VC, Went LN. Color matching in autosomal dominant tritan defect. J Opt Soc Am 1981;71:1327–34.
36. Weitz CJ, Miyake Y, Shinzato K, et al. Human tritanopia associated with two amino acid substitutions in the blue-sensitive opsin. Am J Hum Genet 1992;50: 156.
37. Nathans J, Davenport CM, Maumenee IH, et al. Molecular genetics of human blue cone monochromacy. Science 1989;245:831–8.
38. Barbur J, Harlow A, Plant G. Insights into the different exploits of colour in the visual cortex. Proc Biol Sci 1994;258:327–34.
39. Seshadri J, Christensen J, Lakshminarayanan V, et al. Evaluation of the new web-based "Colour Assessment and Diagnosis" test. Optom Vision Sci 2005;82:882–5.
40. Regan BC, Reffin J, Mollon JD. Luminance noise and the rapid determination of discrimination ellipses in colour deficiency. Vision Res 1994;34:1279–99.
41. Melamud A, Simpson E, Traboulsi EI. Introducing a new computer-based test for the clinical evaluation of color discrimination. Am J Ophthalmol 2006;142:953–60.
42. Mancuso K, Mauck MC, Kuchenbecker JA, et al. A multi-stage color model revisited: implications for a gene therapy cure for red-green colorblindness. Adv Exp Med Biol 2010;664:631–8.
43. Mancuso K, Hauswirth WW, Li Q, et al. Gene therapy for red-green colour blindness in adult primates. Nature 2009;461:784–7.
44. Tyson RK. Principles of adaptive optics. San Diego, CA: Academic Press; 1991.
45. Liang J, Williams DR, Miller DT. Supernormal vision and high-resolution retinal imaging through adaptive optics. J Opt Soc A 1997;14:2884–92.
46. Hofer H, Singer B, Williams DR. Different sensations from cones with the same photopigment. J Vis 2005;5:444–54.
47. Sincich LC, Zhang Y, Tiruveedhula P, et al. Resolving single cone inputs to visual receptive fields. Nat Neurosci 2009;12:967–9.
48. Williams DR. Imaging single cells in the living retina. Vision Res 2011;51: 1379–96.
49. Buck SL. Rod–cone interaction in human vision. In: Chalupa LM, Werner JS, editors. The visual neuroscience. Cambridge, MA: MIT Press; 2004. p. 863–78.
50. Cao D, Pokorny J, Smith VC. Matching rod percepts with cone stimuli. Vision Res 2005;45:2119–28.
51. Pokorny J, Lutze M, Cao D, et al. The color of night: surface color perception under dim illuminations. Vis Neurosci 2006;23:525–30.
52. Willmer EN. Low threshold rods and the perception of blue. J Physiol (Lond) 1949;111:17P.
53. Lie I. Dark adaptation and the photochromatic interval. Doc Ophthalmol 1963;17:411–510.
54. Stabell U, Stabell B. Wavelength discrimination of peripheral cones and its change with rod intrusion. Vision Res 1977;17:423–6.
55. Buck SL, Knight RF, Bechtold J. Opponent-color models and the influence of rod signals on the loci of unique hues. Vision Res 2000;40:3333–44.
56. Volbrecht VJ, Nerger JL, Imhoff SM, et al. Effect of the short-wavelength-sensitive-cone mosaic and rods on the locus of unique green. J Opt Soc Am A 2000;17:628–34.
57. Pokorny J, Smithson H, Quinlan J. Photostimulator allowing independent control of rods and the three cone types. Vis Neurosci 2004;21:263–7.
58. Cao D, Pokorny J, Smith VC, et al. Rod contributions to color perception: linear with rod contrast. Vision Res 2008;48:2586–92.

Visual Acuity and Contrast Sensitivity

Chapter 11

Gary S. Rubin

VISUAL ACUITY TESTS

Introduction

Visual acuity is the most widely used measure of visual function. In fact, visual function is often equated with visual acuity, thereby ignoring other important dimensions of visual stimuli, such as color and contrast. Visual acuity tests have proven to be useful for assessment of refractive error, screening for ocular health, following the course of eye disease, evaluating the effectiveness of medical and surgical treatment, prescribing aids for the visually impaired, and setting vision standards for employment and driving.

Given the variety of its applications, it is not surprising that many different types of visual acuity tests have evolved. Generally, these tests were developed with little concern for standardization. Since the 1980s, several attempts have been made to formulate standards for test design and administration. The Committee on Vision of the National Academy of Sciences-National Research Council (NAS-NRC)[1] has published standards for clinical testing of visual acuity that are widely adopted in the USA, and the British Standards Institution[2] has published similar standards for the UK. The NAS-NRC standards are used as the basis of this chapter.

Chart design

Optotypes

Most familiar acuity tests require the subject to identify letters arrayed in rows of decreasing size. The so-called Snellen acuity test is the prime example, although Snellen acuity now usually refers to a way of reporting test results rather than to any particular type of chart. To facilitate testing of young children and people unfamiliar with the Latin alphabet, other optotype tests based on the tumbling E, Landolt C, numerals, or simple pictures of familiar objects are also used. Visual acuity can also be assessed with grating patterns, but grating acuity often overestimates Snellen acuity in patients with age-related maculopathy,[3] typically by a factor of 2 or more.

The NAS-NRC recommends that the Landolt C test be used as the standard by which other acuity tests are compared. The Landolt C is a broken circle in which the width of the break and the stroke width are both equal to one-fifth the height of the C. The ring is shown with the break at one of four locations, and the subject responds by saying "right," "down," "up," or "left," or by pointing in the appropriate direction.

There are several advantages to the Landolt C test, including equal difficulty of all targets (unlike letters that vary in degree of difficulty), sensitivity to astigmatic refractive error, and suitability for use with illiterate subjects. However, the Landolt C test is not widely used because it has a guessing rate of 25%, so an alternative is to standardize another optotype set by comparing acuities obtained with it to Landolt C test acuities. The Sloan letters,[4] a set of 10 upper-case sans serif letters, are the most popular substitute. An acuity chart based on Sloan letters was developed for the Early Treatment Diabetic Retinopathy Study (ETDRS)[5] and is illustrated in Fig. 11.1. The original ETDRS chart has been replaced by the 2000 series revised ETDRS chart that more accurately equates the difficulty of letters on all lines. The ETDRS charts are the most widely used acuity charts for clinical research.

Chart layout

Careful attention must be paid to the layout of the acuity chart. The chart should follow a uniform progression of letter sizes, typically a 0.1 log unit (or 26%) reduction in size from line to line. The uniform progression ensures that a one-line loss will have the same meaning at any point on the chart and at any viewing distance. The same number of letters should appear on each line, and the spacing should be uniform, both within and between lines. The spacing requirement results in a large chart, with the letters forming an inverted triangle. The NAS-NRC recommends 8–10 letters per line, but studies[6] suggest that as few as three letters are required for an accurate estimate of visual function. The ETDRS chart uses five letters per line.

Concern about uncontrolled "crowding" effects has led to further modifications of the ETDRS chart. Crowding refers to the reduced visibility of letters when they are surrounded by other letters. Crowding has a larger effect in some types of visual dysfunction, notably amblyopia[7] and macular degeneration.[8] For most acuity charts, letters at either the end of a line or at the top or bottom of the chart are less subject to crowding than are internal letters. To equalize crowding effects, contour interaction bars may be added around the perimeter of the chart.[9]

Testing procedure

Acuity test distance

ETDRS charts are available for a range of test distances from 4 meters (13 feet) to 2 meters (6.5 feet) and when used at the designated distance can measure acuities from 20/10 to 20/200. However, given the logarithmic progression of letter sizes, they can be used at any distance with an appropriate correction of the reported results. For patients with very poor acuity, the clinician may resort to finger counting or hand motion. This strategy is strongly discouraged by low-vision practitioners because it can be demeaning and depressing for the patient to be left with the

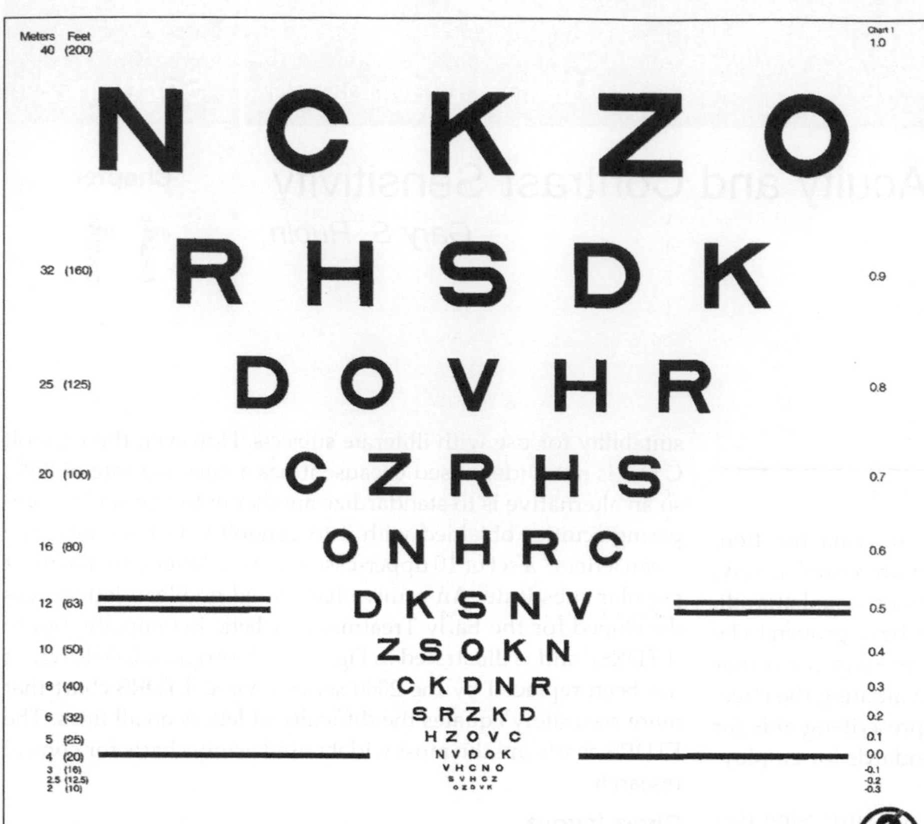

Fig. 11.1 The Early Treatment Diabetic Retinopathy Study (ETDRS) acuity chart. (Reproduced with permission from Ferris FL III, Kassof PA, Bresnick GH, et al. New visual acuity charts for clinical research. Am J Ophthalmol 1982;94:91–6.)

impression that their vision is so poor it cannot even be measured with an eye chart. Instead, it is recommended that the patient be moved closer to the chart. Using a test distance of 50 cm and appropriate refractive correction it is possible to reliably measure "counting finger" acuity with an ETDRS chart (approximately 20/1460 ± 10%).[10] "Hand motions" can be measured with some electronic acuity tests (see below). Distance itself should have little effect on visual acuity, provided that the subject's accommodative state and pupil size are controlled. However, one study[11] found that acuity changed by as much as seven letters (more than one ETDRS line) when the test distance was reduced to less than 2 meters. The reason for this discrepancy remains unexplained.

Luminance and contrast

Whatever the test distance, the chart must be adequately illuminated and of high contrast. Illumination standards vary from 100 cd/m^2 in the USA to 300 cd/m^2 in Germany. Increasing chart luminance improves visual acuity in normal subjects, but reaches a plateau at about 200 cd/m^2.[12] Various types of visual dysfunction can change the effects of luminance on acuity. For example, patients with retinitis pigmentosa may show a decrease in acuity at higher luminance, whereas patients with age-related macular degeneration often continue to improve at luminances well above the normal plateau.[13] A luminance standard of 100 cd/m^2 can be justified because it represents good room illumination for ordinary reading material. Furthermore, most of the currently proposed standards would yield the same acuity scores, plus or minus one letter (assuming five letters per line and a 0.1 log unit size progression) in normal subjects.

The relationship of visual acuity to letter contrast follows a square-root law.[14] For example, decreasing contrast by a factor of 2 would decrease acuity by roughly a factor of 1.4. The NAS-NRC recommends that letter contrast be at least 0.85. Transilluminated, projection, and reflective charts (wall charts) can all meet these standards, but some transilluminated charts are deficient in luminance, and some projection systems lack sufficient luminance and contrast. Accurate calibration requires a spot photometer, for which procedures are described in the NAS-NRC document.[1]

Test administration

Administration of visual acuity tests is simple and straightforward. However, one detail often overlooked in clinical testing is that the test must be administered in a "forced-choice" manner. Rather than allowing the patient to decide when the letters become indistinguishable, the patient should be required to guess the identity of each letter until a sufficient number of errors are made to justify terminating the test. People differ in their willingness to respond to questions when they are not confident about the answers. A person with a conservative criterion answers only when absolutely certain about the identity of the letter, whereas a person with a liberal criterion ventures a guess for any letter that is even barely discernible. These two people may receive different acuity scores because of differences in their criteria rather than because of variations in visual function. This is not merely a theoretical concern. Several studies[15,16] have shown that criterion-dependent test procedures lead to inaccurate and unreliable test results. Forced-choice procedures are criterion-free because the examiner, rather than the observer, determines whether the letter is correctly identified.

Scoring

Until recently, visual acuity tests were usually scored line by line with the patient being given credit for a line when a criterion number of letters were identified correctly. The NAS-NRC recommends that at least two-thirds of the letters on a line be correctly identified to qualify for passing. Allowing a small proportion of errors improves test reliability.[17] For tests that follow the recommended format of an equal number of letters on each line and a constant progression of letter sizes, it is preferable to give partial credit for each letter correctly identified. This is commonly done by counting the number of letters read correctly on the entire chart and converting this to an acuity score by means of a simple formula that values each letter as L/N, where L = difference in acuity between adjacent lines and N = number of letters per line. So for a chart with five letters per line and a 0.1 logMAR (see below) progression from line to line (such as the standard ETDRS chart) each correct letter is worth 0.1/5 = 0.02 logMAR. Although differences between scoring methods are usually small, it has been shown[2,6,18] that letter-by-letter scoring is more reproducible than line-by-line scoring.

The most familiar method for reporting visual acuities is the Snellen fraction. The numerator of the Snellen fraction indicates the test distance, and the denominator indicates the relative size of the letter, usually in terms of the distance at which the stroke width would subtend a visual angle of 1 minute. Thus "20/40" indicates that the actual test distance was 20 feet and that the strokes of the letters would subtend 1 minute of arc at 40 feet.

To simplify comparison of acuities measured at different distances, the minimum angle of resolution (MAR) should be used. The MAR is the visual angle corresponding to stroke width in minutes of arc and is equal to the reciprocal of the Snellen fraction. Visual acuities are frequently converted to log10 and reported as "logMAR." For example, 20/20 acuity corresponds to a MAR of 1 minute of arc, or a logMAR of 0, and 20/100 acuity corresponds to a MAR of 5 minutes of arc, or a logMAR of 0.7 (as does an acuity of 2/10 or 6/30). The MAR and logMAR scales increase with worsening acuity. One often sees visual acuities reported as the decimal equivalent of the Snellen fraction. However acuities are more normally distributed when converted to logMAR rather than decimal values. Moreover, decimals give the false impression that acuity scores can be equated with overall loss of visual function. For example, an acuity of 0.1 (the decimal equivalent of 20/200) may misleadingly suggest that the patient has retained 10% of residual visual function.

Near and reading acuity tests

Near acuity is usually tested to evaluate reading vision. These tests are particularly important for prescribing visual aids for persons with low vision. Near acuity has been shown to be a better predictor of the optimal magnification needed by visually impaired readers than traditional distance acuity.[19]

Although some near acuity tests are simply reduced versions of distance acuity charts, most tests consist of printed text, either unrelated words or complete sentences or paragraphs, covering a range of sizes. Near acuity tests are even less standardized than distance acuity tests.

Specifying letter size

As with all acuity tests, the most critical parameter is the visual angle subtended by the optotype. Many systems have been devised for specification of print size. One of the most common is the Jaeger J notation. Jaeger notation is based on a numeric scale (J1, J2, and so on) that follows no logical progression except that larger numbers correspond to larger print sizes. Furthermore, print with the same J specification can vary by as much as 90% from one test manufacturer to another.[20]

Alternatives to the Jaeger notation are the typesetter's point system, the British N system, and the M notation introduced by Sloan. The typesetter's point is commonly used to specify letter size for printed text and is equal to 0.32 mm (1/72 inch). However, the measurement refers to the size of the metal slug that contains the letter and varies from one font to another. A study[21] of the effect of font on reading speed showed that the nominal sizes of printed text can be very misleading. Of four fonts, all labeled as 12 point, one was much more legible than the other three. But it turned out that the more legible font was actually larger than the others and when equated for real size there was no difference in legibility.

The British N system standardized the point size specification by adopting the Times Roman font. Sloan's M notation,[4] widely used in the USA, is standardized according to the height of a lower-case "x." A lower-case 1M letter subtends 5 minarc at a 1-meter viewing distance and corresponds roughly to the size of ordinary newsprint. None of the print size specifications can be used for quantitative comparisons unless viewing distance is also specified. For example, 1M print read at a distance of 40 cm would be recorded as 0.40/1.00M.

Words versus continuous text

One issue that remains unresolved is whether near acuity tests should be based on unrelated words or meaningful text. An argument in favor of unrelated words is that contextual information promotes guessing and may lead to an overestimate of near acuity.[22] In addition, the presence of semantic context introduces variability because of cognitive intellectual factors that may mask the visual factors of primary concern.[23] On the other side it is argued that the main reason for measuring near acuity is to gain information about reading performance. Since context is normally available to the reader, a reading test that includes meaningful text will be a better indicator of everyday performance. Fortunately, reading speed for meaningful text is highly correlated with reading speed for unrelated words.[24]

The MNREAD test[25] uses meaningful text to evaluate near acuity. The test is composed of 19 standardized sentences in a logarithmic progression of sizes. Each sentence is 55 characters and the words are drawn from a controlled vocabulary. The test can be used to measure reading acuity (the smallest print size that can be read), maximum reading speed, and critical print size (the smallest print size for maximum reading speed). The test-retest variability for the MNREAD test has been assessed in patients with macular disease[26] and the coefficient of repeatability was found to be greater than 65 words/minute. The high level of variability may be due, in part, to the short sentences. The International Reading Speed Test (IReST)[27] uses 150-word paragraphs of continuous text to measure reading speed, which should yield more reproducible measures. The IReST is available in 17 languages.

Electronic acuity tests

Video-based acuity tests have been available since the 1980s, but did not become popular until the introduction of inexpensive LCD monitors in recent years. These electronic tests include computer software that can be used with the experimenter's own computer hardware (such as the Freiburg Acuity and Contrast Test (FrACT)), devices that display optotypes under operator control (such as the Test Chart 2000) and systems that administer, score, and store the results of the acuity measurement (such as the E-ETDRS and COMPlog systems).

Electronic tests offer several potential advantages over paper-based tests:

1. multiple types of test, such as acuity, contrast sensitivity, and stereoacuity, with one instrument
2. better randomization of optotypes. Each test administration can use a different arrangement of letters instead of being constrained to two or three printed charts
3. easier standardization of luminance and contrast, although if calibration instructions are ignored, luminance and contrast errors can be greater than for paper tests
4. the promise of advanced testing algorithms that reduce testing time and/or increase measurment accuracy and precision. So far the electronic systems have not lived up to this promise with test times as long as or longer and measurement accuracy and precision no better than conventional chart tests.[28] One test, the E-ETDRS system used in clinical trials for treatment of central retinal vein occlusion,[29] is reported to take longer without any increase in reliability.[28]

CONTRAST SENSITIVITY TESTS

Introduction

Visual acuity has been and will probably continue to be the most often used clinical measure of visual function. However, contrast sensitivity testing has been widely promoted as an important adjunct or even replacement for visual acuity testing. Acuity measures the eye's ability to resolve fine detail but may not adequately describe a person's ability to see large low-contrast objects such as faces. Contrast sensitivity testing was originally developed as a research tool by engineers and vision scientists interested in characterizing normal visual function. For theoretical reasons, most investigators have used sine-wave grating stimuli, patterns consisting of alternating light and dark bars, which have a sinusoidal luminance profile. Sine-wave gratings vary in spatial frequency (bar width) and contrast. A contrast sensitivity function (CSF) is derived by measuring the lowest detectable contrast across a range of spatial frequencies.

Utility of contrast sensitivity tests

For people with normal vision, contrast sensitivity and visual acuity are correlated. However, various types of visual dysfunction, including cerebral lesions,[30] optic neuritis related to multiple sclerosis,[31] glaucoma,[32] diabetic retinopathy,[33] and cataract,[34] may cause a reduction in contrast sensitivity despite near-normal visual acuity. This led to the suggestion that contrast sensitivity might serve as a tool for differential diagnosis and screening. However, there is no pattern of CSF loss that is unique to any particular vision disorder. The types of CSF measured in patients with macular disease or glaucoma can be similar to the CSFs measured in cataract patients, although detailed analyses with targets of different size or at different retinal eccentricities may help distinguish between various causes of the loss. It is argued that contrast sensitivity tests are more sensitive to early eye disease than visual acuity. While this may be true, much of the apparent difference in sensitivity is due to careless measurement of visual acuity (poorly designed charts and test procedures). Even if the test were more sensitive, its lack of specificity for distinguishing between ocular and retinal/neural disorders limits its usefulness as a screening test.[35]

The real value of clinical contrast sensitivity testing is to gain a better understanding of the impact of visual impairment on functional ability. Several studies have demonstrated that contrast sensitivity is useful for understanding the difficulties in performing everyday visual tasks faced by older people with essentially normal vision[36] and by patients with retinal disease.[37,38] Studies have shown that contrast sensitivity loss leads to mobility problems and difficulty recognizing signs or faces,[39] even when adjusted for loss of acuity.[40]

The association of contrast sensitivity with functional ability argues in favor of including contrast sensitivity measurements in clinical trials. Although visual acuity is the most common primary visual outcome measure, several studies have included contrast sensitivity as a secondary outcome. Considering both visual acuity and contrast sensitivity when assessing the outcomes of clinical trials may provide a more complete picture of the effects of treatment on vision than either measure alone. Examples where contrast sensitivity has been used as a secondary outcome include the Optic Neuritis Treatment Trial,[41] the TAP study of photodynamic therapy for age-related macular degeneration (AMD),[42] and the ABC trial of bevacizumab for AMD.[43]

Methods

Common contrast sensitivity tests

Traditional methods for measuring contrast sensitivity require relatively expensive and sophisticated equipment – typically a computer-controlled video monitor – and employ time-consuming psychophysical procedures. However, several simpler contrast sensitivity tests have been developed primarily for clinical use. These include the Functional Acuity Contrast Test[44] (FACT, replacement for the popular Vistech VCTS chart) and the CSV-1000,[45] sine-wave grating tests in chart form, and various low-contrast optotype tests such as the Lea test,[46] the Pelli–Robson letter chart,[17] the Melbourne Edge Test[47] and the Mars Letter Contrast Sensitivity Test.[48] Examples of three of the most commonly used clinical contrast sensitivity tests are illustrated in Fig. 11.2.

Gratings versus optotypes

A thorough discussion of the relative merits of the various tests is beyond the scope of this chapter; however, a few salient points are worth noting. Various investigators disagree about whether measurement of an entire CSF is necessary or whether a single measure of contrast sensitivity is adequate for clinical purposes. Proponents of the sine-wave grating tests argue that visual dysfunction can cause reductions in contrast sensitivity over a limited range of spatial frequencies, which would be missed by more global measures of contrast sensitivity. On the other hand, advocates of global measures note that contrast sensitivities at specific spatial frequencies tend to be highly correlated with one another, and they maintain that overall changes in contrast sensitivity are clinically more important than subtle bumps and wiggles in the CSF. Data

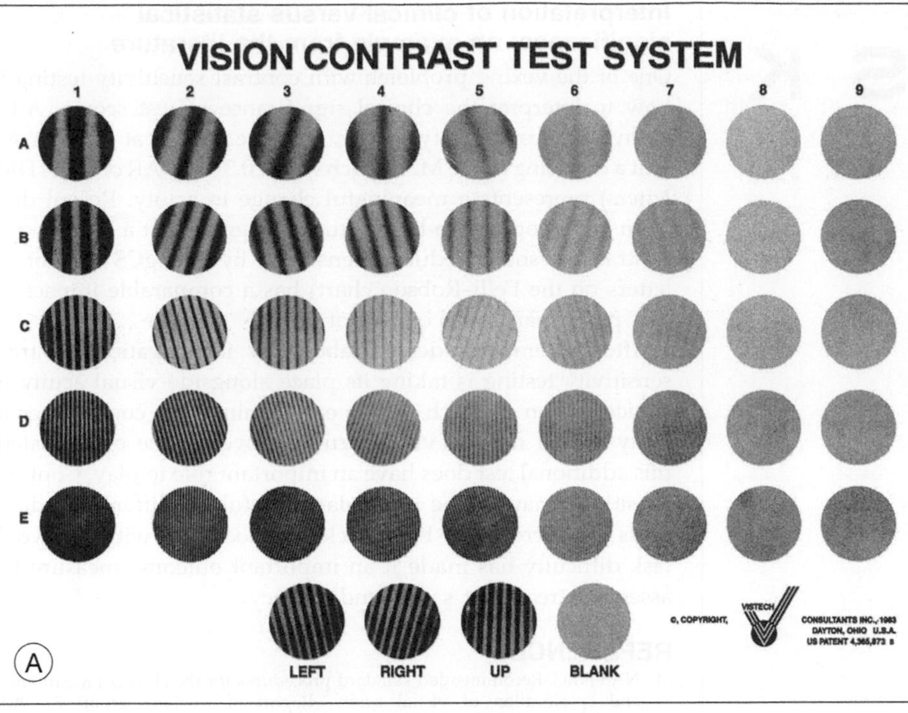

Fig. 11.2 Commonly used clinical contrast sensitivity tests. (A) Vistech VCTS 6500. (Courtesy of Vistech Consultants, Dayton, OH.) (B) Lea numbers low-contrast acuity test. (Courtesy of Good-Lite, Streamwood, IL.)

Continued

N R K Z S K

(C)

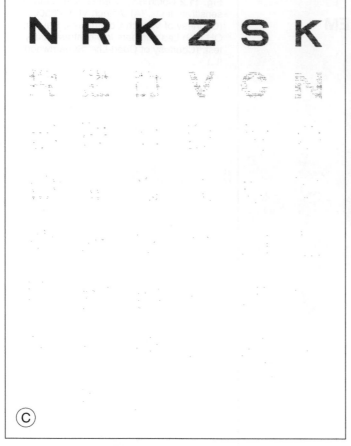

Fig. 11.2 Cont'd (C) Pelli–Robson letter sensitivity chart. (Reproduced with permission from Pelli DG, Robson JG, Wilkins AJ. The design of a new letter chart for measuring contrast sensitivity. Clin Vis Sci 1988;2:187–200.)

from large-scale studies of vision impairment indicate that global measures of contrast sensitivity are valuable predictors of difficulty in everyday life.[39]

Test design and procedure

In order to be useful, contrast sensitivity must be measured accurately and reliably. Many of the same principles of test design previously discussed for visual acuity tests apply to contrast sensitivity tests. Most important, the test should employ a criterion-free procedure, a uniform progression of contrasts, and an adequate number of trials at each contrast to make a reliable estimate of sensitivity. Most of the optotype tests conform to good design principles and produce reliable results, with the Mars test outperforming the very popular Pelli–Robson test.[49] Sine-wave grating charts tend to be less reliable because they have a limited number of trials to make measurements at several spatial frequencies.[50]

Some of the electronic acuity testing systems can also measure contrast sensitivity, including the Vision Test 2000 and FrACT. However, it is difficult to display a wide-enough range of contrasts to measure normal thresholds, and accurate calibration of the display monitor is critical. One study found that the computer-based test was less reliable than paper charts,[49] presumably due to problems generating low-contrast patterns with LCD displays.

Interpretation of clinical versus statistical significance: an example from the literature

One of the vexing problems with contrast sensitivity testing is how to interpret the clinical significance of test scores. After many decades of acuity testing, we have arrived at a consensus that a doubling of the MAR (increase of 0.3 logMAR or 15 ETDRS letters) represents a meaningful change in acuity. Recent data from large population-based studies suggest that a doubling of contrast threshold (reducing sensitivity by 0.3 logCS units or six letters on the Pelli–Robson chart) has a comparable impact on task performance and quality of life.[36,39]

After several decades of laboratory investigation, contrast sensitivity testing is taking its place alongside visual acuity in clinical vision research. While early claims that contrast sensitivity would replace visual acuity proved to be exaggerated, this additional test does have an important role to play. Contrast sensitivity may not be particularly useful for differential diagnosis and screening, but its close association with everyday task difficulty has made it an important outcome measure for assessing treatment safety and efficacy.

REFERENCES

1. NAS-NRC. Recommended standard procedures for the clinical measurement and specification of visual acuity. Report of working group 39. Adv Ophthalmol 1980;41:103–48.
2. British Standards Institution. Specification for test charts determining distance visual acuity. London: British Standards House.
3. White JM, Loshin DS. Grating acuity overestimates Snellen acuity in patients with age-related maculopathy. Optom Vis Sci 1989;66:751–5.
4. Sloan LL, Rowland WM, Altman A. Comparison of three types of test target for the measurement of visual acuity. Q Rev Opthalmol 1952;8:4–16.
5. Ferris FL, Kassoff A, Bresnick GH, et al. New visual acuity charts for clinical research. Am J Ophthalmol 1982;94:91–6.
6. Raasch T, Bailey I, Bullimore M. Repeatability of visual acuity measurement. Optom Vis Sci 1998;75:342–8.
7. Flom MC, Bedell HE. Identifying amblyopia using associated conditions, acuity, and nonacuity features. Am J Optom Physiol Opt 1985;62:153–60.
8. Kitchin JE, Bailey I. Task complexity and visual acuity in senile macular degeneration. Aust J Optom 1981;64:235–42.
9. Strong G, Woo GC. A distance visual acuity chart incorporating some new design features. Arch Ophthalmol 1985;102:44.
10. Schulze-Bonsel K, Feltgen N, Burau H, et al. Visual acuities "hand motion" and "counting fingers" can be quantified with the Freiburg visual acuity test. Invest Ophthalmol Vis Sci 2006;47:1236–40.
11. Dong LM, Hawkins BS, Marsh MJ. Consistency between visual acuity scores obtained at different test distances: theory vs observations in multiple studies. Arch Ophthalmol 2002;120:1523–33.
12. Sheedy JE, Bailey IL, Raasch TW. Visual acuity and chart luminance. Am J Optom Physiol Opt 1984;61:595–600.
13. Sloan LL, Habel A, Feiock K. High illumination as an auxiliary reading aid in diseases of the macula. Am J Ophthalmol 1973;76:745–57.
14. Legge GE, Rubin GS, Luebker A. Psychophysics of reading. V. The role of contrast in normal vision. Vision Res 1987;27:1165–77.
15. Higgins KE, Jaffe MJ, Coletta NJ, et al. Spatial contrast sensitivity. Importance of controlling the patient's visibility criterion. Arch Ophthalmol 1984;102: 1035–41.
16. Rubin GS. Reliability and sensitivity of clinical contrast sensitivity tests. Clin Vis Sci 1988 1988;2:169–77.
17. Pelli DG, Robson JG, Wilkins AJ. The design of a new letter chart for measuring contrast sensitivity. Clin Vis Sci 1988;2:187–99.
18. Arditi A, Cagenello R. On the statistical reliability of letter-chart visual acuity measurements. Invest Ophthalmol Vis Sci 1993;34:120–9.
19. Lovie-Kitchin JE, Whittaker SG. Prescribing near magnification for low vision patients. Clin Exp Optom 1999;82:214–24.
20. Jose RT, Atcherson RM. Type-size variability for near-point acuity tests. Am J Optom Physiol Opt 1977;54:634–8.
21. Rubin GS, Feely M, Perera S, et al. The effect of font and line width on reading speed in people with mild to moderate vision loss. Ophthalm Physiol Opt 2006;26:545–54.
22. Sloan LL, Brown DJ. Reading cards for selection of optical aids for the partially sighted. Am J Ophthalmol 1963;55:1187–99.
23. Baldasare J, Watson GR, Whittaker SG, et al. The development and evaluation of a reading test for low vision individuals with macular loss. J Visual Impairment Blindness 1986;1986:785–9.
24. Legge GE, Ross JA, Luebker A, et al. Psychophysics of reading. VIII. The Minnesota Low-Vision Reading Test. Optom Vis Sci 1989;66:843–53.
25. Mansfield JS, Legge GE, Bane MC. Psychophysics of reading. XV: Font effects in normal and low vision. Invest Ophthalmol Vis Sci 1996;37:1492–501.

26. Patel PJ, Chen FK, Da Cruz L, et al. Test–retest variability of reading performance metrics using MNREAD in patients with age-related macular degeneration. Invest Ophthalmol Visual Sci 2011;52:3854–9.
27. Hahn GA, Penka D, Gehrlich C, et al. New standardised texts for assessing reading performance in four European languages. Br J Ophthalmol 2006;90:480–4.
28. Laidlaw DA, Tailor V, Shah N, et al. Validation of a computerised logMAR visual acuity measurement system (COMPlog): comparison with ETDRS and the electronic ETDRS testing algorithm in adults and amblyopic children. Br J Ophthalmol 2008;92:241–4.
29. Scott IU, Ip MS, VanVeldhuisen PC, et al. A randomized trial comparing the efficacy and safety of intravitreal triamcinolone with standard care to treat vision loss associated with macular edema secondary to branch retinal vein occlusion: the Standard care vs Corticosteroid for Retinal Vein Occlusion (SCORE) study report 6. Arch Ophthalmol 2009;127:1115–28.
30. Bodis-Wollner I. Visual acuity and contrast sensitivity in patients with cerebral lesions. Science 1972;178:769–71.
31. Regan D, Silver R, Murray TJ. Visual acuity and contrast sensitivity in multiple sclerosis-hidden visual loss: an auxiliary diagnostic test. Brain 1977;100: 563–79.
32. Bron AJ. Contrast sensitivity changes in ocular hypertension and early glaucoma. Surv Ophthalmol 1989;33(Suppl):405–6; discussion 9–11.
33. Howes SC, Caelli T, Mitchell P. Contrast sensitivity in diabetics with retinopathy and cataract. Aust J Ophthalmol 1982;10:173–8.
34. Rubin GS, Adamsons IA, Stark WJ. Comparison of acuity, contrast sensitivity, and disability glare before and after cataract surgery. Arch Ophthalmol 1993;111:56–61.
35. Legge GE, Rubin GS. The contrast sensitivity function as a screening test: A critique. Am J Optom Physiol Opt 1986;63:265–70.
36. West SK, Rubin GS, Broman AT, et al. How does visual impairment affect performance on tasks of everyday life? The SEE project. Salisbury Eye Evaluation. Arch Ophthalmol 2002;120:774–80.
37. Lennerstrand G, Ahlström CO. Contrast sensitivity in macular degeneration and the relation to subjective visual impairment. Acta Ophthalmol (Copenh) 1989;67:225–33.
38. Rubin GS, Legge GE. Psychophysics of reading. VI. The role of contrast in low vision. Vision Res 1989;29:79–91.
39. Rubin GS, Bandeen-Roche K, Huang GH, et al. The association of multiple visual impairments with self-reported visual disability: SEE project. Invest Ophthalmol Vis Sci 2001;42:64–72.
40. Rubin GS, Bandeen-Roche K, Prasada-Rao P, et al. Visual impairment and disability in older adults. Optom Visual Sci 1994;71:750–60.
41. Beck RW, Cleary PA, Anderson Jr MM, et al,. A randomized, controlled trial of corticosteroids in the treatment of acute optic neuritis. N Engl J Med 1992;326:581–8.
42. Rubin GS, Bressler NM. Effects of verteporfin therapy on contrast on sensitivity: results from the Treatment of Age-related macular degeneration with Photodynamic therapy (TAP) investigation – TAP report no 4. Retina 2002;22: 536–44.
43. Patel PJ, Chen FK, Da Cruz L, et al. Contrast sensitivity outcomes in the ABC trial: a randomized trial of bevacizumab for neovascular age-related macular degeneration. Invest Ophthalmol Vis Sci 2011;52:3089–93.
44. Ginsburg A. Next generation contrast sensitivity testing. In: Rosenthal BP, Cole R, editors. Functional assessment of low vision. St Louis: Mosby Year Book; 1996. p. 77–88.
45. Pomerance GN, Evans DW. Test–retest reliability of the CSV-1000 contrast test and its relationship to glaucoma therapy. Invest Ophthalmol Vis Sci 1994;35: 3357–61.
46. Jarvinen P, Hyvarinen L. Contrast sensitivity measurement in evaluations of visual symptoms caused by exposure to triethylamine. Occup Environ Med 1997;54:483–6.
47. Verbaken JH, Johnston AW. Population norms for edge contrast sensitivity. Am J Optom Physiol Opt 1986;63:724–32.
48. Arditi A. Improving the design of the letter contrast sensitivity test. Invest Ophthalmol Vis Sci 2005;46:2225–9.
49. Thayaparan K, Crossland MD, Rubin GS. Clinical assessment of two new contrast sensitivity charts. Br J Ophthalmol 2007;91:749–52.
50. Pesudovs K, Hazel CA, Doran RM, et al. The usefulness of Vistech and FACT contrast sensitivity charts for cataract and refractive surgery outcomes research. Br J Ophthalmol 2004;88:11–6.

Chapter 12

Visual Fields in Retinal Disease

Rajeev S. Ramchandran, Steven E. Feldon

One need only review the classic atlas by Dr J. Donald M. Gass[1] to recognize that most retinal diseases are readily diagnosed by careful ophthalmoscopic examination. However, for the ophthalmologist to understand and document visual consequences of retinal disease, qualitative and quantitative assessment is critical. In particular, visual field testing helps with the correlation of structural changes in the retina or elsewhere in the visual pathway with deficits in function. For example, AM is a 70-year-old woman diagnosed as having an old central retinal vein occlusion (CRVO) in the left eye and surface wrinkling retinopathy in both eyes. She also had been treated for elevated intraocular pressure. Fluorescein angiography of the left eye showed shunting vessels around the optic nerve head, thought to be consistent with the old vein occlusion. However, progressive bilateral visual field loss (Fig. 12.1) over 2 years suggested the need for further investigation. A computed tomography (CT) scan demonstrated a large subfrontal meningioma compressing both optic nerves (Fig. 12.2).

Visual field tests can be qualitative or quantitative. They span multiple formats from the simplest confrontation field or Amsler grid to the most advanced quantitative kinetic, static, and microperimetry. For all visual field tests, reliability and reproducibility are important. There are currently three main uses for visual field tests in patients with retinal pathology: (1) to determine the current level of visual field loss and monitor progression; (2) to evaluate the effects of treating retinal pathology on visual function; and (3) to correlate functional and structural changes in the retina.

This chapter reviews the use of visual fields and the principles of perimetry relevant to retinal disease. Visual field defects corresponding to common retinal diseases are described, with an emphasis on clinical situations for which perimetry is useful diagnostically. The value of specialized visual field testing in clinical research is also reviewed.

PRINCIPLES OF PERIMETRY

The island of Traquair

The single most important concept in understanding the visual field is depicted by the island of Traquair, which is defined as a "hill of vision" surrounded by a "sea of blindness."[2] The shape of the normal visual field is oval. There is decreasing sensitivity with increasing eccentricity in the field, as the elevation corresponds to the sensitivity of the field, and the flat plane corresponds to location within the field (Fig. 12.3). From the point of fixation, the field extends 60° superiorly, 60° nasally, 70–75° inferiorly, and 100–110° temporally. The blind spot is represented by a hole in the "hill" about 15° temporal to the foveal "peak."

Perimetric tests have been developed that systematically measure the level of light sensitivity in the visual field. Two basic types exist: kinetic perimetry and static perimetry. In kinetic perimetry a target is moved from outside the potentially seeing area toward the seeing area until it is detected. In static perimetry a target located within a potentially seeing area can be increased in size or intensity until it is detected. With either method a region of vision can be defined in relation to a test stimulus of given size, hue, brightness, and uniform level of background illumination. For instance, under standardized conditions, the central visual field of about 30° can be mapped with a moving white target of 3 mm at a distance of 2 meters.[3]

METHODS OF VISUAL FIELD TESTING

There is no single best test for the evaluation of visual fields in retinal disease. Depending on the location and extent of the disease, the examiner must choose from an ever-increasing selection of sensitive qualitative and quantitative perimetric techniques.

Qualitative techniques

Vision may be extremely poor in many patients with widespread visual dysfunction resulting from retinal disease. In such instances visual fields may be obtained only by confrontation testing. However, this technique also may be used to detect even subtle relative field defects and scotomata. Confrontation testing is performed with the examiner facing the patient, usually at about arm's length. The peripheral vision of the patient is evaluated in relation to that of the examiner's. To test the patient's right eye, the examiner occludes the right eye and aligns the left eye so that both patient and examiner share a common visual axis. The examiner then moves the hand or test object from outside the visual field toward fixation. Relative preservation of peripheral vision can be established if the examiner places both hands or two test objects in different seeing quadrants for the patient and asks the patient to identify the clearer object. Central visual function is estimated by having the patient look toward the examiner's nose or, if vision is very poor, toward the direction of the examiner's voice. The patient describes which parts of the examiner's face are missing or most clearly seen. Results are recorded either descriptively or with a simple drawing.

Although the tangent screen can be used quantitatively, it is most effective as a qualitative tool for estimation of visual loss in the central field. A 1-meter screen can be used to evaluate

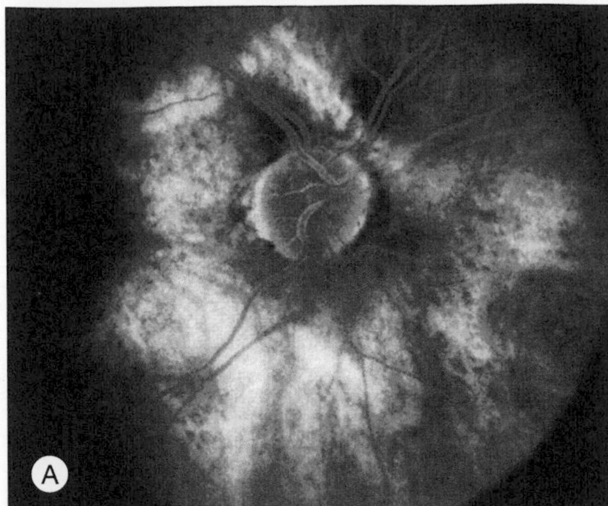

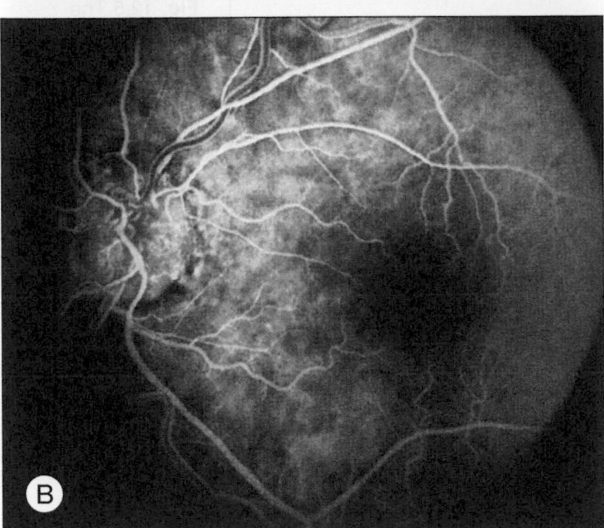

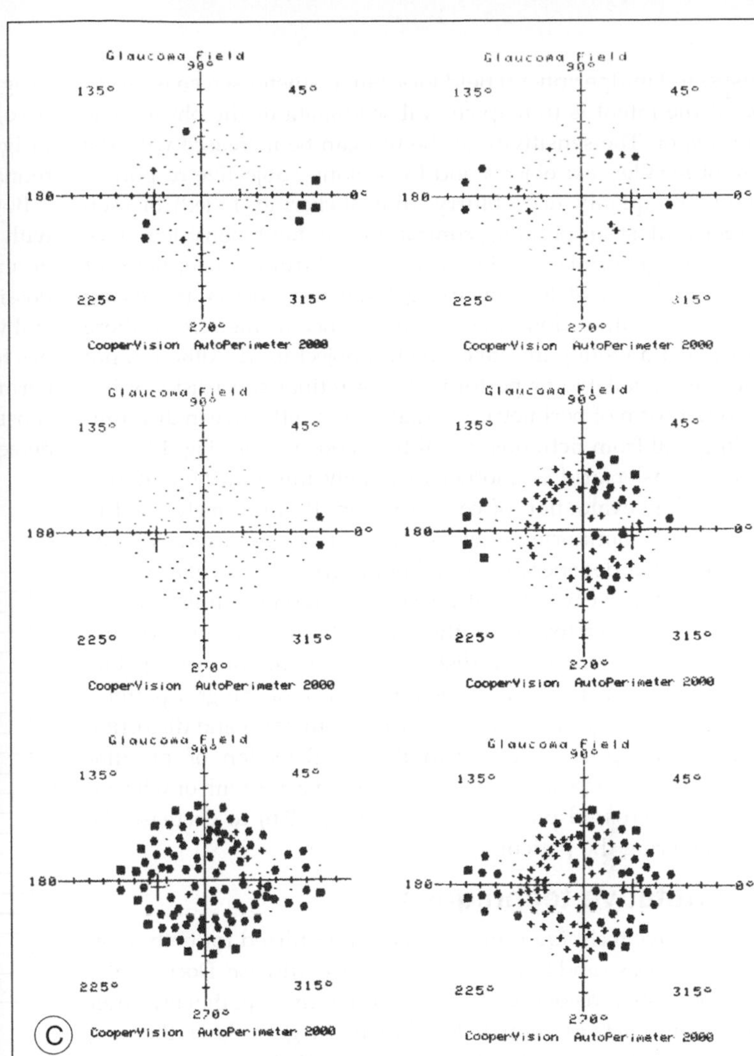

Fig. 12.1 (A, B) Fluorescein angiograms of a 70-year-old woman who has had progressive loss of vision in both eyes over 2 years. She has controlled ocular hypertension and surface-wrinkling retinopathy. The history of an old central retinal vein occlusion in the left eye is supported by the slightly dilated and tortuous retinal veins and the multiple shunting capillaries on the surface of the disc (B). (C) Progressive field loss, documented in both eyes over 3 years, is inconsistent with the ophthalmoscopic appearance. A computed tomographic scan was ordered, the results of which are shown in Fig. 12.2.

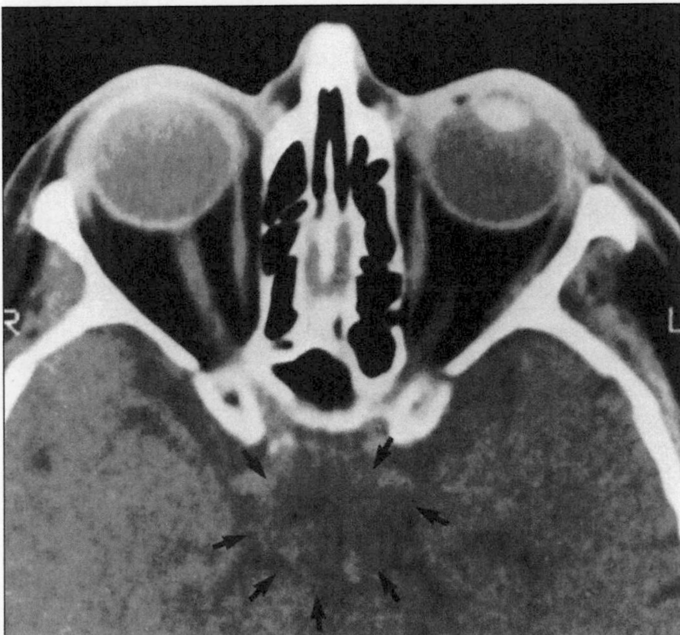

Fig. 12.2 Computed tomographic scan from the patient described in Fig. 12.1 demonstrates a large subfrontal meningioma with bilateral optic nerve compression. Surgical resection improved sensorium but not vision.

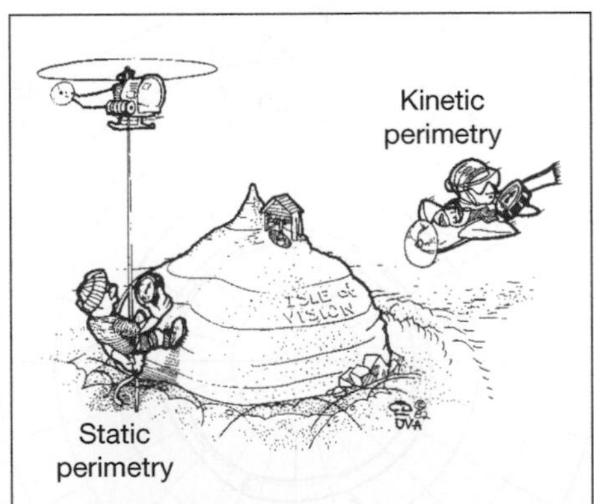

Fig. 12.3 The "island," or "hill of vision," proposed by Traquair is surrounded by a "sea of blindness." The height of the island represents increasing sensitivity. Using kinetic perimetry, the island is intercepted by a moving target of fixed size. Using static perimetry, a target's visibility is increased in size or luminosity until it descends on to the island. The blind spot located 15° temporal to fixation is absolute, creating a small "well" in the sensitivity contour. (Courtesy of Steven Newman, MD.)

suspected midperipheral field loss, but a 2-meter screen is essential if the intent is to map central scotomata or the physiologic blind spot. The sensitivity of the test can be increased with the use of smaller test objects and by seeking subjective responses about the quality (e.g., blurry, dim, flickering, faded) of seen targets. Most important, conical visual field constriction of retinal origin can be readily distinguished from tubular fields of nonorganic visual loss by using large test objects at varying distances. With a doubling of the distance to the screen, there must be a doubling in size of the test object used. Although not routinely available or performed in a retinal specialist's office, no other form of perimetric evaluation is as effective in discriminating real from fictitious visual field constriction (Fig. 12.4).

The Amsler grid is another extremely important qualitative tool for the evaluation of central vision. It is routinely used in regular self-monitoring of vision between eye exams by patients with macular degeneration or other progressive macular pathology to detect early signs of disease progression. In its original form, the patient fixates on the center dot of a white grid on a black background from a distance of 35.5 cm (14 inches) (Fig. 12.5). The patient describes the appearance of the grid pattern, especially in regard to missing areas (scotomata) and distortion (metamorphopsia). The sensitivity for detection of macular lesions can be increased with the use of red grids with or without the use of crossed polarizing lenses (Fig. 12.6) to decrease the light entering the patient's eye.[4]

Quantitative techniques

Quantitative techniques of perimetry are utilized for both diagnosis of disease and following the course of disease. Documentation of visual recovery in eyes with retinal pathology after treatment, such as retinal detachment surgery, laser therapy, anti-inflammatory and antivascular endothelial growth factor drug therapy is becoming an important aspect of patient care. Also, quantitative records are invaluable for achieving new insights into the types of visual disturbances found in various retinal diseases.

Both Goldmann and Tübinger perimetry require examiners with a high degree of training. The Goldmann visual field (GVF) perimeter uses a kinetic strategy, although static perimetry is possible (Fig. 12.7). It is especially useful for monitoring peripheral visual field loss and large scotomata. It has limited capabilities for the evaluation of small central scotomata. The Tübinger perimeter uses a static strategy. It is a sensitive but time-consuming technique for identifying small or large relative field defects once the approximate region of the field loss has been

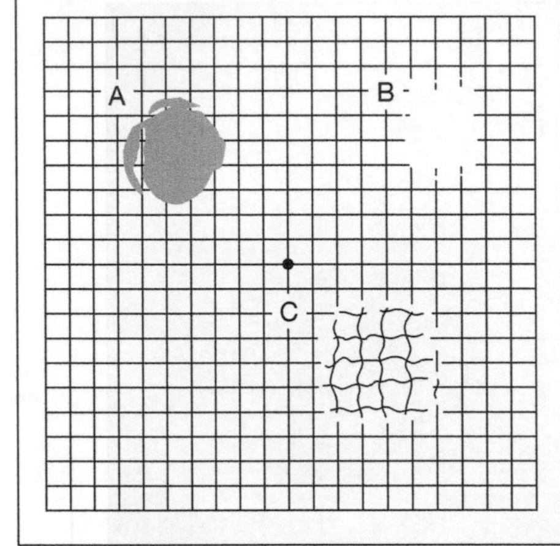

Fig. 12.5 The Amsler grid is viewed at 35.5 cm (14 inches), using the central dot for fixation. Regions of metamorphopsia (C), scotoma (B), and blur (A) are noted.

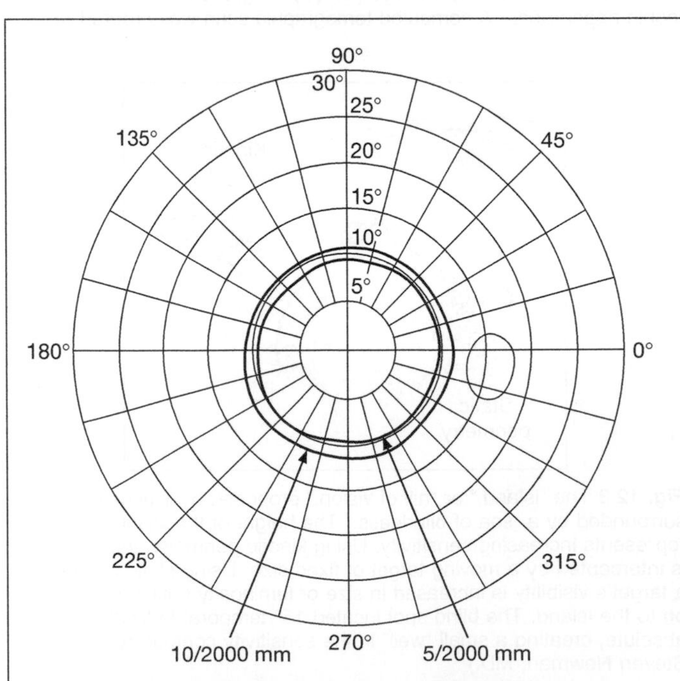

Fig. 12.4 A tangent screen field from a hysterical or malingering patient fails to show expansion of the visual field with doubling of both test object size and distance.

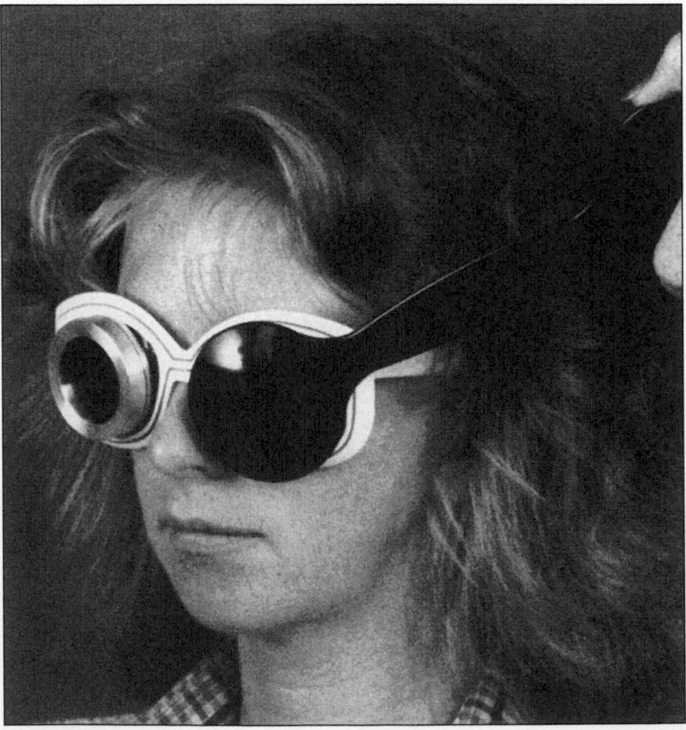

Fig. 12.6 The sensitivity of the Amsler grid test can be increased by using red lines on a black background rather than black or white lines on contrasting backgrounds. Further sensitivity may be achieved by using crossed-polarizing glasses that decrease the amount of light entering the eye. (Courtesy of Alfredo Sadun, MD.)

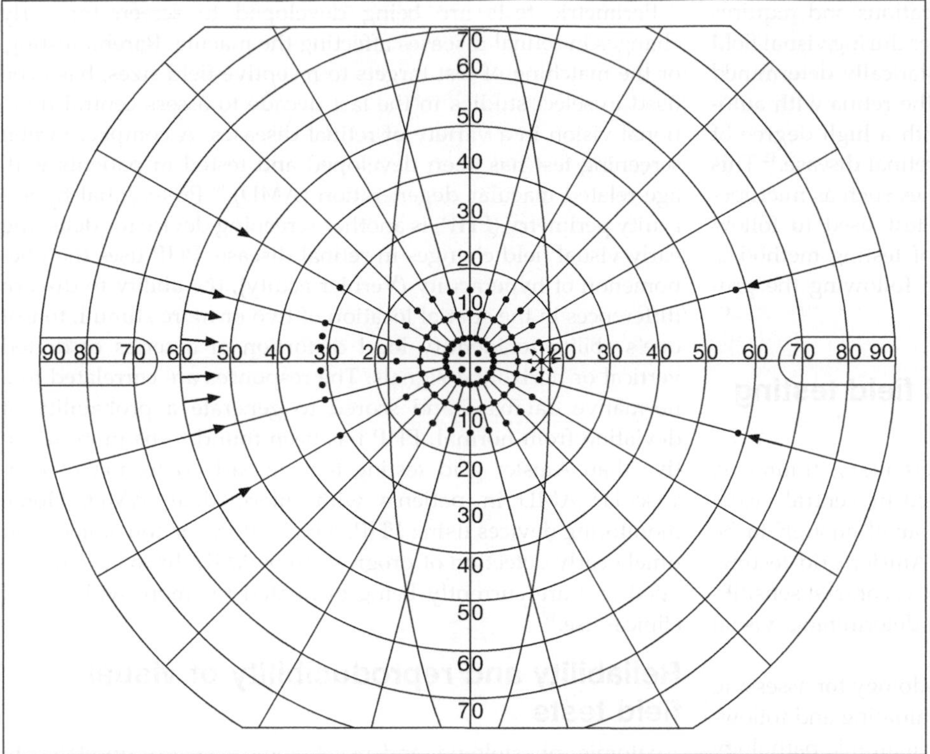

Fig. 12.7 The Goldmann visual field strategy developed by Armaly and Drance uses kinetic targets (arrows) to map the peripheral isopters and suprathreshold static targets (dots) to check central visual field function. (Reproduced with permission from Rock WJ, Drance SM, Morgan RW. Visual field screening in glaucoma. An evaluation of the Armaly technique for screening glaucomatous visual fields. Arch Ophthalmol 1973;89: 287–90.)

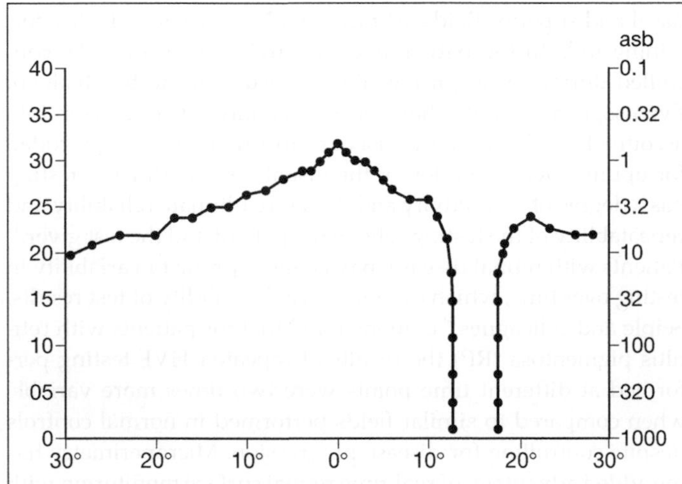

Fig. 12.8 The Tübinger perimeter produces a static profile of visual sensitivity through any chosen meridian. (Reproduced with permission from Harrington DO. The visual fields: a textbook and atlas of clinical perimetry. St Louis: Mosby, 1981.)

determined. Laborious Tübinger profiles are usually made only across a single meridian of the visual field, limiting its screening capabilities (Fig. 12.8).

Quantitative perimetry received a tremendous boost with the advent of automated, computerized methodology. Suprathreshold automated visual screeners, such as the Fieldmaster 101 and the Dicon units, did much to popularize visual field testing in the ophthalmic community. Pseudothreshold algorithms have been developed for these machines to enhance their quantitative capabilities.[5] However, threshold perimeters, such as the Octopus and the Humphrey visual field (HVF) analyzer, have surpassed the capabilities of even the Tübinger instrument. Automated, quantitative threshold perimetry is ideal for the evaluation of retinal disease. Randomized sequences for stimulus presentation within the visual field enhance the possibility of detecting small or irregular field defects. Density of points can be varied to characterize fully field losses that are either focal or diffuse. Although the HVF has the ability to test 60° of visual field, this protocol is very time-consuming. The standard protocols used are the 30-2, 24-2, and 10-2, which measure the central 30, 24, and 10° respectively. The choice of field is based on the region of pathology in the visual field. The dash 2 (-2) refers to protocol 2, the analysis which points on either side of the vertical and horizontal meridians rather than just on the vertical and horizontal axis as performed in protocol 1. Thus, both the 24-2 and 30-2 protocols test points 3° from the horizontal and vertical axis as well as points at 6° intervals beyond this region in the central 24 or 30° respectively. A 10-2 protocol tests points 1° from the horizontal and vertical meridian as well as points at 2° beyond this region in the central 10° and thus is more sensitive for detecting subtle field losses in the macular region.[6]

Newer algorithms such as the Swedish interactive threshold algorithm (SITA) have been developed to increase efficiency and decrease variability in the standard Humphrey strategy. This strategy uses normative and real-time data from patients during the test to update estimates of thresholds and adjust presentation times of stimuli continually. Short-wavelength automated perimetry (SWAP) is a variant on the usual white light stimulus used in standard threshold testing. SWAP isolates the S-cone system (blue–yellow pathway), using a blue stimulus on a yellow background. Normal, age-corrected retinal sensitivity values have been established, increasing the utility in clinical testing.[7,8] Care must be taken when using this technique to correct for chromatic filtering effects from the crystalline lenses.[9] Longer test duration, increased variability, and learning effects make SWAP most applicable to conditions for which early detection has important therapeutic implications and requires careful supervision of the patient by the tester during visual field testing.[10] In each case, the ability to map statically determined threshold retinal sensitivity directly on to the retina with automated quantitative threshold perimetry with a high degree of accuracy is important in the evaluation of retinal disease.[11] This ability has further been refined by techniques such as microperimetry. However, as with any repeated test used to follow changes over time, consistency in choice of testing method is important in accurately characterizing and following the progression of retinal diseases.

Other methodologies of visual field testing in retinal disease

Macular diseases may be degenerative, hereditary, traumatic, toxic, or inflammatory. All are characterized by central visual field defects or distortion, which may be small enough to be undetected without detailed perimetry or Amsler grid testing. Ancillary psychophysical tests of visual acuity, contrast sensitivity, and color vision may be helpful in determining visual function.

Microperimetry is a relatively new methodology for assessing visual fields that is especially helpful for evaluating and following macular disease. It is used to correlate anatomic pathology with function of the visual system by integrating fundus imaging and computerized threshold perimetry at specific locations in the fundus. One technique of microperimetry uses a scanning laser ophthalmoscope (SLO) (e.g., Rodenstock, Ottobrunn, Germany) to plot field defects within geographically defined regions of the retina. A modulated helium-neon laser beam of variable intensity (0–21 dB) at 633 nm projects stimuli on to the retina during ophthalmoscopy performed with an infrared diode laser at 780 nm.[7,12] Another type of microperimetry is Micro Perimeter 1 (MP 1, Nidek Instruments, Padova, Italy) which uses an infrared fundus camera that provides a 45° view and performs perimetry using a liquid crystal display with a special software. The MP-1 allows for eye tracking and real-color fundus image acquisition. Images from other tests, such as fluorescein angiogram, can be overlaid on to the microperimetry, which is not possible in SLO microperimetry. Moreover, as SLO microperimetry is also restricted to red laser light, comparison with standard perimetry or MP-1 is difficult.[12]

Both the SLO and MP-1 microperimetry devices allow for kinetic and static perimetric testing of the macula and permit simultaneous observation of the retina during perimetric testing. Similar to conventional perimetry, stimulus sizes range from Goldmann size I to V and the central 15–20° of visual field can be tested in both devices, although the MP-1 allows for a slightly larger field for testing. Rohrschneider and colleagues determined that for patients with retinal disease both the SLO and MP-1 microperimetry devices provided comparable results, with the SLO devices providing better-resolution fundus images and the MP-1 providing better fixation analysis with more accurate real-time image alignment.[13] As efforts to correlate better anatomic and functional changes in the retina have advanced, more refined devices are being developed that combine techniques of visualizing the ultrastructure of the retina, such as three-dimensional spectral optical coherence tomography (OCT) and adaptive optics, with corresponding perimetric functional assessment.[14,15]

Perimetric tests are being developed to screen for early changes in retinal diseases affecting the macula. Rarebit testing, or the matching of test targets to receptive field sizes, has been used in select studies in the last decade to assess central functional vision in a variety of retinal diseases. A compact rarebit screening test has been developed and tested in patients with age-related macular degeneration (AMD).[16] Preferential hyperacuity perimetry (PHP) is another screening device for detecting early visual field changes in retinal disease. PHP uses the phenomenon of hyperacuity (Vernier acuity), the ability to discern differences in the spatial location of two or more stimuli, to test one's ability to identify local distortion of a series of dotted vertical or horizontal signals. The responses are correlated to a normative database and scored to generate a probability of deviation from normal. PHP has been found to be more sensitive than Amsler grid testing for the early detection of neovascular AMD in patients with intermediate AMD. Home monitoring devices using PHP, which allow for convenient and timely early detection of progression of AMD, have been developed and are currently being evaluated for more widespread clinical use.[17]

Reliability and reproducibility of visual field tests

Anatomic, physiologic, and psychological factors unrelated to the pathology in question can significantly affect measurement of the visual field. The nose, brow, and lid may constrict the nasal and superior fields artifactually. Numerous variables pertaining to both the patient and the environment must be controlled during testing if meaningful results are to be obtained. Even so, considerable short-term variability must be taken into account. Box 12.1 outlines a list of factors that must be controlled for optimal determination of the visual field. Perimetric testing has a degree of subjectivity and therefore ultimate reliability and repeatability of the testing rely on the patient and the test giver.[18] Patients with retinal disease may be more prone to variability in testing over time, which can influence the validity of test results. Seiple and colleagues[19] demonstrated that for patients with retinitis pigmentosa (RP) the results of repeated HVF testing performed at different time points were two times more variable when compared to similar fields performed in normal controls despite controlling for disease progression. Microperimetry has the added advantage of real-time retinal surface monitoring with

Box 12.1 Variables affecting measurement of the visual field

- Environmental
- Illumination
- Equipment
- Examiner
- Technique
- Ocular
- Retinal adaptation
- Refractive state
- Media
- Pupil size
- Global
- Age
- Fixation
- Reaction time
- Fatigue

eye tracking to correct for eye movements during testing. Weingessel and colleagues have demonstrated good interexaminer and intraexaminer reliability of microperimetry using the MP-1 device in eyes with and without retinal disease.[20]

PERIMETRY IN SPECIFIC RETINAL DISEASES

The visual fields tests described are used in patients with retinal disease to assess and catalog progression of functional visual field loss, to determine the outcomes of treatment on visual function, and to correlate functional and structural changes in the retina.

Retinal dystrophies

Visual fields have traditionally been used to characterize and monitor the progression of visual field loss in RP. The earliest field defect in RP is reported to be a group of isolated scotomata 20–25° from fixation.[3] Eventually these isolated defects coalesce into a "ring scotoma" affecting the midperiphery of the visual field. Usually the peripheral field loss progresses and leaves a small, central island of vision. Eventually, complete visual loss may occur (Fig. 12.9).

Characterization and comparison of specific patterns of visual field loss in genotypically and phenotypically different forms of RP such as X-linked, dominant, pericentral, and Usher syndrome

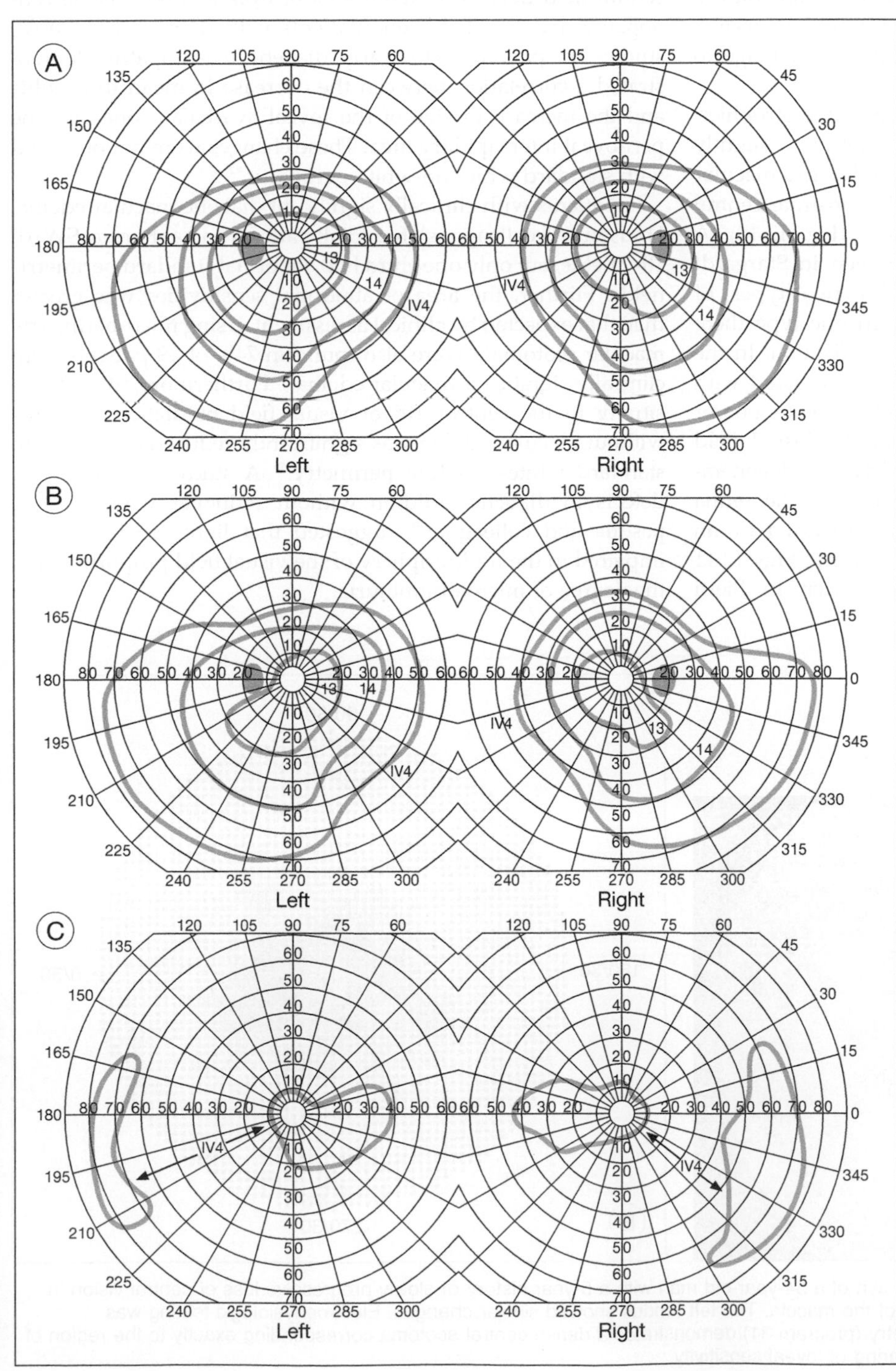

Fig. 12.9 Classic development of a ring scotoma with focal sparing of a peripheral temporal island seen in retinitis pigmentosa and cone–rod dystrophies. (A) Progressive depression of peripheral visual field in a patient with cone–rod degeneration at presentation. (B) Same patient after 1 year. (C) Same patient during fourth year of follow-up. (Reproduced with permission from Krauss HR, Heckenlively JR. Visual field changes in cone–rod degenerations. Arch Ophthalmol 1982;100:1784–90.)

using GVF perimetry have been attempted to differentiate better subgroups of RP based on visual prognosis and genotype.[21–23] Association of degree of visual field loss with different genotypes in syndromic associations of RP, including Bardet–Biedl syndrome 1, has also been studied.[24] In addition, HVF measurements have been correlated with contrast sensitivity in RP and were found to be a sensitive predictor for central visual function in advanced RP.[25,26] Visual field perimetry has been used to test outcomes of treatments for varieties of RP, including fundus albipunctatus.[27]

Visual fields have also been used in correlating photoreceptor anatomy and visual function in RP. Decreased retinal sensitivity on electroretinogram has been linked to visual field loss demonstrated by perimetry in RP.[28] Recently, changes in GVF, HVF, and microperimetry have been correlated with anatomical changes at the cellular level using OCT and autofluorescence to identify abnormal photoreceptor morphology and damage to retinal pigment epithelial (RPE) cells.[29–35]

Perimetric changes occur in a variety of retinal dystrophies. Cone dystrophy produces progressive symmetric to slightly asymmetric central visual loss. This is associated with a macular pigmentary disturbance. The visual fields demonstrate central scotomata with relative sparing of the fovea (Fig. 12.10). A central or paracentral scotoma can also be seen in Stargardt disease. However, microperimetry identifies two types of scotoma in patients with Stargardt disease. In one type there is a dense ring scotoma associated with stable fixation. In the second type there is a dense central scotoma associated with fixation shift. The second type is also correlated with poorer acuity.[36] In contrast, there is constriction of the visual field corresponding to the progressive peripheral retinal degeneration with scalloped margins in gyrate atrophy of the retina and choroid, a rare tapetoretinal degeneration caused by an inborn error of ornithine aminotransferase activity (Figs 12.11 and 12.12). Constricted GVF tests are also seen in Bietti crystalline dystrophy.[37] Correlations between HVF sensitivity and multifocal electroretinogram (mERG) have been documented for eyes with central areolar choroidal dystrophy and North Carolina macular dystrophy.[38,39] Functional changes as evidenced by perimetry and mERG have also been correlated with morphological changes documented by fundus autofluorescence in adult vitelliform macular dystrophy.[40]

Diabetic retinopathy

The diffuse retinal ischemia associated with diabetic retinopathy would seem to make visual field assessment an ideal method for follow-up of the disease. However, visual fields are not routinely used to evaluate this retinal disease, even though field defects may exist in the absence of observable retinopathy. Roth[41] found central field defects in about 40% of eyes without visible retinopathy and in all diabetic patients with retinopathy. SWAP studies on patients with early diabetic maculopathy demonstrated a correlation between the decrease in mean thresholds and the increase in size of the foveal avascular zone and the perifoveal intercapillary area. These changes were not observed with standard white-on-white perimetry.[42]

In patients with clinically significant diabetic macular edema, Hudson and colleagues[43] found all patients had abnormal SWAP 10–2 fields, but only one-third had abnormal standard perimetric fields. Further, the area of abnormal sensitivities was greater than that expected by clinical assessment. Using microperimetry, macular scotomata were also found in 74% of 19 patients with clinically significant macular edema.[44] Furthermore, SWAP sensitivity in the central 10° of visual field of diabetic patients without macular edema was significantly reduced compared to standard white-on-white perimetry.[45] A study of visual field defects in diabetic children without retinopathy by Mastropasqua and colleagues[46] suggested that light sensitivity was impaired in the midperiphery of the visual field proportional to the degree of microalbuminuria.

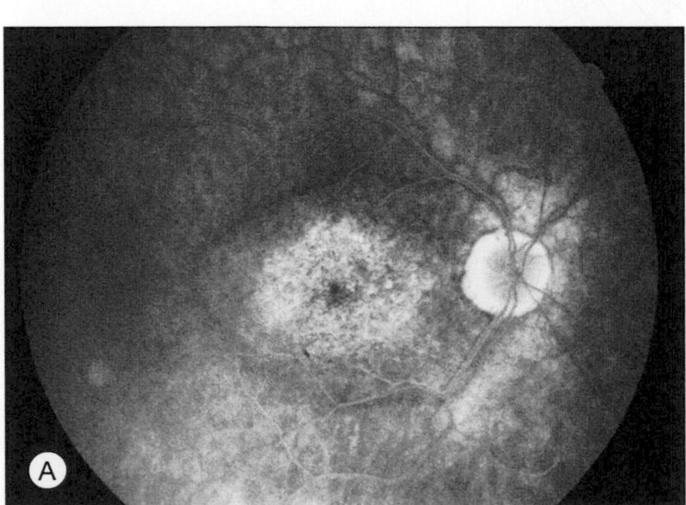

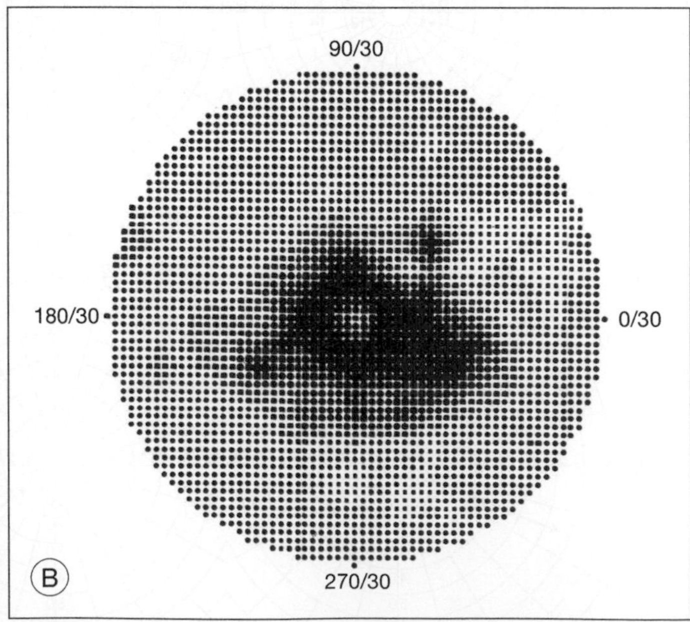

Fig. 12.10 (A) Fluorescein angiogram of the right eye of a 54-year-old man with a 5-year history of slowly progressive loss of central vision in each eye shows marked pigmentary disturbance of the macula. The left fundus showed similar changes. Electrophysiologic testing was diagnostic of cone dystrophy. (B) Octopus perimetry (program 31) demonstrates a dense central scotoma corresponding exactly to the region of macular pigmentary change. Note the relative sparing of foveal sensitivity.

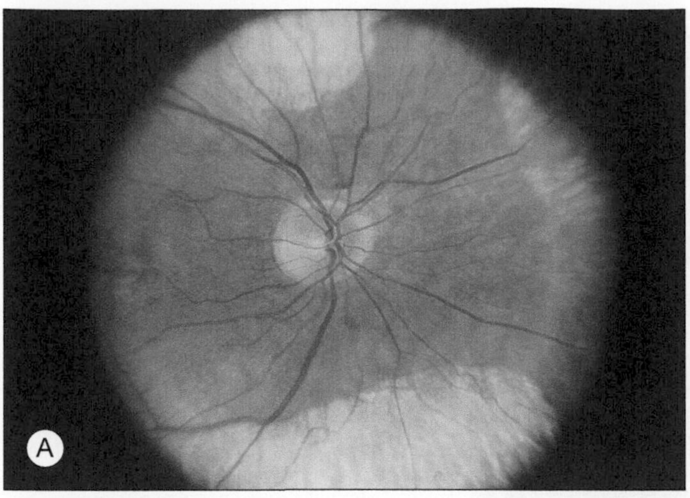

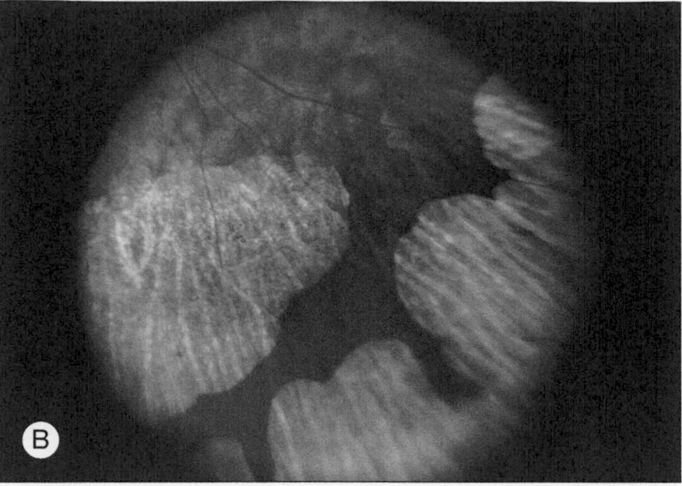

Fig. 12.11 Central (A) and peripheral (B) fundus appearance of a patient with gyrate atrophy of the retina. The visual field of this patient is shown in Fig. 12.12.

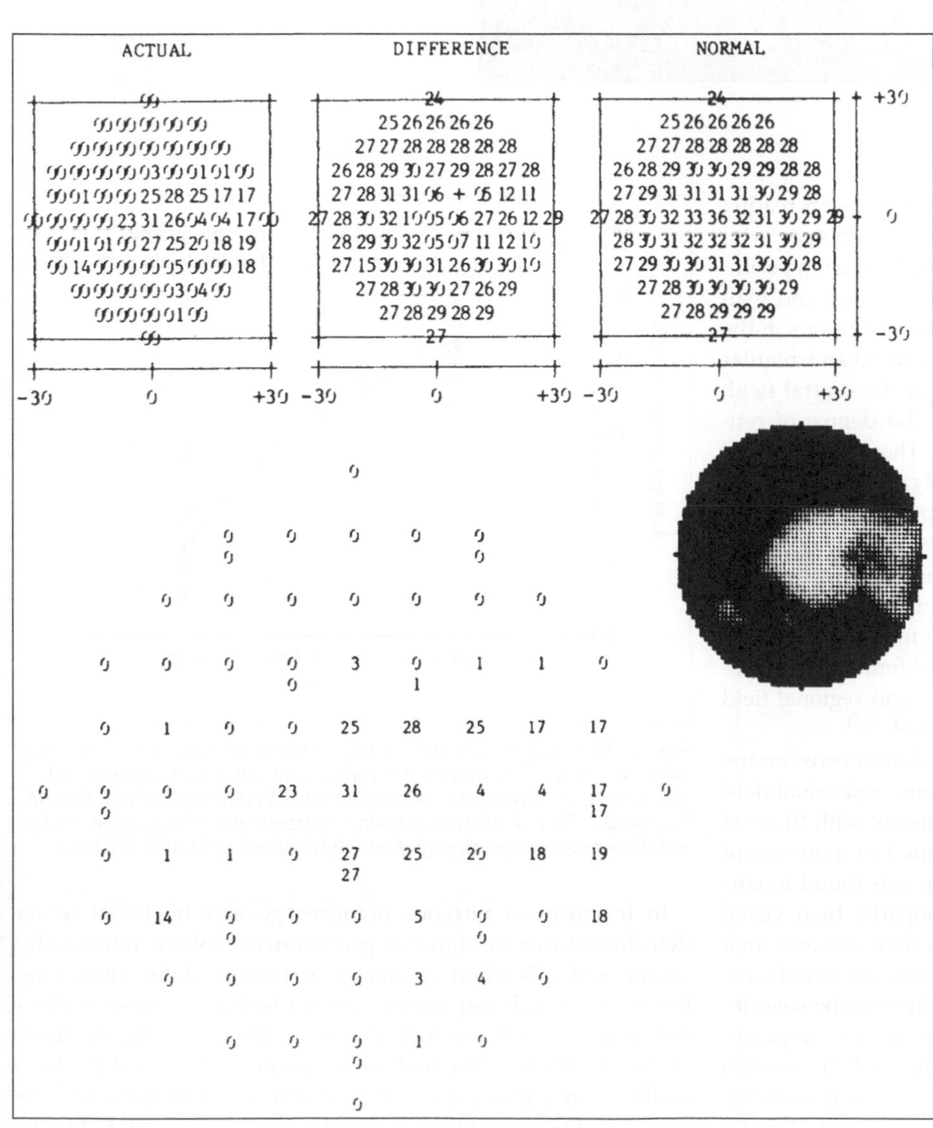

Fig. 12.12 Thirty-degree Octopus visual field (program 31) demonstrates marked peripheral constriction, with relative sparing in the centrocecal region. In addition, there are a few more peripheral islands of reduced sensitivity. (Reproduced with permission from Feldon SE. Computerized perimetry in selected disorders of the retina. In: Whalen WR, Spaeth GL, editors. Computerized visual fields: what they are and how to use them. Thorofare, NJ: Slack; 1985.)

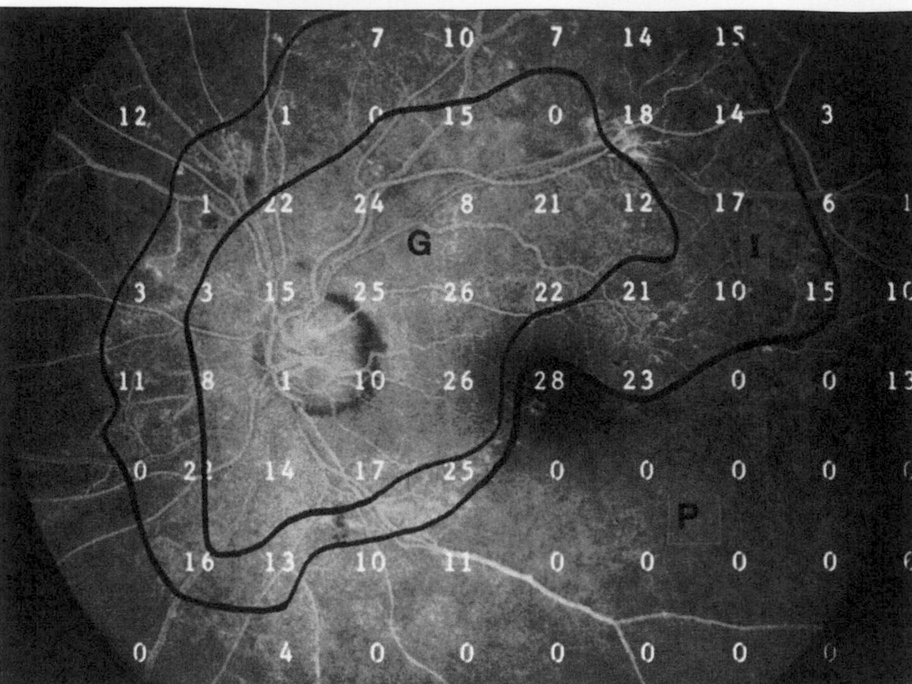

Fig. 12.13 Fluorescein angiogram of a patient with preproliferative diabetic retinopathy. Static sensitivities from Octopus perimetry are superimposed. Areas of good perfusion (G) have normal visual function. Areas of intermediate perfusion (I) have a moderate decrease of visual function, and nonperfused areas (P) have complete loss of visual function. (Reproduced with permission from Bell JA, Feldon SE. Retinal microangiopathy: correlation of Octopus perimetry with fluorescein angiography. Arch Ophthalmol 1984;102:1294–8.)

Once diabetic retinopathy is present, visual field loss is readily documented. Gandolfo and colleagues[47] studied 85 eyes with preproliferative diabetic retinopathy using the Goldmann perimeter. They were able to identify retinal hemorrhages and exudates of at least 3–4° in diameter as localized depressions in the visual field. Macular exudation and edema caused an irregular depression and flattening of static profiles of the central field. Wisznia and colleagues[48] tried to correlate the degree of retinopathy with the amount of visual field loss. They hypothesized that a correlation might exist between retinal capillary perfusion and field loss. Bell and Feldon[11] used Octopus static perimetry to show that visual sensitivity is quantitatively correlated with retinal perfusion in preproliferative diabetic retinopathy (Figs 12.13 and 12.14). Utilizing standard perimetry, Federman and Lloyd[49] found the degree of perfusion to be more important in predicting field loss than the amount of proliferative retinopathy. This relationship between nonperfusion and regional field loss has been confirmed in other studies as well.[47,50]

Lutze and Bresnick[51] demonstrated a correlation between the degree of retinopathy in type I diabetic patients and visual field loss using SWAP. These findings were consistent with those of Zwas and coworkers and have been confirmed in more recent studies.[9,52] In addition, automated perimetry was found to correlate better with severity of diabetic retinopathy than visual acuity.[53] A study by Agardh and colleagues demonstrated that SWAP sensitivity of visual field loss was correlated to ischemic changes in areas of macular edema, rather than to the severity of macular edema.[54] SWAP analysis also demonstrated a greater decrease in mean sensitivity in menstruating diabetic women who were in the luteal phase, which was not seen in menstruating control patients.[55] In a study by Stavrou and Wood,[56] flicker perimetry appeared to be more sensitive than static perimetry in documenting early visual field changes in diabetic retinopathy, especially in a region of clinically significant diabetic macular edema.

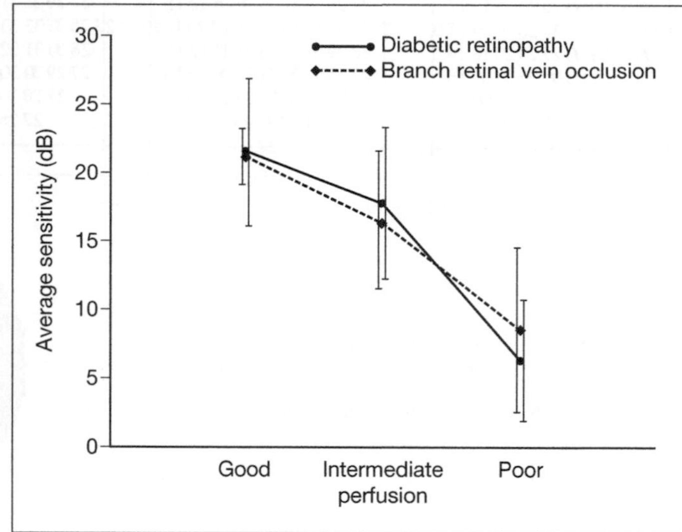

Fig. 12.14 Average sensitivity of the retina decreases with decreasing perfusion, both for diabetic retinopathy (dots) and for branch retinal vein occlusion (diamonds). (Reproduced with permission from Bell JA, Feldon SE. Retinal microangiopathy: correlation of Octopus perimetry with fluorescein angiography. Arch Ophthalmol 1984;102:1294–8.)

In instances of vitreous hemorrhage and tractional retinal detachment due to high-risk proliferative diabetic retinopathy, visual acuity is often dramatically improved by vitrectomy; however, severely impaired visual fields due to extensive retinal ischemia may still preclude driving.[57] Moreover, the treatment of diabetic retinopathy with either panretinal or focal photocoagulation may produce visual field defects, a fact that should be considered in overall patient management.[58,59] In a study by Zingirian and colleauges,[60] isolated photocoagulation of diabetic retinopathy results in small scotomata that are difficult to isolate by kinetic perimetry. Confluent lesions measuring one to two disc diameters cause correspondingly sized scotomata with sloping margins. Panretinal photocoagulation produces a marked concentric contraction of the visual field. Yoon et al.[61] demonstrate preservation of retinal sensitivity in central visual field after panretinal photocoagulation in diabetic patients. At 1 week after treatment, there is significant depression, but recovery of up to 95% occurred within the ensuing 3 months. They attribute these encouraging findings to the use of burn sizes of 200 μm or less, as recommended by Hulbert and Vernon.[62]

Using automated perimetry, an initial loss of sensitivity seen after grid laser for diabetic macular edema was seen followed by improvement.[63] Hudson and colleagues[64] followed 24 diabetic patients with macular edema before grid laser treatment and up to 12 weeks following treatment with microperimetry. They found correlation between the edema index and visual function in some, but not all, patients. In another study of 30 patients, 8 eyes remained stable, 15 improved mean deviation after treatment, and laser scars corresponded to marked loss of function.[65]

Thus, retinal sensitivity tested by microperimetry appears to increase after micropulse diode laser, but to decrease after modified Early Treatment Diabetic Retinopathy Study focal laser in eyes with clinically significant diabetic macular edema. These perimetric changes are observed even though there is no difference in visual acuity or retinal thickness after either treatment.[66] Recent studies highlight associations between morphological and functional alterations in diabetic macular edema using microperimetry. Microperimetry sensitivities are reduced in eyes with diabetic macular edema, and direct correlations have been made between decreased microperimetry sensitivity and increased cystoid edema, as evidenced by OCT and increased fundus autofluorescence.[67–70]

Other vascular diseases and nondiabetic macular edema

Many other vascular abnormalities of the choroid and retina have been evaluated with perimetry. For example, visual field defects corresponded to retinal vascular occlusions in sickle-cell disease.[71] GVF perimetry showed a slight constriction of peripheral visual fields, thought to be visually insignificant, a decade after diode laser retinal ablative therapy for retinopathy of prematurity. This field construction was similar to peripheral field changes observed years after cryotherapy for retinopathy of prematurity.[72] Mean deviation improvement recorded with automated static Octopus 500 perimetry was noted following carotid endarterectomy for clinically significant carotid stenosis.[73]

Microperimetry has been used to document functional improvement with resolution of absolute scotomata and improvement in vision to baseline in the setting of Purtscher's retinopathy after treatment with oral steroids.[74] Recovery of visual field loss was also seen using HVF and microperimetry after central and branch artery occlusions.[75,76] In addition, greater decrease in scotopic macular sensitivity was shown with microperimetry fine matrix mapping of the macula in eyes with type 2 idiopathic macular telangiectasia. In similar eyes, Wong and colleagues[77] demonstrated correlations between microperimetry sensitivities, OCT retinal morphology, and fundus autofluorescence.

After injection of intravitreal triamcinolone for treatment of branch retinal vein occlusion, improvement in macular sensitivity by microperimetry correlates with improvement in macular edema.[78] According to the Branch Vein Occlusion Study guidelines, microperimetry is useful in assessing the benefit of laser treatment. Regression of the scotoma from the foveal avascular zone is observed in one-third of patients, but in one-half of treated patients an increase in total scotoma size occurs.[79] In branch vein occlusions, Bell and Feldon[11] show good correlation between residual capillary perfusion and threshold retinal sensitivity (Figs 12.14 and 12.15).

Visual fields may effectively document the effects of treatments for CRVO.[80] For instance, microperimetry improves central fixation and retinal sensitivity following resolution of

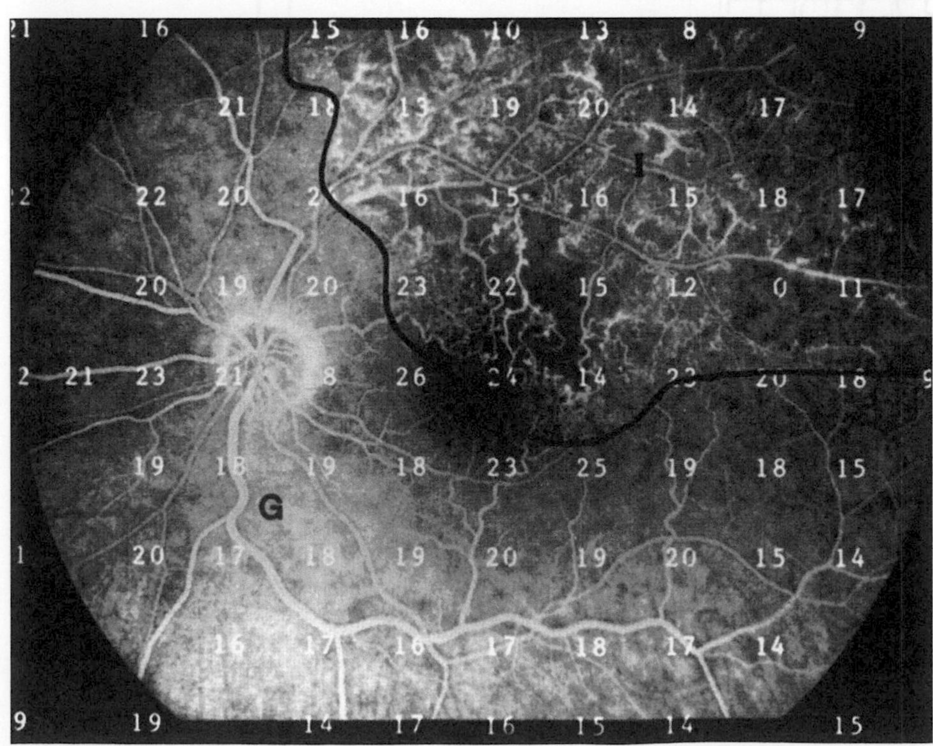

Fig. 12.15 Fluorescein angiogram from a patient with a superior branch retinal vein occlusion. Retinal sensitivities from Octopus perimetry are superimposed to show depressed function in the area of intermediate retinal perfusion (I). G, Area of good perfusion. (Reproduced with permission from Bell JA, Feldon SE. Retinal microangiopathy: correlation of Octopus perimetry with fluorescein angiography. Arch Ophthalmol 1984;102:1294–8.)

macular edema due to CRVO after treatment with intravitreal triamcinolone acetonide. Though microperimetry shows a benefit in macular function and field after radial optic neurotomy for CRVO, according to Tsujikawa and colleages,[81] persistent peripheral field defects are documented by full-field perimetry corresponding to the incision site on the optic nerve head in similar eyes with CRVO that underwent the same treatment.[82]

Metamorphopsia on Amsler grid testing is characteristic of central serous retinopathy, but there is an accompanying mild central depression which varies in size from 2 to 5° (Fig. 12.16). The scotoma is usually substantially larger using SWAP relative to that detected with white-on-white perimetry.[83] HVF and microperimetry central retinal sensitivity is reduced as subretinal fluid in central serous retinopathy increases, documented by OCT.[84,85] Even after resolution of edema, the majority of patients have residual Amsler and perimetric defects[86–88] (Fig. 12.17). Similar changes may result from other causes of fluid accumulation in the macula, such as diabetic retinopathy, Irvine–Gass syndrome, trauma (Berlin's edema), and retinal vasculitis.[3,89]

Age-related macular degeneration and other maculopathies

Macular drusen are not usually associated with any reduction of retinal sensitivity using standard techniques. However, in a prospective study using SWAP, the mean sensitivity of patients with soft drusen and early AMD is significantly lower compared to patients without drusen.[90,91] In this study the presence or absence of focal hyperpigmentation does not affect mean sensitivity. Microperimetry of macular drusen shows decreased overlying sensitivity in some, but not all, studies.[92,93] Microperimetry is used to assess retinal sensitivities for a variety of other diseases affecting retinal function in the macula, including X-linked retinoschisis, S-cone syndrome, retinopathy of membranoproliferative glomerulonephritis type II, and atrophic maculopathy associated with spinocerebellar ataxia type 7.[94–97]

AMD of the pigmentary type usually causes irregularly shaped central scotomata with sloping margins and variable density. Field defects may be bilateral but often are asymmetric. Microperimetry retinal sensitivity correlates with alterations in fundus autofluorescence even in early stages of AMD.[98] Perimetry is also used to evaluate macular retinal sensitivity after novel treatments for nonexudative AMD.[99–101]

Disciform subfoveal scarring from subretinal neovascularization, hemorrhage, and gliosis due to exudative AMD causes a dense central scotoma,[3] as shown in Fig. 12.18. Detailed studies of subfoveal choroidal neovascularization in exudative AMD have been performed by microperimetry (Fig. 12.19). Of 179 eyes evaluated by Fujii and colleagues,[102] 135 (75%) had central fixation, 42% had stable fixation, and in 28% there was a dense central scotoma. The authors found that both central and stable fixation deteriorated over time. These fixational patterns were felt to be important in the selection of patients for macular translocation surgery.[103] When microperimetry was utilized to

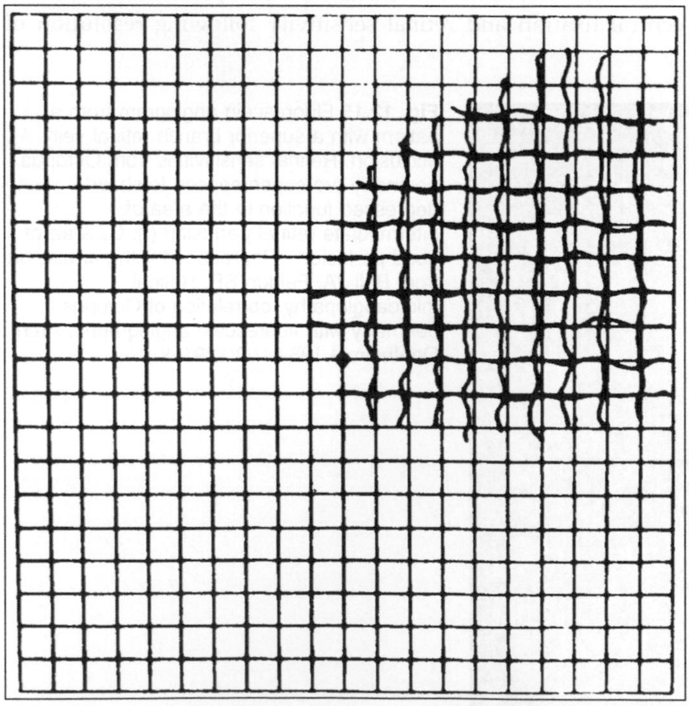

Fig. 12.16 An Amsler grid from a patient with long-standing metamorphopsia caused by central serous retinopathy. (Reproduced with permission from Natsikos VE, Hart JCD. Static perimetric and Amsler chart changes in patients with idiopathic central serous retinopathy. Acta Ophthalmol 1980;58:908–17.)

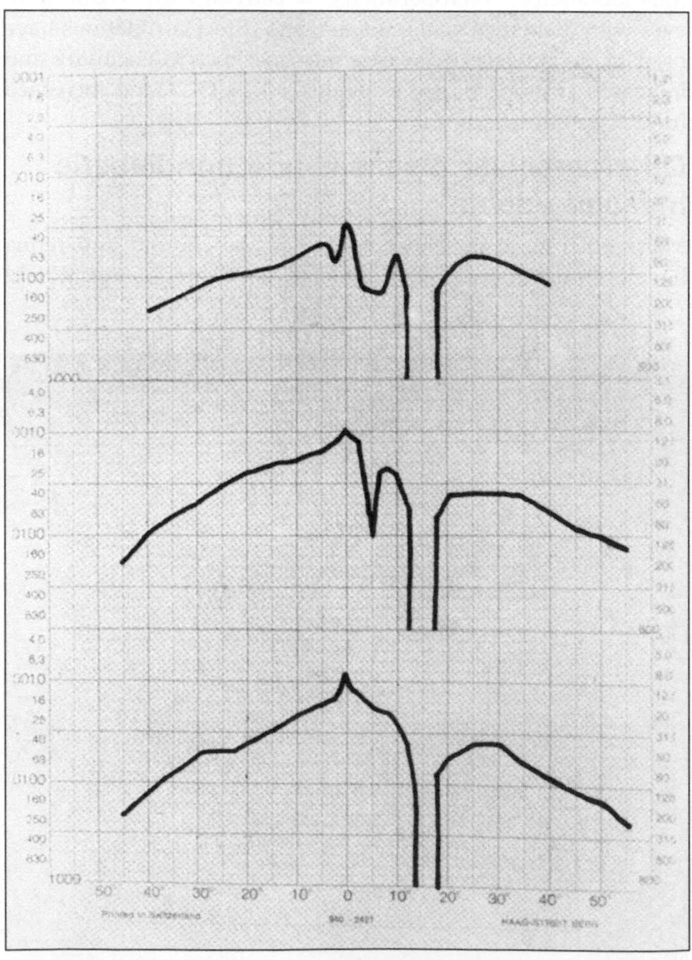

Fig. 12.17 A set of Tübinger static perimetric profiles showing pattern of recovery over 7 months in a patient with central serous retinopathy. (Reproduced with permission from Natsikos VE, Hart JCD. Static perimetric and Amsler chart changes in patients with idiopathic central serous retinopathy. Acta Ophthalmol 1980;58:908–17.)

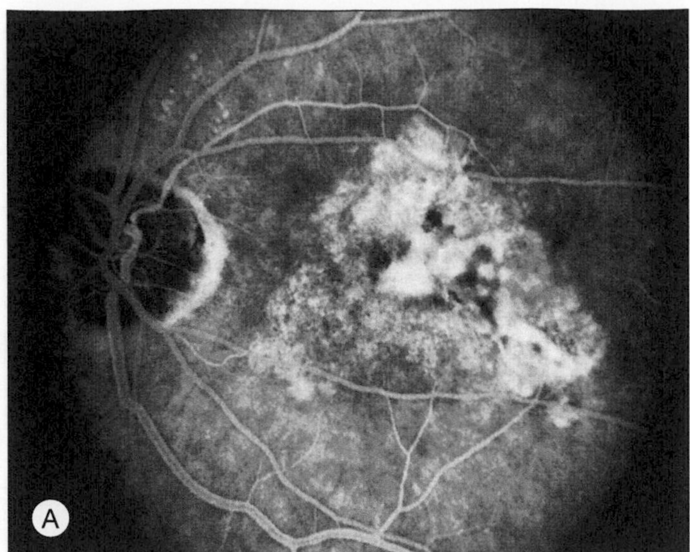

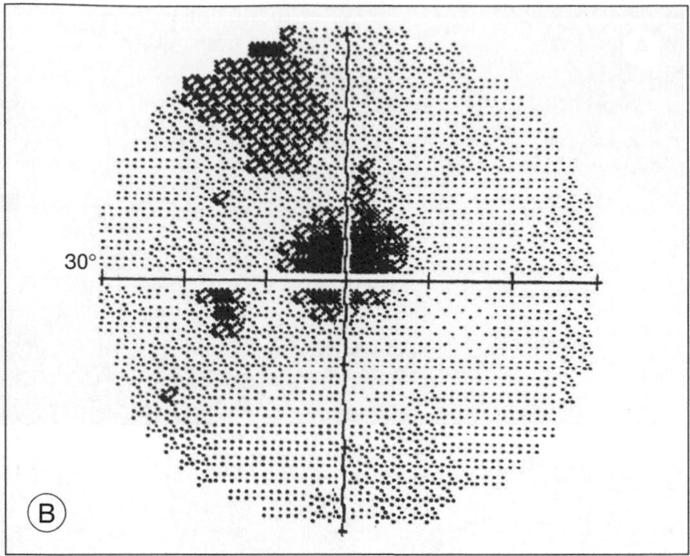

Fig. 12.18 (A) Fluorescein angiogram of a 60-year-old patient referred for evaluation of transient right homonymous hemianopia documents disciform macular degeneration of the left eye. (B) Dense central scotoma corresponding to the fundus lesion is shown by gray-scale printout from Humphrey perimeter (program 30–2).

evaluate the anatomic abnormalities associated with an absolute scotoma in subfoveal choroidal neovascularization, Tezel and associates found that the relative risk (RR) was highest in areas of chorioretinal scar (RR = 107.61) compared to areas of RPE atrophy (RR = 9.97), subretinal hemorrhage (RR = 2.88), and neovascular membrane (RR = 1.86).[104] The majority of patients with stable fixation preferred an area of RPE hyperplasia. Using the HVF macular threshold protocol, improvement in macular visual field sensitivity occurred after treatment with intravitreal bevacizumab for exudative AMD, even in cases where visual acuity has not improved.[105] Microperimetry has shown similar improvement in central retinal sensitivity after intravitreal ranibizumab treatment for exudative AMD.[106,107] HVF 10-2 and microperimetry have also demonstrated improvements in macular visual fields after photodynamic therapy for exudative AMD and subfoveal polypoidal choroidal vasculopathy.[108–110] Microperimetry has also been used to assess retinal sensitivity after autologous RPE choroid graft for exudative AMD.[111]

Patients with AMD or other macular pathology are routinely instructed to monitor their visual field in each eye with an Amsler grid regularly. Comparison of the original white lines on a black background Amsler grid proved to be superior at detecting metamorphopsia and central vision changes than the modified grid, which displays black lines on a white background.[112] This is likely because of the increased contrast provided by the white lines on black background. However, due to ease in photocopying, the grid with black lines on a white background is most commonly used in the office setting and provided to patients for home use.

With the increasing prevalence of AMD and the ability to treat early neovascular AMD effectively, new perimetric tests that allow for patient self-monitoring of visual fields are being devised to detect early deficits. Nazemi and colleagues[113] developed a three-dimensional automated computer-based threshold Amsler grid test that maps the visual field and records steep slopes in areas of nonexudative AMD and shallow slopes in regions corresponding to exudative AMD. As discussed at the beginning of this chapter, the psychophysical property of hyperacuity has been used to develop a device which detects progressive maculopathy and the early onset of exudative disease in AMD.[114,115] The device, PreView PHP (Carl Zeiss Meditec, Dublin, CA), was evaluated as a home-based device in a multicenter trial and found to have a sensitivity and specificity of 85% to detect alterations in hyperacuity corresponding to exudative and intermediate nonexudative AMD.[17] Other home-based perimetric devices for patients to monitor their vision routinely are expected in the near future. With the development of better algorithms to detect early disease progression, these home devices will hopefully ensure timely sight-saving treatment.

Macular holes and epiretinal membrane

Cysts may develop in the macula without producing appreciable scotomata. Macular holes, however, result in dense scotomata with steep margins (Figs 12.20 and 12.21). Microperimetry may be helpful in predicting the outcome of macular hole surgery. In a study by Amari and associates, visual outcome correlated with the maximum sensitivity adjacent to the hole.[116] In another study, absolute scotomata disappeared completely in 18 of 28 eyes that achieved complete closure, became relative in five of six eyes with partial closure, and remained absolute in four eyes with atrophic closure.[117] Ozedemir and colleagues[118] suggested that MP-1 microperimetry may be more sensitive than visual acuity in measuring retinal function following closure of a macular hole with pars plana vitrectomy and internal limiting membrane (ILM) peeling. Increases in retinal sensitivity by microperimetry have also been correlated with the degree of fundus autofluorescence after macular hole closure.[119] Perimetry has also been used to evaluate visual fields in eyes with epiretinal membrane (ERM). Binocular correspondence perimetry, a method akin to PHP, but which uses the principle of retinal correspondence and requires binocular testing, was used to quantify metamorphopsia in eyes with ERM.[120] This study demonstrated focal areas of abnormal retinal correspondence in eyes with ERM compared to the normal fellow eye. Increased microperimetry retinal sensitivity

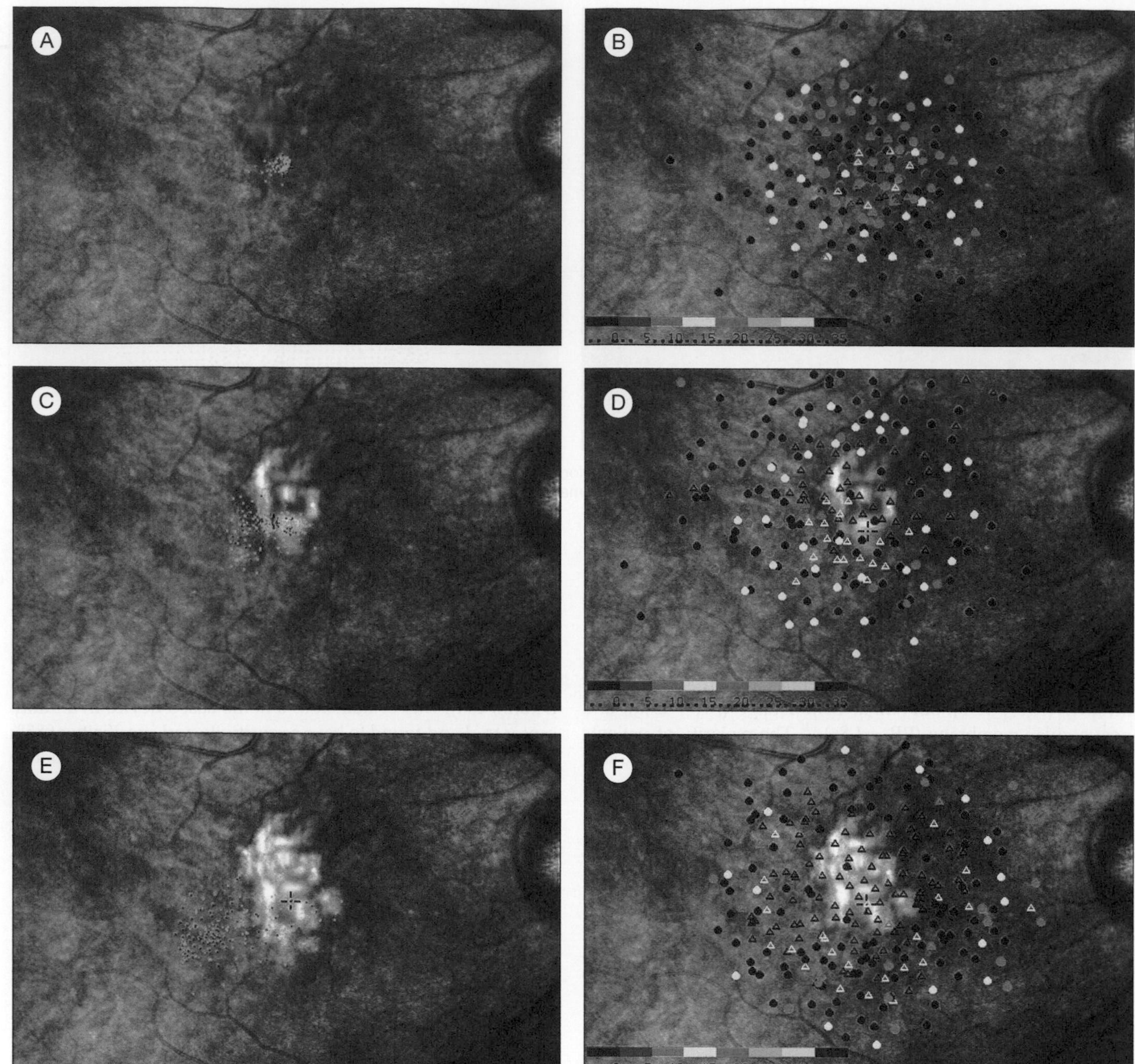

Fig. 12.19 A sequence of scanning laser ophthalmoscope (SLO) microperimetry shows the progressive functional deterioration in one eye with subfoveal choroidal neovascularization (CNV) secondary to age-related macular degeneration (AMD). The SLO testing demonstrated that eyes with subfoveal CNV secondary to AMD experienced a predictable and progressive loss of fixation stability, decreased central retinal sensitivity, and loss of central fixation location. A 65-year-old man presented with 20/150 vision and a 1-month history of decreased vision due to a predominantly classic subfoveal CNV secondary to AMD. (A) The SLO testing performed at presentation disclosed a pattern of predominantly central and stable fixation. (B) The balls indicate the areas where the patient could perceive the stimulus; the triangles indicate the areas where the patient could not perceive the stimulus. Each ball and triangle is color-coded to indicate the intensity of the stimulus. The SLO microperimetry also showed a mild decrease in central retinal sensitivity. The patient elected not to receive any treatment and had a follow-up visit 4 months after initial visual symptoms. (C) An SLO test was performed and demonstrated that the fixation pattern became poor central and relatively unstable. (D) The microperimetry also showed that retinal sensitivity was markedly affected with some central areas of dense scotoma. Best-corrected visual acuity at this visit was 20/200. Twelve months after onset of initial visual symptoms and no treatment, SLO microperimetry was performed and disclosed further functional deterioration. (E) The fixation became predominantly eccentric and unstable. (F) Retinal sensitivity testing demonstrated a large central area of dense central scotoma. (Reproduced with permission from Wong WT, Kam W, Cunnigham D, et al. Treatment of geographic atrophy by the topical administration of OT-551: results of a phase II clinical trial. Invest Ophthalmol Vis Sci 2010;51:6131–9.)

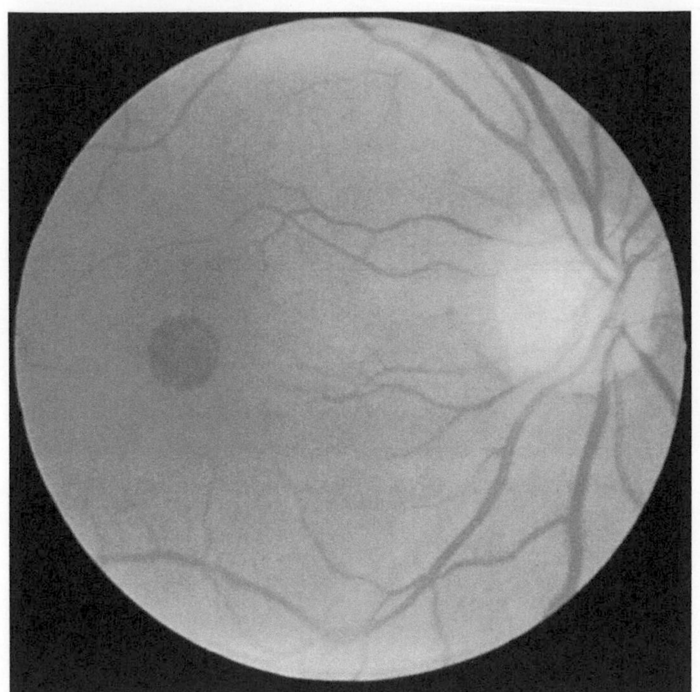

Fig. 12.20 Fundus photograph of an eye with a full-thickness macular hole. The visual field defect is shown in Fig. 12.21.

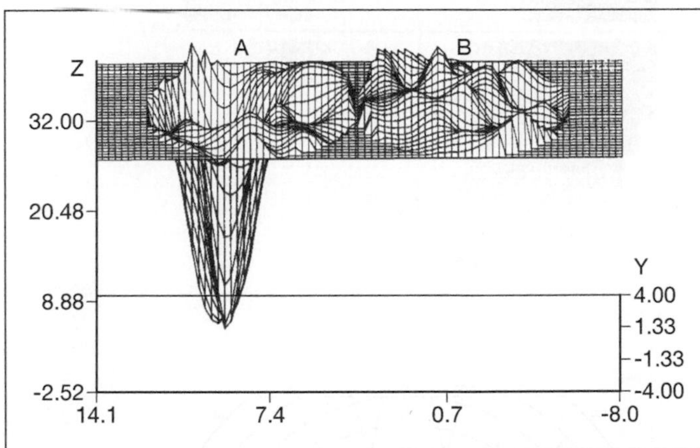

Fig. 12.21 Three-dimensional reconstruction of high-density macular grid (1° spacing) documenting steep absolute central scotoma of the left eye (A) and unaffected right eye (B). Retinal sensitivity is noted on the vertical axis and position is noted on the horizontal axis. (Copyright 1983, Wesley K. Herman, MD and Joseph M. DeFaller, Alcon Laboratories, Inc. Courtesy of Dr Herman.)

without change in metamorphopsia as quantified by PHP following vitreoretinal surgery for ERM and macular hole was reported by Richter-Mueksch and colleagues.[121]

After uncomplicated repair of macular holes and ERM and using pars plana vitrectomy and ILM peeling, several investigators reported a high incidence of peripheral field defects infringing on the central visual field[122–128] (Fig. 12.22). A majority of studies documented postoperative field defects only after patients complained of perceived field loss. Tsuiki and colleagues[129] specifically compared pre- and postoperative GVF tests and found new peripheral field defects in 17 of 140 eyes postoperatively. In the majority of eyes, indocyanine green (ICG) was used to enhance visualization of the ILM during peeling. In vitro studies demonstrated the toxicity of ICG exposure to human retinal cell lines.[130] The postsurgical visual defects are probably due to: (1) toxic effects of ICG; (2) alterations in the retina, such as damage to the peripapillary nerve fibers, during the pars plana vitrectomy; or (3) mechanical damage incurred with peeling of the ILM. Damage to the nerve fiber layer from intraocular gas tamponade in cases of macular hole repair must also be considered.[121] Further studies that systematically and more accurately compare pre- and postoperative visual fields in eyes undergoing retinal surgery are needed to understand better the effects of the procedure and the adjuvant dyes or agents used to assist in the procedure on visual function.

Toxic retinopathies

Toxic maculopathy is epitomized by chloroquine and hydroxychloroquine retinopathy. The most characteristic field defect caused by macular involvement is a ring-like central scotoma with a small island of slightly less visual loss in its center, commonly referred to as a "bull's eye" (Fig. 12.23).[131] GVF and HVF perimetry document visual field changes that can persist and worsen for decades even after stopping the medicines.[132–134] Threshold Amsler grid testing, which uses variable light transmission through two cross-polarizing filters, and PHP hyperacuity may be useful in screening for early functional changes due to chloroquine and hydroxychloroquine.[135,136]

To screen for chloroquine and hydroxychloroquine toxicity HVF, 10-2 white-on-white protocol is recommended. mERG is a helpful adjunct when early perimetric changes are seen, but may not be readily available in all retina practices. Recent screening guidelines advocate the addition of high-resolution imaging, such as spectral domain OCT and fundus autofluorescence, to correlate functional changes with structural alterations in the photoreceptor and RPE layers.[137] In concert with other testing modalities, early perimetric changes that may be nonspecific for macular toxicity can be validated to allow for timely changes in medication with ultimate preservation of vision.

A number of medications are associated with retinal toxicity resulting in visual field loss. Thioridazine, a phenothiazine derivative, is a cause of pigmented maculopathy with associated central scotoma. Even in the absence of clinical tamoxifen retinopathy, SWAP fields show depressed mean deviations which correlated with duration of therapy.[138] Peripheral visual field loss is detected in about 30% of patients using the antiepileptic drug vigabatrin.[139–142] Sildenafil (Viagra) has been associated with nonarteritic ischemic optic neuropathy in individuals with pre-existing cardiovascular disease.[143] Although visual field defects can occur in these cases, sildenafil has not been proven to cause retinal toxicity.[144]

Infectious and inflammatory retinopathies

Infectious and inflammatory retinopathies exhibit visual field defects corresponding to the area of pathology. Toxoplasmosis commonly produces focal chorioretinal destruction that causes corresponding dense, irregular, steep-margined, isolated scotomata.[145] More disseminated types of inflammation, such as syphilitic choroiditis, produce a more diffuse depression of visual field function. In a patient with idiopathic retinal vasculitis, the inferior arcuate field defect corresponds to leakage from the superior temporal branch vein (Fig. 12.24). One unusual case report describes the use of microperimetry to determine the focal visual loss associated with nematode-induced unilateral subacute neuroretinitis.[146]

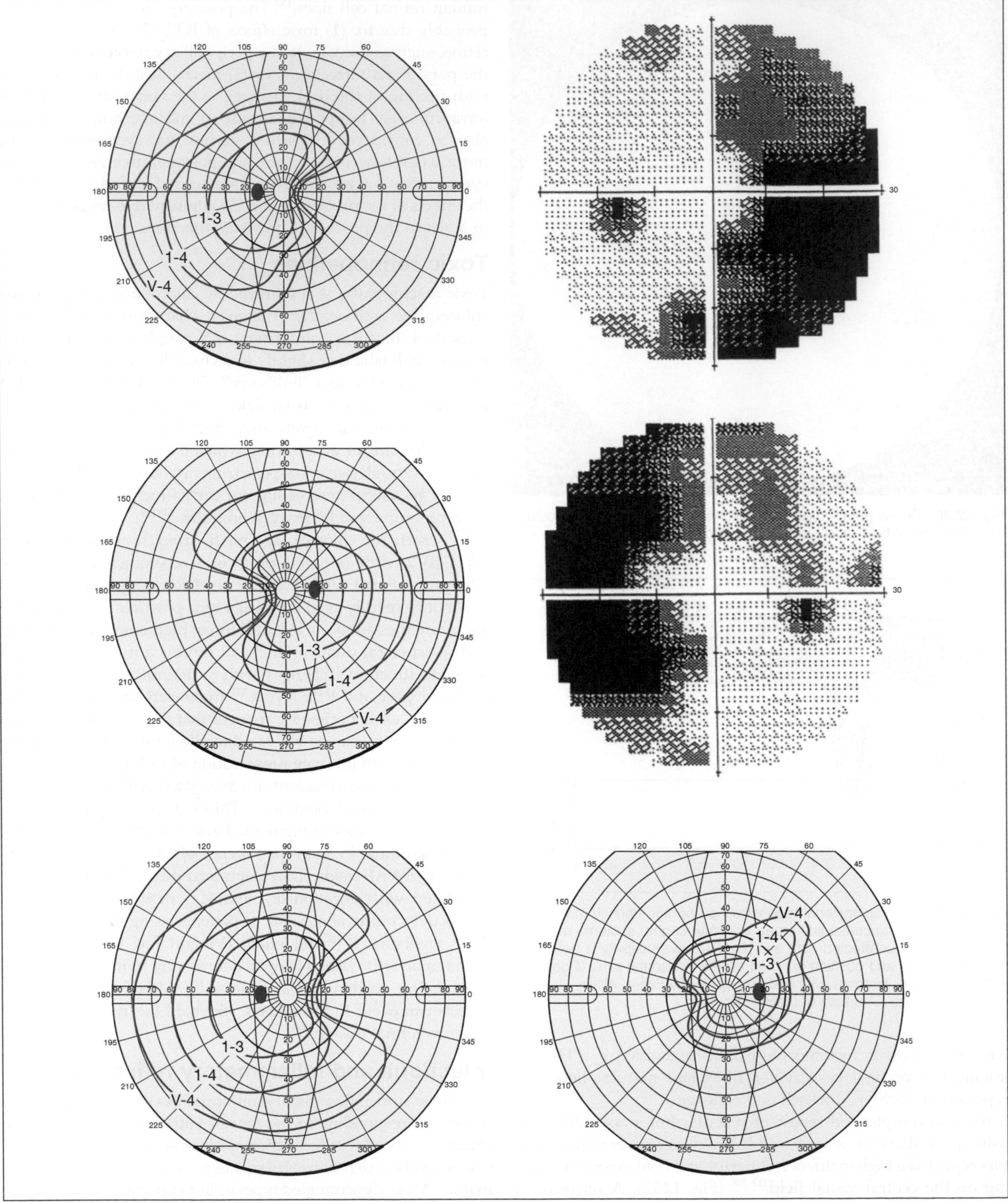

Fig. 12.22 Goldmann and Humphrey 30–2 visual field perimetry depicting peripheral wedge-like visual field loss encroaching on the central visual field in the eyes of 3 patients after pars plana vitrectomy, internal limiting membrane (ILM) peeling assisted by indocyanine green staining of the ILM for external limiting membrane. (Reproduced with permission from von Jagow B, Hoing A, Gandorfer A, et al. Functional outcome of indocyanine green-assisted macular surgery: 7-year follow-up. Retina 2009;29:1249–56.)

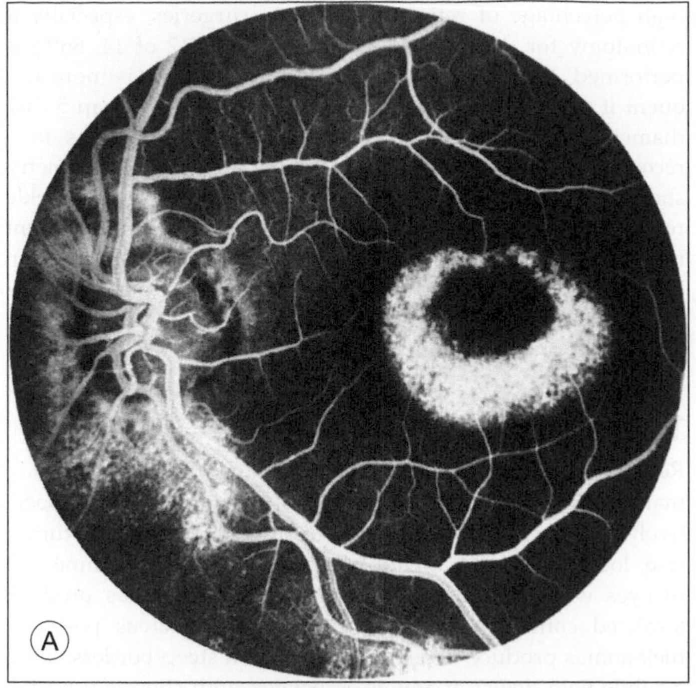

0.0	4.3	13.5	11.2	2.5	5.5
6.5	3.8	8.5	2.5	5.5	3.0
6.5		11.5		8.5	
3.5	9.2	20.5	19.5	19.5	16.8
11.5	4.9	17.5		17.5	3.1
12.5		20.5		13.5	
16.5	18.8	14.5	17.8	22.5	23.8
19.5	1.7	16.5	1.7	23.5	1.5
19.5		22.5		25.5	

Fluctuations (RMS): 3.1 DB Lum interval: 2

B

Fig. 12.23 (A) Fluorescein angiogram of a patient with perifoveal atrophy of the pigment epithelium corresponding to a bull's eye maculopathy, typical of chloroquine retinopathy. (B) Central retinal sensitivities (Octopus program 11) at 3° spacing show depression superiorly and temporally, corresponding to areas of fluorescein angiogram with more marked depigmentation of the macula. Each cluster of five numbers represents a single test location. The three numbers at the left of each cluster are independently determined thresholds. The number at the upper right in each cluster is the mean of the three thresholds. The number at the lower right in each cluster is the standard deviation of the mean threshold value. (Reproduced with permission from Feldon SE. Computerized perimetry in selected disorders of the retina. In: Whalen WR, Spaeth GL, editors. Computerized visual fields: what they are and how to use them. Thorofare, NJ: Slack, 1985.)

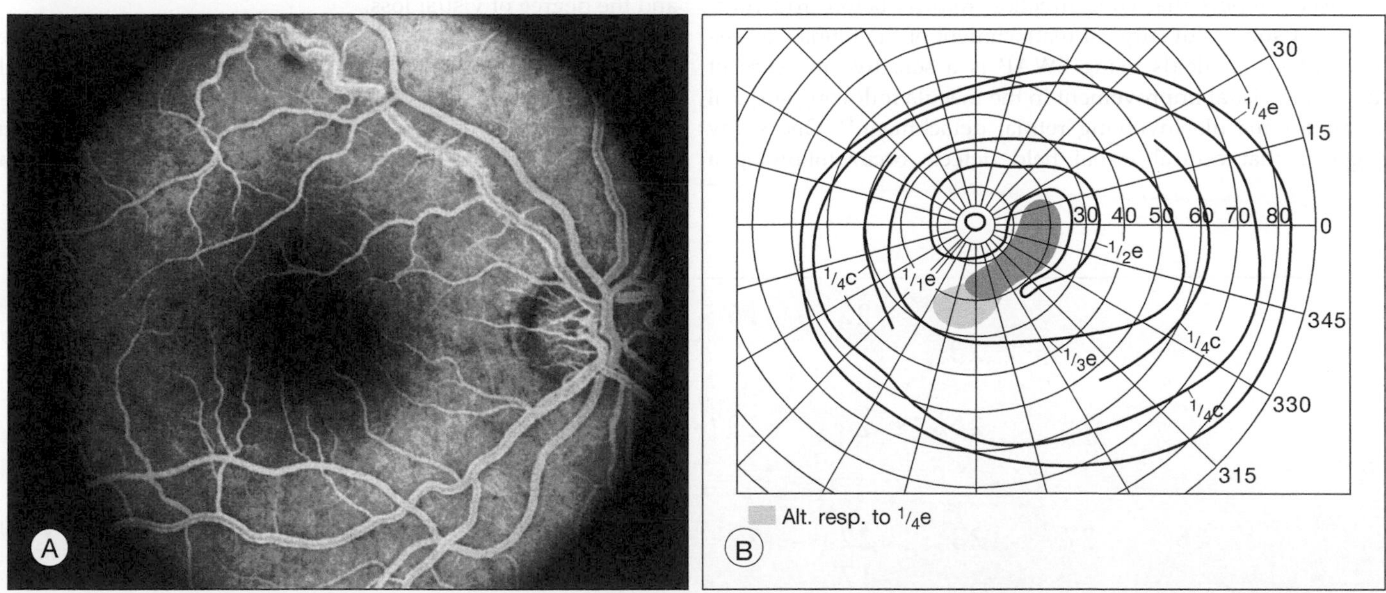

Fig. 12.24 (A) Fluorescein angiogram from a patient with idiopathic retinal vasculitis demonstrates leakage from the superotemporal retinal branch vein of the right eye. (B) Goldmann perimetry shows an inferior arcuate field defect that corresponds to the affected region of the retina.

Even in patients with no clinically evident infectious retinopathy, human immunodeficiency virus (HIV)-positive patients demonstrated significant localized as well as mean defects. These defects were more apparent in SWAP than in white-on-white automated perimetry.[147] Correlation of HVF perimetry with mERG in similar eyes demonstrated involvement of the inner retina and sparing of the outer retina.[148] Perimetric changes may also be related to HIV-related brain dysfunction.[149] More marked changes in retinal sensitivity have been found in HIV-positive patients with low CD4 counts.[149]

In a small case series of patients with multiple evanescent white-dot syndrome, areas of decreased microperimetric sensitivity were shown to correlate with focal regions of inner and outer photoreceptor segment disruption documented by spectral domain OCT. Both the microperimetry and OCT findings changed location in keeping with the resolution and presence of new lesions during the disease course, and returned to normal by the end of clinical recovery.[150,151] Similar correlation between function and structure was seen in eyes with acute posterior multifocal placoid pigment epitheliopathy.[152] Microperimetry retinal sensitivity was also found to correlate with visual acuity in both serpiginous choroiditis and birdshot chorioretinopathy. Gordon and colleagues[153] documented and analyzed HVF in patients with birdshot chorioretinopathy, in an attempt to determine characteristic patterns of field loss. The visual fields of this small series of patients exhibited diffuse loss, central sparing, and blind-spot enlargement. In addition, assessment of outcomes after valacyclovir treatment for acute zonal occult outer retinopathy using GVF demonstrated improved peripheral visual function.[154]

Retinal detachment

Typically, rhegmatogenous retinal detachments have sloping isopters on kinetic perimetry. Occasionally, this feature helps to differentiate a retinal detachment from a retinoschisis, which is characterized by dense defects with steep margins, usually located supranasally. However, long-standing retinal detachments may develop steep isopters. In the case of a shallow detachment, assessment of the visual field may be more accurate than ophthalmoscopy in identifying the border of detached retina.[3]

If the detachment is long-standing, recovery of visual field sensitivity is incomplete.[155] Performing visual fields under conditions of both light and dark adaptation, Alexandridis and Janzarik[156] report that cone function returns before rod function after successful surgical reattachment of the retina. Assessment of visual fields using SWAP is a sensitive measure of functional visual improvement in the macula following surgical repair for macula involving retinal detachment.[157] One study suggests that central visual field defects occur following a high percentage of retinal detachment surgeries, especially if retinotomy for drainage of subretinal fluid (12 of 14, 86%) is performed. In this study, risk of visual field loss is more frequent if the retinotomy is relatively posterior (less than 5 disc diameters from fixation).[158] Although visual field loss may recover initially after retinal detachment repair, GVF perimetry shows persistent decreased visual field following scleral buckle repair of retinal detachment despite continued improvement in visual acuity.[159] In a recent report, microperimetry used in conjunction with spectral domain OCT and fundus autofluorescence demonstrates good correlation of visual function with retinal morphology after rhegmatogenous retinal detachment repair.[160]

Tumors

Retinoblastoma and choroidal melanoma are the most common malignant intraocular tumors in children and adults respectively. Long-term visual field defects that correspond to tumor size, location, and treatment modality have been documented in eyes with retinoblastoma.[161] Anterior melanomas produce localized constriction of the visual field, whereas posterior melanomas produce dense scotomata with steep borders. Only a subtle field defect, if any, is associated with choroidal nevus. Thus fields may be important in distinguishing between these entities.

In Fig. 12.25 the Octopus visual field is superimposed on the fundus photograph of a patient with a small melanoma of the posterior pole. In this instance, loss of sensitivity is found only in the center of the mass. Use of a finer grid pattern would have facilitated a better correlation between the pathologic process and the degree of visual loss.

Like melanomas, choroidal metastases also produce dense scotomata with steep borders. However, in a study by Rahhal and colleagues,[162] HVF depression does not consistently correspond with tumor size or location. The visual fields shown in Fig. 12.26 are obtained from a patient with breast carcinoma

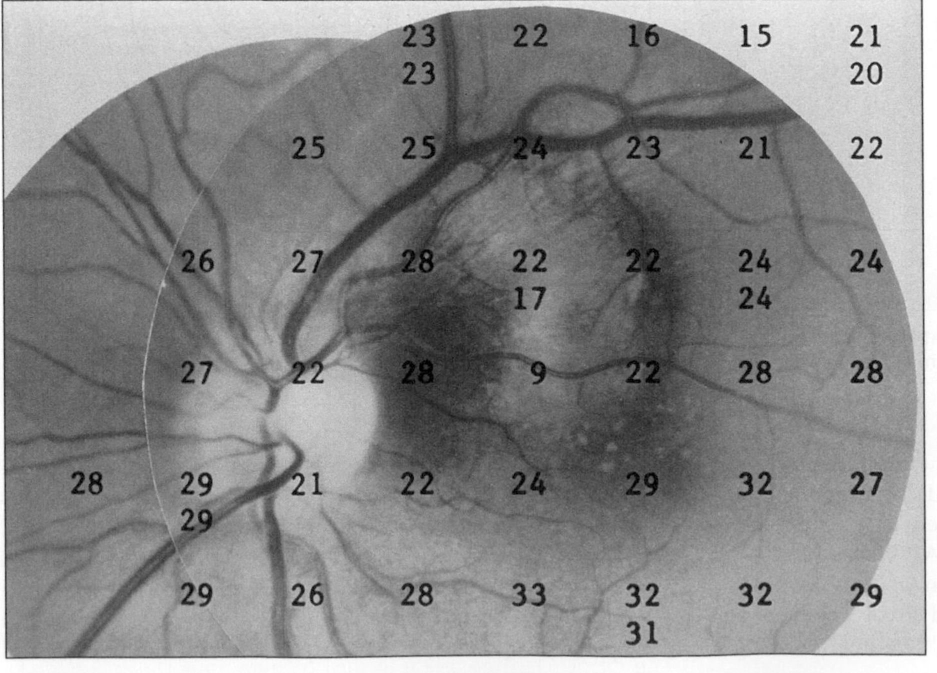

Fig. 12.25 A fundus photograph of a patient with a small malignant melanoma of the posterior pole has been superimposed on the visual field obtained by Octopus perimetry. Because of the relatively coarse (6°) grid pattern of the perimeter, sensitivity is markedly reduced only at the center of the lesion. (Reproduced with permission from Feldon SE. Computerized perimetry in selected disorders of the retina. In: Whalen WR, Spaeth GL, editors. Computerized visual fields: what they are and how to use them. Thorofare, NJ: Slack, 1985.)

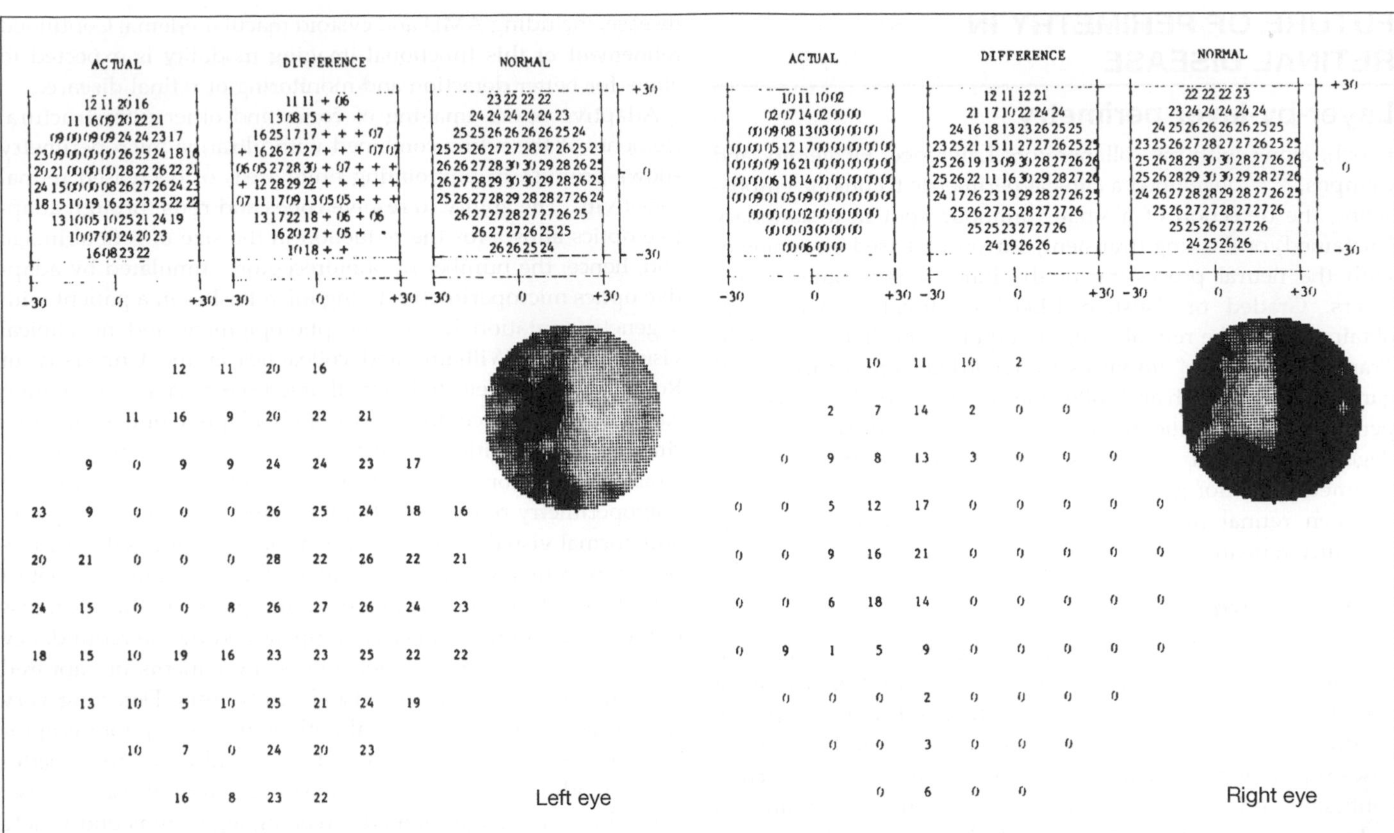

Fig. 12.26 Octopus perimetry (program 32) on the same patient as in Fig. 12.27. An inferonasal field defect in the right eye corresponds to the choroidal metastasis. There is also an unexpected dense bitemporal hemianopsia. A computed tomographic scan was requested for further evaluation. (Reproduced with permission from Feldon SE. Computerized perimetry in selected disorders of the retina. In: Whalen WR, Spaeth GL, editors. Computerized visual fields: what they are and how to use them. Thorofare, NJ: Slack, 1985.)

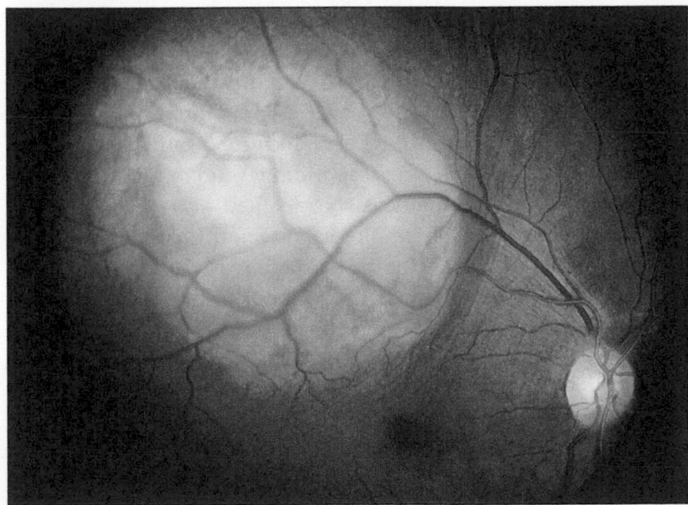

Fig. 12.27 A 50-year-old patient with known breast carcinoma is referred for evaluation of a mass in the posterior pole of the right eye. The visual fields are shown in Fig. 12.26. (Reproduced with permission from Feldon SE. Computerized perimetry in selected disorders of the retina. In: Whalen WR, Spaeth GL, editors. Computerized visual fields: what they are and how to use them. Thorofare, NJ: Slack, 1985.)

whose fundus photograph is shown in Fig. 12.27. This patient demonstrates not only a dense inferonasal field defect corresponding to the choroidal metastasis, but also a bitemporal field defect. Subsequent CT scan demonstrated a suprasellar mass consistent with either a pituitary adenoma or metastasis (Fig. 12.28).

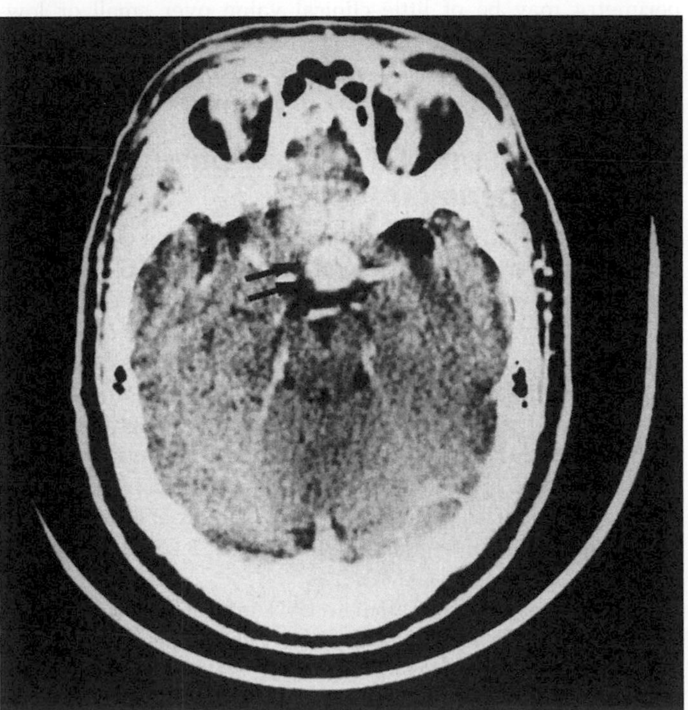

Fig. 12.28 Computed tomographic scan from the patient whose visual field and fundus photograph are shown in Figs 12.26 and 12.27. A suprasellar mass is shown that is consistent with either pituitary tumor or metastasis. (Reproduced with permission from Feldon SE. Computerized perimetry in selected disorders of the retina. In: Whalen WR, Spaeth GL, editors. Computerized visual fields: what they are and how to use them. Thorofare, NJ: Slack, 1985.)

FUTURE OF PERIMETRY IN RETINAL DISEASE

Layer-by-layer perimetry

Enoch, along with his collaborators Lawrence, Fitzgerald, and Campos,[163-165] developed a clinical perimetric technique emphasizing the detection of a small luminous spot in a stationary (sustained) or flashing (transient) surround, based on analogies with the neural processing of the inner versus outer retinal layers. Graded or "sustained-like" electrical responses are obtained from the retinal receptor, bipolar, and horizontal cells. Transient or "spike" impulses are recorded from amacrine and ganglion cells. Enoch and colleagues investigated layer-by-layer perimetry in diabetic retinopathy, macular drusen, macular degeneration, and angioid streaks. However, layer-by-layer perimetry has not gained clinical acceptance. The relationship between retinal function and the testing parameters of this modality remains unconfirmed.

Color perimetry

Assessment of color vision may be helpful in screening for retinal disease and in separating neural from retinal causes of visual loss. Acquired diseases of the retina and choroid typically produce a tritan-like pattern of color confusion, and neural diseases typically produce a protan or deutan-like pattern of color confusion on Farnsworth–Munsell 100-hue discrimination testing.[166] Thus color perimetry might be used to advantage in the identification and quantitative description of certain retinal and choroidal diseases. Although color contrast might be more sensitive in finding visual field defects, Hart and Burde[167] demonstrate that colored test objects used in standard techniques of perimetry may be of little clinical value over small or low-contrast white test objects for detecting scotomata in a number of optic nerve and retinal disorders. Currently, there is no commercially available, standardized color perimeter.

High-resolution OCT and adaptive optics with microperimetry

Although innovative, both layer-by-layer and color perimetry do not appear to add new basic or clinical information relevant to the etiology, localization, or treatment of retinal diseases beyond that already available from more standard clinical tests, such as electroretinography, electro-oculography, contrast sensitivity, and fluorescein angiography. Anatomical imaging of the retina at the ultrastructural level has advanced to a high degree of sophistication, allowing correlations of structure and function at the microscopic level. Hopefully, these new research strategies will result in clinical applications that will allow earlier detection and treatment of potentially debilitating and widely prevalent retinal diseases such as AMD.

The combined spectral domain OCT and SLO, introduced in 2006 (Spectral OCT/SLO; OPKO/OTI, Miami, FL, USA) is a significant achievement in advancing retinal imaging. The enhancement in accurate and real-time image capture with this system allows for integration with microperimetry. Thus, a functional spectral OCT/SLO allows assessment of retinal morphology and function at specific retinal loci. Landa and colleagues[14] demonstrate the effectiveness of a three-dimensional spectral OCT/SLO topography and microperimetry in assessing functional and structural changes of the macula in a variety of retinal disease, including AMD and cystoid macular edema. Continued refinement of this functional imaging modality is expected to allow for better detection and monitoring of retinal disease.

Adaptive optics imaging of cones and other ultrastructural elements of the retina combined with ultrafine microperimetry shows promise in pinpointing finite areas of decreased retinal sensitivity. The ability to resolve cones and rods through adaptive optics allows for the reduction in the size of retinal image and, hence, the number of photoreceptors stimulated by adaptive optics microperimetry. Using microflashes in a patient with a genetic mutation for a cone photopigment and no clinical visual deficits, Williams and colleagues at the University of Rochester have detected retinal microscotomata representing early cone photoreceptor loss through adaptive optics microperimetry.[168] In addition, Roorda and colleagues[15] have demonstrated correlations between healthy and unhealthy RPE and microperimetry retinal sensitivity in patients with maculopathy and normal visual acuity. The precision of testing cellular function in the retina with this modality highlights its ability to detect early loss of function of a few photoreceptors. As this focal loss of retinal function is clinically compensated by the redundancy in the visual system, it is not noticed by patients or captured by standard perimetry and visual acuity tests. Detecting very early functional and structural pathology at the photoreceptor level before its clinical manifestation would allow for a better understanding of early pathophysiology and disease course. With this knowledge, refined screening algorithms and timely interventions for vision-threatening retinal disease might be developed.

CONCLUSIONS

Achromatic and static SWAP provides a cost-efficient, standardized, and reliable way to evaluate and follow visual fields in patients with retinal disease. Microperimetry seems to be a valuable clinical research tool that has been used more frequently to quantify macular function in a variety of retinal diseases. The clinical value of determining very localized retinal sensitivity and correlating it with corresponding retinal microstructure remains uncertain. Nonetheless, a detailed knowledge of how the underlying retinal pathology and morphology impact on vision is crucial in developing and delivering effective treatments for retinal disease to preserve and restore eyesight.

REFERENCES

1. Gass JDM. Steroscopic atlas of macular diseases: diagnosis and treatment. 4th ed. St Louis: Mosby; 1997.
2. Traquair HM. Introduction to clinical perimetry. London: Kimpton; 1927.
3. Harrington DO. The visual fields: a textbook and atlas of clinical perimetry. 5th ed. St Louis: Mosby; 1981.
4. Wall M, Sadun AA. Threshold Amsler grid testing: cross-polarizing lenses enhance yield. Arch Ophthalmol 1986;104:520–3.
5. Keltner JL, Johnson CA, Balestrery FG. Suprathreshold static perimetry: initial clinical trials with the Fieldmaster automated perimeter. Arch Ophthalmol 1979;97:260–72.
6. Wiggins MN, Dersu I. Understanding visual fields, part III: Which field should be performed? J Ophthalm Med Techno [Internet] 2007;3 [cited 2011 Jun 18]. Available from: www.JOMTonline.com.
7. Rohrschneider K, Becker M, Schumacher N, et al. Normal values for fundus perimetry with the scanning laser ophthalmoscope. Am J Ophthalmol 1998; 126:52–8.
8. Mojon DS, Zulauf M. Normal values of short-wavelength automated perimetry. Ophthalmologica 2003;217:260–4.
9. Zwas F, Weiss H, McKinnon P. Spectral sensitivity measurements in early diabetic retinopathy. Ophthalm Res 1980;12:87–96.
10. Wild JM, Cubbidge RP, Pacey IE, et al. Statistical aspects of the normal visual field in short-wavelength automated perimetry. Invest Ophthalmol Vis Sci 1998;39:54–63.
11. Bell JA, Feldon SE. Retinal microangiopathy: correlation of Octopus perimetry with fluorescein angiography. Arch Ophthalmol 1984;102:1294–8.

12. Rohrschneider K, Bultmann S, Springer C. Use of fundus perimetry (microperimetry) to quantify macular sensitivity. Prog Retinal Eye Res 2008;27: 536–48.
13. Rohrschneider K, Springer C, Bultmann S, et al. Microperimetry – comparison between micro perimeter 1 and scanning laser ophthalmoscope – fundus perimetry. Am J Ophthalmol 2005;139:125–34.
14. Landa G, Rosen RB, Garcia PM, et al. Combined three-dimensional spectral OCT/SLO topography and microperimetry: steps toward achieving functional spectral OCT/SLO. Ophthalm Res 2010;43:92–8.
15. Roorda A, Zhang Y, Duncan JL. High-resolution in vivo imaging of the RPE mosaic in eyes with retinal disease. Invest Ophthalmol Vis Sci 2007;48: 2297–303.
16. Winther C, Frisen L. A compact rarebit test for macular diseases. Br J Ophthalmol 2010;94:324–7.
17. Lowenstein A, Ferencz JR, Lang Y, et al. Toward earlier detection of choroidal neovascularization secondary to age-related macular degeneration. Retina 2010;30:1058–64.
18. Norden LC. Reliability in perimetry. J Am Optom Assoc 1989;60:880–90.
19. Seiple W, Clemens CJ, Greenstein VC, et al. Test–retest reliability of the multifocal electroretinogram and Humphrey visual fields in patients with retinitis pigmentosa. Doc Ophthalmol 2004;109:255–72.
20. Weingessel B, Sacu S, Vecsei-Marlovits PV, et al. Interexaminar and intraexaminer reliability of the microperimeter MP-1. Eye 2009;23:1052–8.
21. Sandberg MA, Gaudio AR, Berson EL. Disease course of patients with pericentral retinitis pigmentosa. Am J Ophthalmol 2005;140:100–6.
22. Sandberg MA, Rosner B, Weigel-DiFranco C, et al. Disease course of patients with X-linked retinitis pigmentosa due to RPGR gene mutations. Invest Ophthalmol Vis Sci 2007;48:1298–304.
23. Schwartz SB, Aleman TS, Cideciyan AV, et al. Disease expression in Usher syndrome caused by VLGR1 gene mutation (USH2C) and comparison with USH2A phenotype. Invest Ophthalmol Vis Sci 2005;46:734–43.
24. Azari AA, Aleman TS, Cideciyan AV, et al. Retinal disease expression in Bardet–Biedl syndrome-1 (BBS1) is a spectrum from maculopathy to retina-wide degeneration. Invest Ophthalmol Vis Sci 2006;47:5004–10.
25. Gerth C, Wright T, Heon E, et al. Assessment of central retinal function in patients with advanced retinitis pigmentosa. Invest Ophthalmol Vis Sci 2007; 48:1312–8.
26. Lodha N, Westall CA, Brent M, et al. A modified protocol for the assessment of visual function in patients with retinitis pigmentosa. Adv Exp Med Biol 2003;533:49–57.
27. Rotenstreich Y, Harats D, Shaish A, et al. Treatment of a retinal dystrophy, fundus albipunctatus, with oral 9-*cis*-β-carotene. Br J Ophthalmol 2010;94: 616–21.
28. Iarossi G, Falsini B, Piccardi M. Regional cone dysfunction in retinitis pigmentosa evaluated by flicker ERGs: relationship with perimetric sensitivity losses. Invest Ophthalmol Vis Sci 2003;44:866–74.
29. Fischer MD, Fleischhauer JC, Gillies MC, et al. A new method to monitor visual field defects caused by photoreceptor degeneration by quantitative optical coherence tomography. Invest Ophthalmol Vis Sci 2008;49:3617–21.
30. Rangaswamy NV, Patel HM, Locke KG, et al. A comparison of visual field sensitivity to photoreceptor thickness in retinitis pigmentosa. Invest Ophthalmol Vis Sci 2010;51:4213–9.
31. Jacobson SG, Roman AJ, Aleman TS, et al. Normal central retinal function and structure preserved in retinitis pigmentosa. Invest Ophthalmol Vis Sci 2010; 51:1079–85.
32. Aizawa S, Mitamura Y, Hagiwara A, et al. Changes of fundus autofluorescence, photoreceptor inner and outer segment junction line, and visual function in patients with retinitis pigmentosa. Clin Exp Ophthalmol 2010;38: 597–604.
33. Genead MA, Fishman GA, Stone EM, et al. The natural history of Stargardt disease with specific sequence mutation in the ABCA4 gene. Invest Ophthalmol Vis Sci 2009;50:5867–71.
34. Wakabayashi T, Sawa M, Gomi F, et al. Correlation of fundus autofluorescence with photoreceptor morphology and functional changes in eyes with retinitis pigmentosa. Acta Ophthalmol 2010;88:e177–83.
35. Popovic P, Jarc-Vidmar M, Hawlina M. Abnormal fundus autofluorescence in relation to retinal function in patients with retinitis pigmentosa. Graefes Arch Clin Exp Ophthalmol 2005;243:1018–27.
36. Mori F, Ishiko S, Kitaya N, et al. Scotoma and fixation patterns using scanning laser ophthalmoscope microperimetry in patients with macular dystrophy. Am J Ophthalmol 2001;132:897–902.
37. Gaucher D, Saleh M, Sauer A, et al. Spectral OCT analysis in Bietti crystalline dystrophy. Eur J Ophthalmol 2010;20:612–4.
38. Gundogan FC, Dinc UA, Erdem U, et al. Multifocal electroretinogram and central visual field testing in central areolar choroidal dystrophy. Eur J Ophthalmol 2010;20:919–24.
39. Szlyk JP, Paliga J, Seiple W, et al. Comprehensive functional vision assessment of patients with North Carolina macular dystrophy (MCDR1). Retina 2005; 25:489–97.
40. Renner AB, Tillack H, Kraus H, et al. Morphology and functional characteristics in adult vitelliform macular dystrophy. Retina 2004;24:929–39.
41. Roth JA. Central visual field in diabetes. Br J Ophthalmol 1969;53:16–25.
42. Remky A, Arend O, Hendricks S. Short-wavelength automated perimetry and capillary density in early diabetic maculopathy. Inv Ophthalmol Vis Sci 2000;41:274–81.
43. Hudson C, Flanagan JG, Turner GS, et al. Short-wavelength sensitive visual field loss in patients with clinically significant diabetic macular oedema. Diabetologia 1998;41:918–28.
44. Mori F, Ishiko S, Kitaya N, et al. Use of scanning laser ophthalmoscope microperimetry in clinically significant macular edema in type 2 diabetes mellitus. Jpn J Ophthalmol 2002;46:650–5.
45. Remky A, Weber A, Hendricks S, et al. Short-wavelength automated perimetry in patients with diabetes mellitus without macular edema. Graefes Arch Clin Exp Ophthalmol 2003;241:468–71.
46. Mastropasqua L, Verrotti A, Lobefalo L, et al. Visual field defects in diabetic children without retinopathy: relation between visual function and microalbuminuria. Acta Ophthalmol Scand 1995;73:125–8.
47. Gandolfo E, Zingirian M, Corrallo G, et al. Diabetic retinopathy: perimetric findings. In: Greve EL, Heijl A, editors. Fifth International Visual Field Symposium. The Hague: Dr W Junk; 1983.
48. Wisznia KI, Lieberman TW, Leopold IH. Visual fields in diabetic retinopathy. Br J Ophthalmol 1971;55:183–8.
49. Federman JL, Lloyd J. Automated static perimetry to evaluate diabetic retinopathy. Trans Am Ophthalmol Soc 1984;82:358–70.
50. Pahor D Automated static perimetry as a screening method for evaluation of retinal perfusion in diabetic retinopathy. Int Ophthalmol 1997–1998;21: 305–9.
51. Lutze M, Bresnick GH. Lens-corrected visual field sensitivity and diabetes. Invest Ophthalmol Vis Sci 1994;35:649–55.
52. Remky A, Weber A, Hendricks S, et al. Short-wavelength automated perimetry in patients with diabetes mellitus without macular edema. Graefes Arch Clin Exp Ophthalmol 2003;241:468–71.
53. Bengtsson B, Heijl A, Agardh E. Visual fields correlate better than visual acuity to severity of diabetic retinopathy. Diabetologia 2005;48: 2494–500.
54. Agardh E, Stjernquist H, Heijl A, et al. Visual acuity and perimetry as measures of visual function in diabetic macular oedema. Diabetologia 2006;49: 200–6.
55. Apaydin KC, Akar Y, Akar ME, et al. Menstrual cycle dependent changes in blue-on-yellow visual field analysis of young diabetic women with severe non-proliferative diabetic retinopathy. Clin Exp Ophthalmol 2004;32: 265–9.
56. Stavrou EP, Wood JM. Central visual field changes using flicker perimetry in type 2 diabetes mellitus. Acta Ophthalmol Scand 2005;83:574–80.
57. Barsam A, Laidlaw A. Visual fields in patients who have undergone vitrectomy for complications of diabetic retinopathy. A prospective study. BMC Ophthalmol 2006;6:5.
58. Frank RN. Visual fields and electroretinography following extensive photocoagulation. Arch Ophthalmol 1975;93:591–8.
59. Wessing A, Meyer-Schwickerath G. Die Behandlung der Retinopathia diabetica mit Lichtkoagulation. Diabetologia 1969;5:312–7.
60. Zingirian M, Pisano E, Gandolfo E. Visual field damage after photocoagulative treatment for diabetic retinopathy. In: Greve EL, editor. Second International Visual Field Symposium. The Hague: Dr W Junk, 1977.
61. Yoon YH, Lee J, Kim YJ. Preservation of retinal sensitivity in central visual field after panretinal photocoagulation in diabetics. Korean J Ophthalmol 1996;10:48–54.
62. Hulbert MFG, Vernon SA. Passing the DVLC field regulations following bilateral panretinal photocoagulation in diabetics. Eye 1992;6:456–60.
63. Hudson C, Flanagan JG, Turner GS, et al. Correlation of a scanning laser derived oedema index and visual function following grid laser treatment for diabetic macular oedema. Br J Ophthalmol 2003;87:455–61.
64. Hudson C, Flanagan JG, Turner GS, et al. Correlation of a scanning laser derived oedema index and visual function following grid laser treatment for diabetic macular oedema. Br J Ophthalmol 2003;87:455–61.
65. Rohrschneider K, Bultmann S, Gluck R, et al. Scanning laser ophthalmoscope fundus perimetry before and after laser photocoagulation for clinically significant diabetic macular edema. Am J Ophthalmol 2000;129:27–32.
66. Vujosevic S, Bottega E, Casciano M, et al. Microperimetry and fundus autofluorescence in diabetic macular edema: subthreshold micropulse diode laser versus modified early treatment diabetic retinopathy study laser photocoagulation. Retina 2010;30:908–16.
67. Deak GG, Bolz M, Ritter M, et al. A systematic correlation between morphology and functional alterations in diabetic macular edema. Invest Ophthalmol Vis Sci 2010;51:6710–4.
68. Okada K, Yamamoto S, Mizunoya S, et al. Correlation of retinal sensitivity measured with fundus-related microperimetry to visual acuity and retinal thickness in eyes with diabetic macular edema. Eye 2006;20:805–9.
69. Vujosevic S, Midena E, Pilotto E, et al. Diabetic macular edema: correlation between microperimetry and optical coherence tomography findings. Invest Ophthalmol Vis Sci 2006;47:3044–51.
70. Vujosevic S, Casciano M, Pilotto E, et al. Diabetic macular edema: fundus autofluorescence and functional correlations. Invest Ophthalmol Vis Sci 2011;52:442–8.
71. Cusick M, Toma HS, Hwang TS, et al. Binasal visual field defects from simultaneous bilateral retinal infarctions in sickle cell disease. Am J Ophthalmol 2007;143:893–6.
72. McLoone E, O'Keefe M, McLoone S, et al. Effect of diode laser retinal ablative therapy for threshold retinopathy of prematurity on the visual field: results of goldmann perimetry at a mean age of 11 years. J Pediatr Ophthalmol Strabismus 2007;44:170–3.
73. Kozobolis VP, Detorakis ET, Georgiadis GS, et al. Perimetric and retrobulbar blood flow changes following carotid endarterectomy. Graefes Arch Clin Exp Ophthalmol 2007;245:1639–45.
74. Meyer CH, Callizo J, Schmidt JC, et al. Functional and anatomical findings in acute Purtscher's retinopathy. Ophthalmologica 2006;220:343–6.

75. Imasawa M, Tsumura T, Kikuchi T, et al. Humphrey perimetry as a predictor of visual improvement after photodynamic therapy. Jpn J Ophthalmol 2009;53:281–2.
76. Chalam KV, Agarwal S, Gupta SK, et al. Recovery of retinal sensitivity after transient branch retinal artery occlusion. Ophthalm Surg Lasers Imaging 2007;38:328–9.
77. Wong WT, Forooghian F, Majumdar Z, et al. Fundus autofluorescence in type 2 idiopathic macular telangiectasia: correlation with optical coherence tomography and microperimetry. Am J Ophthalmol 2009;148:573–83.
78. Yamaike N, Kita M, Tsujikawa A, et al. Perimetric sensitivity with the micro perimeter 1 and retinal thickness in patients with branch retinal vein occlusion. Am J Ophthalmol 2007;143:342–4.
79. Barbazetto IA, Schmidt-Erfurth UM. Evaluation of functional defects in branch retinal vein occlusion before and after laser treatment with scanning laser perimetry. Ophthalmology 2000;107:1089–98
80. Ageno W, Cattaneo R, Manfredi E, et al. Parnaparin versus aspirin in the treatment of retinal vein occlusion. A randomized, double blind, controlled study. Thromb Res 2010;125:137–41.
81. Tsujikawa A, Hangai M, Kikuchi M, et al. Visual field defect after radial optic neurotomy for central retinal vein occlusion. Jpn J Ophthalmol 2006;50: 158–60.
82. Barak A, Kesler A, Gold D, et al. Visual field defects after radial optic neurotomy for central retinal vein occlusion. Retina 2006;26:549–54.
83. Afrashi F, Erakgun T, Uzunel D, et al. Comparison of achromatic and blue-on-yellow perimetry in patients with resolved central serous chorioretinopathy. Ophthalmologica 2005;219:202–5.
84. Sekine A, Imasawa M, Iijima H. Retinal thickness and perimetric sensitivity in central serous chorioretinopathy. Jpn J Ophthalmol 2010;54:578–83.
85. Dinc UA, Yenerel M, Tatlipinar S, et al. Correlation of retinal sensitivity and retinal thickness in central serous chorioretinopathy. Ophthalmologica 2010; 224:2–9.
86. Baran NV, Gurlu VP, Esgin H. Long-term macular function in eyes with central serous chorioretinopathy. Clin Experiment Ophthalmol 2005;33: 369–72.
87. Ozdemir H, Karacorlu SA, Senturk F, et al. Assessment of macular function by microperimetry in unilateral resolved central serous chorioretinopathy. Eye 2008;22:204–8.
88. Natsikos VE, Hart JCD. Static perimetric and Amsler chart changes in patients with idiopathic central serous retinopathy. Acta Ophthalmol 1980;58:908–17.
89. Kiss CG, Barisani-Asenbauer T, Simader C, et al. Central visual field impairment during and following cystoid macular oedema. Br J Ophthalmol 2008;92:84–8.
90. Remky A, Lichtenberg K, Elsner AE, et al. Short wavelength automated perimetry in age related maculopathy. Br J Ophthalmol 2001;85:1432–6.
91. Remky A, Elsner AE. Blue on yellow perimetry with scanning laser ophthalmoscopy in patients with age related macular disease. Br J Ophthalmol 2005;89:464–9.
92. Takamine Y, Shiraki K, Moriwaki M, et al. Retinal sensitivity measurement over drusen using scanning laser ophthalmoscope microperimetry. Graefes Arch Clin Exp Ophthalmol 1998;236:285–90.
93. Iwama D, Tsujikawa A, Ojima Y, et al. Relationship between retinal sensitivity and morphologic changes in eyes with confluent soft drusen. Clin Exp Ophthalmol 2010;38:483–8.
94. Sohn EH, Chen FK, Rubin GS, et al. Macular function assessed by microperimetry in patients with enhanced S-cone syndrome. Ophthalmology 2010;117:1199–206.e1.
95. Biswas S, Funnell CL, Gray J, et al. Nidek MP-1 microperimetry and Fourier domain optical coherence tomography (FD-OCT) in X linked retinoschisis. Br J Ophthalmol 2010;94:949–50.
96. Shenoy R, McCilvenny S. Microperimetric evaluation of macula in retinopathy of membranoproliferative glomerulonephritis type II: a case report. Eur J Ophthalmol 2006;16:634–6.
97. Ahn JK, Seo JM, Chung H, et al. Anatomical and functional characteristics in atrophic maculopathy associated with spinocerebellar ataxia type 7. Am J Ophthalmol 2005;139:923–5.
98. Midena E, Vujosevic S, Convento E, et al. Microperimetry and fundus autofluorescence in patients with early age-related macular degeneration. Br J Ophthalmol 2007;91:1499–503.
99. Remky A, Weber A, Arend O, et al. Topical dorzolamide increases pericentral visual function in age-related maculopathy: pilot study findings with short-wavelength automated perimetry. Acta Ophthalmol Scand 2005;83:154–60.
100. Feher J, Kovacs B, Kovasc I, et al. Improvement of visual functions and fundus alterations in early age-related macular degeneration treated with a combination of acetyl-L-carnithine, n-3 fatty acids, and coenzyme Q10. Ophthalmologica 2005;219:154–66.
101. Wong WT, Kam W, Cunnigham D, et al. Treatment of geographic atrophy by the topical administration of OT-551: results of a phase II clinical trial. Invest Ophthalmol Vis Sci 2010;51:6131–9.
102. Fujii GY, de Juan Jr E, Humayun MS, et al. Characteristics of visual loss by scanning laser ophthalmoscope microperimetry in eyes with subfoveal choroidal neovascularization secondary to age-related macular degeneration. Am J Ophthalmol 2003;136:1067–78.
103. Fujii GY, de Juan Hr E, Sunness J, et al. Patient selection for macular translocation surgery using the scanning laser ophthalmoscope. Ophthalmology 2002; 109:1737–44.
104. Tezel TH, Del Priore LV, Flowers BE, et al. Correlation between scanning laser ophthalmoscope microperimetry and anatomic abnormalities in patients with subfoveal neovascularization. Ophthalmol 1996;103:1829–36.
105. Lavinsky F, Tolentino MJ, Lavinsky J. The macular threshold protocol of the Humphrey visual field analyzer: a superior functional outcome of intravitreal bevacizumab for the treatment of neovascular age-related macular degeneration. Arq Bras Oftalmol 2010;73:111–5.
106. Squirrel DM, Mawer NP, Moody CH, et al. Visual outcome after intravitreal ranibizumab for wet age-related macular degeneration: a comparison between best-corrected visual acuity and microperimetry. Retina 2010;30:436–42.
107. Parravano M, Oddone F, Tedeschi M, et al. Retinal functional changes measured by microperimetry in neovascular age-related macular degeneration treated with ranibizumab: 24-month results. Retina 2010;30:1017–24.
108. Schmidt-Erfurth UM, Elsner H, Terai N., et al. Effects of verteporin therapy on central visual field function. Ophthalmology 2004;111:931–9.
109. Yodoi Y, Tsujikawa A, Kameda T, et al. Central retinal sensitivity measured with the micro perimeter 1 after photodynamic therapy for polypoidal choroidal vasculopathy. Am J Ophthalmol 2007;143:984–94.
110. Imasawa M, Tsumura T, Kikuchi T, et al. Humphrey perimetry as a predictor of visual improvement after photodynamic therapy. Jpn J Ophthalmol 2009;53:281–2.
111. Chen FK, Uppal GS, MacLaren RE, et al. Long-term visual and microperimetry outcomes following autologous retinal pigment epithelium choroid graft for neovascular age-related macular degeneration. Clin Exp Ophthalmol 2009;37:275–85.
112. Augustin AJ, Offermann I, Lutz J, et al. Comparison of the original Amsler grid with the modified Amsler grid: result for patients with age-related macular degeneration. Retina 2005;25:443–5.
113. Nazemi PP, Fink W, Lim JI, et al. Scotomas of age-related macular degeneration detected and characterized by means of a novel three-dimensional computer-automated visual field test. Retina 2005;25:446–53.
114. Loewenstein A, Malac R, Goldstein M, et al. Replacing the Amsler grid: a new method for monitoring patients with age-related macular degeneration. Ophthalmology 2003;110:966–70.
115. Preferential Hyperacuity Perimetry Research Group. Preferential hyperacuity perimeter (PreView PHP) for detecting choroidals neoavascularization study. Ophthalmology 2005;112:1758–65.
116. Amari F, Ohta K, Kojima H, et al. Predicting visual outcome after macular hole surgery using scanning laser ophthalmoscope microperimetry. Br J Ophthalmol 2001;85:96–8.
117. Hikichi T, Ishiko S, Takamiya A, et al. Scanning laser ophthalmoscope correlations with biomicroscopic findings and foveal function after macular hole closure. Arch Ophthalmol 2000;118:193–7.
118. Ozdemir H, Karacorlu M, Senturk F, et al. Retinal sensitivity and fixation changes 1 year after triamcinolone acetonide assisted internal limiting membrane peeling for macular hole surgery – a MP-1 microperimetric study. Acta Ophthalmol 2010;88:e222–7.
119. Chung H, Shin CJ, Kim JG, et al. Correlation of microperimetry with fundus autofluorescence and spectral-domain optical coherence tomography in repaired macular holes. Am J Ophthalmol 2011;151:128–36.e3.
120. Kroyer K, Jensen OM, Larsen M. Objective signs of photoreceptor displacement by binocular correspondence perimetry: a study of epiretinal membranes. Invest Ophthalmol Vis Sci 2005;46:1017–22.
121. Richter-Mueksch S, Vecsei-Marlovits PV, Sacu SG, et al. Functional macular mapping in patients with vitreomacular pathologic features before and after surgery. Am J Ophthalmol 2007;144:23–31.
122. Ezra E, Arden GB, Riordan-Eva P, et al. Visual field loss following vitrectomy for stage 2 and 3 macular holes. Br J Ophthalmol 1996;80:519–25.
123. Hutton WL, Fuller DG, Snyder WB, et al. Visual field defects after macular hole surgery: a new finding. Ophthalmology 1996;103:2152–9.
124. Melberg NS, Thomas MA. Visual field loss after pars plana vitrectomy with air/fluid exchange. Am J Ophthalmol 1995;120:386–8.
125. Hillenkamp J, Saikia P, Gora F, et al. Macular function and morphology after peeling of idiopathic epiretinal membrane with and without the assistance of indocyanine green. Br J Ophthalmol 2005;89:437–43.
126. von Jagow B, Hoing A, Gandorfer A, et al. Functional outcome of indocyanine green-assisted macular surgery: 7-year follow-up. Retina 2009;29:1249–56.
127. Uemura A, Kanda S, Sakamoto Y, et al. Visual field defects after uneventful vitrectomy for epiretinal membrane with indocyanine green-assisted internal limiting membrane peeling. Am J Ophthalmol 2003;136:252–7.
128. Tari SR, Vidne-Hay O, Greenstein VC, et al. Functional and structural measurement for the assessment of internal limiting membrane peeling in idiopathic macular pucker. Retina 2007;27:567–72.
129. Tsuiki E, Fujikawa A, Miyamura N, et al. Visual field defects after macular hole surgery with indocyanine green-assisted internal limiting membrane peeling. Am J Ophthalmol 2007;143:704–5.
130. Balaiya S, Brar VS, Murthy RK, et al. Comparative in vitro safety analysis of dyes for chromovitrectomy. Retina 2011;31:1128–36.
131. Hart WM Jr, Burde RM, Johnston GP, et al. Static perimetry in chloroquine retinopathy: perifoveal patterns of visual field depression. Arch Ophthalmol 1984;102:377–80.
132. Michaelides M, Stover NB, Francis PJ, et al. Retinal toxicity associated with hydroxychloroquine and chloroquine: risk factors, screening, and progression despite cessation of therapy. Arch Ophthalmol 2011;129:30–9.
133. Salu P, Uvijls A, van den Brande P, et al. Normalization of generalized retinal function and progression of maculopathy after cessation of therapy in a case of severe hydroxychloroquine retinopathy with 19 years follow-up. Doc Ophthalmol 2010;120:251–64.
134. Xiaoyun MA, Dongyi HE, Linping HE. Assessing chloroquine toxicity in RA patients using retinal nerve fibre layer thickness, multifocal electroretinography and visual field test. Br J Ophthalmol 2010;94:1632–6.

135. Almony A, Garg S, Peters RK, et al. Threshold Amsler grid as a screening tool for asymptomatic patients on hydroxychloroquine therapy. Br J Ophthalmol 2005;89:569–74.
136. Anderson C, Pahk P, Blaha GR, et al. Preferential hyperacuity perimetry to detect hydroxychloroquine retinal toxicity. Retina 2009;29:1188–92.
137. Rodriguez-Padilla JA, Hedges 3rd TR, Monson B, et al. High-speed ultra-high-resolution optical coherence tomography findings in hydroxychloroquine retinopathy. Arch Ophthalmol 2007;125:775–80.
138. Eisner A, Austin DF, Samples JR. Short wavelength automated perimetry and tamoxifen use. Br J Ophthalmol 2004;88:125–30.
139. Toggweiler S, Wieser HG. Concentric visual field restriction under vigabatrin therapy: extent depends on the duration of drug intake. Seizure 2001;10: 420–3.
140. Jensen H, Sjo O, Uldall P, et al. Vigabatrin and retinal changes. Doc Ophthalmol 2002;104:171–80.
141. Hosking SL, Hilton EJ. Neurotoxic effects of GABA-transaminase inhibitors in the treatment of epilepsy: ocular perfusion and visual performance. Ophthalm Physiol Optics 2002;22:440–7.
142. Hilton EJ, Cubbidge RP, Hosking SL, et al. Patients treated with vigabatrin exhibit central visual function loss. Epilepsia 2002;43:1351–9.
143. McGwin G, Vaphiades MS, Hall TA, et al. Non-arteritic anterior ischaemic optic neuropathy and the treatment of erectile dysfunction. Br J Ophthalmol 2006;90:154–7.
144. Jagle H, Jagle C, Serey L, et al. Visual short-term effects of Viagra: double-blind study in healthy young subjects. Am J Ophthalmol 2004;137:842–9.
145. Stanford MR, Tomlin EA, Comyn O, et al. The visual field in toxoplasmic retinochoroiditis. Br J Ophthalmol 2005;89:812–4.
146. Moraes LR, Cialdini AP, Avila MP, et al. Identifying live nematodes in diffuse unilateral subacute neuroretinitis by using the scanning laser ophthalmoscope. Arch Ophthalmol 2002;120:135–8.
147. Plummer DJ, Sample PA, Arevalo JF, et al. Visual field loss in HIV-positive patients without infectious retinopathy. Am J Ophthalmol 1996;122:542–9.
148. Falkenstein I, Kozak I, Kayikcioglu O, et al. Assessment of retinal function in patients with HIV without infectious retinitis by multifocal electroretinogram and automated perimetry. Retina 2006;26:928–34.
149. Plummer DJ, Marcotte TD, Sample PA, et al. Neuropsychological impairment-associated visual field deficits in HIV infection. HNRC Group, HIV Neurobehavioral Research Center. Invest Ophthalmol Vis Sci 1999;40:435–42.
150. Hangai M, Fujimoto M, Yoshimura N. Features and function of multiple evanescent white dot syndrome. Arch Ophthalmol 2009;127:1307–13.
151. Forooghian F, Stetson PF, Gross NE, et al. Quantitative assessment of photoreceptor recovery in atypical multiple evanescent white dot syndrome. Ophthalmic Surg Lasers Imaging 2010;41(Suppl):S77–80.
152. Souka AA, Hillenkamp J, Gora F, et al. Correlation between optical coherence tomography and autofluorescence in acute posterior multifocal placoid pigment epitheliopathy. Graefes Arch Clin Exp Ophthalmol 2006;244: 1219–23.
153. Gordon LK, Goldhardt R, Holland GN, et al. Standardized visual field assessment for patients with birdshot chorioretinopathy. Ocul Immunol Inflamm 2006;14:325–32.
154. Mahajan VB, Stone EM. Patients with an acute zonal occult outer retinopathy-like illness rapidly improve with valacyclovir treatment. Am J Ophthalmol 2010;150:511–8.
155. Ozgur S, Esgin H. Macular function of successfully repaired macula-off retinal detachments. Retina 2007;27:358–64.
156. Alexandridis E, Janzarik BI. Restitution of the retinal sensitivity after cured retinal detachment. In: Greve EL, editor. Second International Visual Field Symposium. The Hague: Dr W Junk; 1977.
157. Sakai T, Iida K, Tanaka Y, et al. Evaluation of S-cone sensitivity in reattached macula following macula-off retinal detachment surgery. Jpn J Ophthalmol 2005;49:301–5.
158. Bourke RD, Dowler JG, Milliken AB, et al. Perimetric and angiographic effects of retinotomy. Aust NZ J Ophthalmol 1996;24:245–9.
159. Sasoh M, Ito Y, Wakitani Y, et al. 10-year follow-up of visual functions in patients who underwent scleral buckling. Retina 2005;25:965–71.
160. Lai WW, Leung GY, Chan CW, et al. Simultaneous spectral domain OCT and fundus autofluorescence imaging of the macula and microperimetric correspondence after successful repair of rhegmatogenous retinal detachment. Br J Ophthalmol 2010;94:311–8.
161. Abramson DH, Melson MR, Servodidio C. Visual fields in retinoblastoma survivors. Arch Ophthalmol 2004;122:1324–30.
162. Rahhal FM, Abramson DH, Servodidio CA, et al. Automated perimetry in patients with choroidal metastases. Br J Ophthalmol 1996;80:309–13.
163. Enoch JM. Quantitative layer-by-layer perimetry: Proctor lecture. Invest Ophthalmol Vis Sci 1978;17:208–57.
164. Enoch JM, Fitzgerald CR, Campos EC. Quantitative layer-by-layer perimetry: an extended analysis. New York: Grune & Stratton, 1980.
165. Enoch JM, Lawrence B. A perimetric technique believed to test receptive field properties: sequential evaluation in glaucoma and other conditions. Am J Ophthalmol 1975;80:734–58.
166. Dubois Poulsen D. Acquired dyschromatopsias. Mod Probl Ophthalmol 1972;11:84–93.
167. Hart Jr WM, Burde RM. Color contrast perimetry: the spatial distribution of color defects in optic nerve and retinal diseases. Ophthalmology 1985;92: 768–76.
168. Makous W, Carroll J, Wolfing JI, et al. Retinal microscotomas revealed with adaptive-optics microflashes. Invest Ophthalmol Vis Sci 2006;47: 4160–7.

Index

Page numbers followed by "f" indicate figures, "t" indicate tables, and "b" indicate boxes.

Printed and bound by CPI Group (UK) Ltd, Croydon, CR0 4YY
03/10/2024
01040378-0020